CANCER

Proceedings of the
1980 International Symposium on Cancer

Presented by
Memorial Sloan-Kettering Cancer Center

Cosponsored by
the National Cancer Institute and
the American Cancer Society

September 14–18, 1980

Grune & Stratton Rapid Manuscript Reproduction

CANCER
Achievements, Challenges, and Prospects for the 1980s
Volume 1

Edited by

Joseph H. Burchenal, M.D.
Memorial Sloan-Kettering Cancer Center
New York, New York

Herbert F. Oettgen, M.D.
Memorial Sloan-Kettering Cancer Center
New York, New York

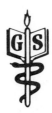

Grune & Stratton
A Subsidiary of Harcourt Brace Jovanovich, Publishers
New York   London   Toronto   Sydney   San Francisco

Grune & Stratton, Inc.
111 Fifth Avenue
New York, New York 10003

Distributed in the United Kingdom by
Academic Press Inc. (London) Ltd.
24/28 Oval Road, London NW 1

Library of Congress Catalog Number 80-85158
International Standard Book Number 0-8089-1351-4
Printed in the United States of America

Contents

Advances in Diagnosis

Preface

Much has been achieved in the years since the Panel on Cancer of the United States Senate began the deliberations that led to the National Cancer Act, passed in 1971, and the subsequent development of the National Cancer Program, a unique event in the history of biology and medicine in this country. Knowledge about the epidemiology, etiology and prevention of cancer has increased, many types of disseminated cancer are no longer completely incurable and great strides have been made in the area of multidisciplinary therapy, particularly adjuvant chemotherapy. At the ten-year mark it seemed appropriate to assess the accomplishments of the past decade, to define current challenges and to gauge the prospects of meeting them during the next decade. To that end, an international conference, presented by Memorial Sloan-Kettering Cancer Center and cosponsored by the National Cancer Institute and the American Cancer Society, entitled "Cancer 1980: Achievements, Challenges, Prospects," was held September 14–18, 1980, in New York City.

The Program Committee, composed of members from the sponsoring institutions, selected 26 major basic and clinical topics for discussion. Leading experts from all over the world were asked to present overviews of these topics in plenary sessions and to select additional speakers to develop important aspects of their particular area in more detail in complementary symposia. The response to these invitations was most gratifying. Up-to-date manuscripts of the presentations were received at the time of the conference, and they have been arranged so that each overview paper is followed by the corresponding symposium papers.

We are grateful to Dr. Edward J. Beattie, Jr., General Chairman, and Dr. William S. Howland, Vice Chairman, for conceiving this conference, to the members of the Program Committee for shaping it, to the speakers who made it a success, to Ms. Leslie Anton for coordinating the entire program, to Steven K. Herlitz, Inc., for organizing the conference, and to the staff at Grune & Stratton for assembling these volumes for rapid publication.

Joseph H. Burchenal
Herbert F. Oettgen

Contributors

Donald F. Austin, M.D.
Chief, Resources for Cancer Epidemiology Section
California State Department of Health Sciences
Oakland, California

Michael A. Bean, M.D.
Member and Associate Director
Virginia Mason Research Center
Seattle, Washington

Gilbert W. Beebe, M.D.
Clinical Epidemiology Branch
National Cancer Institute
National Institutes of Health
Bethesda, Maryland

Thomas L. Benjamin, Ph.D.
Professor, Department of Pathology
Harvard Medical School
Boston, Massachusetts

Klaus Bister, M.D.
Research Associate, Virus Laboratory
University of California
Berkeley, California

Baruch S. Blumberg, M.D.
Associate Director for Clinical Research
The Institute for Cancer Research
The Fox Chase Cancer Center
Philadelphia, Pennsylvania

John D. Boice, M.D.
Environmental Epidemiology Branch
National Cancer Institute
National Institutes of Health
Bethesda, Maryland

H. Worth Boyce, Jr., M.D.
Professor of Medicine
Director, Division of Digestive Diseases and Nutrition
University of South Florida College of Medicine
Tampa, Florida

W. R. Bruce, M.D.
Research Scientist
Physics Division
The Ontario Cancer Institute
Toronto, Ontario, Canada

John Cairns, M.D.
Imperial Cancer Research Fund
London, England

Chu Yuan-yun, M.D.
Vice Director
Qidong Liver Cancer Institute
Kiangsu, China

Philip Cole, M.D.
Professor and Director
Division of Epidemiology
Department of Public Health
University of Alabama in Birmingham
Birmingham, Alabama

Sir Richard Doll
Honorary Director
Imperial Cancer Research Fund
Cancer Epidemiology and Clinical Trials Unit
Oxford, England

Peter H. Duesberg, M.D.
Professor of Molecular Biology
Department of Molecular Biology
University of California
Berkeley, California

M. Essex, D.V.M., Ph.D
Professor of Virology
Department of Microbiology
Harvard University School of Public Health
Boston, Massachusetts

E. S. Fiala, Ph.D
Associate Chief
Division of Molecular Biology and Pharmacology
American Health Foundation
Valhalla, New York

William D. Hardy, Jr., D.V.M.
Laboratory of Veterinary Oncology
Memorial Sloan-Kettering Cancer Center
New York, New York

Frederick Hecht, M.D.
Director, The Cancer Research and Genetics Centers
Southwest Biomedical Research Institute
Tempe, Arizona

Brian E. Henderson, M.D.
Professor and Chairman
Family and Preventive Medicine
University of Southern California
Los Angeles, California

Gertrude Henle, Ph.D
Professor of Virology in Pediatrics
University of Pennsylvania School of Medicine
The Joseph Stokes, Jr., Research Institute
Children's Hospital of Philadelphia
Philadelphia, Pennsylvania

Werner Henle, M.D.
Professor of Virology in Pediatrics
University of Pennsylvania School of Medicine
The Joseph Stokes, Jr., Research Institute
Children's Hospital of Philadelphia
Philadelphia, Pennsylvania

John Higginson, M.D.
Director, International Agency for Research on Cancer
Lyon, France

Robert N. Hoover, M.D.
Environmental Epidemiology Branch
National Cancer Institute
National Institutes of Health
Bethesda, Maryland

Barbara Kaiser-McCaw, Ph.D
Associate Director
The Cancer Research and Genetics Centers
Southwest Biomedical Research Institute
Tempe, Arizona

Ann R. Kennedy, M.D.
Assistant Professor of Radiobiology
Laboratory of Radiobiology
Harvard University School of Public Health
Boston, Massachusetts

Mary-Clare King, Ph.D
Assistant Professor of Epidemiology
School of Public Health
University of California
Berkeley, California

George Klein, M.D.
Department of Tumor Biology
Karolinska Institute
Stockholm, Sweden

Alfred G. Knudson, Jr., M.D., Ph.D
Director, The Institute for Cancer Research
The Fox Chase Cancer Center
Philadelphia, Pennsylvania

Susan E. Krown, M.D.
Assistant Attending Physician
Clinical Immunology Service
Memorial Sloan-Kettering Cancer Center
New York, New York

Frederick P. Li, M.D.
Clinical Epidemiology Branch
National Cancer Institute
National Institutes of Health
Bethesda, Maryland, and
Department of Biostatistics and Epidemiology
Sidney Farber Cancer Institute
Boston, Massachusetts

Frank Lilly, M.D.
Genetics Department
Albert Einstein College of Medicine
Bronx, New York

John B. Little, M.D.
Professor of Radiobiology
Laboratory of Radiobiology
Harvard University School of Public Health
Boston, Massachusetts

Kenneth O. Lloyd, Ph.D
Associate Member
Memorial Sloan-Kettering Cancer Center
New York, New York

W. Thomas London
Senior Research Physician
Institute for Cancer Research
Fox Chase Cancer Center
Philadelphia, Pennsylvania

Brian MacMahon, M.D.
Professor, Department of Epidemiology
Harvard University School of Public Health
Boston, Massachusetts

Genevieve M. Matanoski, M.D., Dr.P.H.
Professor, Department of Epidemiology
School of Hygiene and Public Health
Johns Hopkins University
Baltimore, Maryland

Daniel Medina, M.D.
Department of Cell Biology
Baylor College of Medicine
Houston, Texas

Donald Metcalf, M.D.
Head, Cancer Research Unit
Walter and Eliza Hall Institute of Medical Research
Melbourne, Australia

Anthony B. Miller, M.D.
Director, NCIC Epidemiology Unit
University of Toronto
Toronto, Ontario, Canada

Daniel G. Miller, M.D.
Director, Preventive Medicine Institute
Strang Clinic
New York, New York

Elizabeth C. Miller, M.D.
WARF Professor of Oncology
McArdle Laboratory for Cancer Research
University of Wisconsin Medical School
Madison, Wisconsin

Sidney S. Mirvish, Ph.D
Epply Institute for Research in Cancer
University of Nebraska Medical Center
Omaha, Nebraska

Dianne L. Newton, M.D.
Laboratory of Chemoprevention
National Cancer Institute
National Institutes of Health
Bethesda, Maryland

Garth L. Nicolson, M.D.
Professor and Chairman
Department of Tumor Biology
University of Texas System Cancer Center
M.D. Anderson Hospital and Tumor Institute
Houston, Texas

Herbert F. Oettgen, M.D.
Member, Sloan-Kettering Institute
Chief, Clinical Immunology Service
Memorial Sloan-Kettering Cancer Center
New York, New York

Robert Pollack, Ph.D
Professor, Department of Biological Sciences
Columbia University
New York, New York

David P. Rall, M.D., Ph.D
Director, National Institute of Environmental Health Sciences
Research Triangle Park, North Carolina

B. S. Reddy, Ph.D., D.V.M.
Member and Associate Chief
Division of Nutrition
American Health Foundation
Valhalla, New York

Benno C. Schmidt, M.D.
Chairman, President's Cancer Panel 1972–1980
J. H. Witney and Company
New York, New York

Morton K. Schwartz, Ph.D
Chairman, Department of Biochemistry
Memorial Sloan-Kettering Cancer Center
New York, New York

Michael B. Shimkin, M.D.
Professor of Community Medicine and Oncology
Department of Community Medicine
University of California San Diego
School of Medicine
La Jolla, California

N. E. Spingarn, Ph.D
University of California
Los Angeles, California

Michael B. Sporn, M.D.
Chief, Laboratory of Chemoprevention
National Cancer Institute
National Institutes of Health
Bethesda, Maryland

Sun Tsung-tang, M.D.
Chairman, Department of Immunology
Cancer Institute
Chinese Academy of Medical Science
Beijing, China

Jeffrey C. Theiss, M.D.
Associate Professor of Environmental Sciences
Health Science Center at Houston
School of Public Health
University of Texas
Houston, Texas

Walter Troll, Ph.D
Professor, Department of Environmental Medicine
New York University Medical Center
New York, New York

Arthur C. Upton, M.D.
Director and Chairman
Institute of Environmental Medicine
New York University Medical Center
New York, New York

L. L. Vuolo, M.D.
Division of Nutrition
American Health Foundation
Valhalla, New York

Henry N. Wagner, Jr., M.D.
Professor, Departments of Medicine, Radiology and Environmental Health
  Sciences
The Johns Hopkins Medical Institutions
Baltimore, Maryland

Y. Y. Wang, Ph.D
Division of Nutrition
American Health Foundation
Valhalla, New York

Lee W. Wattenberg, M.D.
Professor of Pathology
Department of Laboratory Medicine and Pathology
University of Minnesota
Minneapolis, Minnesota

J. H. Weisburger, Ph.D
Vice President for Research
American Health Foundation
Valhalla, New York

Elizabeth D. Woodard, M.D., M.P.H.
Assistant Professor of Oncology
Preventive Medicine and Radiology
University of Rochester Medical Center
Rochester, New York

E. L. Wynder, M.D.
President, American Health Foundation
Valhalla, New York

Jorge J. Yunis, M.D.
Professor, Laboratory Medicine and Pathology
University of Minnesota
Minneapolis, Minnesota

Aims of The Conference

BENNO C. SCHMIDT

Chairman
President's Cancer Panel
1972-1980

Dr. Burchenal, distinguished guests from around the world,
ladies and gentlemen.

On behalf of the Trustees, the professional staff, and all
of those connected with Memorial Sloan-Kettering Cancer
Center, it is a great pleasure to welcome all of you in this
distinguished assemblage to the 1980 International Symposium
on Cancer. You are here to take stock of where we are and
where we have been in cancer research and thus to provide
both the scientific community and the public a better perspective, not only of where we are today, but, more importantly, of where we are going in the years immediately
ahead.

Since I am speaking to an audience that is uniquely and
profoundly familiar with the general pattern and, in individual instances, with the fullest details of the research
that has occurred, this is not the place for me to undertake
to highlight the accomplishments of the past ten years in
basic science, in clinical science, or in epidemiology, nor
is it appropriate for me to attempt to assess the implications of those accomplishments in increased knowledge,
improved clinical care, or advances in prevention or in our
ability to deal with environmental carcinogens. That will
be done by the outstanding scientists and physicians who
are gathered here as this great program unfolds over the
next five days. That is the true purpose of this Conference.

Perhaps you will permit me to leave it for your speakers
to unfold the scientific picture and allow me to present a
few reflections by an outsider who found himself catapulted
into the middle of your business.

It was just ten years ago that I was minding my own
business, unknown to and largely unknowing of the national
cancer research scene, when I received a letter from Senator

1

Ralph Yarborough asking me to serve on a Senate Panel to
review and make recommendations regarding cancer research.
That invitation set in motion a series of events that has
resulted in my occupying a ringside seat--and sometimes the
hot seat--from which to observe the developments in cancer
research over the past decade--a decade in which expenditures
by the National Cancer Institute for the support of cancer
research have risen from $180 million in 1970 to over $1
billion in 1980, a decade in which the National Cancer
Institute has spent a total of 6 billion, 691 million dollars
on cancer research. The decade of the seventies also saw
the National Institutes of Health budget go from 1 billion
dollars in 1970 to 3 billion, 429 million dollars in 1980,
thus belying the fear so widely expressed in 1970 and 1971
that any increase in the cancer budget would be at the
expense of other institutes within the National Institutes
of Health. I for one was determined that it should not be
so, so I am particularly pleased that the non-cancer portion
of the NIH budget was over $1-1/2 billion higher at the end
of the decade than at the beginning.

As Chairman in 1970 and 1971 of the Senate Panel whose
recommendations led to the passage of the National Cancer
Act, and as Chairman of the President's Cancer Panel from
the beginning of 1972 until this year, I have had a rare
opportunity to see the problems and controversies that have
been a part of the cancer research picture for the past ten
years, both in the scientific community and the broader
arenas of the Congress, the media and the public.

These issues and controversies have dealt with some very
important questions and their resolution has vitally affected
our cancer research programs. I would like to mention a few
of the more important of these issues and give you an assessment of the matter by one disinterested but close observer.

First, was the Congress wise in passing the National Cancer
Act and in stepping up the appropriations in support of
cancer research? I believe that the answer to this question
is an unequivocal "yes." The money has, on the whole, been
well spent and I know of no Federal dollars which have been
put to better use than these. It was charged that we were
simply "throwing money" at a problem whose solution would be
brought no closer by the increased expenditures. However,
the fact is that we had the capacity, without sacrificing
quality, for the increases which were made in our cancer
research activities. As I look at the results ten years
later, I am proud as an American citizen and thankful as a
taxpayer that these expenditures were made.

It has also been charged that the Cancer Act and the
increased expenditures thereunder were obtained by

overpromise, and that the results have not lived up to the expectations. There was some overpromise, both from a few of those who testified and from some members of the Congress, and much has been made of those quotations, but the overwhelming burden of the testimony and the overwhelming sense of the Congress was not a promise of miraculous results but rather of good research, money well spent, and progress. These purposes have been achieved in measures which will appear in detail as this Conference proceeds.

Secondly, it was charged that good basic research would suffer under an expanded and revitalized cancer program. Why on earth would an expanded research budget hurt basic research? Because, it was said, the people running the cancer program didn't understand basic research. They would try to plan where planning was inappropriate; to program research that couldn't be programmed; they would try to target research that couldn't be targeted; they would use contracts when only grants would attract to the program the best of the basic scientists. Well, it just didn't happen that way. Investigator-initiated, peer-reviewed, grant-supported basic research was funded by the National Cancer Institute at unprecedented levels and the proper atmosphere for fundamental basic research was guarded more zealously than perhaps any aspect of the cancer effort. Good basic scientists were always more than adequately represented on the National Cancer Advisory Board and the President's Cancer Panel. Of course, not everyone who wanted support for basic research got it, and few, if any, got all the support they wanted, but one of the outstanding attributes of the National Cancer Institute's support of cancer research during the past ten years has been the high level of support of excellent basic research. I hope this will always be true and it certainly appears that it will be true under the administration of Dr. DeVita. I was delighted to see that he is phasing out what remains of the use of contracts for the support of basic research. I am sure that investigator initiative and stringent and disinterested peer review works best in this area.

Third, there has been much talk of an inordinately high level of support for clinical research--or as it is more popularly put: spending all the money in a fruitless search for a cancer cure when it could be better spent on something else. That something else might be basic research, prevention research, research in chemical carcinogenesis, epidemiology, nutrition research, or whatever happens to be the special interest of the critic. Incidentally, I have not heard any clinicians or clinical researchers who think we are spending too much on clinical research. Nor do I.

We have made great progress in our clinical research programs, as you will hear, and we must do our best for the 25% of our people who have cancer or are destined to have cancer in the years to come.

I have already pointed out that we are not neglecting basic research and, relative to the budget, I do not believe we are neglecting prevention research, research on chemical carcinogenesis, epidemiology, or nutrition research, all of which are vitally important.

One of the most frequently voiced criticisms of the cancer program has been that we are not doing enough about chemical carcinogenesis. This is frequently combined with the criticism that the National Cancer Institute is "lavishly backing the study of a possible viral cause for cancer, while many scientists have come to believe that the real urgency is now the study of environmental causes of cancer." Actually, both areas are extremely important and both areas are being supported in a substantial way. As they must be.

The big mistake about the support of virology that continuously occurs in our press is that the money spent on virology is being spent in the search for a human cancer virus. The fact of the matter is that this money is being spent in the area called virology because that area has turned out to be the focal area for much of the productive research in molecular biology. It is in the area that we call virology that much of the progress in our basic understanding of the transformation of normal cells to cancer cells is taking place. It is this area of research that has produced our understanding of reverse transcriptase, recombinant DNA, gene structure and function, and surface antigens. The new technique that is provided by recombinant DNA is already leading to a deeper understanding of how genes act in both normal and cancer cells. Virology is a most important area of basic research which no knowledgeable scientist ridicules and substantial research in this area must continue to be supported.

However, this in no way detracts from the importance of environmental carcinogenesis and that area of research is also receiving important support. In my opinion, virology and environmental carcinogenesis are not an either/or proposition. They are both important and they are both being importantly supported under the cancer program.

The single most important discovery in environmental carcinogenesis may well come when we understand through basic research the mechanism of action of chemical and environmental carcinogens. This may prove to be the real key to elimination of this source of cancer.

Two other highly controversial areas of support were
mandated directly by the Congress. One was the recognition
and support of 21 Comprehensive Cancer Centers and the other
the support of the Cancer Control Program. I personally
believe that the support of the Comprehensive Cancer Centers
has been one of the important accomplishments under the
National Cancer Act. These centers receive no special
support. Despite a widespread impression to the contrary,
there is no such thing as a "centers grant" in the Cancer
Institute. Comprehensive Cancer Centers like other institutions are supported by individual research grants, program
project grants, core grants, contracts, and control dollars.
For all of these types of support the centers compete under
peer review on equal terms with other institutions. The
centers are making critical contributions in all fields of
research but their contributions have been particularly
crucial in the advances which have been made in the clinical
care of the cancer patients. The centers have been in the
forefront of combining surgery, radiation therapy and chemotherapy in such a way as to produce the best possible results
for the cancer patient.

One of the most controversial and one of the most difficult
areas under the cancer program has been the area of cancer
control. This area of activity was mandated by the Congress
because the Congress was determined that we should get the
benefits of our scientific discoveries to the patients as
quickly as possible. I do not need to tell this audience
that that is easier said than done. I personally believe
that the age-old assumption that good discoveries lie on the
shelf long after they should be available to the public is
more myth than reality. I believe that most biomedical
discoveries get to the patient at least by the time they
should and as soon as our knowledge is sufficient. As for
getting the highest quality cancer care to every patient,
that is a noble objective and one for which we must strive.
However, it is far from simple to disseminate widely the
skills that are involved today in the finest cancer care in
the best institutions.

I think there are good ways in which the control dollars
can and are being spent--dissemination of lay and professional information, training programs, and clinical cooperative
groups for bona fide clinical research--but I believe we
delude ourselves when we assume that in a short time frame we
can, by the expenditure of control dollars, make available
nationwide the excellence that exists in the best centers.
That takes time, and it cannot be pushed as fast as we would
like to think.

On the whole, the allocations that are being made are sound and the money is being well spent. The problem is that, even with a budget of $1 billion, there is not enough money to support all the good basic research, the good clinical research, or the good environmental research for which support is sought. Since each group is principally concerned with its own area of interest, the members of each group are inclined to think that their area of interest is being shortchanged and that somebody else is getting too much. They are often right about the inadequacy of their own support and usually wrong about the excesses in the other fellow's support. Nevertheless, these criticisms are valuable in provoking a continuous reevaluation of the balance in the program. In this respect, the criticism is healthy. If there is an unhealthy aspect of the criticism it is that it produces doubt and discouragement in the minds of the American people and sometimes the Congress about how their research dollars are being spent.

As we look ahead to the decade of the eighties and beyond, we must maintain our faith in and our commitment to good biomedical research. We must not forget how far biomedical research has already brought us in the brief period of time that it has been a part of the human endeavor. Well into this century our major disease burden consisted of diseases we seldom think of today: tuberculosis, diptheria, scarlet fever, typhoid fever, meningitis, measles, pneumonia, rheumatic fever, and polio. Those were the diseases which concerned our society only sixty years ago. We are largely rid of those diseases today because through biomedical research we have come to understand them and understanding them we are able to deal with them. Our goal now is to achieve through continued biomedical research a comparable understanding of the diseases that confront us today. Cancer, heart disease, stroke, diabetes, arthritis, multiple sclerosis, schizophrenia--there are some twenty-five to thirty major, common, life-threatening or incapacitating organic diseases which all of us would accept as our biomedical research agenda for today. Of these, cancer is far and away the disease which concerns the public most. By Thursday we will have reviewed how far we have come. I believe the results which you will hear will eloquently attest to the excellence of the work that has brought us to where we are today.

I thank every participant in this Conference for his or her contribution to that work.

Thank you.

Epidemiology

EPIDEMIOLOGY FOR CLUES TO ETIOLOGY

JOHN HIGGINSON

Director
International Agency for Research on Cancer
150 cours Albert Thomas
69372 Lyon, France

INTRODUCTION

In modern usage, the concept of 'cancer epidemiology' implies a multidisciplinary approach to the study of the disease, and includes not only geographical pathology, but also related metabolic and laboratory studies. Although epidemiological techniques are pertinent to problems of treatment and diagnosis, discussion will be limited to cancer etiology, especially environmental carcinogenesis. Use of the term 'environment' will follow the practice of earlier workers to include all exogenous factors that impinge on man, i.e., the physical, dietary, behavioral and cultural environments (Clemmesen, 1950; Higginson & Oettlé, 1960; Higginson, 1969), and not be limited only to industrial pollutants. This wide concept was promulgated at a meeting in Oxford in 1950, under the chairmanship of Dr Harold Stewart, which established guidelines for the later activities of the Committee on Geographical Pathology of the International Union Against Cancer (UICC). In the 1950s and 1960s, this Committee established most of the research approaches accepted as routine today for studies in environmental carcinogenesis.

Contrary to misconceptions among the public, progress in environmental cancer has been considerable since 1950, as improved data on geographical distribution and temporal and migrant variations in cancer patterns have become available, high- and low-risk populations identified, and a better understanding of the carcinogenic process has increased collaboration between laboratory and field research workers.

Further, it should be emphasized that epidemiological studies have not only identified specific causal factors for certain tumors but have also provided background data from which etiological hypotheses can be postulated for others (Higginson & Muir, 1979). Progress, however, has been as much dependent on exclusion of hypotheses as on development of new concepts. Thus, geographical and temporal differences in cancer patterns and changes in migrants early indicated that most cancers are not predominantly racial or hereditary in origin, but rather are directly or indirectly modulated by the exo-

7

genous environment (physical, cultural, etc.) (Haenszel, 1961, 1968; Higginson & Oettlé, 1960, Higginson, 1969). This view is frequently misinterpreted.

This essay will attempt to provide a general overview of progress and future developments, as an introduction to the more detailed reports of later speakers.

THE CAUSATION OF CANCER

For convenience, cancer can be divided into those of defined origin, and those for which etiological hypotheses can only be deduced (Higginson, 1969; Higginson & Muir, 1979; Conference on the primary prevention of cancer: assessment of risk factors and future directions, 1979).

Group I: Cancers Caused by Defined Exogenous Factors

These are predominantly tumors in adults, arising in the skin, respiratory tract (larynx and lung), upper digestive tract (nasopharynx and esophagus), liver, pancreas, and bladder. It also includes some other tumors of the endometrium and blood-forming organs. Personal habits, notably cigarette smoking, alcoholic beverage consumption, betel quid chewing and sunbathing, are by far the most important stimuli identified, causing from 25% to 50% of all cancers in males in different populations. All studies increasingly emphasize the overwhelming role of cigarette smoking in human cancer, not only *per se* (Hammond & Seidman, 1980) but also as enhancing the effects of other agents, e.g., asbestos and alcohol. Much of the cancer increases reported in most countries since 1950 relate to this habit.

A smaller proportion is related to occupational and iatrogenic exposures (Doll, 1977; Higginson & Muir, 1979; Royal Society, 1978; Wynder & Gori, 1977). The effects in man of over 500 chemicals and related industrial processes have been evaluated by the working groups of the International Agency for Research on Cancer (IARC, 1972-1980). Unfortunately, epidemiological data are unavailable for many chemicals, so that even when human exposures have occurred, evaluations are not always possible (IARC, 1979). This list is obviously not definitive and further iatrogenic and occupational hazards will certainly be identified.

While less adequately documented, primary liver cancer in Africa and Asia is believed to arise in hepatitis B virus carriers exposed to aflatoxin (Larouzé, Blumberg, London, *et al*., 1977; Linsell & Peers, 1977). Studies on the association between Epstein-Barr virus and Burkitt's lymphoma in Africa, and nasopharyngeal cancer in Chinese suggest that other exogenous factors may play a modulating role (de Thé, 1978). It is possible that further discrete carcinogenic stimuli will be identified for certain tumors, e.g., mesothelioma in rural Turkey, and esophageal cancer in China or in Iran. In the latter country, precancerous mucosal lesions are found in nearly all adults, suggesting a powerful exogenous carcinogen (Crespi, Muñoz, Grassi, *et al*., 1979). Almost all our knowledge of the carcinogenic factors identified in this group has been dependent on epidemiological studies in man.

Group II: Cancers of Probable
Environmental Origin

This group is made up predominantly of tumors of the gastrointestinal tract, stomach, large intestine, endocrine-related organs (prostate, ovary, breast, uterus, cervix) and some tumors of the genito-urinary system. This group forms approximately 40% of cancers in males and 60% to 70% in females (Higginson & Muir, 1979). The view that these tumors are of environmental origin is deduced from analysis of geographical and temporal variations in incidence and migrant studies. Only a few of these cancers have been identified with discrete exposures. In view of its size, this group represents the largest immediate challenge to epidemiology.

Two etiological hypotheses have been put forward to explain these and other cancers of probable, but of undefined environmental etiology, with profoundly different implications for public health and research priorities. First, it has been suggested that these cancers predominantly reflect widespread environmental exposures to chemicals of an industrial nature (Epstein, 1979). Alternatively, others have related the majority of these cancers to a predominant role of exogenous and endogenous stimuli inherent in normal living conditions (lifestyle), notably dietary and behavioral factors known to significantly modulate carcinogenesis (Higginson & Oettlé, 1960; Higginson & Muir, 1979; Royal Society Study Group, 1978; Wynder & Gori, 1977).

Possible Role of
General Environmental Pollution

The role of adverse high risk exposures will be discussed by others. However, the fact that high exposures to certain chemicals cause cancer in man has led to natural concern as to the significance of multiple low exposures in the general environment. Numerous natural and synthetic chemicals, including carcinogens, promoters, enhancers, etc., such as polycyclic aromatic hydrocarbons, nitrosamines, mycotoxins, flavones, have been demonostrated in air, water (Kraybill, 1978), food, and alcoholic beverages (Rose, 1977; Wilkins, Reiches & Kruse, 1979). Nitrosamines have also been found in the tissues of normal individuals (Walker, Castegnaro, Griciute & Lyle, 1978). In fact, in many countries most of the population has been exposed to many of the 140 animal carcinogens already evaluated in the IARC Monographs Series. However, esophageal cancer in Brittany appears related to the ethanol content of the alcoholic beverages concerned and not to the level of nitrosamines or other carcinogens identified in such beverages. Accordingly, for those cancers in which powerful confounding variables such as cigarettes in the lung and alcohol in the esophagus, have been demonstrated, evaluation of the etiological role of the myriad of chemicals separately in a person's environment present almost insoluble logistic and technological difficulties from the viewpoint of epidemiological investigation. Thus, determination of the individual effect of each in humans is largely dependent on theoretical mathematical modelling, an approach many believe oversimplified in view of the many unknown variables involved (Coulston, 1980; Fishbein, 1979).

However, epidemiological studies may permit evaluation of the overall impact of all environmental chemicals, in a specific environment, i.e., the total sum of increased risk. The most intensive studies have been in relation to air pollution, but studies on cancers of other sites have shown essentially similar results. Thus, no consistent relationships have been shown between overall cancer patterns or individual sites and probable indices of ambient environmental pollution, such as industrialization and urbanization (Cederlöf, 1978; Higginson, 1979; Lyon, Gardner & West, 1980; Royal Society Study Group, 1978). No significant effect can be demonstrated even for lung cancer, if correction is made for other variables, notably cigarette smoking and occupational exposures (Hammond & Garfinkel, 1980). On the other hand, the overall effect of occupations which tend to be located in towns can be partially evaluated. However, the demonstration of localized cancer 'hot spots' within a country, e.g., United States (Mason, McKay, Hoover, et al., 1975), requires analysis as to whether they reflect localized high exposures, e.g., mesothelioma in shipyard workers, or lifestyle factors, as distinct from general environmental pollution.

Overall cancer patterns have been relatively stable in most western societies over the last 70 to 80 years, most changes being largely explicable by cigarette smoking, alcohol consumption or lifestyle changes. Available epidemiological data do not indicate a significant increase related to ambient pollution, e.g., water. Thus, Garfinkel (personal communication) has found no increase in lung cancer in non-smokers at 2 periods in the large American Cancer Society sample. The interpretation of minor trends requires careful epidemiological examination. No satisfactory explanation is available for the fall in stomach cancer.

It has been argued that the increase in synthetic organic chemicals is too recent to permit any evaluation of their long-term effects. It should be noted, however, that many were already produced in considerable quantities by 1950 (Davis & Magee, 1979). Further, since no accurate measurements exist of the total carcinogen burden before then, and which is reflected in present cancer patterns, the increase in this burden can only be assumed. Further, in many countries, control of the escape of chemicals into the general environment has increased, so that greater production does not necessarily imply an increase in the total burden of a carcinogen exposure, although the number of potential chemicals involved may be much greater.

Doll (1977) concluded that the data 'make it difficult to believe that industrial pollution, in the ordinary sense of the term, can be responsible for any substantial proportion of the total cancer hazard', and similar views were expressed by the Royal Society Study Group (1978). These opinions are consistent with data on individual chemicals, e.g., 3,4 benzopyrene, as indicated by the moderate cancer differences observed between very high and low exposures.

Although the latent period of cancer may be 40 years or longer, it can be as short as 2 years and seven months, e.g., chlornazine (Higginson, 1975). As far as I am aware most strong chemical carcinogenic stimuli usually begin to show their effects after 20 years' exposure, although, of course, tumors may continue to arise many years later. A failure to demonstrate an effect does not mean that present levels of ambient environmental pollution of industrial origin are safe, only that a carcinogenic effect cannot be demonstrated in relation to other factors. Moreover, there are other excellent health and ecological reasons for the control of general air and water pollution.

Lifestyle

This term describes the overall cultural, behavioral and dietary environments as well as such clearly defined habits as cigarette smoking and alcohol ingestion. The concept is not new, being accepted in oncological circles as early as 1950. The necessity to distinguish between industrial and lifestyle factors, recommended by the Oxford meeting, stimulated early studies such as those on urban and rural Bantu in Africa (Higginson & Oettlé, 1960).

In man, certain factors have been associated with an increased or reduced risk of cancer. These include behavioral patterns, e.g., age at first marriage and pregnancy; physiological parameters, e.g., age at menarche or menopause; diet, e.g., quantity and quality of dietary fat, fiber; and socioeconomic gradient. Such parameters form part of an individual's lifestyle and the term 'carcinogenic risk factor' has proven a convenient label for them. Further, there is an increasing body of literature in man and animals indicating that such factors may be associated with biochemical and metabolic changes in man of relevance to cancer. For example, the carcinogenic effects of exogenous estrogens in endometrial cancer and other sites, clearly indicate a possible and causal role for endogenous estrogens (Hulka, Fowler, Kaufman, et al., 1980; Smith, Prentice, Thompson, et al., 1975; Cole, 1980).

Diet and behavior are culturally conditioned and closely interrelated. They are also related to socioeconomic gradient. Socioeconomic gradient has even been associated with pesticide storage in the tissues (Davies, Edmundson, Raffonelli, et al., 1972), and hormonal variations (Trichopoulos, MacMahon & Brown, 1980). Diet is a determinant in menarche, height, obesity, etc., which have been shown to be risk factors for cancers of the breast and endometrium. Diet must be considered not only in terms of food additives, but also as a highly complex mixture that includes carcinogen precursors and factors that inhibit or enhance tumor formation (Wattenberg, 1979). The non-specific role of diet in carcinogen promotion, e.g., fat and high calorie intake, has long been recognized (Miller, 1980; Wynder & Gori, 1977). While diet might be directly involved in stomach and large intestinal cancer, possibly through intraluminal carcinogen formation, e.g., nitrosamines, mechanisms are probably complex and to date epidemiological studies have been equivocal.

Significance of Occupational Studies

There has been a tendency to associate occupational epidemiological studies only with the identification of discrete carcinogens. Recent occupational studies from the United Kingdom and elsewhere have also produced strong supportive evidence for the role of lifestyle factors in influencing cancer patterns in different occupations (Office of Population Censuses and Surveys, 1978). Since individual occupations are recruited from specific segments of the community, the health patterns in such occupations also reflect the community experience. It has been calculated (Fox & Adelstein, 1978) that most of the differences in cancer patterns between occupational groups are likely to be due to lifestyle and not to workplace exposures. Thus, distinction should be made between tumors due to industrialization *per se* and cancers occurring within an industrialized society.

Low Risk Groups

The importance of lifestyle has also been indicated by low cancer risks, not limited to cancers due to alcohol or tobacco, both in Africa and Asia, and in Seventh Day Adventists and Mormons in the United States (Enstrom, 1980; Higginson & Oettlé, 1980).

Group III: Cancer of Unknown Etiology

For a number of tumors of children, bone and soft tissues and blood system, only a few discrete causal factors have been determined and the majority cannot be easily related to exogenous factors as showing little geographical or temporal variations in incidence. Although transplacental carcinogens have been recognised, e.g., diethylstilboestrol and vaginal adenocarcinoma, no effects of parental aromatic hydrocarbon exposure have been found (Zack, Cannon, Loyd, *et al.*, 1980) on childhood patterns.

IMPLICATIONS OF EPIDEMIOLOGICAL OBSERVATIONS IN RELATION TO MECHANISMS OF CARCINOGENESIS

Epidemiological studies can contribute to the understanding of carcinogenesis since putative biological mechanisms, whether deduced from field or laboratory studies, should be consistent, and hopefully provide a rational explanation for the human cancer patterns. The concept of a discrete carcinogenic stimulus, chemical or physical, as a direct cause of cancer is well comprehended, and has been extensively investigated. However, the view first promulgated by Berenblum (1978), and others in the 1940s, that carcinogenesis is multistage and that numerous exogenous or endogenous parameters modulate neoplasia, is now becoming generally accepted (Boyland, 1980). Such parameters include factors influencing carcinogen activation and inactivation (Miller, J. & Miller, E. 1979), DNA repair, inhibition, promotion, immunological status, etc., on which research has considerably increased in the last decade. Many are under both environmental and genetic influence. Furthermore, not all carcinogenic agents are initiators or genotoxic, nor is initiation always extrinsic and complete. Several hypotheses as to nongenotoxic initiating mechanisms for carcinogens have been postulated, such as gene unmasking, modification of DNA repair, enzyme imprinting, etc. (Kroes, 1979).

Thus, clinical cancer should be considered not in terms of a single mechanism but rather as a summation of events, only a few of which have been identified and studied (Higginson, 1980).

The complexity of carcinogenesis has significant implications in developing cancer control and research strategies. First, it illustrates the inherent difficulties in quantitative extrapolation of carcinogenic risk from animals or *in vitro* models to man. This is especially true for weak carcinogenic stimuli where cancer development or inhibition may be largely dependent on strong modulating factors, whether exogenous or endogenous, and the target cell dose cannot be measured.

Secondly, the numerous modulating factors so far identified offer reasonable biological hypotheses to explain the nature of lifestyle influences and associated carcinogenic risk factors, and also individual susceptibility.

Thirdly, prevention may be possible through interference in other phases of carcinogenesis (Berenblum, 1979) such as changes in lifestyle factors or chemoprevention (Cole, 1980).

Epidemiologically, it has not been usual in evaluating discrete chemicals to distinguish between promoters and initiators, nor was this attempted in the IARC Monographs Series (IARC, 1972-1980). This lack of separation is partly due to the epidemiological problems associated with studying mechanisms in humans and partly due to the public health implications. However, the possibility of making this distinction has become increasingly important as illustrated by the recent controversy on the carcinogenic effects of hormones and saccharin. The control of promoters may require very different public health strategies. Thus, it is possible that legislation for promoters may differ from that of initiators. Further, it obviously would be difficult to make a legislative distinction between a hormone promoter and a dietary factor such as fat (Campbell, 1980) with similar actions. It would appear profitable therefore, to examine first the total picture in man, and then analyse the role of individual modulating factors, where appropriate hypotheses or technology are available.

Multistage carcinogenesis has long been accepted in man. Thus, primary liver cancer in Africa was believed to reflect a two-stage mechanism, one component of which was hepatitis virus (Higginson, 1963). However, the hypothesis could only be adequately tested when the technology necessary to measure hepatitis B virus and aflatoxin became available. There is epidemiological evidence indicating that cigarette smoke almost certainly contains a strong promoting agent, and ethanol probably acts as a surface activating agent. Epidemiological and pathological studies in cancers of the breast (Cole & MacMahon, 1969), endometrium (Richardson & MacLaughlin, 1978), prostate (Coffey & Isaacs, 1979), large intestine, etc., provide further support for multifactorial origin, and multistage carcinogenesis.

Individual Susceptibility

Despite numerous attempts to demonstrate environmentally modulated individual susceptibility, few examples are available. The increased susceptibility to lung cancer in migrants from the United Kingdom to South Africa and Asia may be such an example but so far no obvious markers have been found and studies on aryl benzpyrene hydroxylase have been equivocal. Apart from obvious hereditary syndromes, only a few cancers can be attributed to genetic factors. However, genetic polymorphism for example, operating through enzyme induction may play a major role in modulating individual susceptibility, a field which is only beginning to open up and in which epidemiological investigations will play a key role (Del Villano, Miller, Schacter et al., 1980; Schull, 1979). Nonetheless, it must be noted that migrant studies have constantly emphasized the predominant effect of environmental factors. Susceptibility may be age-dependent as illustrated by changing incidences in migrants of breast and prostate cancer, where factors operative *in utero* or in adolescent life appear to modify tumor development and progression. The mechanisms are as yet unidentified but may include sex-linked enzyme induction and imprinting, as suggested by experimental studies (Mori, Nagasawa & Bern, 1979).

The concept of multistage mechanisms and identification of the role of modulating factors explain why few cancers can be attributed to a single cause. However, a single factor may be so predominant that cancer would not occur in its absence. In this sense, it would be accepted as the predominant or practical cause from the public health point of view, irrespective of the role of other factors. Thus, cigarette smoking would be called the practical cause of 80% of lung cancer in males, without excluding the possibility that other initiating or modulating factors may be involved. In this context, there would be no conflict theoretically between those who attribute most cancers to exogenous chemicals in the ambient environment on the grounds that they are responsible for background initiation, and those who emphasize modulating factors, since the nature of the initiating event cannot be analysed in relation to individual exogenous agents. However, the cancer control and public health implications are very different. Lastly, these observations on general environmental pollution and other epidemiological data are relevant to the concept of reversibility and threshold dosage.

SUMMARY OF PAST ACCOMPLISHMENTS

I hope I have satisfactorily demonstrated that research on environmental carcinogenesis has been considerable, although, of course, progress has been slower than wished. Nonetheless, there are today adequate data on the cause of nearly 50% of cancers in males and 20% in females. In parts of Africa and Asia, the figures may be higher, although cancer is less important in terms of the total disease burden. Further, reasonable data are available as to the possible carcinogenicity in man of about 40 chemical, industrial and iatrogenic hazards (IARC, 1979). In addition, we have numerous hypotheses as to the environmental nature of nearly 40% of male and 70% of female cancers related to lifestyle factors (Higginson & Muir, 1979). Lastly, there is increased recognition of the impact of social gradient on cancer patterns.

Less tangible has been the better integration between laboratory and field studies, so that problems today are being investigated through multidisciplinary biological programs. These accomplishments and their implications for public health can be regarded with some pride and should allay public disquiet. On the other hand, successful efforts do not tend to obtain much publicity among the media, as illustrated by the coverage given to the eradication of smallpox throughout the world. That the full potential of prevention has not been realized does not represent a failure of the epidemiologist, but rather a failure of the public and its representatives to accept the facts. Contrary to misconceptions perpetuated in certain circles, experienced epidemiologists have recognized the multifactorial origin of cancer in man since the mid 1940s. This myth was first put forward by those unwilling to accept that cigarettes were the major cause of lung cancer for practical purposes. The developments of epidemiology are summarized in Table 1-1.

TABLE 1-1
Highlights of Epidemiology since 1950

A. Evaluation of the role of:

　　1. Cultural habits
　　　　i)　　Cigarettes
　　　　ii)　 Alcohol
　　　　iii)　Betel quid
　　　　iv)　Sunlight

　　2. Carcinogenic drugs and industrial or chemical processes
　　　　i)　　19 definite hazards
　　　　ii)　 18 probable hazards

　　3. Ionizing radiation

　　4. Biological agents
　　　　i)　　Liver cancer - aflatoxin and hepatitis B
　　　　ii)　 Burkitt's lymphoma - EB virus + malaria?
　　　　iii)　Nasopharyngeal carcinoma - EB virus

　　5. Lifestyle (and related risk factors)
　　　　i)　　Behavior and culture
　　　　ii)　 Diet
　　　　iii)　Age (including transplacental carcinogens)
　　　　iv)　Socioeconomic gradient
　　　　v)　 Multistage and multifactorial carcinogenesis
　　　　vi)　Biochemical markers of carcinogenic risk factors

　　6. Ambient pollution

　　7. Chemoprevention and cancer inhibition

B. Technological progress in:

　　1. Monitoring and surveillance technology
　　　　i)　　National
　　　　ii)　 International
　　　　iii)　Record linkage systems

　　2. Analytical epidemiological techniques

　　3. Integration of laboratory and field studies (metabolic epidemiology)

Implications for Public Health

Cancer as a Socio-Economic Problem

Among the most important recent developments is renewed interest in the association of cancer patterns with social gradient which was recognized over 40 years ago. This would indicate that the problem of cancer in a population has major social ramifications which extend far beyond that of simple occupational exposures. It is now clear that social gradient is significantly associated with many aspects of lifestyle, as well as with occupational and cultural habits. These imply major changes in lifestyle which are reflected by biological and metabolic variations in the corresponding socioeconomic group. Such changes almost certainly are of importance in explaining some of the variations in cancer patterns between such groups (Hill, Wynder, Garbaczewski *et al.*, 1980; Office of Population Censuses and Surveys, 1978; Trichopoulos, MacMahon & Brown, 1980; Wynder & Gori, 1977). Since over 50% of the American working population is employed in offices and since only a very small proportion of workers are likely to be directly exposed to high concentrations of carcinogens, it is clear that occupational cancer has much greater implications in socioeconomic terms than previously anticipated. Such observations offer an immense intellectual and social challenge to the oncologist and epidemiologist for the next decade, but also emphasize the great difficulties to be encountered in preventive strategy from both the scientific and regulatory viewpoints. However, the fact that populations with low risks of lifestyle related cancer exist indicates that prevention is theoretically possible.

It would be impertinent of me to discuss the regulator's almost impossible task in this context. He all too frequently does not receive the sympathy he deserves as he struggles to develop a rational regulatory policy while exposed to great political and scientific pressures, and tries not to present policy as scientific fact. In discussing preventive strategy and the technology of identifying chemical carcinogens the Royal Society Study Group (1978) concluded that while the newer tests for identifying potential hazards by industrial products or wastes should enable some of the hazards to be reduced, it is probable 'that the mass of cancers related to lifestyle would not be affected by these new ways of detecting and legislation on carcinogenic chemicals'. This in no way invalidates the value of such tests in cancer control, but rather indicates their limitations, some of which have been discussed in IARC Monographs, Supplement 2 (1980).

For some reason, these comments on lifestyle and socioeconomic gradient are often interpreted to imply that occupational exposures or general environmental pollution should be neglected. It is certainly not a case of either/or, but a matter of balancing and maximizing research and public health approaches. My view has never been that a major research effort in the control of industrial hazards is not justified. But I have been concerned that excessive fear of ambient chemicals, possibly induced by the media with the best of motives, has led to distortion of research and public health priorities. In consequence, a substantial portion of the problems of cancer causation in man has not received adequate research support. We should remember to what extent excessive emphasis by both scientists as well as industrial and political interests on air pollution and other environmental chemical carcinogens in lung cancer was detrimental to public recognition and appreciation of the dangers of the cigarette habit, with significant public health consequences. We must not permit a similar situation to develop in regard to lifestyle factors.

Epidemiology has an important role to play in providing a balanced picture of the situation in man, since it provides the background data necessary in making scientific choices whether the latter relate to industry, increased quality of life, health risks, etc. These may vary from culture to culture and are of increasing concern to an energy deprived Third World.

Thus, the importance of epidemiology in providing objective data is further emphasized by the fact that cancer affects a community not only directly as a disease, but also by the fears it may engender. Irrational fear has never provided a rational public health policy and creation of cancerphobia has no place in control strategy and is medically unethical. The difficulties of objectively comparing the problems of overpopulation and pollution versus the minor dangers of the pill have been extensively discussed by Djerassi (1979). In industrial societies, the importance of informed choice is further illustrated by asbestos, a well known human carcinogen. Whereas many of us would prefer a world with limited or no exposures whether in the workplace or in the ambient environment, this so far seems impractical and many attempts are being made to find suitable substitutes. Unfortunately, many of the latter are animal carcinogens, and therefore hasty and unconsidered substitution would be imprudent as possibly introducing a greater hazard. Accordingly, it would appear desirable that while proceeding with gradual substitution of asbestos by other fibers, where possible such action should be complemented by appropriate monitoring of the effects of a substitute. It may be better to accept the devil we do know than the devil we don't. This clearly indicates the high degree of scientific objectivity necessary in discussing para-scientific questions and the importance of responsible media reporting.

Modification of Lifestyle

In contrast to conventional wisdom, there is considerable evidence that the public will modify its lifestyle habits if convinced that it will be of value. This is well demonstrated by the changes that have occurred in many Western countries in terms of both diet and cigarette consumption (McMichael, McCall, Hartshorne, *et al.*, 1979). Unfortunately, oncologists have been much more conservative in research effort on lifestyle than their cardiological colleagues, who accepted its importance in the early 1950s, and the recent fall in acute cardiac deaths may be the result.

FUTURE RESEARCH

Cancer Registration and Future Trends

To forecast future research priorities is hazardous. Nonetheless, many of the recommendations of the meeting in Oxford have been fulfilled and the above discussion indicates areas where future epidemiological work should be intensified and where innovative research is required. Priorities will also depend not only on control of existing cancer patterns but also on the future cancer trends. The latter are difficult to forecast in the absence of concrete information on future environmental conditions and the uncertainty as to whether present cancer and lifestyle trends will continue. Nonetheless, it is probable that tobacco- and alcohol-related cancers will continue to rise in most countries, as will possibly cancers of the breast and endometrium which are related to reproductive customs. On the other hand, it is probable that cervical cancer will fall. In view of such uncertainty, it is essential that an appropriate monitoring and surveillance mechanism and complementary analytical studies be established to evaluate adverse effects, and also the possible beneficial effects of intervention through changes in lifestyle, etc.

Unfortunately, few workers understand the principles and limitations of cancer registration as illustrated by the cancer epidemic scare in the mid 1970s due to a registration artefact and which received widespread media publicity. Thus, some might interpret a rise in breast cancer as a warning of the entrance of new carcinogens into the environment; others would consider it a reaction to the diagnosis of breast cancer in the wife of a public figure, indicative of a pool of breast cancer cases in the community in whom earlier diagnosis should be feasible. Unfortunately, our knowledge of past trends has been considerably hindered by changing registration boundaries, modifications in classifications, etc. Nor has there been adequate analysis of birth cohort changes or changes within limited geographical areas. Further, the existence of the large over-hang of comparatively recent synthetic chemicals will naturally remain a cause of prudent concern, which requires surveillance, even though until now no significant impact has been detected. A reasonable balance must be struck between necessary and rational control, and careless and unnecessary exposures, a balance which will largely depend on epidemiological investigation. Lastly, we are living in an ever changing world, the impact of whose changes on health must be evaluated if future generations are to avoid our present confusion and confrontation.

Discrete Carcinogens

It is necessary to distinguish between potential carcinogens which have only recently been discovered on the basis of animal or *in vitro* studies, and stimuli present in the environment for a significant period. Epidemiology will be essential in monitoring and evaluating such exposures where they occur.

Where long-standing human exposures are present, epidemiology is of great value in the identification and evaluation of risks and also in determining the effects of control strategy, as well illustrated by occupational studies in the United Kingdom (Baxter, 1980; Peto, Doll, Howard *et al.*, 1977). Further, they will provide background data in developing more rational extrapolation through an understanding of basic mechanisms and the effects of modulating factors. The limitations of such data are well recognized by epidemiologists but experience indicates that they should not be overestimated in relation to other techniques. Thus, even an imperfect negative study may provide estimates as to potential risk which may be of greater valididy than more elegant biomathematical calculations with their many uncertainties. Such a view in no way implies using man as a guinea pig.

Lifestyle Factors

Another area of research will obviously be related to lifestyle factors along the lines indicated above. In contrast to discrete chemical carcinogens, with certain major exceptions (Cole & MacMahon, 1969; Hill & Wynder, 1980; MacMahon, Cole & Brown, 1973), research on this has been relatively limited, partly due to inadequate technological methods for extensive population studies and partly due to general lack of interest. Today, it is possible to measure very low levels of carcinogens within the body as well as in the diet and ambient environment. Further, Conney (Conney, Pantuck, Hsiao et al., 1977) and others have introduced techniques whereby variations in carcinogen metabolism and compounds can be studied in man and in animals under different conditions. In addition, many of the mutagenic tests may also be of value in measuring metabolic variations between tissues. Thus, the study of the biochemical nature of lifestyle, formerly considered only a theroretical possibility, is now proving feasible.

Data are already sufficient to provide enough hypotheses for testing through intensified, if sometimes tedious systematic programs in different environmental settings. Such studies not only permit better understanding of mechanisms of risk extrapolation and *in vitro* models, but also an understanding of lifestyle factors in terms of human physiology. I do not agree with those epidemiologists who consider the study of carcinogenic mechanisms unimportant, nor, conversely, with those who believe that an understanding of mechanisms alone is adequate without considering the total biology of human cancer.

CONCLUSIONS

Epidemiology is an observational science based on probabilities, with an inherent uncertainty. Nonetheless, the human experience represents the ultimate criterion against which all etiological hypotheses must be judged. Attempts to deal with such uncertainties by statistical models are essentially policy decisions and cannot be regarded as a substitute for scientific investigation. Since during the last decade, gross misconceptions of the nature of human cancer and its causes have been widespread among the public, and also in governmental and scientific circles it is important that epidemiology has access to the best scientific brains in view of the challenges that lie ahead.

The problem has been discussed recently by Passmore (1978). This author emphasizes that in the past the observational sciences have not been attractive to aristoscience. Accordingly, not only have they been deprived unnecessarily of the best brains, but this gap has led to the field being left open to many wellintentioned individuals who, through lack of knowledge, approach the problem with limited vision and the arrogance of certainty. Further, it has left the scientific community open to the charge of ignoring human needs. It is easy to direct public action to single objectives, but more difficult to direct opinion towards a broad policy of the type needed. Few academic epidemiologists enjoy involvement in public controversy, preferring to address themselves to their peers and to operate within the 'old-boy' scientific network, thus increasing the possibilities of misinterpretation by media and public interest groups. It is essential that epidemiology as a science address itself more adequately to public communication, in view of its public health implications. Experience from Sweden on nuclear power has shown that the more the public is informed, the less ready it is to put forward easy and simplistic solutions (Ashby, 1980).

Nonetheless, opinion is changing and I think that all branches of science recognize the challenge involved in evaluating human disease. However, research will depend on adequate long-term funding and the creation of an appropriate academic milieu. Innovative young scientists will not be attracted to a field requiring long-term planning if governed by short-term objectives and fear of failure resulting from insecure funding, nor will they develop the width of biological knowledge required for complex problems. The creation of the appropriate milieu should have a high priority among those responsible for the direction of future cancer research. Many of the problems, especially in regard to lifestyle and extrapolation from animals, will probably require at least a further decade for solution.

Developments will take place slowly by trial and error. Attempts by managers, politicians, etc., to make research more efficient are unlikely to be more effective than a system governed by a responsible scientific community, in which the public has trust. As Passmore has pointed out, the reputation of biomedical science in terms of honesty and incorruptibility is consistently high. There have been few instances of personal abuse of public money. The fact that certain work has been pedestrian and non-productive must be regretted but it certainly does not mean that scientists have tried to distort research priorities for personal gain. To assume, however, that all scientists are objective in terms of research priorities is naive, as each has his own bias as to what is important. However, we must guard against raising false hopes and making promises about prevention. As Lavater has stated, the public seldom forgives twice. There has been a tendency in certain governmental and scientific circles to constantly present a pessimistic approach to developments in environmental carcinogenesis and prevention. Such an approach cannot but be detrimental to the image of the scientist as seen by the public and is unfair to the past accomplishments of epidemiology. It certainly leads to the belief that little has been done and that past support and effort have been wasted. The public must learn that our present optimism is based both on an ever-growing body of scientific fact, which will permit better intellectual approaches to future research, and cancer control strategy.

In conclusion, I have attempted to show that epidemiological research certainly justifies further support. However, we and the public must accept that the road will be long and uncertain and that future research will largely benefit our children.

REFERENCES

Ashby, Lord Eric, Participating in planning: the public needs better information. Nature, 1980, 283(5749), 712-713.
Baxter, P. J., & Warner, J. B. Mortality in the British rubber industries 1967-76. London: Her Majesty's Stationery Office, 1980.
Berenblum, I. Historical perspective. In T. J. Slaga, A. Sivak, & R. K. Boutwell (Eds.), Carcinogenesis - a comprehensive survey, volume 2, mechanisms of tumor promotion and cocarcinogenesis. New York: Raven Press, 1978, 1-10.
Boyland, E. Some implications of tumour promotion in carcinogenesis. International Research Communications System Medical Sciences, 1980, 1-4.
Bulbrook, R. D. Urinary androgen excretion and the etiology of breast cancer. Journal of the National Cancer Institute, 1972, 48(4), 1039-1042.
Campbell, T. C. Chemical carcinogens and human risk assessment. Federation Proceedings, 1980, 39(8), 2467-2484.
Cederlöf, R., Doll, R., Fowler, B. et al. (Eds.), Air pollution and cancer: risk assessment of methodology and epidemiological evidence (report of a task group). Environmental Health Perspectives, 1978, 22, 1-12.
Clemmesen, J. (Ed.), Symposium on Geographical Pathology and Demography of Cancer, Oxford, England, 1950. Paris, Council for International Organizations of Medical Sciences, 1950.
Coffey, D. S., & Issacs, J. T. (Eds.), Prostate Cancer. UICC Technical Report Series, Volume 48. Geneva: International Union Against Cancer, 1979.
Cole, P. Oral contraceptives and endometrial cancer. New England Journal of Medicine, 1980, 302(10), 575-576.
Cole, P., & MacMahon, B. Oestrogen fractions during early reproductive life in the aetiology of breast cancer. Lancet, 1969, 1(7595), 604-606.
Conference on the primary prevention of cancer: assessment of risk factors and future directions. In Preventive Medicine, 1980, 9(2).
Conney, A. H., Pantuck, E. J., Hsiao, K. C., et al. Regulation of drug metabolism in man by environmental chemicals and diet. Federation Proceedings, 1977, 36(5), 1647-1652.
Coulston, F. (Ed.), Regulatory Aspects of Carcinogenesis and Food Additives: The Delaney Clause. New York, San Francisco, London: Academic Press, 1979.
Crespi, M., Muñoz, N., Grassi, A., et al. Oesophageal lesions in northern Iran: a pre-malignant condition? Lancet, 1979, 2(8136), 217-221.
Davies, J. E., Edmundson, W. F., Raffonelli, A., et al. The role of social class in human pesticide control. American Journal of Epidemiology, 1972, 96(5), 334-341.
Davis, D. L., & Magee, B. H. Cancer and industrial chemical production. Science, 1979, 206(4425), 1356-1358.
Del Villano, B. C., Miller, S. I., Schacter, L. P., et al. Elevated superoxide dismutase in Black alcoholics. Science, 1980, 207(4434), 991-993.
de Thé, G., Geser, A., Day, N. E., et al. Epidemiological evidence for causal relationship between Epstein-Barr virus and Burkitt's lymphoma from Ugandan prospective study. Nature, 1978, 274(5673), 756-761.

Djerassi, C. *The Politics of Contraception.* New York, London: W. W. Norton & Company, 1979.

Doll, R. Introduction. In H. H. Hiatt, J. D. Watson, & J. A. Winsten. *Origins of Human Cancer (Book A: Incidence of Cancer in Humans).* Cold Spring Harbor Laboratory, 1977, 1-12.

Enstrom, J. E. Health and dietary practices and cancer mortality among California Mormons. Banbury Report 4: Cancer Incidence in Defined Populations. Cold Spring Harbor, New York: Cold Spring Harbor Laboratory, 1980, 69-72.

Epstein, S. S. *The Politics of Cancer.* San Francisco: Sierra Club Books, 1978.

Fishbein, L. *Potential industrial carcinogens and mutagens (studies in environmental science 4).* Amsterdam: Elsevier Scientific Publishing Company, 1979.

Fox, A. J., & Adelstein, A. M. Occupational mortality: work or way of life? Journal of Epidemiology and Community Health, 1978, *32,* 73-78.

Haenszel, W. Cancer mortality among the foreign-born in the United States. Journal of the National Cancer Institute, 1961, *26*(1), 37-132.

Haenszel, W., & Kurihara, M. Studies of Japanese migrants. I. Mortality from cancer and other diseases among Japanese in the United States. Journal of the National Cancer Institute, 1968, *40*(1), 43-68.

Hammond, E. C., & Garfinkel, L. General air pollution and cancer in the United States. Preventive Medicine, 1980, *9*(2), 206-211.

Hammond, E. C., & Seidman, H. Smoking and cancer in the United States. Preventive Medicine, 1980, *9*(2), 169-173.

Higginson, J. The geographical pathology of primary liver cancer. Cancer Research, 1963, *23*(10), 1624-1633.

Higginson, J. Present trends in cancer epidemiology. In J. F. Morgan (Ed.), *Proceedings of the Eighth Canadian Cancer Conference, Honey Harbour, Ontario, Canada, 1968.* Toronto: Pergamon Press, 1969, 40-75.

Higginson, J. Cancer etiology and prevention. In J. F. Fraumeni, Jr. (Ed.), *Persons at high risk of cancer (an approach to cancer etiology and control).* New York: Academic Press, 1975, 385-398.

Higginson, J. Perspectives and future developments in research on environmental carcinogenesis. In A. C. Griffin, & C. R. Shaw (Eds.), *Carcinogens: identification and mechanisms of action.* New York: Raven Press, 1979, 187-208

Higginson, J. Implications for future studies in humans. Environmental chemicals, enzyme function and human disease (Ciba Foundation Symposium 76), 1980 (in press).

Higginson, J., & Muir, C. S. Environmental carcinogenesis: misconceptions and limitations to cancer control. Journal of the National Cancer Institute, 1979, *63*(6), 1291-1298.

Higginson, J., & Oettlé, A. G. The incidence of cancer in the Bantu and Cape Colored population of Johannesburg, South Africa. Report of a Cancer Survey in the Transvaal (1953-55). Journal of the National Cancer Institute, 1960, *24*(3), 589-671.

Hill, P., Wynder, E. L., Garbaczewski, L., et al. Diet and menarche in different ethnic groups. European Journal of Cancer, 1980, 16, 519-525.

Hulka, B. S., Fowler, W. C., Kaufamn, D. G., et al. Estrogen and endometrial cancer: cases and two control groups from North Carolina. American Journal of Obstetrics and Gynecology, 1980, 137(1), 92-101.

IARC Monographs on the Evaluation of the Carcinogenic Risk of Chemicals to Humans, Volumes 1-22. Lyon: International Agency for Research on Cancer, 1972-1980.

IARC Monographs on the Evaluation of the Carcinogenic Risk of Chemicals to Humans, Supplement 1, Chemicals and Industrial Processes Associated with Cancer in Humans, IARC Monographs, Volumes 1-20. Lyon: International Agency for Research on Cancer, 1979.

IARC Monographs on the Evaluation of the Carcinogenic Risk of Chemicals to Humans, supplement 2, Long-term and short-term screening assays for carcinogens: a critical appraisal. Lyon: International Agency for Research on Cancer, 1980.

Kraybill, H. F. Origin, classification and distribution of chemicals in drinking water with an assessment of their carcinogenic potential. In R. L. Jolley (Ed), Water chlorination: environmental impact and health effects. Ann Arbor, Michigan: Ann Arbor Science Publishers, 1978, 211-228.

Kroes, R. Animal data, interpretation and consequences. In P. Emmelot, & E. Kriek (Eds.), Environmental carcinogenesis - occurrence, risk evaluation and mechanisms. Amsterdam: Elsevier/North-Holland Biomedical Press, 1979, 287-302.

Larouzé, B., Blumberg, B. S., London, W. T., et al. Forecasting the development of primary hepatocellular carcinoma by the use of risk factors: studies in West Africa. Journal of the National Cancer Institute, 1977, 58(6), 1557-1561.

Linsell, C. A., & Peers, F. G. Aflatoxin and liver cell cancer. Transactions of the Royal Society of Tropical Medicine and Hygiene, 1977, 71(6), 471-473.

Lyon, J. L., Gardner, J. W., & West, D. W. Cancer in Utah - risk by religion and place of residence. Journal of the National Cancer Institute, 1980 (in press).

MacMahon, B., Cole, P., & Brown, J. Etiology of human breast cancer: a review. Journal of the National Cancer Institute, 1973, 50(1), 21-42.

Mason, T. J., McKay, F. W., Hoover, R., et al. Atlas of Cancer Mortality for U.S. Counties: 1950-1969. Washington, D.C.: U.S. Government Printing Office, 1975.

Miller, A. B. Nutrition and cancer. Preventive Medicine, 9(2), 189-196.

Miller, J. A., & Miller, E. C. Perspectives on the metabolism of chemical carcinogens. In P. Emmelot, & E. Kriek (Eds.), Environmental carcinogenesis - occurrence, risk evaluation and mechanisms. Amsterdam: Elsevier/North-Holland Biomedical Press, 1979, 25-50.

McMichael, A. J., McCall, M. G., Hartshorne, J. M., et al. Patterns of gastrointestinal cancer in European migrants to Australia: the role of dietary change. International Journal of Cancer, 1980, 25, 431-437.

Mori, T., Nagasawa, H., & Bern, H. A. Long-term effects of perinatal expo-
    sure to hormones on normal and neoplastic mammary growth of ro-
    dents: a review. Journal of Environmental Pathology and Toxicology,
    1979, 3, 191-205.
Office of Population Censuses and Surveys, Occupational mortality. The
    Registrar General's decennial supplement for England and Wales, 1970-
    72, series DS No. 1. London: Her Majesty's Stationery Office, 1978.
Passmore, J. Science and its critics. New Brunswick, New Jersey: Rutgers
    University Press, 1978.
Peto, J., Doll, R., Howard, S. V., et al. A mortality study among workers in
    an English asbestos factory. British Journal of Industrial Medicine, 1977,
    34(3), 169-173.
Preventive Medicine, New York, London: Academic Press, 1980, 9(2).
Richardson, G. S., & MacLaughlin, D. T. (Eds.), Hormonal biology of endo-
    metrial cancer. UICC Technical Report Series, Volume 42. Geneva:
    International Union Against Cancer, 1978.
Rose, A. H. (Ed.), Alcoholic beverages (economic microbiology volume 1).
    London, New York, San Francisco: Academic Press, 1977.
Royal Society, Long-term toxic effects. Final report of a Royal Society Study
    Group. London: The Royal Society, 1978.
Schull, W. J. Genetic structure of human populations. Journal of Environ-
    mental Pathology and Toxicology, 1979, 2, 1305-1312.
Smith, D. C., Prentice, R., Thompson, D. J., et al. Association of exogenous
    estrogen and endometrial carcinoma. New England Journal of Medicine,
    1975, 293(23), 1164-1167.
Trichopoulos, D., MacMahon, B., & Brown, J. Socioeconomic status, urine
    estrogens, and breast cancer risk. Journal of the National Cancer Insti-
    tute, 1980, 64(4), 753-755.
Walker, E. A., Castegnaro, M., Griciute, L., & Lyle, R. E. (Eds.), Environ-
    mental aspects of N-nitroso compounds. IARC Scientific Publications No.
    19. Lyon: International Agency for Research on Cancer, 1978.
Wattenberg, L. W. Inhibitors of chemical carcinogens. In P. Emmelot, & E.
    Kriek (Eds.), Environmental carcinogenesis - occurrence, risk evaluation
    and mechanisms. Amsterdam: Elsevier/North-Holland Biomedical Press,
    1979, 241-263.
Wilkins, J. R., Reiches, N. A., & Kruse, C. W. Organic chemical contaminants
    in drinking water and cancer. American Journal of Epidemiology, 1979,
    110(4), 420-448.
Wynder, E. L., & Gori, G. B. Contribution of the environment to cancer inci-
    dence: an epidemiologic excercise. Journal of the National Cancer Insti-
    tute, 1977, 58(4), 825-832.
Zack, M., Cannon, S., Loyd, D., et al. Cancer in children of parents exposed
    to hydrocarbon-related industries and occupations. American Journal of
    Epidemiology, 1980, 111(3), 329-336.

Analytic Epidemiology[1,2]

PHILIP COLE[3]

Professor and Director, Division of Epidemiology
Department of Public Health
University of Alabama in Birmingham
Birmingham, Alabama

The topic I am to discuss is analytic epidemiology and, in keeping with the title of this Symposium, I shall deal primarily with "Achievements" and "Prospects". I have elected to deal with only one "Challenge" but it is an important one and I will describe it in the context of the relationship of saccharin and bladder cancer.

I should explain first what I understand the term "analytic epidemiology" to mean. The epidemiologic study of the chronic diseases was pioneered in the late 1940's but it was only in the late 1950's that it started to become an organized science. At about that time the term analytic epidemiology came into use to designate epidemiologic research which was intended specifically to elucidate causes of disease. The intent was to contrast analytic epidemiology with descriptive epidemiology which related to the gathering of statistics on the temporal and spatial distributions of disease. There are other views as to what comprises analytic epidemiology and how it differs from descriptive epidemiology. However, debate over the meaning of these terms long ago passed the point of diminished returns and, I suspect, would not greatly interest you. I propose to discuss epidemiology in relation to the search for the causes of cancer.

First, I will describe some of the many successes of cancer epidemiology during the past decade. I would suggest that epidemiology has made a contribution to the development

[1]From the Epidemiology Program, Comprehensive Cancer Center, University of Alabama in Birmingham.
[2]Presented at the 1980 International Symposium on Cancer, New York, NY, September, 1980.
[3]Supported by a grant, 2 P30 CA13148, from the National Cancer Institute, USPHS.

of virtually all of the available knowledge regarding means
of preventing cancer. But, even in so stating, I emphasize
that few of these contributions were solely epidemiologic.
In fact, epidemiology in isolation is a sterile science, and
I am referring to epidemiology in conjunction with other sciences and with medical practice.

By way of "Achievements" I have selected four examples,
successes I would call them, of the contributions of epidemiology to the search for causes of cancer, to our understanding of mechanisms of carcinogenesis and, I hope, to the for-
mulation of rational public policy. All of these examples
come from the past decade and most of the information to
which I will refer is not more than a few years old.

In the mid-1970's two case-control studies showed an association between the use of exogenous estrogens and the risk
of endometrial cancer[1,2]. The studies suggested that the association was causal because it was strong, with relative
risks of five or more, because it was consistent with respect
to a dose-response relationship and in other ways, and because it had high biologic credibility. Nonetheless, a number of criticisms were offered of these studies, perhaps the
most important one being that the association was invalid due
to a selection bias. The suggested bias rested on the proposal that many of the cases in these studies might have had
a lesion which morphologically mimicked endometrial cancer
but which had no (or only very low) potential to behave as a
cancer. The bias becomes plausible if it is also considered
that such lesions, these proposed pseudocancers, would be
made to bleed or otherwise cause symptoms and come to attention if exogenous estrogens were administered. Even initially there were a number of reasons to reject the idea that
such a proposed bias was of importance. However, one research group which considered the bias to be real conducted
a study designed to obviate the bias, or so it was contend-
ed[3]. This study indeed appeared to be negative but in a
carefully-reasoned argument other epidemiologists[4] have demonstrated that this study is far less acceptable than the
original work which it was supposed to correct. In recent
years it has come to be generally accepted that exogenous estrogens can cause endometrial cancer. The most recent
study[15] of this issue should overcome the last traces of
skepticism as it relates, at least in part, to women with endometrial cancer who had stopped using estrogens one year or
more before the diagnosis was made. Some of the findings
from that study (Table 1) show that when a women stops using
exogenous estrogens, her excess risk of endometrial cancer
gradually declines; nonetheless, even among women who ceased

TABLE 1
Rate Ratio Among Women Who Used Estrogens for Five
Years or Longer According to Time Since Last Use

Time Since Last Use	Rate Ratio
< 1 yr.	8.8
1-	3.6
2-	3.3
3-	2.7
4-	2.7
5+	2.6

(Modified from Shapiro et al; 1980)

use for three or more years the rate ratio remains elevated
at about 2.7 (relative to a value of 1.0 for women who never
used estrogens). Among such women the proposed selection
bias could not operate for vaginal bleeding due to exogenous
estrogens would not occur long after estrogen use has ceased.
This explanation of the association can now be categorically
rejected. In accepting as causal the relationship between
exogenous estrogens and endometrial cancer we should keep in
mind that we are not necessarily incriminating estrogens in
general as causes of endometrial cancer but only estrone, the
specific estrogen which accounts for 80 percent or more of
the biological activity of conjugated estrogens.

For my second example I will deal again with cancer of the
endometrium but switch attention to oral contraceptives
(OCs). This example will show how epidemiology exploits situations that develop in order to evaluate and to quantify
clinical observations and to extend them. It was reported,
on the basis of uncontrolled clinical observations, that wom-
en who used sequential OCs, and especially the particular
preparation named Oracon, had an elevated risk of endometrial
cancer[6,7]. For a number of reasons[8] until recently other interpretations could have been placed on the information which
was available. But, this year a controlled epidemiologic
study[9] showed that, indeed, users of Oracon do have an increased risk of endometrial cancer (Table 2). However, the

TABLE 2
Distribution of Cases and Controls and Endometrial
Cancer Rate Ratio According to Oracon Use

Oracon Use	Cases	Controls	Rate Ratio
Yes	6	8	7.3
No	110	376	1.0

(Modified from Weiss and Sayvetz; 1980)

TABLE 3
Distribution of Cases and Controls and
Endometrial Cancer Rate Ratio According
to Use of Combined Oral Contraceptives

Use of Combined Agents	Cases	Controls	Rate Ratio
Yes	17	76	0.5
No	93	173	1.0

(Modified from Weiss and Sayvetz; 1980)

most provocative finding in this new study is the suggestion
in the data that women who used the usual combined OCs have
a risk of endometrial cancer below that of nonusers of OCs
(Table 3). While this latter finding of a protective effect
cannot yet be considered firm, it is likely to be correct
and, in any event, it is clear that combined OCs do not cause
endometrial cancer. Thus, we can appreciate that some specific feature of sequential agents, which is absent from combined agents, is a cause of endometrial cancer. We can also
suggest that some feature of combined agents may be protective against the disease. The causal agent in Oracon almost
certainly was the uniquely high dose of estrone which was incorporated into the monthly regimen. The fact that this is
exactly the same hormone as is incriminated in the causation
of endometrial cancer by exogenous estrogens makes the two
findings mutually supportive. And, in turn, and of considerable importance both findings support a fundamental underlying hypothesis, for which there is also some direct evidence,
that an excess of endogenous estrone is also a carcinogen for
the endometrium[10]. It is not evident what aspect of the combined OCs is protective; it could be the progestational agent
they contain or the relatively low dose of estrogen or the
specific estrogen used. Therefore, insofar as I can see, endometrial cancer has joined the ranks of those malignancies
whose cause is known. The cause is estrone whether of exogenous or endogenous origin.

    For our third example, I turn to one of the most intrigu-
ing cancer research stories of our era, that of the relationship of in utero exposure to diethylstilbestrol (DES) and
clear cell adenocarcinoma of the vagina among young women[11].
This story is too well known to bear repeating here. But
three important aspects of the association[12] seem not to be
well known and do warrant emphasis. The first of these is
the rarity of this cancer even among young women who were exposed to DES. It seems to be thought that these women are at
high risk but, in fact, their risk is high only in relative
terms. In absolute terms their risk, at least through age

TABLE 4

Distribution of Cases and Controls and the
Rate Ratio of Vaginal Cancer According to
Gestational Age at First Exposure

Gestational Age (wks.)	Cases (%)	Controls (%)	Rate Ratio
1-4	3.1	1.3	2.2
5-6	14.3	4.3	3.1
7-8	30.6	15.2	1.8
9-12	33.7	30.7	1.0
13-16	16.3	18.7	0.8
17+	2.0	29.8	0.1
Total	100.0%	100.0%	-
No. of subjects	98	1418	

(Modified from Herbst, et al; 1979)

25, is less than 1 in 1,000. A second refinement of the DES-vaginal cancer association is shown in Table 4 which displays the rate ratio of vaginal cancer among DES-exposed females according to their gestational age at first exposure. It is evident that the brunt of the disease is borne by girls exposed during the first two months of fetal life. And, for exposures sustained after the fourth month the risk is so low it cannot be estimated with validity; there may be no excess risk at all. A third recent observation from analytic epidemiology relating to the question of DES and vaginal cancer is that the disease virtually does not occur prior to age 14 but then the incidence rate rises rapidly, plateaus through the late teenage years and then probably declines (Figure 1). This age-incidence curve poses a problem to the epidemiologist as it implies that the average induction period of the disease is about 19 years but that the range of the induction period is only about 10 years. The difficulty is that, usually, the range of an induction period is much greater than its average value. The findings can be reconciled with what we expect to see if we propose that DES is not acting as a carcinogen or is acting as an incomplete carcinogen. It may be that DES sets the stage for another element in the causal web of this cancer, one which acts during puberty. Were this so then the median induction period would be only about 8 years and the rapid rise in the incidence rate would seem more reasonable. Of course, the idea that DES is an incomplete carcinogen is supported by the observation I described a moment ago, that is by the fact that vaginal cancer is quite rare even among exposed girls. While the proposal that DES is not a complete carcinogen has little public health significance, it has a profound scientific one: an

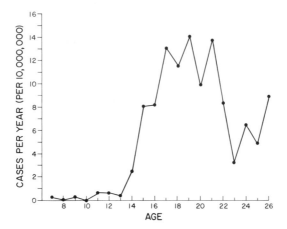

<u>Figure 1</u>. Incidence of clear cell adenocarcinoma by age at
diagnosis among native-born, White, resident female subjects.
(Taken from Herbst et al; 1979)

important part of the causation of this disease is unknown to
us but might be susceptible to discovery if we could study
girls of the appropriate age.

Up to now I have been describing situations in which the
epidemiologic findings are clear, positive, of considerable
scientific and public health importance and demonstrate the
crucial contribution of epidemiology to cancer prevention.
I turn now to an area which is contentious and where there is
more concern with regulatory and public policy issues than
with the scientific ones - and perhaps rightly so. I refer
to the relationship, I would prefer to say the non-relation-
ship, of saccharin and bladder cancer. The issue arose because it was found that when male rats were subjected to massive doses of saccharin, both <u>in</u> <u>utero</u> and throughout life,
they experienced an excess of bladder cancer. A generalization of this finding to human beings was abetted by an epidemiologic study with some positive results[13] and the Food
and Drug Administration proposed successively more stringent
restrictions on saccharin. This proposal elicited massive
public resistance and the FDA was enjoined by Congress
against implementing its ban on saccharin. Later, a Working
Group of the FDA acknowledged that the then available information permitted no judgement as to whether saccharin
caused bladder cancer among people and recommended that further research, especially epidemiologic research, be done.

I would like to suggest what may ultimately prove to be
the principal issue raised by the controversy over saccharin

and the challenge to us; it is a challenge to establish criteria or standards whereby epidemiology or any other science
should be acknowledged to have provided persuasive evidence
that a substance is not a human carcinogen. At present there
are no such criteria. I believe there are two major reasons
for this. First the history of medical research and, in
fact, of science in general, shows that it is positive, not
negative results that attract interest and reward. And
second, there is an asymmetry in the current logic of science
which seems to suggest that safety, or non-carcinogenesis,
could not be established. It is the old "You can prove a
positive but not a negative" argument. But, I contend that
the argument is wrong as is the logic on which it rests.
I do not have the time to present my reasoning here. Nonetheless, whether you agree with my concerns or not, most of
you will agree with the need for the criteria to which I
refer. Now, I return to the subject at hand. A number of
older epidemiologic studies and three excellent new ones
[14,15,16] provide evidence that saccharin as used by people is
not a human bladder carcinogen or, if so, is a carcinogen to
an immeasurably weak extent. The data from one of the recent
studies (Table 5) shows that there is no excess risk of bladder cancer even among heavy users of saccharin. Which evidence is to provide a basis for regulating human choices?
That from a number of large well-controlled studies of human
beings or that from studies in animals designed to maximize
the likelihood of a positive outcome by the use of exposure
conditions which can have no equivalent in human experience.
It is because this is the issue that I consider the epidemi-

TABLE 5
Distribution of Cases and Controls and
Rate Ratio of Bladder Cancer According
to Duration of Use of Sugar Substitutes.
Men and Women Separately.

Duration of Use (Years)	Cases	Controls	Rate Ratio
Men			
None	224	193	1.0
<5	53	66	0.7
5-9	23	25	0.8
10+	17	14	1.0
Women			
None	74	80	1.0
<5	28	20	1.3
5+	22	17	1.3

(From Morrison and Buring; 1980)

ologic studies of saccharin and bladder cancer to constitute
a major success. For, the controversy is only whether saccharin has been completely exonerated as a human bladder carcinogen or whether its heavy use may impose a very slight increase in risk. This being the controversy, I would suggest
that the epidemiologic evidence is crucial and the available
animal evidence irrelevant.

The recent past of cancer epidemiology has been bright.
The near future is brighter still and to suggest what the
"Prospects" are I will indicate three areas where exciting
things will happen over the next several years. First, I
have already suggested that OC use may be protective against
endometrial cancer. It is possible that OC use will turn out
to be protective against cancer of the ovary as well. This
is an idea which could be defended on theoretical grounds but
there is already some epidemiologic evidence[17] -- inconclu-
sive though it may be -- that this is so. Several large epidemiologic studies of cancer of the ovary are now nearing
completion and we may hope to have this issue clarified
within the next two years. Second, several studies which
combine epidemiology and virology are underway to refine our
understanding of the relationship between the chronic Hepa-
titis-B Virus carrier state and cancer of the liver. This
association, which has only relatively recently been appreciated, is moving rapidly toward resolution and already
appears to be the leading candidate for demonstrating a
virus-human cancer relationship. The public health implications of this are not great for the United States and other
Western countries, where liver cancer is quite rare, but are
of tremendous importance for vast populations elsewhere in
the world among which liver cancer is quite common. A third
cancer with respect to which we may anticipate important
advances in the next five years or so is breast cancer. To
elucidate the causes of this disease two important lines of
research need to be brought together now. It is almost certainly true that breast cancer is largely hormonally determined, perhaps in young adulthood. In addition, recent studies[18,19] suggest that a woman's breast cancer risk may, at
least to some extent, be predictable from the appearance of
the structure of her breasts on the mammogram. If this is
so, we can expect an acceleration in epidemiologic research
on breast cancer in order to define the relationship of the
breast structure to the hormonal milieu. This, in turn, may
lead to an appreciation of the specific hormonal aberration
which causes the disease and, possibly, to a preventive
approach.

REFERENCES

1. Ziel HK, Finkle WD. Increased risk of endometrial car-
    cinoma among users of conjugated estrogens. N Engl J
    Med. 1975; 293:1167-70.
2. Smith DC, Prentice R, Thompson DJ, Herrmann WL. Asso-
    ciation of exogenous estrogens and endometrial carci-
    noma. N Engl J Med. 1975; 293:1164-7.
3. Horwitz RI, Feinstein AR. Alternative analytic methods
    of case-control studies of estrogens and endometrial
    cancer. N Engl J Med. 1978; 299:1089-94.
4. Hutchison GB, Rothman KJ. Correcting a bias? N Engl J
    Med. 1978; 299:1129-30.
5. Shapiro S, et al. Recent and past use of conjugated
    estrogens in relation to adenocarcinoma of the endo-
    metrium. N Engl J Med. 1980; 303:485-90.
6. Silverberg SG, Makowski EL. Endometrial carcinoma in
    young women taking oral contraceptive agents. Obstet
    Gynecol. 1975; 46:503-6.
7. Silverberg SG, Makowski EL, Roche WD. Endometrial car-
    cinoma in women under 40 years of age: comparison of
    cases in oral contraceptive users and non-users.
    Cancer. 1977; 39:592-8.
8. Cole P. Oral contraceptives and endometrial cancer.
    N Engl J Med. 1980; 302:575-6.
9. Weiss NS, Sayvetz TA. Incidence of endometrial cancer
    in relation to the use of oral contraceptives. N Engl
    J Med. 1980; 302:551-4.
10. MacDonald PC, Edman CD, Hemsell DL, Porter JC, Siiteri
    PK. Effect of obesity on conversion of plasma andro-
    stenedione to estrone in postmenopausal women with and
    without endometrial cancer. Am J Obstet Gynecol. 1978;
    130:448-55.
11. Herbst AL, Ulfelder H, Poskanzer DC. Adenocarcinoma of
    the vagina: association of maternal stilbestrol therapy
    with tumor appearance in young women. N Engl J Med.
    1971; 284:878.
12. Herbst AL, Cole P, Norusis MJ, Welch WR, Scully RE.
    Epidemiologic aspects and factors related to survival in
    384 registry cases in clear cell adenocarcinoma of the
    vagina and cervix. Am J Obstet Gynecol. 1979; 135:876-
    83.
13. Howe GR, Burch JD, Miller AB, et al. Artificial sweete-
    ners and human cancer. Lancet. 1977; ii:578-81.
14. Hoover RN, Strasser PH. Artificial sweeteners and
    human bladder cancer. Lancet. 1980; 8173:837-40.

15. Morrison AS, Buring JE. Artificial sweeteners and can-
     cer of the lower urinary tract. N Engl J Med. 1980;
     302:537-41.
16. Wynder EL, Stellman SK. Saccharin usage and bladder
     cancer. Science. 1980; 207:1214-16.
17. Newhouse ML, Pearson RM, Fullerton JM, Boesen EA,
     Sharron HS. A case control study of carcinoma of the
     overy. Br J Prev Soc Med. 1977; 31:148-53.
18. Wilkinson E, Clopton C, Gordonson J, Green R, Hill A,
     Pike MC. Mammographic parenchymal pattern and the risk
     of breast cancer. J Natl Cancer Inst. 1977; 59:1397-
     400.
19. Brisson J, Merletti F, Sadowsky NL, Twaddle JA,
     Morrison AS, Cole P. Mammographic features of the
     breast and breast cancer risk. 1980. Submitted for
     publication.

The Interface between Epidemiology
and Cancer Control Policy

Richard Doll
Honorary Director

Imperial Cancer Research Fund
Cancer Epidemiology and Clinical Trials Unit
9 Keble Road, Oxford OX1 3QG

Strategic Planning

It is perhaps not surprising that some individuals and committees, faced with the problem of deciding which chemicals should be restricted in their use, tend to discount epidemiological evidence when they find that few of the several thousand on their agenda have been studied by epidemiologists in sufficient depth for them to be able to draw firm conclusions about their effects. But to condemn epidemiology, in consequence, as not being a valid tool for the purpose of cancer control is to condemn it for failing to achieve ends that it does not have. An epidemiological perspective starts, not with the 10,000 chemicals that pollute an area, but with the 10,000 deaths that occur in it each year and seeks to determine the major causes of these actual deaths. It is much more likely to overlook a large number of small effects than laboratory science; but much less likely to overlook the chief determinants of current mortality rates and trends, especially if these are not simple direct effects of individual chemicals on D.N.A.

When our knowledge of the mechanisms of carcinogenesis and of the metabolism of chemicals in man and laboratory animals is much more complete than it is today, it may be possible to predict the precise effect on the incidence of human cancer of different forms of behaviour and different degrees of exposure to different chemicals under different conditions. In this ideal future, there will be no need for men and women to suffer any ill effects inadvertently, and the raison d'etre of cancer epidemiology will disappear - although the practical and ethical problems of how to

assess the relative costs and benefits of different lines of
action will, of course, remain. For the foreseeable future,
however, one principal role for epidemiology is to help
scientists, committees, industry, and government to maintain
a sense of proportion in the face of the myriad, actual or
hypothetical risks to which men and women are exposed; and,
by so doing, to ensure that a reasonable amount of effort
is devoted to controlling the factors that involve the greatest hazards and that a reasonable amount of funds is directed
into the support of research in fields in which work would
seem likely to have the greatest impact on human health.

What these factors and fields are, as far as cancer is
concerned, has been, or will be, discussed by others. I
shall, therefore, confine my remarks to emphasizing the importance of this role for epidemiology, in the development
of a sensible policy for reducing the toll of cancer and
will concentrate, for the rest, on those other contributions
which help by:

(i)   detecting unsuspected hazards,
(ii)   demonstrating the absence of hazards suspected on
       other grounds, and
(iii) providing data necessary for weighing cost and benefit.

Detection of unsuspected hazards

That observations on man have hitherto provided the
first clue to the majority of hazards that have been shown
to cause concern in man is a matter of history which, with
the advance of biological knowledge, should not repeat
itself. We cannot assume, however, that it will be practicable to recognize and eliminate all present and future
hazards before they produce disease in man, just because
the great majority of the agents responsible for these
hazards have subsequently been shown to be mutagenic by one
or other in vitro test or to be carcinogenic when tested
in a particular way in a particular species of laboratory
animal. The question that has to be asked is whether any
series of tests that can be carried out on a routine basis
can reveal all, or nearly all, such hazards without being
focused by knowledge of human experience. So far as we can
tell, the answer is clearly 'no', as is demonstrated by experience of occupational exposure to arsenic, benzene. and
some as yet unknown aspect of the manufacture of hardwood
furniture; of medical treatment with busulphan and phenacetin: and of the social use of alcohol. Furthermore, many

cancer research workers now believe that aspects of diet may contribute to the development of the disease indirectly by leading to or preventing the formation of carcinogens in vivo or by modifying their action: for example, by affecting age at menarche or other hormonal factors, by providing necessary substrates, by inducing enzymes, or by trapping free radicals. Few, if any, of these mechanisms would be discovered by the routine screening of many substances for carcinogenic activity. Epidemiological evidence cannot, of course strictly prove that a substance, a process, or a mode of behaviour causes a particular type of cancer, except in the rare circumstances in which it is possible to do a controlled trial of the effects of withdrawing a suspected agent, as has been attempted in the case of cigarette smoking (1), or a trial in which the carcinogenicity of a drug is tested inadvertently in the course of testing other effects – and even then the evidence must fall short of logical proof as the experiment can hardly be repeated. Experience, however, has shown that if sufficient care is taken in the analysis and interpretation of the data a case can be built up from human evidence that is strong enough to justify preventative action and that the result of this will support or otherwise the validity of the conclusion. This is true, even without the support of laboratory evidence – although, of course, laboratory evidence can make things much easier in several ways.

The kind of evidence required is listed in Table 1. It's nature is being discussed by others and I should like to make only two comments. First, it is not always necessary for the absolute risk to be large, nor for a large number of cases to be observed before a conclusion can be reached.

If the type of cancer produced is normally rare, the relative risk can be increased a hundredfold or more and detection is simple. Angiosarcoma of the liver following the use of thorotrast, adenocarcinoma of the vagina following exposure to diethyl-stilboestrol in utero, squamous carcinoma of the renal pelvis in patients suffering from phenacetin pyelonephritis, nasal sinus cancer following exposure to dust in a nickel refinery or fumes in the manufacture of isopropyl alcohol, and mesothelioma of the pleura following exposure to asbestos are examples of hazards that were detected by observation of less than 10 cases. In some instances the hazard proved to be large, affecting as many as 5% of the exposed population; in others it was as small as 1 in 1000.

Table 1

REQUIREMENTS FOR ESTABLISHING CARCINOGENECITY
FROM EPIDEMIOLOGICAL EVIDENCE

Positive associations in groups of individuals with known

    exposure (case-control or cohort studies)

That is not explained by bias in recording or detection

    "   "   "   " by confounding

    "   "   "   " by chance

That varies appropriately with dose

    "   "   "   " with period of exposure

That is observed repeatedly in different circumstances

Secondly, hazards can be detected that produce only a small relative risk, increasing the risk from other causes by a factor of (say) less than two. In these circumstances, however, interpretation is often exceedingly difficult, even though disease is produced in as many as 3 or 4% of the exposed population. (as would be the case with the production of cancers in the lung or breast). It may be noted,for example, that smoking habits of men in different categories of occupation vary from about 65% of the national average to over 130% and that Fox and Adelstein (2) found that these percentages correlated closely with the mortality ratios in each category for cancer of the lung (r = 0.72), so that confounding with smoking habits may produce artefacts of comparable size. The difficulties may be overcome, but only after detailed study of large numbers of cases. Stewart (3) and MacMahon (4), for example, were able to document the relationship between exposure of the foetus to ionizing radiations in utero and the child's subsequent development of cancer, because some 10% of all pregnant women were customarily X-rayed for obstetric purposes and they were able to study all cases of cancer that occurred in children under 10 years of age in, respectively, a whole country and several States. As a result it was possible to exclude all other explanations (5) and conclude that exposure of the foetus to approximately 1 rad would cause cancer in about 1 child in 2000, increasing the natural incidence of the disease by some 50%. With less material, it would have been extremely difficult to eliminate the possibility that the result could have been due to biased information, confounding, or chance.

The extent of many human studies is, however, strictly limited by the number of people exposed, particularly in those studies concerned with occupational exposure, and, when the number is small, human evidence of the production of small relative risks is seldom strong enough to be conclusive in itself. It is always relevant, as it refers directly to the animal whose cancers we are trying to prevent, but its meaning has to be interpreted in the light of other information. And it is often necessary to wait for a conclusion until more information is obtained by collaboration across national frontiers or the passage of time.

Demonstrating the absence of hazard

Whether, conversely, it is ever possible for negative human evidence to outweigh positive evidence of mutagenicity

in vitro or the production of tumours in laboratory animals
and to justify the conclusion that an agent is not carcinogenic under the conditions in which men and women are exposed
to it, is an important biological question that still has to
be decided. Personally, I believe that this depends on the
character of the laboratory evidence; but whether this is
correct or not, it would, I think, be generally agreed that
human evidence can demonstrate that a risk is negligibly
small in comparison with the normal risks of daily life and
can be properly ignored if the process or substance is of
real value to individuals, either directly or indirectly as
members of a social organization.

It is not practicable, however, to lay down precise
criteria that will justify such a conclusion. It is reasonable enough to tell a laboratory investigator that he must
use so many animals, test in so many species, treat at so
many levels of dose for such and such periods, and observe
the animals for a specified length of time, as these conditions are under his personal control - subject only to the
non-negligible qualification of financial constraint. But
it is self-defeating to lay down the same sort of rules for
the epidemiologist as the conditions of his experiment were
determined by others and often many years in the past. To
suggest, as has been done (6), that human data should be
considered as evidence of the lack of carcinogenicity only
if it refers to groups of subjects who have had at least
20 years exposure, been followed for at least 30 years from
the time of first exposure, and are large enough for a 50%
increase in incidence of the predicted cancers to be statistically significant, is fine in theory, but has no place in
the real world. Had vinyl chloride not caused angiosarcoma
in the human liver it would, on this basis, have required
about 40 million men-years of observation of chloride workers
to demonstrate the lack of effect. While not to consider
negative evidence that was as limited as that considered for
evidence of a positive effect, could lead to the absurd
situation described by Gaffey (personal communication) in
which a positive effect was accepted because one was shown
at the 1 in 20 level of significance in one study, while
evidence from 19 similar studies, which were all negative,
was ignored because it failed to satisfy the criteria for
consideration.

It must be accepted, however, that great difficulties
are created by the length of induction times and the fact

that for at least some types of cancer, the risk appears to increase with the third, fourth, or even the fifth power of the duration of exposure. Human evidence, therefore, increases in weight with the length of time over which the observations are made.

Nearly all risks so far recognized have, however, begun to appear within 15 years of first exposure and exceptionally some have appeared much earlier (non-Hodgkin's lymphoma, for example, reaches a peak incidence within 2 years of the start of immuno-suppressive therapy and leukaemia 5 to 8 years after acute irradiation). It is only very few risks (in particular that of nasal sinus cancer in nickel refiners and in manufacturers of hardwood furniture) that have not appeared within 15 years. Judging by past experience the absence of an effect within 10 years of first exposure means very little, but all evidence relating to longer periods of observation is worth having.

Empirically, too, the dependence on duration of exposure is less clear for occupational and iatrogenic hazards than it is for smoking and exposure to ultra-violet light – due perhaps in some cases (e.g. asbestos, nickel, and beryllium) to prolonged half-lives in the tissues at risk. If however, individuals are to be exposed for the whole of their lives, weak carcinogens can become of major importance and little reliance can be placed on negative data relating to exposures of less than 20 years.

The difficulty in basing decisions on negative epidemiological data, but at the same time the importance of doing so, is illustrated by the data on saccharin, which causes cancer of the bladder in rats under defined if rather unusual conditions. It is certainly not a powerful carcinogen for man, since there is not the slightest suggestion of an increase in bladder cancer mortality in national cohorts, corresponding to the great increase in consumption that occurred at the beginning of the war (7), nor is there any increase in the mortality from bladder cancer in diabetics, despite the great use that many of them make of it (8). Indeed, diabetics seem to experience somewhat less bladder cancer than normal, due, possibly, to a less than average consumption of cigarettes. More importantly, there is now evidence from 5 well-conducted case-control studies, covering altogether 5000 affected patients in the USA, the results of which provide estimates of the relative risk of bladder can-

cer in users of artificial sweeteners which range neatly on
either side of 1 for both sexes (Table 2). The largest and
most representative of these studies (11), which was immacu-
lately conducted, has been interpreted by some as suggesting
the existence of a positive effect, because statistically
significant trends in risk were found in a few of the many
subgroups examined. Positive results in subgroups that are
not supported by the overall results are, however, dangerous
to rely on and are better regarded as hypothesis-forming
than conclusive. In this case, moreover, the subgroups in
which one would naturally first look for an effect, i.e.
those of persons who have used the sweeteners longest, show
relative risks that were, if anything, diminished (Table 3).

No guarantee can, of course, be given that an effect
would not be produced by a life-time consumption of the large
amounts that are currently consumed in diet drinks by some
adults in the USA and the extent to which the use of the
substance is controlled will need to take account of this
potential, but limited and unproven, risk against the benefit that many users feel they obtain.

Weighing cost and Benefit

When a risk is eventually established, it cannot always
be eliminated and standards have to be set which will contain
it within acceptable limits. These are always set at the
lowest practicable level; but this is not a precise term and
varies with the availability of money to achieve it. A line
has to be drawn somewhere and the decision where to draw it
is facilitated if it is possible to predict the risk from
known relationships between dose and effect in man. Most
investigators would, I think, agree with the National Research Council's Committee on Prototype Explicit Analyses
for Pesticides (14) that it is not possible to make numerical
estimates of the effect of chemicals on cancer incidence
in man, except when reliable human data are available. At
present, data of this sort are available for relatively few
of the risks to which man is exposed. These include cigarette smoking and ionizing radiations (with some precision)
and the combustion products of fossil fuels, arsenic, and
asbestos.

Each is a topic for discussion in itself and I can
comment now only on the standards applied to general atmospheric pollution, which is generally thought, so far as can-

Table 2

RISK OF BLADDER CANCER WITH USE OF ARTIFICIAL SWEETENERS

| Authors | No. of cases | Relative risk with use of: | | | Sex |
		Table top sweet-eners	Diet bever-ages	Artificial sweeteners, any form	
Howe et al., (9)	480	1.6	0.8	-	
Kessler & Clark (10)	365	0.88	0.95	0.97	
		-	-	1.08*	M
Hoover et al., (11)	2226	1.04	0.95	0.99	
Morrison & Buring (12)	469	0.8	0.8	-	
Wynder & Stellman (13)	302	0.93	0.85	-	
Howe et al., (9)	152	0.6	0.9	-	
Kessler & Clark (10)	154	0.91	1.00	1.00	
		-	-	0.87*	F
Hoover et al., (11)	744	1.04	0.97	1.01	
Morrison & Buring (12)	197	1.5	1.6	-	
Wynder & Stellman (13)	65	0.62	0.60	_	

*specifically saccharin

Table 3

RISK OF BLADDER CANCER IN PERSONS WHO HAVE TAKEN ARTIFICIAL
SWEETENERS FOR 10 YEARS OR MORE

(total study group: patients 3,010, controls 5,783)

| Type of sweetener | Sex | Number of subjects | | Relative risk* in users |
		Patients with bladder cancer	Controls	
Table-top	M	157	314	0.97
	F	62	137	0.96
Diet drink	M[†]	131	248	1.01
	F[†]	56	96	1.14
	M[ø]	84	220	0.75
	F[ø]	33	91	0.77

* Adjusted for race, age, and cigarette smoking

[†] 10-14 years

[ø] 15 years or more

After Hoover et al. (11)

Table 4

MORTALITY FROM LUNG CANCER, STANDARDIZED FOR
SMOKING HABITS AND AGE AMONG MEN NOT OCCUPATIONALLY
EXPOSED TO DUST, FUMES, ETC., EXPRESSED AS
PROPORTION OF THAT EXPECTED: BY PLACE OF RESIDENCE.*

(after Hammond and Garfinkel (18))

Metropolitan area	
population 1,000,000+	0.98
population less than 1,000,000	0.97
Non-Metropolitan area	0.92
Los Angeles, Riverside, and Orange Counties, California	0.96

Cities with air contamination ($\mu g/m^3$):

Particulates		Benzene soluble organic matter	
130-180	0.89	8.5-15.0	1.01
100-129	0.79	6.5- 7.9	0.87
35- 99	1.10	3.4- 6.3	0.93

*All men not occupationally exposed 0.96

All men occupationally exposed 1.09

cer is concerned, to be measured most appropriately by the
benzene soluble organic matter typified by benzo(a)pyrene,
although it also includes radioactive isotopes and many
other constituents (15). Extrapolation from the occupational
experience of men who made coal-gas in Britain and from
roofers working with pitch and asphalt in the United States
(16,17) leads to the conclusion that pollution of city air
with 30 or 40 ng benzo(a)pyrene/m^3 (an amount that used to
be common) might have contributed, in conjunction with cigarette smoke, to some 10% of all cases of lung cancer - a
figure that is closely in line with that estimated at an
international symposium in Sweden in 1977 (15). Pollution
with the combustion products of fossil fuels is now reduced
to perhaps a tenth of this figure and we have been provided
with an opportunity of testing the extent of its cumulative
effect by the results of the American Cancer Society's massive follow-up study of a million Americans (18). Followed
from 1960 to 1972, they have revealed lung cancer mortality
rates among men not occupationally exposed to dust, fumes,
etc. which accord reasonably well with this estimate (since
benzo(a)pyrene contributes some 0.1% to the total benzene
soluble organic matter) and, indeed, with one that could
be even lower.

Conclusion

        I conclude, therefore, as I began; that a rational pol-
icy for the prevention of cancer should start from observations on man and a realistic assessment of the proportion
of deaths attributable to the various causes that are capable
of prevention. In making this assessment, we are greatly
aided by the large-scale studies of the type that have been
carried out by American Cancer Society and the National
Cancer Institute, when they sought information from respectively a million Americans and a quarter of a million American
veterans and followed them up for 12 to 16 years (18, 19, 20,
21, 22) and by large-scale case-control studies of different
types of cancer, like the study of bladder cancer recently
carried out by the National Cancer Institute (11). A rational
policy will, however, need to go further and will seek to
discover sections of the population that suffer abnormally
high risks even though the separate sections may be individually small. In doing this, it will be aided by the use of
epidemiological methods to monitor the effects of occupational and medicinal exposure and of the way that these exposures interact with other aspects of the individual's way

of life. Studies of this sort are not an alternative to the
screening of industrial products by laboratory tests; they
are complementary to it. The results obtained by each method
help to interpret the results obtained by the other and ultimately to make a judgement about what is best for society
as a whole. What this is, is not a matter for scientists
to decide, but for society itself.

References

(1) Rose, G. and Hamilton, P.J.S. (1978)
A randomized controlled trial of the effect on middle-
aged men of advice to stop smoking.
J.Epidemiol.Community Health 32, 275-281

(2) Fox, A.J., and Adelstein,A.M. (1978)
Occupational mortality work or way of life?
J.Epidemiol. Community Health, 32, 73-78

(3) Stewart, A. Webb,J. and Hewitt, D. (1958)
A survey of childhood malignancies.
Brit. med. J., 1, 1495-1508

(4) MacMahon,B. (1962)
Prenatal X-ray exposure and childhood cancer.
J. nat. Cancer Inst., 28, 1173-91

(5) Mole, R.H. (1974)
Antenatal irradiation and childhood cancer, causation or
coincidence?
Brit. J.Cancer, 30, 199-208

(6) Occupational Safety and Health Administration (1980)
Documentation of epidemiological studies
Federal Register 45, January 18, 1980, Part B IV
Sections A, B, C, pp 34-59

(7) Armstrong,B. and Doll,R. (1974
Bladder cancer mortality in England and Wales in
relation to cigarette smoking and saccharin consumption.
Brit.J. prev.soc. Med. 28, 233-240

(8) Armstrong,B., Lea,A.J., and Adelstein,A.M. et al.,(1976)
Cancer mortality and saccharin consumption in diabetics.
Brit.J. prev.soc. Med., 30, 151-157

(9) Howe, G.R., Burch, J.D., Miller, A.B. et al (1977)
Artificial sweeteners and human bladder cancer.
Lancet, 1977, 2 578-581

(10) Kessler,I.I. and Clark,J.P. (1978)
Saccharin, cyclamate, and human bladder cancer.
J.Amer.med.Ass. 240, 349-355

(11) Hoover,R., et al (1980)
Progress report to the Food and Drug Administration
from the National Cancer Instute concerning the
national bladder cancer study.
National Cancer Institute, unpublished.

(12) Morrison,A.S. and Buring,J.E. (1980)
Artificial sweeteners and cancer of the lower urinary
tract.
New Engl.J.Med., 302, 537-581

(13) Wynder,E.L. and Stellman,S.D. (1980)
Artificial sweetener use and bladder cancer.
Science,

(14) COMMITTEE ON PROTOTYPE EXPLICIT ANALYSES FOR
PESTICIDES (1980)
Regulating Pesticides
National Academy of Sciences, Washington, D.C.

(15) Cederlöf,R., Doll,R., Fowler,B., et al. (1978)
Air pollution and cancer: risk asse ssment methodology
and epidemiological evidence.
Environ.Hlth.Perspect.,22 1-12.

(16) Pike,M.C. Gordon,R.J., Henderson,B.E., et al (1975)
Air pollution
in Persons at high risk of cancer: an approach to
cancer etiology and control.
Ed. Fraumeni, J.F. pp 225-238.
Academic Press, New York.

(17) Hammond,E.C., Selikoff,I.J., and Lawther,P.L. (1976)
Inhalation of benzpyrene and cancer in man.
Ann. N.Y. Acad.Sci. 271, 116-124.

(18) Hammond,E.C. and Garfinkel,L. (1980)
General air pollution and cancer in the United States.
Prev. Med., 9, 206-211

(19) Hammond,E.C. (1966)
Smoking in relation to the death rates of one million
men and women in Epidemiological approaches to the
study of Cancer and other Chronic Diseases, in
National Cancer Institute Monograph No. 19 pp 127-204.
U.S. Department of Health, Education & Welfare, U.S.
Public Health Service, Washington.

(20) Kahn,H.A. (1966)
The Dorn study of smoking and mortality among U.S.
veterans: report on eight and one half years of
observation, in Epidemiological study of cancer and
other chronic diseases. National Cancer Institute
monograph 19 pp 1-125
U.S. Government Printing Office, Washington

(21) Hammond,E.C. and Seidman, H. (1980)
Smoking and cancer in the United States.
Prev. Med. 9, 169-173

(22) Rogot,E. and Murray,J.L. (1980)
Smoking and causes of death among U.S. veterans: 16
years of observation.
Public Health Reports, 95, 213-222

Descriptive Epidemiology and
Geographic Pathology*

BRIAN E. HENDERSON, M.D.

Professor and Chairman
Family & Preventive Medicine
University of Southern California
Los Angeles, California 90032

It is the purpose of this brief paper to provide some examples of the uses of descriptive epidemiology in generating and testing etiological hypotheses. Because of the brevity of time only a few examples can be discussed and even these must be dealt with superficially. However, it is hoped that the breadth of this area of research can be appreciated even given the limitation of time.

Descriptive epidemiology is concerned primarily with counting cancer cases and collecting readily available information on age at diagnosis, sex, race, county of birth, socioeconomic class, marital status and the like. Using population data on such descriptors it is then possible to calculate and compare incidence and mortality rates.

It is immediately obvious that the usefulness and reproducibility of such descriptive information on cancer will be determined by the accuracy and consistency by which new cases are counted either

*Supported by a Grant No. 2PO1-CA-17054 from the National Cancer Institute. Reprint requests should be addressed to Dr. B.E. Henderson, Family & Preventive Medicine, University of Southern California, 1840 North Soto Street, Los Angeles, California 90032.

at diagnosis or at death. As we shall see in the
examples that follow, accurate case-counting is
fraught with hazards occasioned by variations in
1) case ascertainment methods, 2) methods of diagnosis, 3) awareness of potential diagnosis and
4) clarity of histopathological criteria. One
recent example of these difficulties in accurately
and reproducibly defining cancer cases has come
from attempts to monitor secular trends in cancer
incidence and mortality in the United States[14].

Site by site cancer mortality rates among males
and females have been relatively stable over the
past several decades with three notable exceptions.
Lung cancer rates have steadily risen first in
males and more recently in females. Consistent
with current data on age and cohort specific
cigarette smoking rates, the recent cohort of
white males seems to show no further increase
while female mortality rates continue to rise. At
the current rate of increase lung cancer will be
the first cause of cancer deaths for females by
the mid-1980's. Mortality rates of uterine,
primarily cervix cancer, have steadily fallen over
the past several decades. This fall preceded the
introduction of the PAP smear and presumably is
due to improvements in vaginal hygiene, alterations
in sexual practices, as well as improved methods
of detection and treatment.

One of the most extraordinary changes in cancer
mortality has been the steady decline in stomach
cancer. Ranked as the leading cause of cancer
death in 1930, stomach cancer rates have fallen
not only in the United States but in virtually
every population under surveillance. This remarkable achievement in cancer control has been
"unconscious" as the reasons behind the change
remain unknown. In analyzing changes in diet
composition, food preservation methods, and smoking
and alcohol consumption no consistent etiological
hypothesis emerges.

TABLE 1.

FOOD CONSUMPTION (LBS) PER CAPITA PER YEAR
BY FOOD GROUP 1909-13 TO 1975*

Food Group	1909-1913	1975	Total	% Change 1909-1975 Per year
Meat	141	158	12	0.2
Dairy Products	177	216	22	0.3
Total fats and oils	41	57	39	0.5
Fruit-citrus	17	74	335	2.3
Vegetables-yellow & green	14	25	79	0.9
Vegetables-other	172	125	-27	0.5
Potatoes	205	84	-59	-1.4
Flour and cereals	291	139	-52	-1.1
Sugars	89	114	28	0.4
Calories (per day)	3480	3220	- 7	-0.1
Vitamin A (I.U. per day)	7600	8000	5	0.0
Ascorbic Acid (mgm per day)	104	118	13	0.2
Dietary fiber (lbs)	25	15	-40	-0.8

*From Page and Friend[12].

A favorite hypothesis implicates nitrosamines, ingested preformed or formed in-vivo from nitrite and secondary amines. The presence of vitamin C protects by blocking this in-vivo synthesis. However, while fresh fruit consumption, which provides vitamin C, has steadily risen over the past several decades, total vitamin C consumption has remained unchanged as intake of other vitamin C rich foods such as potatoes has declined[12]. It is unclear whether the levels of nitrite in stomach contents has risen since the intake of nitrate-containing vegetables has clearly increased (nitrate being converted readily to nitrite by saliva) while data on secular changes in the small amounts of preformed nitrosamines in preserved meats is not readily available. Finally one other hypothesis suggests

milk consumption might protect against stomach
cancer but there has been only a slight increase
in dairy product consumption since 1909.

In their recent paper, Pollack and Horm[14] used
cancer mortality data for 1969-76 to calculate an
incremental annual change in rates. Using these
figures we have calculated the expected mortality
rates for 1990, a decade from now.

TABLE 2.
TRENDS IN CANCER MORTALITY 1975-1990
(Rates per 100,000, Age-Adjusted)*

		Mortality		
		1975	1990	%
Stomach	M	8.8	5.7	-35
	F	4.3	2.5	-42
Lung	M	64.8	95.2	+47
	F	15.5	43.4	+180
Breast	F	26.8	28.0	+ 4
Prostate	M	20.3	24.3	+20
Colon-Rectum	M	25.9	27.1	+ 5
	F	19.5	18.9	- 3
All Sites	M	206.6	242.1	+17
	F	131.9	155.7	+18
All Sites	M	141.8	141.1	0
(Exc. Lung)	F	116.4	112.3	- 4

*Calculation based on tables in Pollock & Horm[14]

By that time the total cancer mortality among men
and women will have risen 17% and 18% respectively.
However, excluding the expected continued rise in
lung cancer due to cigarette smoking, total cancer
mortality in men will remain unchanged and in
women will fall by 4%. The rise in prostate cancer
mortality will offset the decline in stomach cancer
among men. However, this projected increase in
prostate is probably an artifact. Using age-

specific cancer mortality rates for the past three
decades one could argue that among age groups up
to 74 the rate is actually falling and that over
75 the rate is variable but not definitely increasing. Thus, total cancer mortality in males may
actually be falling.

Moving now from this review of cancer mortality
trends to the recent studies of cancer incidence
trends, a somewhat different picture emerges.
Comparing cancer incidence rates from the Third
National Cancer Survey (1969-71) and the SEER
program (1973-76) Pollack and Horm conclude that
overall cancer incidence rates are increasing at
between 1.3% (males) and 2% (females) per year[14].
Again projecting ahead one decade, and even excluding lung cancer, leads one to the alarming conclusion that cancer rates will increase by about 25%.

TABLE 3.

TRENDS IN CANCER INCIDENCE 1975-1990
(Rates per 100,000, Age-Adjusted)*

| | | Incidence | | |
		1975	1990	%
Stomach	M	12.7	9.0	-29
	F	5.4	3.1	-43
Lung	M	76.4	94.1	+23
	F	21.8	75.1	+244
Breast	F	86.2	112.6	+31
Prostate	M	64.8	91.1	+41
Colon-Rectum	M	53.8	66.3	+23
	F	42.6	48.0	+13
All Sites	M	365.8	444.0	+21
	F	301.8	435.3	+44
All Sites	M	289.4	349.9	+21
(Exc. Lung)	F	280.0	360.2	+29

*Calculations based on tables in Pollack and Horm[14].

Most of the difference between the projected
mortality and incidence rates is due to large
projected increases in the incidence of certain
cancers with relatively good survival, e.g. breast,
colon-rectum, and prostate. A major potential
flaw in this report is the comparison of cancer
counting during the national surveys with that of
the on-going cancer monitoring SEER program. Even
a cursory examination of the published data leads
to suspicions that methods of case ascertainment
and definition could produce the artifact of
increasing incidence. No major clinical advances
have been made which could explain the discrepancy
between morbidity and mortality trends. Furthermore, comparison of rates from the Second and
Third National Cancer Surveys indicated no change
in breast and colon-rectum cancer incidence
rates over this 20 year period[4]. In addition, our
Cancer Surveillance Program shows no overall change
in the incidence of breast, colon-rectum and
prostate cancer over the period 1972-77. Thus,
the combined mortality and morbidity data over the
past several years in the United States does not
suggest that we are entering a general epidemic
which some have suggested might be due to general-
ized industrial or other chemical carcinogens.
Rather, variations in case ascertainment methods
within the TNCS and SEER program appear to have
produced an artifactual increase in cancer incidence
in several sites.

While a suggested increasing trend for breast,
colon-rectum and prostate cancer may be difficult
to substantiate in the United States such is not
the case in some other countries where these
cancers have traditionally been of low incidence
and mortality. It might be instructive at this
time to digress somewhat to describe in detail the
international variation in breast cancer and how
this can be explained by understanding the biology
of breast cancer.

There is remarkable variation in breast cancer
rates between different countries. Figure 1 shows
that, as of 1970, rates were some 6 times higher
in the U.S. and Canada than in Asia or Black
Africa.

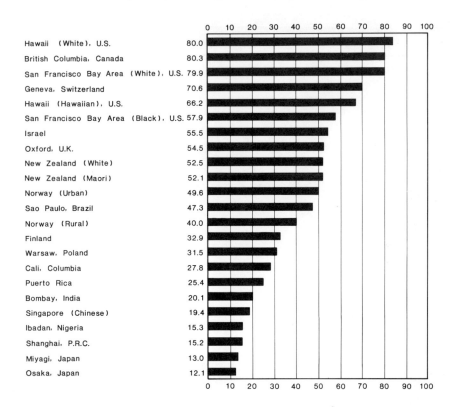

		0	10	20	30	40	50	60	70	80	90	100
Hawaii (White), U.S.	80.0											
British Columbia, Canada	80.3											
San Francisco Bay Area (White), U.S.	79.9											
Geneva, Switzerland	70.6											
Hawaii (Hawaiian), U.S.	66.2											
San Francisco Bay Area (Black), U.S.	57.9											
Israel	55.5											
Oxford, U.K.	54.5											
New Zealand (White)	52.5											
New Zealand (Maori)	52.1											
Norway (Urban)	49.6											
Sao Paulo, Brazil	47.3											
Norway (Rural)	40.0											
Finland	32.9											
Warsaw, Poland	31.5											
Cali, Columbia	27.8											
Puerto Rica	25.4											
Bombay, India	20.1											
Singapore (Chinese)	19.4											
Ibadan, Nigeria	15.3											
Shanghai, P.R.C.	15.2											
Miyagi, Japan	13.0											
Osaka, Japan	12.1											

Figure 1. Age-adjusted Breast Cancer Incidence Rates for Different Countries (From Waterhouse et al[15]).

Rates nearly as high as those of North America are seen in Switzerland, while rates 4 times higher than in Japan are seen in many Western European countries and in New Zealand. The rates in South America, the Caribbean and Eastern Europe are intermediate.

These differences in breast cancer rates are not determined by variation in genetic susceptibility. Furthermore, studies of Japanese migrants to Hawaii[6] and California[3] show that Japanese-Americans are likely soon to have the high breast cancer rates of U.S. women.

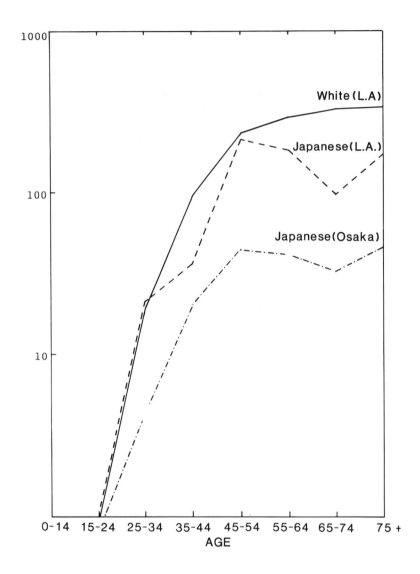

Figure 2. Age-specific Incidence Rates for Japanese
women (Osaka and Los Angeles)[7] and White
Women (Los Angeles)[7].

Figure 2, for example, compares the rates of breast cancer in Japanese women in Los Angeles and Osaka. Under age 55, the incidence of breast cancer in Japanese women in Osaka is about one-fifth that of White women in Los Angeles, whereas Japanese women in Los Angeles have rates that are within 20% of the White rates. Over age 55, the Japanese-Osaka rates are one-eighth that of Los Angeles White rates, with Japanese-Los Angeles rates some 4-fold higher than the Osaka rates, but still only half the Los Angeles White rates. This latter gap will presumably continue to decrease as more Japanese women born in the U.S. enter the older age groups.

Calculations based on data on age at first birth in different countries suggest that this factor could only explain a small amount of differences observed in breast cancer rates. Data on age at menopause is sparse but from the studies available and MacMahon's detailed analysis of U.S. data[1] it appears likely that there are not very large international differences. However, the age at menarche of women born as late as 1940 differ widely from one country to another, and differences in body weight between the U.S. and Japan are also still substantial. In 1960 at age 20, U.S. women weighed some 10 kg more than Japanese women and for 60 year old women, the difference was double this at 20kg[8,16]. The combined effect of these two factors can account for much of the difference between U.S. and Japanese breast cancer rates.

There have been major changes in the dietary habits of Japanese since 1945. In 1950 Japanese girls aged 15 were some 9 kg lighter and had menarche 2.4 years later than U.S. girls (Table 4): these differences have existed at least as far back as 1900.

TABLE 4.

AGE AT MENARCHE, AND HEIGHT AND WEIGHT AT AGE 12
OF GIRLS IN JAPAN AND THE U.S.*

	Birth Year			
	+1885	+1935	+1945	+1955
Japan				
Height (cm)	133	137	144	148
Weight (kg)	30	32	37	40
Menarche (years)	16.5	15.2	13.9	12.5
U.S. Whites				
Height (cm)	147	153	151	155
Weight (kg)	39	41	43	45
Menarche (years)	14.2	12.8	12.8	12.8

*From Henderson, B. and Pike M.[7]

By 1970 the difference in weight had been reduced
to 5 kg and the difference in age at menarche had
disappeared. There has been some recent increase
in breast cancer rates in Japan, and we would
predict on the basis of the data given in Table 4
that current Japanese teenagers will, as a cohort,
have breast cancer rates quite close to U.S. rates.
How close the rates will be will depend on at
least two factors. Firstly, for postmenopausal
women on whether, as a group, the Japanese gain a
substantial amount of weight after age 20; contrary
to U.S. experience, such adult weight gains have
not been a feature of Japanese women[8]. Secondly,
on whether the precise constitution of the diet
producing the near equality of age at menarche has
an independent effect: we do not expect this to be
of major importance.

To return to an analysis of secular trends in
cancer in the United States, there is good evidence
that there have been recent secular increases in
cancer of the endometrium and malignant melanoma
that are not so clearly seen in mortality data.
Endometrial or corpus uteri cancer rates were

stable between the Second and Third National Cancer Surveys[4] but these increased in the early-to-mid 1970's[17]. This increase was largely confined to post-menopausal women and consistently related to prolonged use of menopausal estrogens[11]. There is some recent evidence that the rate of increase has slowed, presumably because prescribing practices for menopausal estrogens have moved towards lower dosages and perhaps shorter duration of use[9].

There appears to be a real secular increase in malignant melanoma that was already discernible among White males and females between the Second and Third National Cancer Surveys[4]. In a careful analysis of data from the Cancer Surveillance Program in Los Angeles County, Mack[10] has shown that the increase in rates is particularly true for lesions of the body. There were substantial increases in risk for those with professional occupations and no specific evidence of occupational disease.

TABLE 5

AVERAGE ANNUAL AGE-ADJUSTED* INCIDENCE RATE (AAIR)
AND FREQUENCY (F) OF MALIGNANT MELANOMAS
BY OCCUPATION**

Whites Aged 25-64, Los Angeles County, 1972-1977

Occupation***	Males		Females	
	AAIR	(F)	AAIR	(F)
White Collar:				
Professional, Technical and Kindred Workers	22.8	(303)	15.4	(135)
Managers and Administrators	21.8	(236)	27.4	(70)
Sales Workers	17.0	(100)	6.6	(28)
Clerical and Kindred Workers	11.8	(59)	9.1	(188)
Blue Collar:				
Craftsmen and Kindred Workers	10.3	(148)	7.4	(7)
Operatives, Except Transport	7.3	(47)	2.6	(16)
Transport Equipment Operatives	11.3	(31)	16.7	(3)
Laborers	11.1	(23)	0	(0)

  * 1970 US Census age distribution standard. [10]
 ** From Mack, T.
*** Miscellaneous Occupation of low frequency excluded.

Those born in California experience higher risk
than those born elsewhere particularly when compared
to those born in the Northern and Midwestern United
States. Those born outside California showed
consistent increases in risk on migration to Los
Angeles when compared to appropriate non-immigrant
populations in the U.S. and abroad. A comparison
of a subset of invasive and/or fatal melanomas
with the total suggests that none of these observations is due to misclassification of benign lesion.
These data are interpreted to constitute good

evidence that the major risk for malignant melanoma
consists of an accumulation of intermittent,
intense recreational exposure to solar radiation
rather than small doses acquired on a routine
basis.

Two final problems that I would like to briefly
address illustrate the importance of careful histopathological diagnosis particularly when evaluating
reports of rare cancers.

Mesothelioma

We noticed an apparent increase in the reported
number of male mesotheliomas in Los Angeles from
1972 to 1977.

TABLE 6.
NUMBER OF MESOTHELIOMA CASES IN
LOS ANGELES COUNTY, 1972-1977

Year	Male	Female
1972	10	7
1973	12	4
1974	17	10
1975	20	3
1976	37	8
1977	23	7

Such an increase could be expected because of the
increased asbestos exposure during WWII and the
long latent period for mesothelioma. However,
there has been considerable speculation in the
professional and lay press over this potential
"epidemic" with one widely circulated estimate
that there would be 280,000 mesothelioma deaths
from WWII exposure[2]. We thus considered that at
least some of the reported increase in cases in
Los Angeles County could result from misclassification of lung cancers of uncertain histology to
mesothelioma if a history of possible asbestos
exposure was available. Therefore, we have undertaken a careful review of occupational history and
the histopathological diagnosis (Dr. Russell Sherwin
- University of Southern California School of
Medicine) of all our cases. Although this review
is still in process it is already evident that
considerable misclassification has occurred. Of

57 patients with no convincing history of direct
or indirect asbestos exposure, 50 (88%) were not
diagnosed by Dr. Sherwin as mesotheliomas. Five of
the remaining seven patients were female who presumably have mesothelioma not etiologically related to
asbestos exposure. It is less certain whether the
two males were not exposed to asbestos without a more
detailed history than was available.

In contrast, of the 34 patients with a positive
history of asbestos exposure so far studied, about
50% have a histopathological diagnosis consistent
with mesothelioma. Dr. Sherwin has found benign
mesothelial tumors and malignant lung cancers are
most frequently misclassified as malignant
mesotheliomas.

Since the occupational exposure history correctly
classifies a malignant mesothelioma at least 50%
of the time, and assuming that perhaps an equal
number of asbestos-caused mesotheliomas are
incorrectly labelled as lung cancer, it is possible
to attempt a prediction of the number of mesothelioma cases that might be seen nationally from the
WWII exposure to asbestos. These calculations have
been done by J. Peto (Oxford, England) using the
age at first exposure and age at diagnosis of the
male mesothelioma cases for Los Angeles County
with a positive asbestos exposure history for
1974-1978[13]. The total number of cases among men
first exposed between 1935 and 1945, both past and
future, is likely to be about 30 to 40 times the
number diagnosed in 1976. If Los Angeles County
is typical of the rest of the United States this
would imply an eventual total of about 10,000
cases among men first exposed during WWII. The
number of cases by 5 year period of diagnosis is
shown in Table 7, assuming that 1400 cases occur
between 1974-1978.

TABLE 7.

NUMBER OF MESOTHELIOMA CASES IN THE UNITED STATES
DUE TO WWII EXPOSURE*

Period	No. Cases
1949-	30
1954-	110
1959-	290
1964-	600
1969-	980
1974-	1400
1979-	1750
1984-	1950
1989-	1850
1994-	1440
1999-	800
	11200

*Calculations based on a projected positive history
of asbestos exposure during WWII in 1400 (35%) of
approximately 4000 mesothelioma cases diagnosed in
United States between 1974-1978 (Peto, J. and
Henderson, B.)[13]

From these calculations one-third of the expected
cases has already occurred and the actual number
of cases will fall at the end of the decade as the
last of the exposed cohort dies. Further studies
are needed to define the degree of post-WWII
asbestos exposure - we have no pathologically
confirmed cases of mesothelioma out of 5 cases
reviewed with date of first possible exposure
after 1950.

Liver Tumors

A final word about liver tumors. An eminent liver
pathologist at our institution, Dr. Hugh Edmondson,
noted a sudden increase in referred cases of a
previously rarely seen benign liver tumor. These
liver adenomas were exclusively diagnosed in women of
reproductive age and after careful inquiry into their
past history, he noted that many of these women were
long-term users of oral contraceptives. Subsequently, we published a case-control study confirming this association[5].

A less rare benign liver tumor known as focal
nodular hyperplasia (FNH) has also been associated
with oral contraceptive use although this has not
been confirmed in an analytical study.
Recently we reviewed all liver cancers in women
15-50 years of age reported in Los Angeles County
between 1972-1977.

TABLE 8.

LIVER TUMORS IN WOMEN 15-50 YEARS OF AGE
LOS ANGELES COUNTY 1972-1977

	YEAR		
	1972-73	1974-75	1976-77
Benign			
Hamartoma	2	1	1
Adenoma	2	4	4
FNH	3	2	1
Malignant			
Cholangiocarcinoma	2	3	1
Hepatoma	3	7	11
Total	12	17	18

Two points are worth stressing as a result of this
review. First, a number of pathologically diagnosed
liver cancers are, in fact, benign, resectable
liver tumors. Secondly, there appears to be an
increase, although the numbers are very small, in
hepatomas between 1972-73 and 1976-77. We have
observed three frankly malignant hepatomas apparently
arising in benign liver adenomas in women with a
history of oral contraceptive use. We are currently
conducting a case-control study of these rare
malignant neoplasms to examine this possible
association.

The lesson from these studies of mesotheliomas and
liver cancers in young women is that careful histopathology is a vital part of descriptive epidemiology.
In countries where histopathology is infrequent,
such studies are difficult if not impossible.

Conclusion

This somewhat rambling discourse hopefully conveys
some of the richness as well as the problems inherent
in studies of descriptive epidemiology. Many other
examples could have been used but most of those
chosen came from our experience with the population
based Cancer Surveillance Program in Los Angeles
County. We have a tremendous population resource
of 7 million people of diverse ethnic background to
serve as a laboratory. Equally important we have
been able to assemble a talented group of
biostatistians, epidemiologists, pathologists and
laboratory scientists who have begun to exploit the
numerous etiological clues emerging from the descriptive data. Hopefully the ensuing decade will provide a wealth of additional information derived
from programs such as ours which can lead to new
etiological associations and methods of cancer
prevention.

REFERENCES

1. Age at menopause: United States 1960-1962. Vital and Health Statistics, Series 11, No. 19. National Center for Health Statistics, Washington, D.C., 1966.

2. Bridbord, K., Decoufle, P., Fraumeni, J.F., et al. Estimates of the fraction of cancer in the United States related to occupational factors. Manuscript, September 15, 1978.

3. Buell, P.: Changing incidence of breast cancer in Japanese-American women. J. Natl. Cancer Inst., 51, 147, 1973.

4. Devesa, S.S. and Silverman, D.T.: Cancer incidence and mortality trends in the United States: 1935-1974. J. Natl. Cancer Inst., 60, 545, 1978.

5. Edmondson, H.A., Henderson, B.E. and Benton, B.: Liver-cell adenomas associated with use of oral contraceptives New Engl. J. of Med., 294, 470, 1976.

6. Haenszel, W., and Kurihara, M.: Studies of Japanese I. Mortality from cancer and other diseases among Japanese in the United States. J. Natl. Cancer Inst., 40, 43, 1968.

7. Henderson, B.E. and Pike, M.C.: The epidemiology of breast cancer. (In press) CRC press.

8. Hirayama, T.: Epidemiology of breast cancer with special reference to the role of diet. Prev. Med., 7, 173, 1978.

9. Jick, H., Watkins, R.N., Hunter, J.R., et al.: Replacement estrogens and endometrial cancer. N. Engl. J. Med., 300, 218, 1979.

10. Mack, T.: Malignant melanoma in Los Angeles (Manuscript).

11. Mack, T.M., Pike, M.C., Henderson, B.E., et al.: Estrogens and endometrial cancer in a retirement community. N. Engl. J. Med., 294, 1262, 1976.

12. Page, L. and Friend, B.: The changing United States diet. Bio. Science, 28, 102, 1978.

13. Peto, J. and Henderson, B.: Trends in mesothelioma incidence in the U.S. and the forecast "epidemic" due to exposure during World War II. (Manuscript).

14. Pollack, E.S. and Horm, J.W.: Trends in cancer incidence and mortality in the United States, 1969-76. J. Natl. Cancer Inst., 64, 1091, 1980.
15. Waterhouse, J., Muir, C., Correa, P., et al. Cancer incidence in five continents. Volume III. Intern. Agency for Research on Cancer, 1976, Lyon. IARC Scientific Publications No. 15.
16. Weight, height, and selected body dimensions of adults. Vital and Health Statistics, Series 11, No. 8. National Center for Health Statistics, Washington, D.C., 1965.
17. Weiss, N.S., Szekely, D.R. and Austin, D.F.: Increasing incidence of endometrial cancer in the United States. N. Engl. J. Med., 294, 1259, 1976.

Lifestyle Factors in Human Cancer

ANTHONY B. MILLER

Director
NCIC Epidemiology Unit
University of Toronto
Toronto, Ontario M5S 1A8 Canada

INTRODUCTION

Over the last few years it has been increasingly appreciated that the factors encompassed by the term "lifestyle" are of substantial importance in the etiology of human cancers. These factors include those rather loosely covered by the term "socio-economic status", specific agents such as tobacco and alcohol, a large number of different agents in diet, sexual and reproductive habits, drug and exogenous hormone use, and exposure to sunlight. In this presentation I shall first consider some recent insights into socio-economic status, then discuss dietary factors and sexual and reproductive habits. I shall not consider tobacco, alcohol, drugs, exogenous hormones or exposure to sunlight because the need for control measures when such specific factors are identified is largely understood.

SOCIO-ECONOMIC STATUS

The effect of differences in socio-economic status on the incidence of a number of human cancers is well recognised, though it is understood that differences in social class and income are directly and indirectly related to a number of factors including all the lifestyle factors already mentioned as well as differences in occupation, and that these factors are those causally responsible for the incidence differentials. The Register-General's Decennial Supplement for England and Wales[1] and the report by Fox and Adelstein[2] have thrown further light on the relative importance of lifestyle and occupational factors in these

associations. Social class standardisation, whereby
comparisons are made between people within strata made up by
those of the same social class with subsequent summarization
over all classes, has shown that nearly all occupational
groups with standardised mortality ratios significantly
different from expectation are reduced once account is taken
of social class. Fox and Adelstein[2] have calculated that
work accounts for approximately 12% of the variation in
mortality between orders for cancer, with way of life or
lifestyle accounting for 88%, the corresponding proportions
for all causes of death are 18% and 82%. A recent
publication from the Finnish Cancer Registry[3] also points
to the association of social class with a number of sites,
with negative correlations of high social class with lip and
stomach cancer in males and the reverse correlation with
colon cancer in both sexes, and breast and lung cancer in
females.

Studies within single social classes or occupational groups
such as British Doctors have confirmed the reduction in
smoking associated diseases such as coronary heart disease
and lung cancer, but have shown little change for other
malignancies. Other alcohol and or stress related diseases
such as cirrhosis of the liver and suicide, have, however,
shown an increase.[4]

Specific groups with lifestyles demonstrably different from
others such as Mormons[5] and Seventh Day Adventists[6] have
also pointed to the importance of lifestyle in cancer
etiology.

DIET AND NUTRITION

Although there had been a number of attempts to evaluate
the potential importance of dietary and nutritional factors,
a major advance was made with the bringing together of
laboratory workers and epidemiologists in a symposium on
Nutrition and Cancer held by the National Cancer Institute
with the collaboration of the American Cancer Society in May,
1975, with the proceedings published in Cancer Research in
November 1975. Since then, the collaboration of epidemiology
with laboratory investigations has continued to be fruitful,
as exemplified by the term "Metabolic Epidemiology", though
some of the studies encompassed by this term have
unfortunately not had a defined population base and, because
of the complexity of the laboratory investigations,
conclusions have of necessity been based on small numbers of
subjects studied. In addition studies that have continued in

laboratory animals and on the biochemical processes involved have increased our understanding of the issues.

Diet could exert an effect on human cancers in a number of different ways: through carcinogens as components or contaminants of food, either naturally or as additives or preservatives; through carcinogens produced in food by processing or cooking; through carcinogens produced in the body, especially in the stomach, small or large intestine, from food constituents; through the indirect effects of undernutrition, malnutrition or overnutrition; through the protective effect of certain dietary factors.

A number of dietary factors have been associated with increased risk of carcinogenesis. These include high intakes of total fat, though experimental studies in animals have pointed to the importance of a small proportion of polyunsaturated fat to exert the potentiating action of high fat levels in mammary carcinogenesis.[7] High intakes of animal protein, possibly particularly beef in Hawaii[8] and pork in Japan[9] have been implicated, though in view of the high correlation with total fat[10] and the high fat content of such meats, the effect may well be almost entirely mediated through fat. Mutagenic studies in various foods, especially those preserved by smoking or the use of spices, and those broiled or barbecued, have pointed to the potential importance of food processing and possibly cooking particularly in the etiology of stomach cancer.[11] Similarly a role for endogenously produced carcinogens, especially nitrosamines, has been suggested in the etiology of colo-rectal[12] as well as stomach cancer.[13]

Other dietary factors have been associated with protection from carcinogenesis. These include dietary fiber, particularly associated with protection from colon cancer,[14] though it is not clear whether all components of dietary fiber are equally protective. Vitamins that may be protective include vitamin A with an effect possibly on lung[15,16] and bladder cancer,[17] vitamin C with an effect in inhibiting the intra-gastric[11] and possibly intra-colonic production of nitrosamines, the latter effect possibly also being exerted by vitamin E.[12] Possibly linked with the protective effect of vitamin A on lung cancer is the observation of Hirayama of the protective effect of green-yellow vegetables.[18] Wattenberg[19] has pointed to the effect of dietary constituents on the metabolism of chemical carcinogens by the microsomal mixed function oxidase system. Naturally occuring inducers of increased activity in this system are found in cruciferous vegetables such as brussel sprouts, cabbage and cauliflower. Graham and his colleagues have found a possible protective effect of such vegetables on colon cancer.[20]

In stomach cancer, the possible protective effect of fresh fruit and vegetables and Vitamin C has come largely from experimental studies,[13] but the effect of high nitrate consumption from studies in a number of different areas, especially Britain[21] and Colombia.[22]

Case-control studies in colon and rectal cancer have not produced consistant findings. A study in Hawaiian Japanese pointed to the importance of Western type meals and especially beef intake,[8] but these findings were not replicated in Japan[23] though a negative association with consumption of cabbage was found. A study in Israel with a diet frequency questionnaire suggested the importance of foods low in fiber consumption in the etiology of colon but not rectal cancer.[24] However, a study in Canada has shown an association of both colon and rectal cancer with saturated fat intake but not with estimated consumption of crude fiber.[25] Rectal cancer has been associated with beer consumption in some studies.[26] It has also been pointed out that there is a better correlation of trends in rectal cancer mortality with changes in beer consumption than with saturated fat.[27]

A role for dietary factors in the etiology of breast cancer has been suggested by results of animal experimental studies, by changes in incidence on migration and in various countries possibly associated with changes in nutrition, from studies which have correlated variation of inter and intra national incidence and mortality rates with dietary factors, from the association of indirect correlates of nutrition such as height, weight and age at menarche with breast cancer, and from a small number of case-control studies in which an estimate of the consumption of various dietary constituents has been made.[28] Our case-control study in Canada showed an association between total fat intake and both pre- and post-menopausal breast cancer.[29] However, the overall risk ratio was low, (1.5) and the corresponding attributable risk was small (27%), findings that might however be partially explained by a methodology that concentrated on current diet and over matching with a neighbourhood control series. Nevertheless, the evidence taken as a whole tends to support an etiological role for total fat intake.

Other cancers also associated with total fat intake include endometrial cancer (also associated with obesity and possibly excessive caloric intake), ovarian, pancreatic, renal and prostate cancer, though the evidence for these associations is largely indirect.[10,30]

Liver cancer has been associated with nutritional deficiency, and exposure to mycotoxins (especially aflatoxin).[31]

Although it is not possible to develop specific recommendations for dietary modification on present evidence, it is difficult to avoid some sort of general dietary advice. This should include the avoidance of over-nutrition in western countries to maintain ideal weight at all ages. Further, excess consumption of fat should be avoided, with an adequate (though not necessarily an excess) intake of vitamins such as A and C, and of dietary fiber. Such advice is unlikely to be hazardous and may be beneficial. It should be noted that the evidence suggests that for many cancer sites dietary factors (especially fat intake) may act as promotors of carcinogenesis. This would suggest that the possible effect of dietary intervention of this type is likely to be more immediate than action taken to remove or inhibit initiators of carcinogenesis.

Further work is however required on dietary methodology, and investigation should be pursued of the associations of dietary factors with cancers that are changing in incidence in the population concerned. Cohort studies should be established if possible, and studies pursued of the interaction between dietary factors and other possible causal factors, such as with hormonal factors in the etiology of breast cancer.

SEXUAL AND REPRODUCTIVE HABITS

Cancer of the cervix has been associated in a number of studies with early age at first intercourse and exposure to multiple sexual partners.[32] Further, in spite of the difficulties in such studies, evidence is emerging that appears to suggest an association between cancer of the cervix and cancer of the penis in spouses.[33] Whether this indicates a common dependency on sexual habits or a shared etiological agent (such as a virus) is at present unclear. This evidence, while pointing to the nature of cancer of the cervix as a venereal disease, with a search for a venereally transmitted agent as a possibly necessary but not necessarily a sufficient cause, involves an inevitable association with multiparity. In contrast, cancer of the breast, endometrial and ovarian cancer are all associated with protection from multiparity.[34] The overriding importance of age at first birth in breast but not endometrial or ovarian cancer has now been confirmed in a large number of studies. Although not

found in at least two recent studies, and not universally in
every subgroup studied, it seems likely that failure to
demonstrate the effect may have been due to small numbers or
over-matching cases with controls. There appears to be a
protective effect of high parity over and above that of an
early age at first birth in some populations.[28]

Although the association of age at first birth with breast
cancer does not explain international variation, indeed
changing trends in age at first birth in Iceland are
diametrically opposed to the changes in breast cancer
incidence observed,[35] in Canada, changing mortality rates
for breast cancer may be at least partially associated with
changes in fertility.[36] These associations have led to the
fear that delay in age at first birth in present populations
will be associated with an increasing incidence of breast
cancer in the future. Paradoxically, the changes that are
occurring in sexual habits also seem to be associated with an
increase in at least the presumed precursors of cancer of the
cervix in young women, and a possible increase in invasive
cancer and mortality as well. These changes should not
necessarily be presumed to make it impossible to offer advice
on possible control measures. Thus the increasing incidence
of cancer of the cervix may be averted by avoidance of
promiscuity, encouragement in the use of barrier
contraceptives, and appropriate participation in screening
programs. Further, it is likely that a population which
achieved a 5 year reduction in age at first birth might see a
30% reduction in breast cancer incidence. Thus women should
be informed that if they plan to have children, they should
not delay their first pregnancy unduly (not later than age
25) if this is at all posssible.[28]

In men, cancer of the prostate has been suspected as
related to sexual activity. Several case-control studies are
ongoing currently, but one appears to be producing
preliminary results that supports an etiological role for
"suppressed" sexual activity in this disease.[37]

One further indicator of the importance of lifestyle
factors in cancer of the cervix has come from the association
with cigarette smoking.[38] Although such associations
suggest confounding with sexual activity, in one case control
study, attempts to eliminate confounding support a possible
direct role of cigarette smoking in the etiology of cancer of
the cervix (E.A. Clarke, personal communication, 1980).

CONCLUSION

In conclusion, there now seems little doubt that lifestyle factors, all potentially within the control of the subject, and therefore presumably subject to modification by appropriate education, are of significant importance in the etiology of a number of different cancers. The present discussion has concentrated on factors on which the evidence, though not conclusive, is very substantial. Other possible life-style factors, such as the role of coffee-drinking in the etiology of bladder cancer, still require evaluation.[39] Nevertheless, enough is known to support approaches to prevention on the lines of a "sensible", if not prudent diet, with advice on modification, or at least awareness of the implication, of sexual and reproductive factors. The downturn in the mortality from coronary heart disease in some countries suggests that dietary changes may have an impact on populations. These changes, involving a substitution of polyunsaturated for other fats, should now be supplimented by a reduction in total fat intake and an increase in dietary fiber consumption. The breakfast cereal manufacturers are now helping with fiber consumption upturns. Perhaps other economic changes will help in reducing the consumption of total fat and over nutrition generally.

REFERENCES

1. Office of Population Censuses and Surveys. Occupational
   Mortality. The Registrar General's Decennial Supplement
   for England and Wales 1970-72. Series DS. No. 1
   London. Her Majesty's Stationery office. 1978.
2. Fox, A.J., Adelstein, A.M. Occupational mortality: work
   or way of life? J. Epidemiol. Commun. Hlth. 32: 73-78,
   1978.
3. Teppo, L., Pukkala, E., Hakama, M. et al. Way of life
   and cancer incidence in Finland. Scandinavian Journal of
   Social Medicine. Supplement 19, 1980.
4. Lee, P.N. Has the mortality of male doctors improved
   with the reductions in their cigarette smoking? Brit.
   Med. J. 2: 1538-1540, 1979.
5. Lyon, J.L., Klauber, M.R., Gardner, J.W. et al. Cancer
   incidence in Mormons and non-Mormons in Utah, 1966-1970.
   N. Engl. J. Med. 294: 129-133, 1976.
6. Phillips, R.L. Role of lifestyle and dietary habits in
   risk of cancer among Seventh-Day Adventists. Cancer Res.
   35: 3513-3522, 1975.
7. Carroll, K.K., Hopkins, G.J. Dietary polyunsaturated fat
   versus saturated fat in relation to mammary
   carcinogenesis. Lipids 14: 155-158, 1979.
8. Haenszel, W., Berg, J.W., Segi, M. et al. Large-bowel
   cancer in Hawaiian Japanese. J. Nat. Cancer. Inst. 51:
   1765-1779, 1973.
9. Hirayama, T. Changing patterns of cancer in Japan with
   special reference to the decrease of stomach cancer
   mortality, in Origins of Human Cancer. Cold Spring
   Harbor Laboratory, Cold Spring Harbor, N.Y., 1977 pp
   55-75.
10. Armstrong, B., Doll, R. Environmental factors and cancer
    incidence and mortality in different countries, with
    special reference to dietary practices. Int. J. Cancer
    15: 617-631, 1975.
11. Weisburger, J.H., Marquardt, H. Mower, H.F. et al.
    Inhibition of Carcinogenesis: Vitamin C and the
    prevention of gastric cancer. Preventive Medicine 9:
    352-361, 1980.
12. Bruce, W.R., Varghese, A.J., Wang, S. et al. The
    endogeous production of nitroso compounds in the colon
    and cancer at that site, in Miller, J.A., Miller, E.C.,
    Sugimira, T. et al. (Eds): Naturally occurring
    carcinogens-mutagens and modulators of carcinogenesis.
    Proceedings of the 9th Princess Takamatsu Symposium
    Tokyo. University Park Press, Baltimore, 1975.

13. Weisburger, J.H., Marquardt, H., Hirota, N. et al. Induction of glandular stomach cancer in rats with an extract of nitrite-treated fish. J. Natl. Cancer Inst. 64: 163-167, 1980.
14. IARC Microecology group. Dietary fibre, transit-time, facal bacteria, steroids and colon cancer in two Scandinavian populations. Lancet 2: 207-211, 1977.
15. Bjelke, E. Dietary vitamin A and human lung cancer. Int. J. Cancer. 15: 561-565, 1975.
16. Mettlin, C., Graham, S., Swanson, M. Vitamin A and Lung cancer. J. Natl. Cancer Inst. 62: 1435-1438, 1979.
17. Mettlin, C., Graham, S. Dietary risk factors in human bladder cancer. Am. J. Epidemiol. 110: 255-263, 1979.
18. Hirayama, T. Presentation at the 12th Internatioanl Cancer Congress. Buenos Aires. October, 1978.
19. Wattenberg, L.W. Effects of Dietary Constituents on the Metabolism of Chemical Carcinogens. Cancer Research 35: 3326-3331, 1975.
20. Graham, S., Dayal, H., Swanson, M. et al. Diet in the epidemiology of cancer of the colon and rectum. J. Natl. Cancer Inst. 61: 709-714, 1978.
21. Hill, M.J., Hawkesworth, G., Tattersall, G. Bacteria, Nitrosamines and cancer of the stomach. Brit. J. Cancer 28: 562-567, 1973.
22. Cuello, C., Correa, P., Haenszel, W. et al. Gastric Cancer in Colombia 1. Cancer risk and suspect environmental agents. J. Natl. Cancer Inst. 57: 1015-1026, 1976.
23. Haenszel, W., Locke, F.B., Segi, M. A case-control study of large bowel cancer in Japan. J. Natl. Cancer Inst. 64: 17-22, 1980.
24. Modan, B., Barrell, V., Lubin, F. et al. Low-fiber intake as an etiologic factor in cancer of the colon. J. Natl. Cancer Inst. 55: 15-18, 1975.
25. Jain, M., Cook, G.M., Davis, F.G. et al. A case-control study of diet and colo-rectal cancer. Int. J. Cancer. In Press, 1980.
26. Enstrom, J.E. Colorectal cancer and beer drinking. Brit. J. Cancer 35: 674-683, 1977.
27. McMichael, A.J., Potter, J.D., Hetzel, B.S. Time trends in colo-rectal cancer mortality in relation to food and alcohol consumption: United States, United Kingdom, Australia and New Zealand. Int. J. Epidemiol. 8: 295-303, 1979.
28. Miller, A.B., Bullbrook, R.D. Special report: The epidemiology and etiology of breast cancer. In preparation, 1980.

29. Miller, A.B., Kelly, A., Choi, N.W. et al. A study of diet and breast cancer. Amer. J. Epidemiol 107: 499-509, 1978.

30. Miller, A.B., Gori, G.B., Graham, S. et al. Nutrition and Cancer. Preventive Medicine 9: 189-196, 1980.

31. Higginson, J. Perspectives and future developments in research on enviromental carcinogenesis, in Griffin, A.C., Shaw, C.R., Ed: Carcinogens: Identification and Mechanisms of Action. Raven Press, New York. 1979 pp 187-208.

32. Rotkin, I.D. A comparison review of key epidemiological studies in cervical cancer related to current searches for transmissable agents. Cancer Res. 33: 1353-1367, 1973.

33. Graham, S., Priore, R., Graham, M. et al. Genital cancer in wives of penile cancer patients. Cancer 44: 1870-1874, 1979.

34. Miller, A.B., Barclay, T.H.C., Choi, N.W. et al. A study of cancer, parity and age at first pregnancy. J. Chron. Dis. In press, 1980.

35. Tulinius, H., Day, N.E., Johannesson, G. et al. Reproductive factors and risk for breast cancer in Iceland. Int. J. Cancer 21: 724-730, 1978.

36. Fabia, J., Bernard, P.M., Hill, G. Recent time-trends of age-specific death rates for breast cancer; Quebec and other provinces, 1965 through 1974. CMA Journal 116: 1135-1138, 1977.

37. Schuman, L. Cancer of the prostate. Evidence from a case-control study, in proceedings of the symposium: Trends in Cancer Incidence, Oslo 6-7. August, 1980, In preparation.

38. Winkelstein, W. Smoking and cancer of the Uterine Cervix: Hypothesis. Am. J. Epidemiol 106: 257-259, 1977.

39. Howe, G.R., Burch, J.D., Miller, A.B. et al. Tobacco use, occupation, coffee, various nutrients, and bladder cancer. J. Natl. Cancer Inst. 64: 701-713, 1980.

Viruses

Viruses and Cancer

GEORGE KLEIN

Department of Tumor Biology
Karolinska Institutet
S 104 01 Stockholm, Sweden

HISTORIC BACKGROUND

Few fields in modern biology and certainly no other field
in cancer research can be traced back to the work of one man
in the same way that the foundations in the field of viral
oncology can be traced back to the work of Peyton Rous in
1911 (Rous, 1911). The fact that he was awarded the Nobel
Prize for his work in 1968, as the first nonagenarian to receive this honor, reflects the span of time that was needed
to appreciate the full impact of Rous' discovery. For several
decades, Rous' work was kept on the shelf of curiosa; did it
really matter that some avian tumors could be transmitted
with cell-free filtrates? And yet, Rous' original work showed
more than that. Rous isolated not just one virus (the sole
modern survivor, virus no. 1, now designated as RSV) but at
least half a dozen, derived from different primary tumors
that were brought to him directly by the chicken farmers.
Rous pointed out that the agents were not only competent to
induce tumors, but also imprinted the phenotypic properties
of the original tumor on the recipient transformed cell. Was
this the first observation that reflected the action of src
and other, analogous pieces of the cellular genome that can
be picked up and transduced by the transforming RNA tumor
viruses?
  During the two first decades following Rous' discovery, interest in tumor viruses waned, mainly because of the difficulties to obtain unequivocal evidence of viral oncogenesis
in mammalians. The climate of opinion did not radically
change until Ludwik Gross' discovery of murine leukemia transmission with cell filtrates in 1951 (Gross, 1951). This does
not mean that the four decades between Rous and Gross lacked

important discoveries concerning viral oncogenesis. In the
early 30s, Shope isolated a virus (SPV) that induced benign
papillomas in wild cottontail rabbits (Shope, 1933). The
lesions progressed occasionally to malignant carcinoma, but
the relative rarity of this event indicated that SPV was
responsible for the precancerous rather than the cancerous
change. In retrospect, it is clear that the Shope system has
taught us many important lessons. Papillomas were only induced in wild but not in domestic rabbits, exemplifying the
highly selective host range, characteristic for many tumor
viruses. Virus particles were only made in the keratinizing
cells. This exemplifies the dependence of the viral cycle on
cell differentiation. In the basal layer, the viral DNA is
carried in a "silent", non-productive form (Ito & Evans,
1961). This was the first example of the "moderate" interaction between virus and host cell that was later identified
as a basic characteristic of all oncogenic DNA viruses. The
simultaneous regression of multiple papillomas in the same
rabbit and the subsequent watertight resistance of the host
to new induction by viral DNA (Ito, 1971) was an early example
of the powerful immune surveillance of the host, characteristic for all naturally occurring oncogenic virus/host combinations (Klein, 1979a).

The next important milestone, the discovery of the mammary
tumor virus (MTV) by Bittner in 1936 (Bittner, 1936) was no
less important. This has led not only to the discovery of a
mammalian oncogenic virus, but also to the insight that viral
and host (genetic, hormonal and immunological) factors interact in favoring or counteracting the malignization process.
The virus by itself was neither absolutely necessary nor
sufficient.

In 1951, Gross first transmitted mouse leukemia by inocula-
ting newborn mice of a particularly susceptible strain with
the filtrate of AKR leukemia cells. In retrospect, the Gross
virus and the MTV system are not so different as the difference of their impact on contemporary thinking would indicate.
It was the experimental approach and the emphasis of the investigators that differed, more than the biological systems.

The main points are summarized in Table 1.

The virus is neither necessary nor sufficient in either
system. Host factors are of major importance. In mammary
carcinoma, they are hormonal and genetic; - in mouse leukemia
they are genetic and immunological. For mammary carcinoma,
known genetic mechanisms include genes that influence the
replication of the virus, the hormonal environment, and the
likelihood of the neoplastic change at the target cell level
(Nandi & McGrath, 1973). In the AKR leukemia strain, the

TABLE 1
Involvement of the mammary tumor virus (MTV)
in mouse mammary carcinoma and of murine
leukemia virus (Gross) in leukemia

	MTV/mammary carcinoma	MuLV/leukemia
Is the virus absolutely necessary?	no	no
Is the virus sufficient by itself?	no	no
What conditioning factors?	hormonal, genetic	genetic, immunological
Does the virus induce preneoplastic cells?	yes	yes
What relevant components of the system are known to be under genetic control?	MTV reproduction, hormonal environment, target cell transformability	Integr. virus, Fv-1 amplification, immune unresp. $(Rgv-1^S)$, target cell transformability
Somatic genetics	stepwise progression (focal)	chromosomal change (trisomy 15)

integrated provirus acts as a genetic factor in itself. The
Fv-1 system amplifies viral replication and the Rgv-1 gene
probably modulates the immune responsiveness of the host.
Still other genes act on target cell transformability (Lilly
& Pincus, 1973).

Important parallels can be found at the somatic cell level.
Mammary tumors develop by stepwise progression, a series of
focal (probably clonal) changes (Foulds, 1958). In mouse
T-cell leukemia, trisomy of chromosome 15 is the outstanding
feature, as discussed later.

Thus, the high mammary carcinoma and the high leukemia
strains carry multiple genes that favor the development of
the tumor by a whole variety of mechanisms. Prolonged in-
breeding and selection for a complex phenotypic property
like tumor development tends to fix all available genes that
favor the expression of the selective trait. While the
inbred mouse is an arteficial system, it has provided an un-
parallelled analytical tool for the understanding of these
interactions.

THE MODERN ERA

The discovery of Gross triggered a true explosion of interest in viral oncology. Many new oncogenic viruses were discovered (for detailed history see Gross, 1970). Their main oncogenesis related properties are summarized in Table 2 and in the following sections.

a) Oncogenic DNA viruses

They belong into three taxonomic groups, the papovaviruses (MW of DNA: 3-5 x 10^6), the adenoviruses (20-23 x 10^6) and the herpesviruses (100 x 10^6). They carry very different amounts of genetic information and the strategy of their viral cycle (Wolstenholme & O'Connor, 1971) is based on different principles. Their transforming action shows certain similarities, however, summarized as follows:

Entry into the viral cycle is incompatible with cell survival. Proliferation of the virus-DNA carrying cell is therefore entirely dependent on the suppression of most viral functions. The control mechanisms are not known. Transforming papova- and adenovirus genomes integrate with host cell DNA   (for reviews see Flint, 1980; Howley, 1980; Ito, 1980). Herpesviral transformation is more complex. A few integrated and a larger number of free viral DNA copies are carried in each transformed cell, as a rule (Adams, 1980).

To understand the transforming action of the DNA-viruses, it is essential to define the virally determined function(s) expressed in the transformed cell. Oncogenic DNA viruses of all 3 taxonomic groups induce one or several intranuclear antigens, designated as T antigens for the papova- (Black et al., 1963) and adenoviruses (Pope & Rowe, 1964) and as EBNA (Reedman & Klein, 1973), HUPNA (Ohno et al., 1977) and HATNA (Ohno et al., 1979b) for the lymphotropic herpesviruses (EBV, HVP and HVA).

The small oncogenic papovaviruses, SV40 and polyoma, are best known. Their complete DNA base sequence has been published (for review see Howley, 1980; Ito, 1980). During lytic infection and transformation, the entire early region is represented in a single transcriptional unit, utilized with remarkable efficiency. If read in a single frame, the polyoma early region could only code for 100K protein. There are at least three known protein products, however, large, middle and small T, totalling 170K. This paradox was resolved by the finding that the early messenger is spliced in three different ways. Distal to the splice, all three reading

TABLE 2

Schematic summary of the biological properties
of the three main groups of oncogenic viruses

Taxonomic distribution	a) Oncogenic DNA viruses Broad (papova, adeno, herpes)	b) Transforming oncornaviruses Narrow (C-type)	c) Non-transforming oncornaviruses Narrow (B, C and D-type)
Compatibility between viral replication and cell multiplication	No	Yes	Yes
Integration of proviral DNA with host cell DNA	Yes	Yes	Yes
T-type antigen (intra-nuclear, DNA-binding) in transformed cells	Yes	No	No
Is transforming function required for viral cycle?	Yes	No	No known transforming function
Does the virus carry host-cell derived information, required for transformation?	No (possible exception: middle T of polyoma)	Yes	No
Is the putative transforming protein endowed with kinase activity?	Probably	Yes	No viral transforming protein known
Is the putative transforming protein, or its close homologues, also found in normal cells?	No	Yes	No viral transforming protein known

frames are utilized to a certain extent (Ito, 1980). The
role of the three products was defined by comparing viral
mutants that were defective in large T or in middle + small T.
While large T is not required for transformation, middle +
small T or middle T alone is. Interestingly, middle T is
associated with the cell membrane (Ito, 1979) and has protein
kinase activity (Benjamin & Schaffhausen, 1979). This
suggests possible functional analogies with the sarc products
of the transforming RNA viruses, discussed below.

In SV40, there is no middle T; the role of large T in transformation is controversial (for review see Danna & Haynes,
1980; Howley, 1980). Viral mutant studies suggest that large
T is necessary for initiation and maintenance of transformation. Microinjected T-antigen can trigger DNA synthesis
(Tjian et al., 1978). Large T binds to viral DNA near the
origin of replication (Jessel et al., 1976). It has been
suggested that T antigen can act as a continuous initiator
of DNA synthesis in transformed cells (Martin & Oppenheim,
1977).

The transforming function of the small oncogenic DNA viruses
is an essential part of the viral cycle: temperature sensitive (ts) transformation mutants are also ts for lytic infection. The opposite is true for transforming RNA viruses, as
discussed below.

Much less is known about the transforming function of the
adeno- and herpesviruses. The recent purification of adeno-
viral T-antigen (Biron et al., 1978) and EBNA (Luka et al.,
1978) will permit functional studies. In preliminary experiments, microinjection of EBNA stimulated DNA-synthesis in
contact inhibited cells (Klein et al., in press).

The large T-antigen of SV40 (Lane & Crawford, 1979; Linzer
& Levine, 1979) and EBNA (Klein et al., in press; Luka et al.,
in press) form a complex with a 53–54K protein of cellular
origin. A similar or identical 53K protein occurs in mouse
teratocarcinoma cells and, in much lower quantities, in
normal thymus tissue (Linzer & Levine, 1979). Possibly analogous 53K components were also found in chemically induced
mouse sarcomas (DeLeo et al., 1979) and in EBV-negative
human B-cell lymphomas (Klein et al., in press). It is not
yet clear whether 53K is a "transformation associated" or a
normal cellular protein. Tumor bearing, but not normal mice
form antibodies to 53K (DeLeo et al., 1979), suggesting a
transformation-determined or transformation-modified component. As a possible unifying feature of virally, chemically
and spontaneously transformed cells it is of great current
interest.

b) Oncogenic RNA (oncorna) viruses

All oncornaviruses have two highly unusual features:
i) They can replicate without impairing the viability of
the host cell. This is in contrast to all DNA-viruses, and
virtually all non-oncogenic RNA viruses.
ii) In contrast to non-oncogenic RNA viruses, all oncornaviruses carry reverse transcriptase (RT) and use it to make
a DNA copy of their RNA genome. The DNA provirus integrates
with host cell DNA. Propagation of the oncornaviruses in the
form of integrated proviral DNA provides a common denominator between the oncogenic DNA and RNA viruses.
The oncornaviruses can be subdivided into groups with and
without direct transforming ability in vitro. Transforming
viruses are oncogenic after short latency periods in vivo, as
a rule. Nontransforming oncornaviruses are either not known
to be oncogenic, or induce tumors (mostly leukemias) only
after long latency periods.

b-i) Directly transforming oncornaviruses

The oldest representative, Rous virus (RSV) is still one
of the most interesting tumor viruses. In vitro transformation was first discovered with RSV (Manaker & Groupe, 1956;
Temin & Rubin, 1958). The dependence of the transformed state
on the continued synthesis of a virally coded protein was
also first shown with RSV (Martin, 1970). The corresponding
viral gene, src, is not present in non-transforming oncornaviruses, including RSV mutants. Src is a cell-derived addition to the genome of the sarcoma virus, not required for
viral replication (for review see Hunter, 1980).

The product of the src gene has been recently identified as
a phosphorylated 58K-60K polypeptide, designated pp 60^{src}. It
has protein kinase activity and is associated with the inner,
cytoplasmic portion of the cell membrane (Courtneidge et al.,
1980).

Normal cell DNA contains src-related sequences, designated
sarc (Spector et al., 1978). The sequence is highly conserved over large phylogenetic distances. The protein product of sarc, pp $60^{proto-src}$, is closely related to pp 60^{src}
with regard to antigenic specificity, structure, kinase
activity and localization, but occurs in a hundredfold lower
concentration in normal cells than its counterpart in transformed cells (Oppermann et al., 1979). Since there are also
minor structural differences between the viral and the
cellular product (Collett et al., 1979), it cannot be decided
whether the oncogenic properties of src result from changes

in the genetic information or from a dosage effect.

RSV and other sarcoma viruses are not the only avian representatives of this group. While the non-transforming leukemia viruses have no src-like extra information and are oncogenic only after long latency periods, the acute leukemia viruses can transform in culture. Moreover, they are defective for replication and contain a new class of transforming sequences (onc), analogous to src (Graf & Beug, 1978). Interestingly, each of the 4 subclasses of these viruses transform different target cells and also differ in their transforming sequences. Corresponding sequences are found in normal cellular DNA (Sheiness & Bishop, 1979).

The mammalian sarcoma viruses (of rat, mouse, cat and primate origin) have provided similar information, but different in detail (for review see Shih & Scolnick, 1980). They are also generated by recombination between helper independent C-type viruses and the DNA of the host cell from which they were isolated. Further studies on the sarcoma viruses will provide important information on the mechanisms involved in the generation of highly oncogenic viruses by recombination, the origin of the transforming proteins, and, hopefully, the transformation mechanisms themselves.

Avian sarcoma viruses can be defective or non-defective. The oldest member of the group, Rous sarcoma virus, is the only known non-defective representative. It contains a complete set of genes required for virus replication (gag, pol, env) and, in addition, the src gene, responsible for transformation. In the defective sarcoma viruses, some of the viral genetic information has been replaced by cell derived sequences. All known mammalian sarcoma viruses are defective and require a non-transforming helper for replication. Recently, sarcoma viruses have been generated de novo. Transformation defective mutants were shown to acquire src sequences from the genetic information of the normal chicken (Hanafusa et al., 1977). Transforming murine viruses were derived by growing endogenous (non-transforming) viruses in spontaneously or chemically transformed cells (Rapp & Todaro, 1978; Rasheed et al., 1978).

Do all sarcoma viruses of the same species carry related cell-derived sequences? A large group of avian sarcoma viruses appear to do so, but it is questionable whether they represent truly independent isolates. The known murine sarcoma viruses carry at least 3 different fibroblast-transforming sequences. They are all unrelated to the src gene of avian sarcoma virus.

Most known mammalian leukemia viruses lack transforming

ability in vitro and are oncogenic after long latency periods
in vivo. One notable exception is the Abelson mouse leukemia
virus (Rosenberg & Baltimore, 1980). It is leukemogenic after
a short latency period and can transform immature B-lymphocytes into leukemic cells in vitro. Unlike other mouse
leukemia viruses, it is defective virus: 5.6 kb of the 8.3 kb
viral genome is replaced by a large cellular insert that
codes for a P120 polyprotein, unrelated to known viral
proteins and to the sarc products of the murine sarcoma
viruses. Normal mouse DNA contains a virtually exact counterpart of the viral insert and corresponding proteins are found
in normal hemopoietic mouse cells but in small quantities.

The presence of normal cell derived sequences thus appears
to be a rule for all directly transforming viruses, whether
of avian or mammalian origin, whether sarcomo- or leukemogenic. A study of these sequences provides new opportunities
for the understanding of transformation. As expected, sar-
coma-virus derived cellular sequences were found to transform
by themselves (Blair et al., 1980). The recent finding that
certain DNA segments of chemically transformed (Shih et al.,
1979) and even normal (Cooper et al., 1980) cells can transform is a striking extension of the area that will narrow
down the gap between chemical and viral carcinogenesis. It
may be expected that the two seemingly so different fields
will gradually converge towards an understanding of the
malignant transformation at the level of the cell genome.

b-ii) Oncornaviruses without direct transforming effect

This group includes the slow-acting avian leukosis viruses,
all murine leukemia viruses except the Abelson virus, and
the mammary tumor agent (MTV). MTV is a B-type retrovirus,
while the others are all C-type retroviruses. The leukemia
viruses are non-defective and have no known cell-derived
information. Until recently, the same was believed to be
true for MTV. Bentvelzen and Hilgers have now postulated
that MTV contains cell derived ("mam") sequences, required
for the oncogenic effect (Bentvelzen & Hilgers, 1980). All
these systems are characterized by the accumulation of preneoplastic cells during the long latency period. When the
autonomous tumor finally appears, it is monoclonal (Canaani
& Aaronson, 1979; Neiman et al., 1980; Steffen & Weinberg,
1978) and may show specific cytogenetic changes, as discussed
below. In Table 1, we have summarized some of the complex
host factors that contribute to tumor development in two
prototype systems of this category.

In all likelihood, the oncogenic action of these viruses is less direct than of categories a) and b-i) above. They appear to act by promoting the accumulation of preneoplastic cells; - in some systems this may be their only function. The same or closely similar preneoplastic cells can also be generated in other ways, however. In virally induced murine T-cell leukemia, viremia stimulates the generation of pre-leukemic T-cells by acting as an antigen (Lee & Ihle, 1979) or by binding to cell surface receptors (McGrath & Weissman, 1979). Preleukemic T-cells can also be generated by X-irradiation or chemical carcinogens. Here, abnormal regene-ration of the damaged T-cell system may provide the main pro-liferation inducing stimulus (for review see Haran-Ghera, 1980). Thus, the preleukemic T-cells can be compared to "conditioned" tumors, generated by an imbalance of the host-cell equilibrium, rather than by a specific cellular change (Furth, 1953). The emergence of autonomous leukemic clone would then be the result of some more specific change. Two main alternatives have been suggested: viral recombination and non-random chromosomal changes. The first alternative, recombination between endogenous, xenotropic and ecotropic C-type virus, generating the so called MCF viruses, is re-ceiving attention since recombinants have been isolated from leukemic organs (Hartley et al., 1977) and were shown to accelerate spontaneous leukemia in AKR mice (Cloyd et al., 1980). In low leukemia strains, the MCF viruses are not more oncogenic than the parental viruses, however (Cloyd et al., 1980) and lymphoma lines do not consistently express recom-binant viruses (Nowinski et al., 1977). It would be also difficult to reconcile the postulated direct transforming effect of the recombinant viruses with the monoclonality of the lymphomas.

The non-random cytogenetic changes found in the fully auto-nomous lymphomas provide a more plausible explanation. Thymus-derived leukemias induced by different viruses, chemical carcinogens and X-radiation show the same chromoso-mal aberration in the majority of the cases, chromosome 15 trisomy (Chang et al., 1977; Dofuku et al., 1975; Wiener et al., 1978a,b,c). Translocation studies point to the distal part of chromosome 15 as the critically important region (Spira et al., 1980; Wiener et al., 1978b).

It may be argued that trisomy 15 is a consequence rather than a cause of leukemogenesis. According to this view, a variety of trisomies would be generated by non-disjunction but only trisomy 15 would be viable and/or compatible with continued proliferation. We have found, however, that

virally and chemically induced thymic leukemias arising in
mice that carry Robertsonian translocations, derived from
the centromeric fusion of chromosome 15 and chromosomes 1, 5
or 6, resp., are trisomic for the whole translocation (Spira
et al., 1979). This strongly suggests that trisomy 15 is a
primary (causative) event in lymphoma development.

One of the most interesting aspects of these findings lies
in the fact that the identification of specific chromosomal
regions involved in the malignant transformation of a given
target tissue may shed light on the localization of genetic
determinants that influence the differentiation and/or growth
control responsiveness of the target cell. It is noteworthy
that chromosome 15 trisomy has now also been found in some
B-cell lymphomas (Fialkow, submitted for publ.; Wiener et al.,
submitted for publ.). Moreover, translocations involving
the distal region of one chromosome no. 15 and the Ig-heavy
or kappa light chain determinant carrying chromosomes (nos.
12 and 6) occur regularly in murine plasmocytomas (Ohno et
al., 1979a; Wiener et al., in press). It is likely that the
distal region of chromosome 15 contains a "supergene" area,
regulating the normal differentiation and/or function of
the lymphocyte series.

If the long latency period preceding the appearance of
autonomous leukemias in animals infected with the slow acting
viruses reflects the time required for the occurrence of the
"right" chromosomal change in the virus-stimulated preleukemic cell population, directly transforming viruses of the
category b-i) above, would be expected to induce genetically
unchanged tumors. This expectation was verified on the
Abelson system (Klein et al., 1980). The intriguing question
arises whether the large cellular insert, transduced by the
Abelson virus, represents the same segment (or a functionally
analogous segment) that is duplicated by trisomy in the corresponding leukemias induced by the slow acting viruses. This
question is open for direct studies.

The concept of a "convergent" lymphoma evolution (Klein,
1978a), i.e. common cytogenetic changes in tumors derived
from the same target cell even if induced by different agents,
is also supported by the EBV/human Burkitt lymphoma system,
discussed in the next section.

Viruses involved in the causation of naturally occurring tumors in animals and humans

There are a number of naturally occurring animal tumors
with a firmly established viral etiology. They include the

epizootic Marek's disease, a lymphotropic herpesvirus caused
lymphomatosis in chickens (Nazerian, 1980) that used to be
the economically most important disease problem of the poul-
try industry until the recent development of an effective
vaccine.   Chickens also have a number of naturally occurring
C-type virus induced leukemias.   The majority of feline
(Essex, 1980) and bovine (Burny et al., 1980) leukemias are
caused by exogenous, horisontally transmitted C-type viruses.
There are many important lessons to be learned from the study
of these diseases that cannot be dealt with here in detail.
To mention only one example, a clear correlation was found
between the ability of the feline leukemia virus infected
cats to react against a virally induced cell membrane antigen
(FOCMA) and their resistance to leukemia development after
viral infection (Essex, 1980).
    For obvious reasons, the search for viruses involved in
the causation of human tumors is a most difficult area.   The
lessons of experimental viral oncology and its slow and ar-
duous history should warn against hasty conclusions.   Neither
negative nor positive evidence can be taken at face value.
Virus particles and even viral footprints may be absent in
virus-induced tumors.   In DNA virus transformed cells, the
viral cycle is switched off and the viral genome may be
undetectable in the absence of suitable probes.   Transformation of non-permissive cells by RNA viruses may be equally
elusive.   Contrariwise, the presence of viruses or viral footprints in tumors does not necessarily indicate a causal relationship.   Viruses often grow better in transformed than in
normal cells.   In trying to distinguish between passenger
viruses and etiologically important agents, the consistency
of a given virus-tumor association, and its independence of
geographic and ethnic variation is particularly important
(cp. Klein, 1971).
    Two presently known human tumor-associated viruses are
likely to play an etiological role: Epstein-Barr virus (EBV)
and hepatitis B virus.

Epstein-Barr virus (EBV) and human malignancies
    Originally isolated from Burkitt's lymphoma, EBV is a
lymphotropic herpesvirus that can infect and transform (im-
mortalize) B-lymphocytes of human and some non-human primates
(for reviews see Henle & Henle, 1972; Klein, 1973; Epstein &
Achong, 1979; Miller, 1980).   Transformed cells grow indefinitely as established lines.   They carry multiple viral
genomes and a virally determined nuclear antigen, EBNA
(Reedman & Klein, 1973).   Under certain conditions, they can

grow progressively in immunosuppressed animals. The virus
can cause malignant lymphoproliferative disease in marmosets
and some other monkeys. Primary infection of humans can pass
without detectable symptoms or may lead to a self-limiting
lymphoproliferative disease, infectious mononucleosis.

Only two human tumors carry EBV and with great regularity:
Burkitt's lymphoma (BL) and nasopharyngeal carcinoma (NPC).
The endemic, African form of BL contains EBV genomes in 97%
of the cases. In the EBV-positive tumors, all cells carry
multiple copies of the viral genome and express the EBNA
antigen (Klein, 1975). The sporadically occurring non-
African cases carry EBV in only about one fifth of the cases
(Andersson et al., 1976).

In mononucleosis, the self-limiting proliferation of EBV-
infected B cells is polyclonal. BL is always monoclonal
(Fialkow et al., 1970). Both the EBV carrying and the EBV-
negative forms of BL have the same chromosomal anomaly, a
reciprocal 8;14 translocation with identical breakpoints in
different cases (Manolov and Manolova, 1972; Zech et al.,
1976).

In some immunodeficiency diseases, such as the X-linked
lymphoproliferative syndrome (XLP) (Purtilo et al., 1978), the
progressive lymphoproliferative disease that occurs in renal
transplant patients (Hanto et al., in press) and at least one
"lymphoma" in an ataxia teleangiectasia patient (Saemundsen
et al., submitted for publ.), unchecked proliferation of
EBV-carrying cells appears to be responsible for the disease.
These probably polyclonal proliferations are quite different
from the monoclonal, cytogenetically changed Burkitt's lymphoma that arises in immunocompetent patients.

We have suggested (Klein, 1979a) that the EBV-carrying
African BL arises in at least 3 different steps:

a) EBV-transformation (immortalization) of some B-cells in
the primarily infected African children. The virus load of
the pre-BL child is probably higher than of healthy control
children in the same environment (de-Thé, 1980). This
difference is only statistical, however, and cannot explain
the occurrence of Burkitt's lymphoma by itself.

b) The second phase in the development relates to the geographical (climate) factor. Burkitt suggested chronic holoendemic malaria as the most likely candidate (Burkitt, 1969).
Since chronic malaria is as a potent stimulator of lymphoid
proliferation, its effect may be similar to that of a tumor
promotor. It may force the virally transformed but still
host-controlled preneoplastic cells to continued proliferation. Since EBV-transformation freezes the differentiation

of the B-cell, the latently infected cells would undergo multiple divisions. The risk of genetic error increases with
each division. In the rare case of the BL patient, this
would lead to the third stage:
   c) the reciprocal 8;14 translocation, arising by chance,
or by more specific mechanisms. This would be the decisive
event in generating the autonomous, uniclonal lymphoma.
   In nasopharyngeal carcinoma, the situation is less well
understood. It is clear that the epithelial (carcinoma) cells
carry the viral genomes in this case (for review see Klein,
1979b).
   Great significance must be attributed to the fact that all
adequately studied low differentiated or anaplastic nasopharyngeal carcinomas were found to carry multiple copies of EBV-
DNA, no matter whether they arose in a high-incidence Southern
Chinese population, or a moderate or low risk population.
Nasopharyngeal tumors of other histological types were virus-
free.
   It cannot be excluded that a specific viral subtype may be
responsible for NPC. Alternatively, co-factors could play
a decisive role. Unlike the clearly environmental cofactors
involved in African BL, the development of NPC is more likely
to be influenced by genetic (or cultural) factors.

          Hepatitis B-virus (HBV) and carcinoma of the liver
   Epidemiological evidence (Szmuness, 1980) indicated a correlation between infectious hepatitis, due to HBV, and primary
carcinoma of the liver. Recently, 4 independent groups reported the presence of integrated virus in a hepatoma derived
cell line and in tumor biopsies (Brechot et al., 1980;
Chakraborty et al., 1980; Edman et al., 1980; Marion et al.,
1980).
   While the mere presence of integrated HBV genes and a
parallel limited expression of viral proteins does not prove
a causal association, the findings are at least consistent
with this possibility. There are, however. hepatoma-derived
lines that lack HBV-DNA, and primary hepatocellular carcinoma
also occurs in HBV-negative individuals. On the other hand,
the woodchuck hepatitis virus, a close relative of human HBV,
was found to induce hepatitis and subsequently, hepatocellular carcinoma in a substantial percentage of its natural host
animal (Summers et al., 1978).

                        Epilogue

   The contributions of viral oncology to cancer research may

be considered from two points of view:
  a) Understanding the malignant transformation;
  b) Etiology of naturally occurring tumors.
  Re. a) In the fundamental area, there have been many unexpected turns and surprises. Regarded first as a bizarre
exception on the shelf of curiosa, relevant only for some
birds, tumor viruses were subsequently isolated from all
properly studied mammalians and from some amphibians and rep-
tiles as well. The seemingly unbridgeable dichotomy of the
RNA and DNA tumor viruses has been replaced by the perfect
unity provided by the proviral DNA, integrated with the host
genome. The transforming proteins of the RNA and DNA tumor
viruses, so different at first sight, are presently converging
towards the inner surface of the plasma membrane, possibly
with an unusual type of protein kinase activity as their
common denominator. The extraordinary recombining ability
of the oncogenic RNA viruses, first regarded as a playtoy of
the viral geneticist, was found to endow these agents with
a remarkable facility to pick up "transforming sequences"
from the normal host cell genome, providing the investigator
with specific DNA sequences that bear the responsibility for
transformation. With the recent spectacular advances in
molecular biology, the imminent localization of these sequences in the normal cellular genome and the study of their
function in the normal and neoplastic cell will carry our
understanding much further in the immediate future, both
with regard to the malignant transformation, and the genetic
control of growth functions in the normal cell. As the
latest unexpected turn, the seemingly wide gap between chemical and viral carcinogenesis appears to narrow down and will
perhaps disappear. The direct isolation of transforming
sequences from the genome of the chemically transformed and
even the normal cell shows that the molecular biologists may
learn the art of transformation from the oncogenic viruses
and will be able to apply it to many previously unapproach-
able systems.
  Re. b), there is no doubt that certain naturally occurring
animal tumors, like avian, feline and bovine leukemias,
papillomatosis of many species, and at least one amphibian
carcinoma are due to horisontally spread RNA or DNA tumor
viruses. Studies on the epidemiology, pathogenesis, and
immunology of these diseases has taught us much about the
special circumstances, under which oncogenic viruses of
relatively moderate pathogenicity can cause disease. To the
tumor immunologist, the most interesting tumor virus-host
interactions are those where tumor development is entirely

prevented under natural conditions. I am referring to the
highly transforming, ubiquitous oncogenic viruses that infect
most individuals of a given species; this can be exemplified
by polyoma in the mouse, EBV in man and H. saimiri in the
squirrel monkey. The practically watertight host surveillance shows that a symbiotic balance has evolved, comparable
to the most advanced parasitic adaptations. Tumors only
develop through biological accidents like immunodeficiency
or the escape of an otherwise tightly contained preneoplastic
cell, due to a specific cytogenetic change. The involvement
of EBV in Burkitt's lymphoma is a case in point.

At this time, we cannot tell how many naturally occurring
neoplastic diseases will reveal a viral contribution that
is now hidden from sight; this has been and will remain a
field of surprises. The recent, increasingly persistent claim
of an association between hepatitis B-virus and primary carcinoma of the liver may turn out to be the next surprise and
there may be others in store, even though the concept that
all or even most neoplastic diseases in humans are caused
by viruses is probably as unrealistic as other "all-encom-
passing" claims, an occupational hazard of the cancer re-
searcher.

REFERENCES

Adams, A. Molecular biology of the Epstein-Barr virus. In
    G. Klein (Ed.), Viral Oncology. New York: Raven Press,
    1980, 683-711.
Andersson, M,. Klein, G., Ziegler, J.L. & Henle, W., Nature,
    1976, 260, 357.
Benjamin, T.L. & Schaffhausen, B.S., Cell, 1979, 18, 935.
Bentvelzen, P. & Hilgers, J. Murine mammary tumor virus.
    In G. Klein (Ed.), Viral Oncology. New York: Raven Press,
    1980, 311-355.
Biron, K.K., Morrongiello, M.P., Raskova, J. & Raska, K.,
    Virol., 1978, 85, 464.
Bittner, J.J., Science, 1936, 84, 162.
Black, P,H,. Rowe, W.P., Turner, H.C. & Huebner, R.J., Proc.
    Natl. Acad. Sci. USA, 1963, 50, 1148.
Blair, D.G., McClements, W.L., Oskarsson, M.K., Fischinger,
    P.J. & van de Woude, G.F., Proc. Natl. Acad. Sci. USA,
    1980, 77, 3504.
Brechot, C., Pourzer, Ch., Rain, A.-L.B. & Tiollais, P.,
    Nature, 1980, 286, 533.
Brugge, J.S. & Erikson, R.L., Nature, 1977, 269, 346.

Burkitt, D., J. Natl. Cancer Inst., 1969, 42, 19.

Burny, A., Bruck, C., Chantrenne, H. et al. Bovine leukemia virus: Molecular biology and epidemiology. In G. Klein (Ed.), Viral Oncology. New York: Raven Press, 1980, 231-289.

Canaani, E. & Aaronson, S.A., Proc. Natl. Acad. Sci., 1979, 76, 1677.

Chakraborty, P.R., Ruiz-Opazo, N., Shouval, D. & Shfritz, D.A., Nature, 1980, 286, 531.

Chang, T.D., Biedler, J.L., Stockert, E., & Old, L.J., Proc. Am. Assoc. Cancer Res., 1977, 18, 225.

Cloyd, M.W., Hartley, J.W. & Rowe, W.P., J. Exp. Med., 1980, 151, 542.

Collett, M.S., Erikson, E., Purchio, A.F., Brugge, J.S. & Erickson, R.L., Proc. Natl. Acad. Sci. USA, 1979, 76, 3159.

Cooper, G.M., Okenquist, S. & Silverman, L., Nature, 1980, 284, 418.

Courtneidge, S.A., Levinson, A.D. & Bishop, J.M., Proc. Natl. Acad. Sci. USA, 1980, 77, 3783.

Danna, K.J. & Haynes, F.B. The Genetics of Simian Virus 40. In G. Klein (Ed.), Viral Oncology. New York: Raven Press, 1980, 551-580.

DeLeo, A.B., Jay, G., Appella, E. et al., Proc. Natl. Acad. Sci. USA, 1979, 76, 2420.

Dofuku, R., Biedler, J.L., Spengler, B.A. & Old, L.J., Proc. Natl. Acad. Sci., 1975, 72, 1515.

Edman, J.C., Gray, P., Valenzuela, P., Rall, L.B. & Rutter, W.J., Nature, 1980, 286, 535.

Epstein, M.A. & Achong, B.G. The Epstein-Barr Virus. Springer Verlag, 1979.

Erikson, R.L. Avian sarcoma viruses: Molecular biology. In G. Klein (Ed.), Viral Oncology. New York: Raven Press, 1980, 39-53.

Essex, M. Feline leukemia and sarcoma viruses. In G. Klein (Ed.), Viral Oncology. New York: Raven Press, 1980, 205-229.

Fialkow, P.J., submitted for publ.

Fialkow, P.J., Klein, G., Gartler, S.M. & Clifford, P., Lancet, 1970, 7643, 384.

Flint, S.J. Molecular Biology of adenoviruses. In G. Klein (Ed.), Viral Oncology. New York: Raven Press, 1980, 603-663.

Foulds, L.M.A., J. Chr. Dis., 1958, 8, 2.

Furth, J., Cancer Res., 1953, 13, 477.

Graf, T. & Beug, H., Biochim, Biophys, Acta, 1978, 516, 269.

Gross, L., Proc. Soc. Exp. Biol. Med., 1951, 76, 27.

Gross, L., Oncogenic Viruses, ed. 2. Oxford: Pergamon Press, 1970.

Hanafusa, H., Halpern, C.C., Buchhagen, D.L. & Kawai, S.,
    J. Exp. Med., 1977, 146, 1735.
Hanto, D.W., Frizzera, G., Gajl-Peczalska, K.J. et al.,
    Transpl. Proc., in press.
Haran-Ghera, N. Pathogenesis of murine leukemia. In G. Klein
    (Ed.), Viral Oncology. New York: Raven Press, 1980.
Hartley, J.W., Wolford, N.K., Old, L.J. & Rowe, W.P., Proc.
    Natl. Acad. Sci., 1977, 74, 789.
Henle, W. & Henle, G. Epstein-Barr virus: The cause of
    infectious mononucleosis. A review. In P. Biggs, G. de-Thé
    & L. Payne (Eds.), Oncogenesis and Herpesviruses. Lyon,
    France: IARC, 1972, 269-274.
Howley, P.M. Molecular Biology of SV40 and the human polyoma-
    viruses BK and JC. In G. Klein (Ed.), Viral Oncology.
    New York: Raven Press, 1980, 489-550.
Hunter, E. Avian oncoviruses: Genetics. In G. Klein (Ed.),
    Viral Oncology. New York: Raven Press, 1980, 1-38.
Ito, Y. Papilloma-myxoma viruses. In F.F. Becker (Ed.),
    Cancer. New York: Plenum Publ. Corp., 1971, 2, 323-341.
Ito, Y., Virology, 1979, 98, 261.
Ito, Y., Organization and expression of the genome of polyoma
    virus. In G. Klein (Ed.), Viral Oncology. New York:
    Raven Press, 1980, 447, 480.
Ito, Y. & Evans, C.A., J. Exp. Med., 1961, 114, 485.
Jessel, D., Landau, T., Hudson, J. et al., Cell, 1976, 8, 535.
Klein, G., Israel J. Med. Sci., 1971, 7, 111.
Klein, G. The Epstein-Barr virus. In A.S. Kaplan (Ed.),
    The Herpesviruses, New York: Academic Press, 1973, 521-555.
Klein, G., Cold Spring Harbor Symp. on Quant. Biol., 1975,
    39, 783.
Klein, G., Proc. Natl. Acad. Sci. USA, 1979a, 76, 2442.
Klein, G. The relationship of the virus to nasopharyngeal
    carcinoma. In M.A. Epstein & B.G. Achong (Eds.), The
    Epstein-Barr Virus. Springer Verlag, 1979b, 339-350.
Klein, G., Luka, J. & Zeuthen, J., Cold Spring Harbor Symp.
    for Quant. Biol., 1980, in press.
Klein, G., Ohno, S., Rosenberg, N. et al., Int. J. Cancer,
    1980, 25, 805.
Lane, D.P. & Crawford, L.V., Nature, 1979, 278, 261.
Lee, J.C. & Ihle, J.N., J. Immunol., 1979, 123, 2351.
Lilly, F. & Pincus, T., Adv. Cancer Res., 1973, .7, 231.
Linzer, D.I.H. & Levine, A.J., Cell, 1979, 17, 43.
Luka, J., Jörnvall, H. & Klein, G., J. Virol., in press.
Luka, J., Lindahl, T. & Klein, G., J. Virol., 1978, 27, 604.
Manaker, R.A. & Groupe, V., Virol., 1956, 2, 838.
Manolov, G. & Manolova, Y., Nature, 1972, 237, 33.
Marion, P.L., Salazar, F.H., Alexander, J.J. & Robinson, W.S.,

J. Virol., 1980, 33, 795.
Martin, G.S., Nature, 1970, 227, 1021.
Martin, R.G. & Oppenheim, A., Cell, 1977, 11, 859.
McGrath, M.S. & Weissman, I.L., Cell, 1979, 17, 65.
Miller, G. Biology of Epstein-Barr virus. In G. Klein (Ed.), Viral Oncology. New York: Raven Press, 1980, 713-738.
Nandi, S. & McGrath, C.M., Adv. Cancer Res., 1973, 17, 353.
Nazerian, K. Marek's disease: A herpesvirus-induced malignant lymphoma of the chicken. In G. Klein (Ed.), Viral Oncology. New York: Raven Press, 1980, 665-682.
Neiman, P., Pane, L.N. & Weiss, R.A., J. Virol., 1980, 34, 178.
Nowinski, R.C., Hays, E.F., Doyle, T. et al., Virology, 1977, 81, 363.
Ohno, S., Babonits, M., Wiener, F. et al., Cell, 1979a, 18, 1001.
Ohno, S., Luka, J., Falk, L. & Klein, G., Int. J. Cancer, 1977, 20, 941.
Ohno, S., Luka, J., Klein. G. & Daniel, M.D., Proc. Natl. Acad. Sci. USA, 1979b, 76, 2042.
Oppermann, H., Levinson, A.D., Varmus, H.E., Levinton, L. & Bishop, J.M., Proc. Natl. Acad. Sci. USA, 1979, 76, 1804.
Pope, J.H. & Rowe, W.P., J. Exp. Med., 1964, 120, 577.
Purtilo, D.T., Hutt, L., Bhawan, J. et al., Clin. Immunol. Immunopathol., 1978, 9, 147.
Rapp, U.R. & Todaro, G.J., Science, 1978, 201, 821.
Rasheed, S., Gardner, M.B. & Huebner, R.J., Proc. Natl. Acad. Sci. USA, 1978, 75, 2972.
Reedman, B.M. & Klein. G., Int. J. Cancer, 1973, 2, 499.
Rosenberg, N. & Baltimore, D. Abelson virus. In G. Klein (Ed.), Viral Oncology. New York: Raven Press, 1980, 187-203.
Rous, P., J. Exp. Med., 1911, 13, 397.
Saemundsen, A.K., Berkel, A.I., Henle, W. et al., submitted for publ.
Sheiness, D. & Bishop, J.M., J. Virol., 1979, 31, 514.
Shih, C., Shilo, B.-Z., Goldfarb, M.F., Dannenberg, A. & Weinberg, R.A., Proc. Natl. Acad. Sci. USA, 1979, 76, 5714.
Shih, T.Y. & Scolnick, E.M. Molecular biology of mammalian sarcoma viruses. In G. Klein (Ed.), Viral Oncology. New York: Raven Press, 1980, 135-160.
Shope, R.E., J. Exp. Med., 1933, 68, 607.
Spector, D.H., Varmus, H.E. & Bishop, J.M., Proc. Natl. Acad. Sci. USA, 1978, 75, 4102.
Spira, J., Babonits, M., Wiener, F. et al., Cancer Res., 1980, 40, 2609.

Spira, J., Wiener, F., Ohno, S. & Klein. G., Proc. Natl.
    Acad. Sci., 1979, 76, 6619.
Steffen, D. & Weinberg, R.A., Cell, 1978, 15, 1003.
Summers, J., Smolec, J.M. & Snyder, R., Proc. Natl. Acad.
    Sci., 1978, 75, 4533.
Szmuness, W., Progr. Med. Virol., 1980, 24, 40.
Temin, H.M. & Rubin, H., Virol., 1958, 6, 669.
de-Thé, G. Role of Epstein-Barr virus in human diseases:
    Infectious mononucleosis, Burkitt's lymphoma, and naso-
    pharyngeal carcinoma. In G. Klein (Ed.), Viral Oncology.
    New York: Raven Press, 1980, 769-797.
Tjian, R., Fey, G. & Graessman, A., Proc. Natl. Acad. Sci.
    USA, 1978, 75, 1279.
Wiener, F., Babonits, M., Spira, J. et al., submitted for
    publ.
Wiener, F., Babonits, M., Spira, J., Klein. G. & Potter, M.,
    Somatic Cell Gen., in press.
Wiener, F., Ohno, S., Spira, J., Haran-Ghera, N. & Klein, G.,
    J. Natl. Cancer Inst., 1978a, 61, 227.
Wiener, F., Ohno, S., Spira, J., Haran-Ghera, N. & Klein, G.,
    Nature, 1978b, 275, 658.
Wiener, F., Spira, J., Ohno, S., Haran-Ghera, N. & Klein, G.,
    Int. J. Cancer, 1978c, 22, 447.
Wolstenholme, G.E.W. & O'Connor, M. (Eds.). Strategy of
    the viral genome. Edinburgh and London, Churchill-Living-
    stone, 1971, pp. 406.
Zech, L., Haglund, U., Nilsson, K. & Klein. G., Int. J.
    Cancer, 1976, 17, 47.

CELL TRANSFORMATION BY POLYOMA VIRUS

THOMAS L. BENJAMIN

Professor
Department of Pathology
Harvard Medical School
Boston, Massachusetts 02115

INTRODUCTION

Animal viruses from several taxonomic groups are able to cause cancers in susceptible hosts. These tumor viruses form a diverse collection, exhibiting vastly different structures and life styles. Certain of them are able to infect normal cells in culture and to convert them rapidly and efficiently into malignant cells. This phenomenon of *in vitro* neoplastic transformation has opened the way for investigations into the mechanism of action of tumor viruses at the molecular level. Two groups of viruses have been favored in these studies — the small DNA-containing viruses of the papova group and the RNA-containing retraviruses. A brief account of some of the essential features of virus-host interactions with these two virus groups will serve to illustrate their strong biological differences, as well as some unifying features concerning the modes of action of their respective oncogenes.

It should be noted initially that cancer is not an inevitable consequence of the propagation of either papova or retraviruses under natural conditions, despite the oncogenic potential these viruses have in the laboratory and their occasional association with naturally occurring disease. Members of the retravirus group are enveloped viruses and contain RNA as their genetic material. These viruses exist in nature as DNA proviruses and are present in normal cellular DNA of many, and perhaps all, vertebrate species. Endogenous proviruses are transmitted as DNA from cell to cell during development, and from generation to generation via the germ line. Provirus may become activated to produce infectious virus which can spread "horizontally", i.e., from cell to cell within the host, from animal to animal, and occasionally across species. A single

cycle of infection involves a flow of viral genetic information from RNA to DNA and back to RNA. The virus acquires its
envelope by budding out of RNA core structures through the
plasma membrane of the host. This infectious cycle is usually
non-cytocidal and occurs without detectable consequences in
the whole animal. Some members of the retravirus group are
clearly oncogenic, and these appear to have evolved from their
non-oncogenic relatives. They differ from their progenitors
in having acquired a single new gene from the host (viruses
with different tropisms acquiring different cellular genes),
usually in exchange for one or more of their own essential
replication genes. Most RNA tumor viruses are therefore defective, but can propagate and spread horizontally in the
presence of non-defective helper virus.

Papovaviruses are DNA-containing, non-enveloped, icosahe-
dral viruses which replicate and assemble in the nuclei of the
host cell. They exist in nature apparently without causing
disease. The genetic material of these viruses is not present
as endogenous provirus in their natural hosts. Virus is therefore maintained strictly by replication and horizontal spread.
The infectious cycle of papovaviruses is cytocidal, i.e., the
virus generally cannot replicate without killing the host cell.
How the balance is maintained between virus growth and host
survival, and how the host remains tumor-free while harboring
a potentially oncogenic virus throughout its life, is not understood, although the host immune response clearly must play
a dominant role. In the case of polyoma virus, which is endemic in many wild and domestic populations of mice, the inheritance of maternal anti-viral antibody apparently protects
the newborn which contact the virus early in life. The oncogenic potential of polyoma virus is realized in the laboratory
in an optimal way by injecting large doses of virus in the
first few hours after birth. Newborn hamsters and rats —
species which do not harbor polyoma virus in nature — are
more susceptible than mice to tumor induction by the virus.
In contrast to retroviral oncogenes which are cellular in origin and non-essential to virus replication, the genetic material of polyoma responsible for malignant transformation has
no homologue in the DNA of normal cells but does play an important role in the propagation of the virus. Polyoma, therefore, is bound to express its oncogenic potential in the
course of its replication cycle. Cells become permanently
transformed when, due to absence of host cell factor(s) required by the virus or to a defectiveness of the infecting
virus particle itself, the virus cannot complete its replication cycle. For the host, this necessitates a second kind of
immunity, directed against viral induced neoantigen(s) in the

infected or transformed cells. The existence of such specific transplantation antigens induced by papovaviruses has been demonstrated experimentally. This suggests that another component to the successful symbiosis of polyoma virus and the mouse lies in the induction of cellular immunity directed against the virus specific transplantation antigen, providing an effective anti-tumor immunity. Despite the extensive knowledge we now have of polyoma virus at the molecular level, the identity of the transplantation antigen(s) remains unknown.

Papova and retraviruses seem more akin when one focuses not on the natural histories of the viruses, but rather on the transformed cells and the effects produced by the action of the respective viral oncogenes. Transformation of fibroblasts of the appropriate species by either polyoma virus or avian (Rous) sarcoma virus results in pronounced changes in cell morphology and in altered and less restrictive requirements for cell growth. In each case, the multiple cellular alterations which arise can be traced to the action of a single viral gene which is expressed in a continuous manner by a viral genome that has become integrated into host DNA. This paper will present a brief review of work leading to the identification and partial characterization of the transforming gene of polyoma virus and its products. Other contributions to this symposium volume are concerned with members of the retravirus group.

RESULTS AND DISCUSSION

Step-Wise Approaches to the Overall Problem

Understanding the mechanism of transformation by polyoma virus can begin with the question: How does the emergence of altered properties in neoplastically transformed cells depend on the expression of viral genetic information? The experimental approach to this question begins with attempts to isolate virus mutants that have undergone functional alterations in gene(s) essential to the transformation process. The quest continues with careful studies of the physiological properties of the non-transforming mutants in attempts to discover the precise ways in which they differ from wild type virus. An additional and essential step along the way is the identification of the viral gene product(s) responsible for transformation. As will be illustrated below, the non-transforming mutants themselves provide the tools enabling assignments to be made between specific proteins and viral genes. Substantial progress has been made on these aspects of the overall problem. A major challenge which remains for the future will have to do

with defining the complicated cellular pathways that are triggered by the action of the viral gene products.

Identification of Viral Genes

The genetics of polyoma virus has been probed by two approaches based on isolation of temperature-sensitive and host
range mutants. The former approach has uncovered at least
three distinct complementation groups, of which one, called
ts-a, is involved in transformation. Ts-a mutants transform
rat or hamster fibroblasts with reduced efficiency at 39°C
compared to 33°C. The bulk of the evidence suggests that the
ts-a function is required to initiate stable transformation,
probably by facilitating the integration of viral DNA into the
cell, but that is not essential for maintaining the transformed state.

Host range mutants have been isolated using infectable
transformed cells carrying an integrated polyoma viral genome
as the permissive host, and normal cells as the non-permissive
host. The rationale behind this selection is that mutants
altered specifically in the transformation function might be
isolated by virtue of being complemented in their growth by
the homologous wild type function expressed by the integrated
virus in the transformed host. Mutants isolated in this way
in fact form a single complementation group, and all are
totally defective in transformation. These mutants have been
designated hr-t.

Properties of Ts-a and Hr-t Mutants

Mutants of the ts-a and hr-t groups are distinct by a
variety of criteria. First, complementation tests have been
carried out between the two mutant classes. Cells doubly infected by various pairs of hr-t and ts-a mutants produce progeny virus or become transformed at 39°C, indicating clearly
that the defects are different and 'complementary' in the two
mutant classes.

A key physiological experiment which highlights the major
difference between these mutants is that of abortive transformation. Normal rat or hamster fibroblasts are infected and
incubated at 39°C and their behavior is observed over the
course of 3-4 days. Following infection by either wild type
virus or ts-a mutants, the cells undergo identical patterns of
change. Beginning as early as 24 hours post-infection, cells
undergo dramatic changes in morphology accompanied by decreased adhesion to the solid substratum and loss of well organized microfilament bundles ('stress fibers') in the

cytoplasm. Cell surface changes also occur, as shown by agglutination studies with a variety of lectins. At the same
time, the cells acquire the ability to grow when suspended
in soft agar. The latter phenomenon, termed "loss of anchorage dependence of growth", indicates a relaxation of growth
control that correlates well with the acquisition of malignant growth potential in the animal. If left on a solid substrate, the cells adopt a criss-cross overlapping growth pattern. These changes occur initially in a comparable and usually large fraction of both wild type virus and ts-a mutant
infected cells. However, when the cultures are examined after
a period of 10-14 days, the frequency of stable transformation
— i.e., the per cent of initially transformed cells which have
become fixed in the transformed state and destined to give
rise to transformed progeny — is significantly lower in the
ts-a mutant infected cultures compared to the wild type.
While the major response of cells to both wild type virus and
ts-a mutants is that of initial or abortive transformation,
only the wild type virus is able occasionally to integrate
its DNA into the host to stabilize the transformed state, and
this in only a few per cent of the population. Ts-a mutants
are defective in the stabilization process, intepreted as integration of viral DNA, but retain the capability of eliciting the full range of transformed cell characteristics. Hr-t
mutants, in sharp contrast, fail to alter the cells in any of
the above mentioned ways. The hr-t function, therefore, acts
pleiotropically to induce the whole array of transformation-
related cellular changes.

The Early Region of the Viral Genome and its Products

Application of restriction enzyme and DNA sequencing techniques has lead to the complete sequencing of polyoma virus
DNA. Using defined restriction enzyme fragments of wild type
viral DNA to 'rescue' the genetic lesions in ts-a and hr-t mutants, it has been possible to localize the region of the
viral DNA encoding these two viral functions. Both mutants
map in the early region of the genome, i.e., in the sequences
that are transcribed in transformed cells and during the pre-
DNA replication phase in productively infected mouse cells.
Using sera from polyoma tumor bearing animals, it is possible to specifically precipitate a series of proteins from extracts of either productively infected or transformed cells.
These proteins, operationally defined as "T" or tumor antigens,
are presumably encoded by the viral genome. Proof of this supposition comes from the ability to synthesize the proteins in
cell-free translation systems primed by viral messenger RNAs.

Three discrete species of polyoma T antigen have been defined
by immune precipitation experiments. 1) The large T antigen,
with an apparent molecular weight of 100K, is localized predominantly in the nucleus of productively infected cells, but
is not always found in transformed cells. 2) The middle T
antigen is a 56K protein localized in membrane fractions (most
likely the plasma membrane) of both lytically infected and
transformed cells. 3) The small T antigen is a 22K protein
found predominantly in the cytosol fraction, again in both
infected and transformed cells.

The exact arrangement of coding sequences in the DNA for
these three T antigen species has been arrived at through a
combination of experiments at the DNA, RNA and protein levels.
Peptide maps of ^{35}s-methionine labelled T antigens have been
analyzed to determine which peptides are shared among the
three T antigen species and which are unique. The maps are
also compared to amino acid sequences as deduced from the DNA
sequence. Studies of viral RNAs have revealed 'introns' in
each of the T antigen mRNAs and have indicated their most
likely locations within the DNA sequence. The picture shown
in Figure 1 is based on integrating the information drawn
from these various lines of investigation.

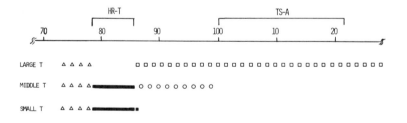

T ANTIGEN CODING SEQUENCES IN POLYOMA VIRUS DNA

Figure 1. The early region of polyoma virus DNA showing the
coding sequences for large, middle and small T antigens and
the locations of Hr-t and Ts-a mutants.

As indicated in the Figure, all three T antigens share a common amino terminal end (△); this sequence of about 80 amino acids is specified by sequences from roughly 74-79 map units on the viral DNA. Sequences from 79-86 map units are spliced out of the large T mRNA, while sequences from 86 to 28 map units code for the long unique carboxy terminal portion of the large T protein (□). The middle and small T antigens share sequences specified by the region spliced out of the large T mRNA, i.e., 79-86 map units (■). Small introns are found in the mRNAs for each of these proteins, roughly at position 86 map units. Downstream of these introns, the two proteins are encoded in different frames, giving rise to a short unique carboxy terminal sequence of just 4 amino acids for small T, and to a much longer carboxy terminal sequence of roughly 200 amino acids for middle T (o). The latter sequence is also unique, being read in a different frame from that of the overlapping large T.

T Antigens as Products of the Ts-a and Hr-t Genes

Figure 1 also indicates the separate regions in which various hr-t and ts-a mutants have been mapped. The lesions in hr-t mutants all map within a small segment in the proximal part of the early region, corresponding precisely to the large T intron. These sequences, from 79-86 map units, encode the amino acid sequences shared by the small and middle T antigens, but which are missing from the large T protein. Ts-a mutants map distally, in the region affecting the unique portion of the large T, and specifically in the carboxy terminal segment lying downstream of the overlap region with middle T.

The predictions that small and middle T antigens are dual products of the hr-t gene and that the large T antigen is the sole product of the ts-a gene have been confirmed experimentally by examining alterations in T antigen patterns induced by different mutants. Ts-a mutants code for large T antigen species which are thermolabile in low-temperature-pulse high-temperature-chase experiments. These mutants show normal patterns and thermolabilities of the small and middle T species. Hr-t mutants on the other hand are affected with respect to the 56K and 22K proteins, in different ways depending on the exact nature of the mutation. Sequencing of various hr-t mutant viral DNAs in the 79-86 map unit region has uncovered three categories of alterations, each giving rise to the predicted change in the small and middle T antigens: 1) The most common class of hr-t mutants consists of those with sizeable deletions that alter the reading frame; these mutants produce no detectable 56K or 22K proteins. 2) A single hr-t

mutant has been found with an in-phase deletion of 141 base
pairs; this mutant induces the synthesis of a ∿50K species,
consistent with the removal of 47 amino acids from the middle
T protein.   3) A group of three hr-t mutants have undergone an
identical change consisting of the insertion of a single trip-
let (ATA) followed by a G to A transition; this change, which
totally inactivates the transforming capacity of the virus,
gives rise to the addition of a single isoleucine residue followed by the change of an aspartic acid to asparagine.   These
three mutants produce detectable middle and small T proteins
which co-migrate with the wild type products.   Mutants of all
three categories produce normal amounts of the large T antigen as expected.

Protein Modification Reactions Affected by the Hr-t Gene

Two protein modification reactions have been observed that
are affected in hr-t mutants.   The first concerns histone
acetylation of encapsidated histones: the H-3 and H-4 species
of histone present in the polyoma virion show extensive
acetylation in the case of wild type virus, but not in the
case of hr-t mutants.   The second reaction is one leading to
phosphorylation of the 56K protein *in vitro*.   This reaction is
carried out by incubating T antigen immune precipitates with
γ-P^{32} labelled ATP.   In the case of wild type virus and ts-a
mutants, this reaction leads to phosphorylation of the middle
T protein.   Hr-t mutants making altered middle T species fail
to show phosphorylation of those species.   It is not yet clear
whether either of the hr-t gene products possesses catalytic
properties capable of carrying out these reactions, or whether
they act in some indirect way to regulate cellular enzymes involved in the modifications.   It is interesting to note that
the src protein encoded by the transforming gene of Rous sarcoma virus also has a protein kinase activity associated with
it, and furthermore that the amino acid undergoing phosphorylation in both virus systems is tyrosine.   The further study
of these modification reactions under control of viral oncogenes is clearly of great interest in view of the well-docu-
mented pleiotropic action these genes have in cells.

REFERENCES

1. Benjamin, T. L.   Host range mutants of polyoma virus.
    PNAS, 1970, 67, 394.
2. Benjamin, T. L. and Burger, M. M.   Absence of a cell mem-
    brane alteration function in non-transforming mutants of
    polyoma virus.   PNAS, 1970, 67, 929.
3. Benjamin, T. L.   Physiological and genetic studies of
    polyoma virus.   Current Topics in Microbiology & Immunol-
    ogy, Springer Verlag, Publ., 1972, 59, 107.
4. Benjamin, T. L., Schaffhausen, B. S. and Silver, J. E.
    Polyoma T (Tumor) antigen species in abortively and stably
    transformed cells.   J. Supramol. Structure, 1979, 12, 127.
5. Carmichael, G. G. and Benjamin, T. L.   Identification of
    DNA sequence changes leading to loss of transforming
    ability in polyoma virus.   J. Biol. Chem., 1980, 255, 230.
6. Collett, M. and Erikson, R.   Protein kinase activity as-
    sociated with the avian sarcoma virus transforming gene
    product.   PNAS, 1978, 75, 2021.
7. Eckhart, W., Hutchinson, M. and Hunter, T.   An activity
    phosphorylating tyrosine in polyoma T antigen immuno-
    precipitates.   Cell, 1979, 18, 925.
8. Feunteun, J., Sompayrac, L., Fluck, M. and Benjamin, T.
    Localization of gene functions in polyoma virus DNA.
    PNAS, 1976, 73, 4169.
9. Fluck, M. M., Staneloni, R. J. and Benjamin, T. L.   Hr-t
    and Ts-a: Two early gene functions of polyoma virus.
    Virology, 1977, 77, 610.
10. Fluck, M. and Benjamin, T. L.   Comparisons of two early
    gene functions essential for transformation in polyoma
    virus and SV40.   Virology, 1979, 96, 205.
11. Friedmann, T., Esty, A., LaPorte, P. and Deininger, P.
    The nucleotide sequence and genome organization of the
    polyoma early region: Extensive nucleotide and amino
    acid homology with SV40.   Cell, 1979, 17, 715.
12. Hattori, J., Carmichael, G. G. and Benjamin, T. L.   DNA
    sequence alterations in hr-t deletion mutants of polyoma
    virus.   Cell, 1978, 15, 485.
13. Hunter, T., Hutchinson, M., Eckhart, W., *et al.*

14. Ito, Y., Brocklehurst, J. R. and Dulbecco, R.   Virus
    specific proteins in the plasma membrane of cells lytic-
    ally infected or transformed by polyoma virus.   PNAS,
    1977b, 74, 4666.

15. Kamen, R., Favaloro, J., Parker, J., *et al.* Cold Spring
    Harbor Symp. Quant. Biol., 1979, *in press.*
16. Schaffhausen, B. S. and Benjamin, T. L. Deficiency in
    histone acetylation in non-transforming host range mutants
    of polyoma virus. PNAS, 1976, 73, 213.
17. Schaffhausen, B. S., Silver, J. and Benjanim, T. L. T
    antigen(s) in cells productively infected by wild type
    polyoma virus and mutant NG-18. PNAS, 1978, 75, 79.
18. Schaffhausen, B. S. and Benjamin, T. L. Phosphorylation
    of polyoma T antigens. Cell, 1979, 18, 935.
19. Schlegel, R. and Benjamin, T. Cellular Alterations de-
    pendent upon the polyoma virus Hr-t function: Separation
    of mitogenic from transforming capacities. Cell, 1978,
    14, 587.
20. Silver, J., Schaffhausen, B. and Benjamin, T. Tumor anti-
    gens induced by non-transforming mutants of polyoma virus.
    Cell, 1978, 15, 485.
21. Smith, A., Smith, R., Griffin, B. and Fried, M. Protein
    kinase activity associated with polyoma virus middle T
    antigen *in vitro.*
22. Soeda, E., Arrand, J. R., Smolar, N., Walsh, J. E. and
    Griffin, B. E. Coding potential and regulatory signals of
    the polyoma virus genome. Nature, 1980, 283, 445.
23. Staneloni, R. J., Fluck, M. M. and Benjamin, T. L. Host
    range selection of transformation defective "Hr-t" mutants
    of polyoma virus. Virology, 1977, 77, 598.

Transforming Genes of Retroviruses: Definition, Specificity and Relation to Cellular DNA[1,2]

PETER H. DUESBERG and KLAUS BISTER

Professor of Molecular Biology and Research Associate
Department of Molecular Biology and Virus Laboratory
University of California
Berkeley, California

ABSTRACT

The oncogenic properties of sarcoma, acute leukemia and lymphatic leukemia viruses are interpreted in terms of their genetic structures. Highly oncogenic sarcoma and acute leukemia viruses are shown to contain transforming onc genes which are different from the three virion genes gag, pol and env essential for replication. Biochemical and genetic approaches to define onc genes are discussed. The hallmark of retroviral onc genes is shown to be a specific RNA sequence, that is unrelated to essential virion genes. On this basis five different classes of onc genes can be distinguished in the avian tumor virus group alone: two of these, the onc genes of Rous sarcoma virus (RSV) and avian myeloblastosis virus (AMV) share one design. Their coding sequence is a specific RNA section which either replaces env [RSV(-), AMV] or maps adjacent to the 3' end of env (RSV). Expression of this class of onc genes is mediated via subgenomic mRNAs containing sequences from the 5' end of viral RNA spliced onto the onc gene coding sequences. The onc gene product of RSV has been identified as a 60,000 dalton phosphoprotein. Three other

[1]With minor variations this paper has been presented at three symposia during the summer of 1980: (1) Proceedings of the Third International Feline Leukemia Meeting, St. Thomas, Virgin Islands; (2) Modern Trends in Human Leukemia IV, Wilsede, Germany; (3) 1980 International Symposium on Cancer, New York.

[2]We thank L. Evans, M. Nunn and G. S. Martin for a critical review of the manuscript and D. Baltimore, J. M. Bishop and M. Essex for communicating results prior to publication. Supported by U.S. Public Health Grant CA 11426.

classes of onc genes, namely those of the myelocytomatosis
(MC29) subgroup of viruses, avian erythroblastosis virus (AEV)
and Fujinami sarcoma virus (FSV) share another design. Their
coding sequences are hybrids consisting of specific as well
as of gag or gag and pol gene-related elements. The products
of these onc genes, translated from full size genomic RNA,
are hybrid proteins carrying gag or gag and pol determinants
in addition to specific sequences. They are phosphorylated
and range in size from 75,000 to 200,000 daltons. Since viruses with totally different onc genes can cause the same
disease (namely RSV, FSV, AEV, and MC29 cause sarcoma and AEV,
AMV or E26 and MC29 cause erythroblastosis) it is concluded
that multiple mechanisms, involving multiple cellular targets,
exist for sarcomagenic and leukemic transformation of the
avian cell. Comparisons between viral onc genes and onc-re-
lated chromosomal DNA sequences of the cell reveal qualitative differences. Hence viral onc genes are not simply transduced cellular genes and cellular sequences related to viral
onc genes appear not directly relevant to cancer. It follows
that viral onc genes are unique and more than the sum of their
parts related to cellular DNA and to replicative genes of
retroviruses. We speculate that onc genes also may play a
role indirectly in cancers caused by lymphatic leukemia viruses although these viruses are not known to contain such
genes. (End of Abstract)

 Retroviruses cause sarcomas, carcinomas, acute and lymphatic leukemias or no disease in animals (Gross, 1970; Beard et
al., 1973; Tooze, 1973; Levy, 1978; Jarrett, 1978; Duesberg,
1980; Essex, 1980). Table 1 shows schematically the pathology of representative retroviruses of the avian, murine and
feline tumor virus groups. The avian, murine and feline sarcoma viruses predominantly cause sarcomas and transform fibroblasts in culture. The Harvey (Ha), Kirsten (Ki) and Moloney (Mo) murine sarcoma viruses (MuSV) and rarely avian
Rous sarcoma virus (RSV) also cause erythroid leukemia (Gross,
1970; Scher et al., 1975; Ostertag et al., 1980; Duesberg,
1980). This has not been observed with avian Fujinami virus
(FSV) (Lee et al., 1980). Feline sarcoma virus (FeSV), in
addition to sarcomas, also causes melanocarcinomas (McCullough et al., 1972; Chen et al., 1980). The avian acute leukemia viruses of the MC29 subgroup and erythroblastosis virus
(AEV) that transform fibroblasts [therefore termed class I
(Duesberg, 1980)] and haematopoietic cells in culture have
broad oncogenic spectra including sarcomas and carcinomas in
addition to acute leukemias in the animal (Purchase and Burmester, 1972; Beard, 1973; Graf and Beug, 1978). However,
the fibroblast-transforming murine Abelson leukemia virus has

TABLE 1
Oncogenic Properties of Retroviruses

| Viruses | Tumors in Animals | | | | Transformation in Culture | |
	Sarcoma	Carcinoma	Acute	Lymphatic	Fibro-blast	blood cell
				Leukemia		
Sarcoma viruses RSV,RSV(-) FSV Mo-MuSV Ki-Ha-MuSV FeSV	+	-/+[a]	+[b]	-/+[c]	+	?
Acute leukemia class I Avian MC29 subgroup: MC29,MH2,CMII,OK10 AEV Abelson MuLV	+[d]	+[d]	+	-/+[c]	+	+
Acute leukemia class II AMV, E26	-[e]	-[e]	+	+	-	+
Lymphatic leukemia Avian leukosis and Rous-associated viruses, tdRSV,RAV(0) MuLV FeLV	-[f]	-[f]	-	+/-	-	-

[a] Liver and kidney metastases have been reported for RSV (Gross, 1970; Purchase and Burmester, 1972). FeSV has been shown to cause melanocarcinomas (McCullough et al., 1972; Chen et al., 1980).

[b] Observed among other non-tumorous diseases with Harvey, Kirsten and Moloney MuSV (see text) (Scher et al., 1975; Ostertag et al., 1980) and rarely with RSV (Gross, 1970; Purchase and Burmester, 1972).

[c] Possibly due to helper virus (Gross, 1970; Purchase and Burmester, 1972; Graf and Beug, 1978).

[d] Not observed with Abelson virus (Rosenberg and Baltimore, 1980).

[e] Some (Beard, 1973; Purchase and Burmester, 1972), but not all (Moscovici, 1975), stocks of AMV have caused carcinomas or sarcomas, perhaps due to other viral or non-viral components.

[f] Lymphatic leukemia viruses have been described to cause sarcomas and carcinomas at low frequency and after long, latent periods (Gross, 1970; Purchase and Burmester, 1972). However, sarcoma- or carcinoma-causing variants have not been isolated.

not been reported to cause sarcomas and carcinomas (Rosenberg and Baltimore, 1980). By contrast the avian acute leukemia viruses AMV and E26, that do not transform fibroblasts
in culture [therefore termed class II (Duesberg, 1980)] have
rather specific oncogenic spectra in the animal, where they
cause myeloid and erythroid leukemias (Beard et al., 1973;
Moscovici, 1975; Graf and Beug, 1978). The viruses listed
thus far have in common that they transform fast, within 1-2
weeks and that transformation is an inevitable consequence of
infection in susceptible animals. This implies that transforming onc genes are integral parts of the genomes of these
viruses.

This appears not to be true for the majority of naturally
occurring retroviruses, the lymphatic leukemia viruses. These
are rather ubiquitous, nondefective viruses, that often cause
viremias but rarely and in particular not simultaneously,
leukemias (Gross, 1970; Tooze, 1973) as for example in chickens (Rubin et al., 1962; Weyl and Dougherty, 1977), mice
(Gardner et al., 1976; Levy, 1978; Cloyd et al., 1980) or cats
(Jarrett, 1978; Essex, 1980). The transformation-defective
(td), src-deletion mutants of RSV have the same biological
(Biggs et al., 1972) and genetic properties (Wang et al.,
1976) as the lymphatic leukemia viruses (Fig. 1). The RNA
genome of these viruses contains all three essential virion
genes in the following 5' to 3' order: gag (for internal
virion proteins or group-specific antigens), pol (for RNA dependent DNA polymerase) and env (for envelope glycoprotein)
and a 3' terminal c-region. The c-region has regulatory functions in the reverse transcription of viral RNA and in the
transcription of proviral DNA (Fig. 1) (Wang et al., 1975;
Wang, 1978; Tsichlis and Coffin, 1980). The endogenous, nondefective (containing all three virion genes) retroviruses of
chicken, such as RAV(0) (Tooze, 1973), and of mice, such as
xenotropic viruses (Levy, 1978; Cloyd et al., 1980) are inherited according to Mendelian genetics. These viruses probably never cause a disease directly and appear to differ from
the more pathogenic lymphatic leukemia viruses in minor genetic elements, including the c-region that influences virus expression (Tsichlis and Coffin, 1980; Lung et al., 1980; Cloyd
et al., 1980). Since transformation is not, or only rarely,
a consequence of replication by any of these viruses and only
occurs after considerable latent periods, these viruses may
not contain authentic onc genes.

In the following we will describe the definition of onc
genes of the rapidly transforming sarcoma and acute leukemia
viruses. On this basis we will then ask whether the oncogen-
genic specificity of some and the lack of specificity by other
viruses is due to distinct onc genes or whether one onc gene

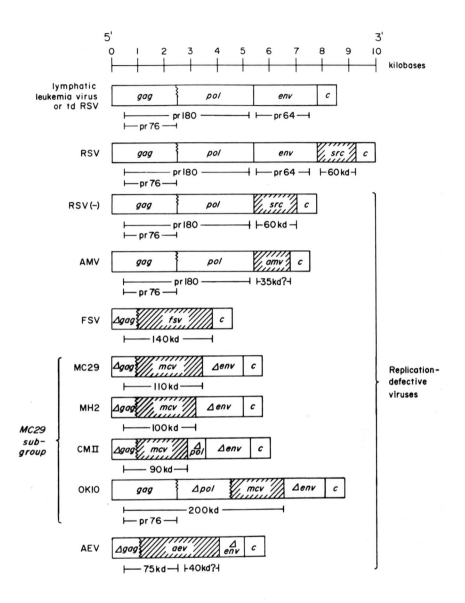

Figure 1. Genetic structures of viruses of the avian tumor virus group: White boxes indicate map locations and complexities in kilobases of complete or partial (Δ) complements of the three essential virion genes gag, pol and env and of the non-coding c region at the 3' end of viral RNAs. Hatched

115

can cause multiple forms of cancer. In addition, we review
the question of the relationship between viral onc genes and
cellular DNA. Finally, the question is addressed of how lymphatic leukemia viruses, which lack known onc genes, may
cause cancer. The focus will be on avian tumor viruses, because their genetic structures are better defined than those
of other viruses. This review extends two previous ones published recently (Duesberg, 1980; Bister and Duesberg, 1980).

Definition of onc Genes

src, the onc gene of RSV. The only onc gene of retroviruses for which nearly complete genetic and biochemical definitions are available is the src gene of RSV. In 1970 the src
gene was formally distinguished from the three essential virion genes of nondefective RSV by the isolation of a mutant
that was temperature-sensitive only in transformation but not
in virus replication (Martin, 1970) and by the isolation of
non-conditional src-deletion mutants (Duesberg and Vogt, 1970;
Martin and Duesberg, 1972). These transformation-defective
src deletion mutants retain all virion genes and are physic-
ally and serologically like wild type RSV (Fig. 1) (Wang et
al., 1975; Wang, 1978). However the RNA of the wild type
measures 10 kb (kilobases) whereas that of the tdRSV measures
only 8.5 kb (Fig. 1) (Duesberg and Vogt, 1970, 1973; Beemon
et al., 1974; Wang, 1978). On the basis of this difference
src gene-specific RNA sequences were first defined by sub-
tracting from the 10 kb RNA of RSV with the genetic structure
5' gag-pol-env-src-c 3', the 8.5 kb RNA of the isogenic src
deletion mutant tdRSV with the genetic structure 5' gag-pol-
env-c 3' (Fig. 1) (Lai et al., 1973). The 1.5 kb that set
apart the wild type RSV from the src-deletion mutant were
shown to be a contiguous sequence that mapped near the 3' end
of viral RNA (Wang et al., 1975).

The src gene was independently defined by recombination

---

*boxes indicate location and complexities of specific sequence
elements which are unrelated to essential virion genes, and
which define five distinct RNA subgroups within the avian tumor virus group. These specific sequences represent all (src,
amv) or part (fsv, mcv, aev) of the coding sequences of the
five different onc genes associated with avian tumor viruses.
Undulated lines indicate that translation crosses and half-
undulated lines that translation may cross borders between
RNA sequence elements of different genetic origin. Lines under the boxes symbolize the complexities in kilodaltons of
the protein products encoded by the respective RNA sequences.*

analysis in which a <u>src</u>-deletion mutant with variant virion genes (5' <u>gag</u>'-<u>pol</u>'-<u>env</u>'-<u>c</u> 3') was allowed to recombine with a nondefective RSV. All sarcomagenic recombinants with variant virion genes had the genetic structure 5' <u>gag</u>'-<u>pol</u>'-<u>env</u>'-<u>src</u>-c 3') and hence had inherited the <u>src</u> gene (Beemon et al., 1974; Wang et al., 1976; Wang, 1978) (see also Fig. 1). It followed that the 1.5 kb sequence of RSV-specific RNA was necessary for transformation.

A first step towards proving that the 1.5 kb <u>src</u>-specific RNA sequence is possibly sufficient for transformation at least in terms of its coding capacity was taken when a 60 kilodalton (kd) protein product was identified in RSV-transformed cells (Brugge and Erikson, 1977) that was serologically unrelated to the <u>gag</u>, <u>pol</u> and <u>env</u> virion proteins. Since the genetic complexity of the 1.5 kb RSV-specific RNA sequence and of the 60 kd <u>src</u> protein are about the same, the 1.5 kb RNA must encode most or all of the protein (Fig. 1). The same <u>src</u>-specific sequence has also been identified in a <u>env</u>-deletion mutant of RSV, termed RSV(-) (Table 1, Fig. 1) (Wang et al., 1976a) and recently also in a <u>gag</u>, <u>pol</u> and <u>env</u>-defective sarcomagenic deletion mutant of RSV (Martin et al., 1980). Transformation by the <u>gag</u>, <u>pol</u> and <u>env</u>-defective RSV is definitive proof that the <u>src</u> gene (but not the <u>src</u>-specific RNA sequence alone) is sufficient for transformation. The fact that expression of the <u>src</u> gene of RSV involves a mRNA which also includes sequences derived from the 5' and 3' ends of virion RNA, that are shared with <u>src</u>-deletions of RSV (Mellon and Duesberg, 1977) first indicated that <u>src</u>-specific RNA may not be sufficient for transformation. It would appear then that the <u>src</u>-specific sequence of RSV defined by deletion and recombination analysis represents most or all of the coding sequences of <u>src</u> but that it does not act independently and is by itself not sufficient for transformation (see below).

Since the definition of the <u>src</u> gene of RSV, most other acutely transforming retroviruses have been shown to contain specific sequences, unrelated to essential virion genes. Such sequences appear to be the hallmark of highly oncogenic viruses and they represent most or at least part of their <u>onc</u> genes (see below). To date the oncogenic retroviruses are the only class of viruses which have <u>onc</u> genes that are non-essential for virus replication. The only known function of these genes is their oncogenicity.

Identification of the Genome and Definition of the onc Genes of Replication-Defective Oncogenic Viruses (a-e):

The definition of the <u>onc</u> genes of highly oncogenic viruses other than RSV is less advanced than that of <u>src</u>. This is because, with the exception of RSV, all other highly oncogenic retroviruses lack essential virion genes and consequently are replication-defective. The genetic phenotype of most defective sarcoma and acute leukemia viruses is: gag^-, pol^-, env^-, onc^+ (Fig. 1) (Tooze, 1973; Bister and Vogt, 1978; Graf and Beug, 1978). Due to this phenotype classical deletion and recombination analysis cannot be used to define onc genes, as was the case with src. An onc deletion of such a virus (i.e. gag^-, pol^-, env^-, onc^-) would obviously be undetectable by classical techniques measuring viral gene expression. Likewise would the lack of secondary markers complicate or prevent recombination analysis of onc genes of defective viruses.

(a) Genome identification. Defectiveness also complicates identification of the viral RNA genomes. The genome of a nondefective retrovirus is essentially identified by extracting the RNA from purified virus. Since the defective virus only replicates if complemented by a nondefective helper virus, usually a lymphatic leukemia virus, it is obtained as a complex containing defective as well as helper viral RNAs. Moreover, the two RNAs are replicated at unpredictable ratios, usually favoring the RNA of nondefective helper virus. The RNA of defective and helper virus were first separated by electrophoretic analysis of viral RNAs, which typically yields one larger RNA species measuring 8 to 9 kb and a smaller one measuring 4 to 7 kb (Maisel et al., 1973; Duesberg et al., 1977). By its absence from nondefective helper viruses, the small RNA species was shown to be necessary for transformation (Maisel et al., 1973; Duesberg et al., 1977). Subsequent biochemical analyses directly identified the smaller RNA species, consistent with its low complexity, as the genome of the defective virus (Duesberg, 1980; Bister and Duesberg, 1980). The larger RNA species was shown to be the RNA of nondefective helper virus, whose size is invariably 8 to 9 kb as dictated by the requirement for complete gag, pol and env genes in nondefective helper viruses (see Fig. 1 for examples).

(b) Defining transformation-specific nucleotide sequences by subtraction from the RNA of defective transforming virus sequences shared with nondefective helper viruses. Given the RNA of defective transforming virus, it can be asked whether a sequence unrelated to essential virion genes is present. Moreover in the avian system it can be asked whether this sequence is related to the genetically defined src. Experimentally this is accomplished by comparing the RNAs (or proviral DNAs) of defective and helper virus by various nucleic acid scopes including hybridization of defective viral RNA with cDNA of helper viruses, comparative fingerprinting of RNase T_1-oligonucleotides or comparison of proviral DNA fragments generated by a given restriction enzyme. By these methods two classes of sequences are distinguished in the RNAs of defective transforming viruses: helper virus-related and specific sequences (Duesberg, 1980). In all cases examined the specific sequences form contiguous internal map segments which are flanked by helper virus-related terminal map segments (Fig. 1) (Mellon et al., 1978; Bister and Duesberg, 1980; Duesberg, 1980).

Although biochemical subtraction of helper virus-related sequences from the RNA of a defective, transforming virus is formally analogous to deletion analysis, the subtracted (shared) RNA is not the genome of a viable deletion mutant (cf. Fig. 1). Therefore, it can only be inferred but cannot be deduced from this type of analysis, that the resulting specific sequence of the defective oncogenic virus (hatched in Fig. 1) is necessary for transformation.

(c) Genetic evidence that specific and gag-related RNA sequences of avian class I acute leukemia and Fujinami sarcoma viruses are necessary for oncogenicity. Genetic evidence was used to determine whether the specific sequences of defective transforming viruses are necessary for transformation. Since due to the absence of selective markers other than onc, suitable recombinants have not as yet been prepared in the laboratory, different isolates of closely and distantly related avian acute leukemia viruses were used as substitutes of recombinants. The RNAs of these viral isolates were compared to each other by electrophoretic size analyses, by hybridization with cDNAs of various avian tumor viruses, and by mapping RNase T_1-resistant oligonucleotides (Duesberg et al., 1977; Bister et al., 1979; Roussel et al., 1979; Duesberg et al., 1979; Bister et al., 1980a; Bister and Duesberg, 1979, 1980).

Such comparisons show that four different isolates of avian acute leukemia viruses, whose oncogenic spectra are closely related (Table 1) (Beard et al., 1973; Graf and Beug, 1978) namely MC29, MH2, CMII and OK10 also have closely related genetic structures (Fig. 1). The hallmark of each viral RNA is an internal, helper virus-unrelated sequence of about 2 kb (Duesberg et al., 1977, 1979; Bister et al., 1979; Bister and Duesberg, 1980; Bister et al., 1980a; Roussel et al., 1979). Because the specific sequences of the four viruses are closely related and because the sequence was first identified in MC29 virus, it is termed here mcv. The mcv sequence is the structural basis for the classification of the four viruses into the MC29 subgroup of avian RNA tumor viruses (Bister et al., 1979; Bister and Duesberg, 1980; Bister et al., 1980a; Duesberg, 1980).

The size and the oligonucleotide composition of the mcv sequences appears to vary between approximately 1.8 and 2.2 kb in different viral strains (Fig. 1) (Duesberg et al., 1979; Bister et al., 1979; Bister et al., 1980a). Based on oligo-

nucleotide complexity the largest mcv sequence appears to be
that of MC29 virus and the smallest one either that of CMII
or of MH2 (Bister et al., 1980a). In MC29, CMII and MH2 the
mcv sequence is flanked at the 5' end by a partial (Δ) gag
gene, termed Δgag and in OK10 by a complete gag followed by a
Δpol (Fig. 1). It is not clear as yet whether the Δgag sequences of MC29, MH2 and CMII have the same complexities.

At the 3' end the mcv sequence of MC29 and OK10 is flanked
by a Δenv gene and that of CMII by Δpol (Fig. 1) [env sequences are present in MH2 RNA, but the RNA has not been analyzed
sufficiently to determine whether its mcv sequence borders at
Δenv (Fig. 1) (Duesberg and Vogt, 1979)].

These comparisons of the four MC29-subgroup viral RNAs
show that: (i) the 5' parts of their Δgag or gag sequences
and most, but not all, of their mcv sequences are highly conserved; (ii) their env-related sequences are related by hybridization but variable if compared at the level of shared
and specific T$_1$-oligonucleotides (Bister et al., 1979; Duesberg et al., 1979; Bister et al., 1980a) and (iii) they may
have optional sequences such as the 3' half of gag and the
Δpol at the 5' end of mcv in OK10, or the Δpol at the 3' end
of mcv in CMII (Fig. 1). There are probably optional parts
of the mcv sequence itself, because its size appears to vary
in different viral strains. It would follow that most of mcv
is an essential specific correlate and Δgag an essential, non-
specific (because it is shared with helper virus and other
defective viruses; Fig. 1) correlate of viral oncogenicity.

These genetic analyses are confirmed and extended if one
includes avian erythroblastosis virus (AEV) (Bister and Duesberg, 1979) and Fujinami sarcoma virus (FSV) (Lee et al.,
1980). Each of these viruses has a genetic structure similar
to the viruses of the MC29 subgroup, with a Δgag sequence at
the 5' end and internal specific sequences termed aev and fsv
which are unrelated to essential virion genes, to src, to mcv
and to each other (Fig. 1). Thus, these viruses form an analogous series of defective transforming viruses. It follows
that the internal, specific sequence of each of these viruses
is necessary, but probably not sufficient for transformation
since oncogenicity of each of these viruses also correlates
with a highly conserved Δgag. Hence the onc genes of these
viruses appear to be genetic units consisting of gag-related
and specific RNA sequences.

(d) Nonstructural, gag-related proteins define genetic
units of helper virus-related and specific RNA sequences in
class I avian acute leukemia and Fujinami sarcoma virus. Each
of the class I avian acute leukemia viruses as well as FSV
code for gag-related nonstructural phosphoproteins ranging in
size from 75 to 200 kd (Fig. 1) (Bister et al., 1977;

Bister et al., 1979; Hayman et al., 1979a, b; Bister and Duesberg, 1980; Lee et al., 1980; Ramsay and Hayman, 1980; Bister
et al., 1980b). That these proteins are coded for by gag-related as well as specific sequences of viral RNA was deduced
from in vitro translation of viral RNAs of known genetic
structure (Mellon et al., 1978; Lee et al., 1980) and from
peptide analyses of these proteins (Hayman et al., 1979a, b;
Kitchener and Hayman, 1980). This directly supports the view
that the specific sequences of these viruses are not independent genetic units (Fig. 1). They function together with at
least the 5' part of gag (or all of gag and part of pol in
OK10) as one genetic unit (Fig. 1) (Mellon et al., 1978; Bister and Duesberg, 1980; Lee et al., 1980; Bister et al.,
1980a). To indicate that translation crosses the border between gag-related or between gag-Δpol-related and specific
sequence elements these borders were drawn as undulated lines
in Fig. 1, also indicating that their exact location is uncertain. Given the very similar oncogenic spectra of these
viruses and assuming transforming function of these proteins,
we deduce that the size differences among the 90, 100, 110
and 200 kd gag-related proteins of CMII, MH2, MC29 and OK10
directly confirm the point made above, on the basis of RNA
analysis, that the Δgag/gag-Δpol-mcv units include optional
elements (see Fig. 1).

Moreover the structure of the genetic unit coding for the
200 kd protein of OK10 which contains a complete gag and a
mcv-sequence which replaces only a part of pol (Fig. 1) is of
particular interest regarding the role of gag-related sequences in these proteins. Based on analogy with pol gene expression by nondefective viruses which proceeds via a gag-pol
precursor protein (Fig. 1), the OK10 protein could also be
processed into a product that contains only Δpol and mcv.
The fact that such a protein is not found in infected cells
(Ramsay and Hayman, 1980) suggests again that the gag-related
portion is essential for the function of this protein. The
optional nature of the pol-sequence in OK10, already evident
from its lack in other MC29 subgroup proteins, is underscored
by the fact that it includes the pol sequences that map at the
3' end of mcv in CMII which are not part of the CMII protein
(Fig. 1) (Bister et al., 1979, 1980a). Because the genetic
units of the MC29 subgroup viruses, that read Δgag-mcv or
gag-Δpol-mcv share conserved 5' gag-elements and most of mcv,
but differ in optional, internal sequences, it has been proposed that these genes and their protein products have two essential domains, one consisting of the conserved gag-related,
the other of the conserved mcv-related sequences (Bister et
al., 1980a).

Since the known proteins coded for by the class I acute

leukemia viruses do not account for genetic information of the
3' half of the viral RNAs it cannot be excluded that 3' terminal sequences are also necessary for transformation. Nevertheless the variability of the 3' terminal sequences, both in
terms of oligonucleotide composition and in relationship to
env and pol genes (Fig. 1) as well as the lack of evidence for
protein products synthesized in infected cells argue that
these sequences may not be translated. It was hypothesized
therefore that these sequences may not play a direct role in
transformation (Duesberg et al., 1979; Bister et al., 1980a;
Bister and Duesberg, 1980).

By contrast all genetic information of Fujinami sarcoma virus, which has a genetic structure that is similar to that of
class I acute leukemia viruses (Fig. 1), can be accounted for
in terms of one known viral protein. Moreover, if one assumes
that transformation requires a viral protein and that the viral RNA is translated in only one reading frame, one may argue that in the case of FSV the Δgag-fsv sequence is not only
necessary but also sufficient for transformation, since the
genetic complexities of the 4.5 kb FSV RNA and of the 140 kd
protein encoded by Δgag-fsv are about the same (Fig. 1).

(e) The onc gene of avian myeloblastosis (AMV) and E26
virus, avian acute leukemia viruses of class II. AMV and E26
are acute leukemia viruses which fail to transform fibroblasts
and cause no sarcomas and possibly no carcinomas, signaling a
unique class of onc genes (Beard et al., 1973; Moscovici,
1975; Graf and Beug, 1978). Until recently the analysis of
AMV and related viruses has been slow, because infectious virus typically contains a large excess of nondefective helper
virus. This has been changed by the discovery of defective
AMV particles which are relased by AMV-transformed, nonproducer myeloblasts. Such particles contain a 7.5 kb viral RNA
and are infectious if fused into susceptible cells together
with helper virus (Duesberg et al., 1980). Consistent with
the ability of AMV to produce defective virus particles, the
RNA was found to contain a complete gag and pol gene and non-
producer cells contain 76 kd gag and 180 kd gag-pol precursor
proteins (Fig. 1). However there is no evidence for gag- or
gag and pol-related nonstructural proteins in AMV-transformed
cells (Duesberg et al., 1980). Between pol and a unique 3'
terminal c-region AMV contains a specific amv sequence of
about 1.5 kb that is unrelated to those of any other acutely
transforming avian tumor virus except E26 (Fig. 1) (Duesberg
et al., 1980). It appears that the genetic structure of AMV
resembles closely that of RSV(-) (Fig. 1). From this genetic
structure it may be expected (see below) that the amv sequence
codes possibly for a specific protein unrelated to gag and pol
genes, by a mRNA similar to that coding for the src protein

of RSV (Mellon and Duesberg, 1977). It would be expected
that this protein has transforming function. Preliminary evidence indicates that a 35 kd protein is translated in vitro
from AMV RNA (Fig. 1) (Lee and Duesberg, unpublished).

Two Distinct onc Gene-Designs
     The onc genes described here have -- as far as defined --
two different designs: those with a coding sequence that is
specific and unrelated to essential virion genes, examples
being the src gene of RSV and possibly the onc gene of AMV,
and those with a coding sequence that is a hybrid of genetic
elements derived from essential virion genes and specific sequences, examples being the onc genes of MC29, AEV, and FSV.
The specific sequences of the hybrid onc genes are all inserted at their 5' ends adjacent to partially deleted gag or pol
genes (Fig. 1). By contrast the specific sequences of the
onc genes, whose coding sequences lack genetic elements of essential virion genes either replace env genes [RSV(-), AMV] or
are inserted between env and the c-region (RSV) (Fig. 1). For
convenient reference one design is referred to as RSV-design
and the other as MC29-design of onc genes according to their
best studied prototypes.
     The two onc gene designs also differ in their mechanism of
gene expression: the hybrid onc genes, whose specific sequences replace gag or pol genetic elements are probably translated from genomic viral RNA into gag- or gag and pol-related
proteins, like the pr76 gag or pr180 gag-pol proteins of non-
transforming viruses that they replace (Fig. 1). However,
there is no evidence that the hybrid gene products are subsequently processed. By contrast the src gene of RSV and probably the amv sequence of AMV, which replace env or are inserted downstream of env, are translated from subgenomic mRNAs
like the env genes of nontransforming viruses (Fig. 1) (Mellon and Duesberg, 1977; Hayward, 1977; Duesberg et al., 1980;
Lee and Duesberg, unpublished; Gonda and Bishop, personal
communication). Hence the mechanism of gene expression of the
two different onc designs closely follows that of the 5' most
virion gene that they partially or completely replace (Fig. 1).
     To determine whether the gag-related elements of the hybrid
onc genes are indeed essential for the probable transforming
function of their proteins, as our analyses suggest, it would
be necessary to find transforming viruses in which the specific sequences of hybrid onc genes are not linked to gag or
pol sequences. Conversely it would be interesting to know
whether src or the amv sequence would have transforming function if inserted into gag or pol genes.
     It is thought that the 60 kd src gene product functions
catalytically, probably as a phosphokinase (Erikson et al.,

1980; Bishop et al., 1980), although there is evidence that
kinase activity may not be the only function of the src gene
product (Rubsamen et al., 1980; Bishop et al., 1980).

By contrast the function of the gag-related proteins of
avian acute leukemia and Fujinami sarcoma viruses, of the
Abelson MuLV and of the feline sarcoma viruses may not be
solely catalytic. Although, again, a kinase activity appears
as a candidate for a catalytic function of these proteins,
this has not been demonstrated in each of these proteins. It
appears associated with the gag-related proteins of some
strains of Abelson virus (Witte et al., 1980) and, with some
uncertainty, also with the proteins of the Gardner and Snyder-
Theilen strains of feline sarcoma virus (Reynolds et al.,
1980), but has not been found in the avian viruses with onc
genes of MC29-design (Bister et al., 1980b) and in the McDonough strain of feline sarcoma virus (Van de Ven et al., 1980).
It is possible that these onc gene products have, in addition
to a possible catalytic function, a structural function involving their gag-related elements. Analogous to the function
of virion gag proteins, the gag portions of the nonstructural
proteins of these viruses may function by binding to specific
cellular and also to intracellular viral nucleic acid sequences. This specific binding may represent a regulatory function of a cellular catalytic activity or perhaps of a yet to
be discovered catalytic activity of the gag-related proteins.
This function would then correspond to one of the two domains
diagnosed in the proteins of the MC29 subgroup viruses, described above.

The consistent difficulties in isolating temperature-sensitive onc mutants of these viruses, that respond fast to
temperature shifts (unpublished experiments and personal com-
muncations), support the view that onc genes of the MC29-de-
sign may have a structural function.

Multiple onc Genes: Multiple Mechanisms and Multiple Targets of Transformation

Despite some insufficiencies in the definition of onc
genes of defective viruses, it is clear that multiple, at
least five different classes of specific sequences (src, mcv,
aev, fsv, and amv) and hence probably five different onc genes
exist in the avian tumor virus group alone. The number will
increase if other viruses are analyzed and if viruses of other
taxonomic groups are included. Some of these onc genes cause
specific cancers in the animal: for example, RSV and FSV
which cause predominantly sarcomas and AMV and E26 which cause
specifically leukemias affecting myeloid or erythroid precursor cells or more primitive stem cells depending on the host
(chicken or quail; Moscovici and Loliger, personal communica-

tion). Other onc genes, like those of MC29 and AEV may, in
addition to acute leukemias, cause sarcomas and carcinomas
(Table 1).

The fact that different onc genes vary in specificity yet
may cause the same cancer argues against a unique mechanism
to transform a given class of differentiated cells. For example RSV, FSV, MC29, AEV [and even Kirsten MuSV (Galehouse
and Duesberg, 1976)] all may cause sarcomas in birds and can
also transform mammalian fibroblasts (not tested for FSV)
(Quade, 1979) although they contain totally different onc
genes. Likewise, AEV, MC29 and E26 and AMV may cause erythroblastosis (Table 1) (Beard et al., 1973; Graf and Beug, 1978)
although their onc genes except for those of AMV and E26
(Duesberg et al., 1980) are different. It is concluded that
multiple mechanisms, involving multiple onc genes and onc
gene products and presumably multiple cellular targets, exist
for sarcomagenic and leukemogenic transformation. The fact
that different onc genes cause the same cancers or that one
onc gene may cause multiple cancers argues against the hypothesis that the transforming proteins of these viruses closely resemble specific cellular differentiation proteins and
that transformation is a consequence of a competition between
a specific viral transforming protein and a specific, related
cellular counterpart (Graf et al., 1980).

The overlap among the oncogenic spectra of different onc
genes suggests that different onc genes either interact with
different specific cellular targets or that onc genes interact with nonspecific targets. A unique target for a given
form of cancer would fail to explain why different onc genes
may cause the same disease and why in some cases one onc gene
may cause different cancers. The nature of cellular targets
for viral transformation remains to be elucidated; it is believed to include factors determining susceptibility to virus
infection and replication as well as intracellular substances
that interact directly with viral transforming proteins.

On the Relationship Between Viral onc Genes and Cellular
Chromosomal Sequences

The helper virus-unrelated, specific sequences of acutely
transforming avian, murine and feline viruses have been shown
to have closely related cellular counterparts (Scolnick et
al., 1973, 1975; Tsuchida et al., 1974; Frankel et al., 1979;
Sheiness and Bishop, 1979; Hughes et al., 1979a, b; Souza et
al., 1980; Oskarsson et al., 1980). This has lent support to
the hypothesis that normal cells contain viral onc genes and
that viral onc genes are transduced cellular genes (Huebner
and Todaro, 1969; Stephenson et al., 1979; Bishop et al.,
1980). If correct, this hypothesis would predict that, para-

doxically, normal cells contain a number of viral or cellular
onc genes that apparently are not subject to negative selection. (At present this number is around a dozen and is going
up as more onc genes are defined.) Thus normalcy would be an
admirable effort of cellular suppression of endogenous onc
genes. Although their cellular relatives are even less well
defined than most viral onc genes themselves, enough is known
about them to deduce that viral onc genes are not in the cell
but that some or most of their coding sequences have related
counterparts in cellular DNA.

(i) One example is src of RSV: The only form in which the
specific sequence of RSV has ever been shown to have transforming function is if it is part of the viral src gene. As
such this sequence is expressed via a mRNA that shares 5'
leader and 3' terminal c-region sequences with other virion
genes (Mellon and Duesberg, 1977). These virion sequences are
not found in all vertebrates said to contain src-related sequences (Spector et al., 1978a) except in some strains of
chicken. However in chicken, src-related and endogenous virion gene-related sequences are not located on the same restriction fragments of cellular DNA (Hughes, 1979b) nor on the
same chromosomes (Hughes, 1979a). Moreover, the cellular src-
related mRNA and DNA sequences appear not to be colinear with
those of RSVs (Wang et al., 1977; Spector et al., 1978b; Hughes
et al., 1979b). Hence concrete qualitative differences set
apart the src of RSV and its relatives in normal vertebrate
cells.

(ii) Another example of a close relationship between a viral onc gene and cellular alleles is the case of MuSV: Most
of the helper virus-unrelated 1.5 kb sequence of MuSV has a
closely related, perhaps identical counterpart in the cell
(Oskarsson et al., 1980; Blair et al., 1980). However, molec-
ularly cloned "MuSV-specific" DNA from the cell or from MuSV
can only transform cultured mouse fibroblasts if it is first
linked with (presumably noncoding) terminal sequences from
MuSV or helper MuLV. Again concrete qualitative differences
exist between the onc gene of MuSV and related DNA sequences
of the cell. Moreover transformation by these modified MuSV-
related sequences from the cell is abortive and no infectious
virus is recovered. Thus transformation by this kind of DNA
and by infectious virus may prove not to be the same, although
they appear indistinguishable based on the fibroblast assay.

(iii) The transforming genes of viruses which appear to be
hybrids of structural and nonstructural viral genetic elements
provide even more convincing evidence that viral onc genes and
their cellular relatives are not the same thing: Although it
has been shown that most but not all vertebrate cells contain
sequences related to the helper virus-unrelated part of MC29

and AEV, the helper virus-related, in particular, gag-related
elements of these viruses do not have the same distribution
and are not found in the same cells (Sheiness and Bishop,
1979; Roussell et al., 1979). Hence gag-related sequences,
thought to be an essential element of the onc genes of MC29
and AEV are not part of the cellular sequences related to
those genes. Moreover, the cellular sequences related to the
3 kb AEV-specific RNA sequence have recently been shown to be
distributed over a 15 kb-DNA segment that includes AEV-relat-
ed and AEV-unrelated sequences (J. M. Bishop, personal communication). Likewise has the cellular DNA sequence, related
to the Abelson murine leukemia virus-specific RNA sequence of
3 kb (Shields et al., 1979) been shown to be distributed over
a 12 kb DNA segment that must include Abelson virus-unrelated
sequences (D. Baltimore, personal communication). Hence in
these cases proviral DNA and related cellular DNA sequences
are not colinear. It follows that the genetic units of class
I acute leukemia viruses, that consist of gag-related and
specific RNA sequences (Fig. 1), have no known counterparts in
normal cells.

It is concluded that viral onc genes of the RSV- and in
particular those of the MC29-design are different from related sequences present in the cell. The onc genes of the RSV-
design, like src, and possibly amv (Fig. 1) may share most,
but possibly not all their coding sequences with cellular
homologs but differ from cellular relatives in essential regulatory elements. The onc genes of the MC29-design differ
from cellular counterparts in coding (gag and pol-related sequences) as well as regulatory elements. Consequently the
cellular relatives of most viral onc genes are probably not
present in the cell as functional onc genes as has been postulated (Huebner and Todaro, 1979; Bishop et al., 1980) and
hence are probably not directly relevant to transformation.

Instead these cellular sequences may be relevant to the
archaeology of viral onc genes. Viral onc genes probably
have been generated by rare transductions of cellular sequences by nondefective viruses. To generate onc genes of the
RSV-design transduction must have involved illegitimate recombination with nondefective virus. In the case of Moloney
MuSV, specific deletions of the parental nondefective virus
also had to occur (Dina et al., 1976; Donoghue et al., 1979;
Chien et al., 1979; Blair et al., 1980). Until the cellular
src-related sequence is characterized directly, it remains
unclear whether in the case of RSV the coding sequence of src
was transduced unchanged or after alteration when RSV was
generated.

Both transduction involving again illegitimate recombination , as well as specific deletions of virion genes (see

Fig. 1), must have been necessary to generate the onc genes
of the MC29-design from cellular and viral genetic elements.
Such events are much less likely to occur than for example
the transduction by phage lambda of a functional galactosidase
gene. It is noted that experimental evidence for the transduction of cellular sequences has led to the hypothesis that
viral transformation is the product of enhancing the dosage
of endogenous cellular onc genes by homologous equivalents
from exogenous viruses (Bishop et al., 1980). We submit that
sequence transduction is not synonymous with the transduction
of unaltered gene function which would be a necessary corollary of the gene dosage hypothesis. It would appear that viral onc genes are unique and more than the sum of their parts
related to cellular DNA and replicative genes of retroviruses.

The Role of onc Genes in Carcinogenesis

Highly oncogenic viruses, with onc genes such as those
described here, have only been isolated in relatively few
cases from animal tumors (reviewed in Gross, 1970; Tooze,
1973; Duesberg, 1980). By contrast leukosis and lymphatic
leukemia viruses have been isolated from many viral cancers
in particular from leukemias (see above) (Gross, 1970; Tooze,
1973). Thus paradoxically the lymphatic leukemia viruses
which lack known onc genes appear to be more relevant to viral carcinogenesis than retroviruses with known onc genes.

However it has been argued that onc genes also play a role
in carcinogenesis caused by lymphatic leukemia viruses (Duesberg, 1980). These onc genes may derive from endogenous, defective retrovirus-like RNAs known to exist in some normal
cells (Duesberg and Scolnick, 1977; Scolnick et al., 1979) or
from cellular genes acquired by processes involving illegitimate recombination and specific deletions (compare genetic
structures shown in Fig. 1). The necessity for such a secondary event to occur would explain the poor correlation between the distribution of lymphatic leukemia viruses and cancers in animals (see above). The failure to find onc genes
in most retroviral cancers may then reflect technical difficulties. These include the lack of suitable probes to detect
viral RNA as the only characteristic viral structural component, or nonstructural proteins as the only characteristic
products of defective transforming viruses. Moreover detection of a putative, defective transforming virus will be complicated by the fact that the ratio of defective transforming
to nondefective helper virus is low in typical stocks of de-
fective-helper virus complexes (Duesberg et al., 1977; Bister
and Duesberg, 1979; Duesberg et al., 1979; Lee et al., 1980).
Thus the analysis of viral onc genes may prove to be less academic than it appears at present -- it may provide the tools
and concepts necessary to understand all retroviral cancers.

REFERENCES

1. Beard, J. W., Langlois, A. J., & Beard, D. Etiological
    strain specificities of the avian tumor virus. In R. M.
    Dutcher and L. Chieco-Bianchi (Ed.), Unifying concepts of
    leukemia, Bibl. Haemat. 39. Basel: Karger, 1973, 31-44.
2. Beemon, K., Duesberg, P. H., & Vogt, P. K. Evidence for
    crossing over between avian tumor viruses based on analy-
    sis of viral RNAs. Proc. Nat. Acad. Sci., 1974, 71, 4254-
    4258.
3. Biggs, P. M., Milne, B. S., Graf, T., & Bauer, H. Oncogen-
    icity of nontransforming mutants of avian sarcoma virus.
    J. Gen. Virol., 1972, 18, 399-403.
4. Bishop, J. M., Courtneidge, S. A., Levinson, A. D., Op-
    permann, H., Quintrell, N., Sheiness, D. K., Weiss, S. R.,
    & Varmus, H. E. The origin and function of avian retrovi-
    rus transforming genes. Cold Spring Harbor Symp. Quant.
    Biol., 1980, 44, 919-930.
5. Bister, K., Hayman, M. J., & Vogt, P. K. Defectiveness of
    avian myelocytomatosis virus MC29: Isolation of long-term
    nonproducer cultures and analysis of virus-specific poly-
    peptide synthesis, Virology, 1977, 82, 431-448.
6. Bister, K., & Vogt, P. K. Genetic analysis of the defec-
    tiveness in strain MC29 avian leukosis virus. Virology,
    1978, 88, 213-221.
7. Bister, K., & Duesberg, P. H. Structure and specific se-
    quences of avian erythroblastosis virus RNA: Evidence for
    multiple classes of transforming genes among avian tumor
    viruses. Proc. Nat. Acad. Sci., 1979, 76, 5023-5027.
8. Bister, K., Löliger, H.-C., & Duesberg, P. H. Oligoribo-
    nucleotide map and protein of CMII: Detection of con-
    served and nonconserved genetic elements in avian acute
    leukemia viruses CMII, MC29 and MH2. J. Virol., 1979, 32,
    208-219.
9. Bister, K., & Duesberg, P. H. Genetic structure of avian
    acute leukemia viruses. Cold Spring Harbor Symp. Quant.
    Biol., 1980, 44, 801-822.
10. Bister, K., Ramsay, G., Hayman, M. J., & Duesberg, P. H.
    OK10, an avian acute leukemia virus of the MC29 subgroup
    with a unique genetic structure. Proc. Nat. Acad. Sci.,
    1980a, in press.
11. Bister, K., Lee, W.-H., & Duesberg, P. H. Phosphorylation
    of the nonstructural proteins encoded by three avian
    acute leukemia viruses and by avian Fujinami sarcoma vi-
    rus. J. Virol., 1980b, in press.

12. Blair, D. G., McClements, W. L., Oskarsson, M. K., Fisch-
    inger, P. J., & VandeWoude, G. F. Biological activity of
    clones Moloney sarcoma virus DNA: Terminally redundant
    sequences may enhance transformation efficiency. Proc.
    Nat. Acad. Sci., 1980, 77, 3504-3508.
13. Brugge, J. S., & Erikson, R. L. Identification of a trans-
    formation-specific antigen induced by an avian sarcoma
    virus. Nature, 1977, 269, 346-348.
14. Chen, A., Essex, M., Shadduck, J. A., Niederkorn, J. Y.,
    & Albert, D. Retravirus encoded transformation-specific
    polyproteins: Expression coordinated with malignant phen-
    otype in cells from different germ layers. Science, 1980,
    in press.
15. Chien, Y.-S., Verma, I. M., Duesberg, P. H., & Davidson,
    N. Heteroduplex analysis of the RNA of clone 3 Moloney
    murine sarcoma virus. J. Virol., 1979, 32, 1028-1032.
16. Cloyd, M. W., Hartley, J. W., & Rowe, W. P. Lymphomagen-
    icity of recombinant mink cell focus-inducing murine leu-
    kemia viruses. J. Exp. Med., 1980, 151, 542-552.
17. Dina, D., Beemon, K., & Duesberg, P. H. The 30S Moloney
    sarcoma virus RNA contains leukemia virus nucleotide se-
    quences. Cell, 1976, 9, 299-309.
18. Donoghue, B. J., Sharp, P. A., & Weinberg, R. A. Compara-
    tive study of different isolates of murine sarcoma virus.
    J. Virol., 1979, 32, 1015-1027.
19. Duesberg, P. H., & Vogt, P. K. Differences between the
    ribonucleic acids of transforming and nontransforming
    avian tumor viruses. Proc. Nat. Acad. Sci., 1970, 67,
    1673-1680.
20. Duesberg, P. H., & Vogt, P. K. RNA species obtained from
    clonal lines of avian sarcoma and from avian leukosis
    virus. Virology, 1973, 54, 207-219.
21. Duesberg, P. H., & Scolnick, E. M. Murine leukemia virus-
    es containing a ~30S RNA subunit of unknown biological
    activity, in addition to the 38S subunit of the viral
    genome. Virology, 1977, 83, 211-216.
22. Duesberg, P. H., Bister, K., & Vogt, P. K. The RNA of
    avian acute leukemia virus MC29. Proc. Nat. Acad. Sci.,
    1977, 74, 4320-4324.
23. Duesberg, P. H., & Vogt, P. K. Avian acute leukemia virus-
    es MC29 and MH2 share specific RNA sequences: Evidence for
    a second class of transforming genes. Proc. Nat. Acad.
    Sci., 1979, 76, 1633-1637.
24. Duesberg, P. H., Bister, K., & Moscovici, C. Avian acute
    leukemia virus MC29: Conserved and variable RNA sequences
    and recombination with helper virus. Virology, 1979, 99,
    121-134.
25. Duesberg, P. H. Transforming genes of retroviruses. Cold

Spring Harbor Symp. Quant. Biol., 1980, 44, 13-29.
26. Duesberg, P. H., Bister, K. & Moscovici, C. Genetic structure of avian myeloblastosis virus released as defective
virus particle from transformed myeloblasts. Proc. Nat.
Acad. Sci., 1980, in press.
27. Erikson, R. L., Collet, M. S., Erikson, E., Purchio, A.
F., & Brugge, J. S. Protein phosphorylation mediated by
partially purified avian sarcoma virus transforming gene
product. Cold Spring Harbor Symp. Quant. Biol., 1980, 44,
907-917.
28. Essex, M. Etiology and epidemiology of leukemia and lymphoma in outbred animal species. In D. S. Yohn, B. A.
Lapin and J. R. Blakeslee (Ed.), Advances in comparative
leukemia research. New York: Elsevier North-Holland, 1980,
423-430.
29. Frankel, A. E., & Fischinger, P. J. Nucleotide sequences
in mouse DNA and RNA specific for Moloney sarcoma virus.
Proc. Nat. Acad. Sci., 1976, 73, 3705-3709.
30. Frankel, A. E., Gilbert, P. M., Porzig, K. J., Scolnick,
E. M., & Aaronson, S. A. Nature and distribution of feline
sarcoma virus nucleotide sequences. J. Virol., 1979, 30,
821-827.
31. Galehouse, D., & Duesberg, P. H. RNA and proteins of Kirsten sarcoma xenotropic leukemia virus complex propagated
in rat and duck cells. Virology, 1976, 70, 97-104.
32. Gardner, M. B., Henderson, B. E., Estes, J. D., Rongey,
R. W., Casagrande, J., Pike, M., & Huebner, R. J. The
epidemiology and virology of C-type virus-associated hematological cancers and related diseases in wild mice.
Cancer Res., 1976, 36, 574-581.
33. Graf, T., & Beug, H. Avian leukemia viruses. Interaction
with their target cells in vivo and in vitro. Biochim.
Biophys. Acta, 1980, 516, 269-299.
34. Graf, T., Beug, H., & Hayman, M. J. Target cell specificity of defective avian leukemia viruses: Haematopoietic
target cells for a given virus type can be infected but
not transformed by strains of a different type. Proc. Nat.
Acad. Sci., 1980, 77, 389-393.
35. Gross, L. Oncogenic viruses. New York-Oxford-London-
Paris: Pergamon Press, 1970.
36. Hayman, M. J., Royer-Pokora, B., & Graf, T. Defectiveness
of avian erythroblastosis virus: Synthesis of a 75k gag-
related protein. Virology, 1979, 92, 31-45.
37. Hayman, M. J., Kitchener, G., & Graf, T. Cells transformed
by avian myelocytomatosis virus strain CMII contain a 90K
gag-related protein. Virology, 1979, 98, 191-199.
38. Hayward, W. S. The size and genetic content of viral RNAs
in avian oncovirus-infected cells. J. Virol., 1977, 24,

47-64.

39. Huebner, P. J., & Todaro, R. J. Oncogenes of RNA tumor viruses as determinants of cancer. Proc. Nat. Acad. Sci., 1969, 64, 1087-1091.

40. Hughes, S. H., Payvar, F., Spector, D., Schimke, R. T., Robinson, H., Payne, G. S., Bishop, J. M., & Varmus, H. E. Heterogeneity of genetic loci in chickens: Analysis of endogenous viral and nonviral genes by cleavage of DNA with restriction endonuclease. Cell, 1979, 18, 347-359.

41. Hughes, S. H., Stubblefield, F., Payvar, F., Engel, J. D., Dodgson, J. B., Spector, D., Cordell, B., Schimke, R. T., & Varmus, H. E. Gene localization by chromosome fractionation: Globin genes are on at least two chromosomes and three estrogen-inducible genes are on three chromosomes. Proc. Nat. Acad. Sci., 1979, 76, 1348-1352.

42. Jarrett, O. Infectious leukemias in domestic animals. In R. Neth, R. C. Gallo, P.-H. Hofschneider, and K. Mannweiler (ED.), Modern trends in human leukemia III. Berlin: Springer, 1978, 439-444.

43. Kitchener, G., & Hayman, M. J. Comparative tryptic peptide mapping studies suggest a role in cell transformation for gag-related proteins of avian erythroblastosis virus and avian myelocytomatosis virus strains CMII and MC29. Proc. Nat. Acad. Sci., 1980, 77, 1637-1641.

44. Lai, M. M. C., Duesberg, P. H., Horst, J., & Vogt, P. K. Avian tumor virus RNA. A comparison of three sarcoma viruses and their transformation-defective derivatives by oligonucleotide fingerprinting and DNA-RNA hybridization. Proc. Nat. Acad. Sci., 1973, 70, 2266-2270.

45. Lee, W.-H., Bister, K., Pawson, A., Robins, T., Moscovici, C., & Duesberg, P. H. Fujinami sarcoma virus: An avian RNA tumor virus with a unique transforming gene. Proc. Nat. Acad. Sci., 1980, 77, 111-213.

46. Levy, J. H. Xenotropic type C viruses. Curr. Top. Microbiol. Immunol., 1980, 79, 111-213.

47. Lung, M. L., Hering, C., Hartley, J. W., Rowe, W. P., & Hopkins, N. Analysis of the genomes of mink cell focus-inducing murine type C viruses: A progress report. Cold Spring Harbor Symp. Quant. Biol., 1980, 44, 1260-1274.

48. Maisel, J., Klement, V., Lai, M. M. C., Ostertag, W., & Duesberg, P. H. Ribonucleic acid components of murine sarcoma and leukemia viruses. Proc. Nat. Acad. Sci., 1973, 70, 3536-3540.

49. Martin, G. S. Rous sarcoma virus: A function required for the maintenance of the transformed state. Nature, 1970, 227, 1021-1023.

50. Martin, G. S., & Duesberg, P. H. The a subunit in the RNA

of transforming avian tumor viruses: I. Occurrence in different virus strains. II. Spontaneous loss resulting in non-transforming variants. Virology, 1972, 47, 494-497.

51. Martin, G. S., Lee, W.-H., & Duesberg, P. H. Generation of non-defective Rous sarcoma virus by recombination between deletion mutants. J. Virol., 1980, in press.

52. McCullough, B., Schaller, J., Shadduck, J. H., & Holin, D. S. Induction of malignant melanomas associated with fibrosarcomas in cats inoculated with Gardner-feline fibrosarcoma virus. J. Nat. Cancer Inst., 1972, 48, 1893-1896.

53. Mellon, P., & Duesberg, P. H. Subgenomic, cellular Rous sarcoma virus RNAs contain oligonucleotides from the 3' half and the 5' terminus of virion RNA. Nature, 1977, 270, 631-634.

54. Mellon, P., Pawson, A., Bister, K., Martin, G. S., & Duesberg, P. H. Specific RNA sequences and gene products of MC29 avian acute leukemia virus. Proc. Nat. Acad. Sci., 1978, 75, 5874-5878.

55. Moscovici, C. Leukemic transformation with avian myeloblastosis virus: Present status. Curr. Top. Microbiol. Immunol., 1975, 71, 79-101.

56. Oskarsson, M. K., McClements, W. L., Blair, D. S., Maizel, J. V., & VandeWoude, G. S. Properties of a normal mouse cell DNA sequence (sarc) homologous to the src sequence of Moloney sarcoma virus. Science, 1980, 207, 1222-1224.

57. Ostertag, W., Vehmeyer, K., Fagg, B., Pragnell, I. B., Paetz, W., Le Bourse, M. C., Smadja-Joffe, F., Klein, B., Jasmin, C., & Eisen, H. Myeloproliferate virus, a cloned murine sarcoma virus with spleen focus-forming properties in adult mice. J. Virol., 1980, 33, 573-582.

58. Quade, K. Transformation of mammalian cells by avian myelocytomatosis virus and avian erythroblastosis virus. Virology, 1979, 98, 461-465.

59. Ramsay, G., & Hayman, M. J. Analysis of cells transformed by defective leukemia virus OK10: Production of non-infectious particles and synthesis of pr76 gag and an additional 200,000 dalton protein. Virology, 1980, in press.

60. Reynolds, F. W., Van de Ven, W. J. M., & Stephenson, J. R. Feline sarcoma virus polyprotein P115 binds a host phosphoprotein in transformed cells. Nature, 1980, 286, 409-412.

61. Rosenberg, N., & Baltimore, D. Abelson virus. In G. Klein (Ed.), Viral oncology. New York: Raven Press, 1980, 187-203.

62. Roussel, M., Saule, S., Lagrou, C., Rommens, C., Beug, H., Graf, T., & Stehelin, D. Three new types of viral oncogenes of cellular origin specific for haematopoietic cell transformation. Nature, 1979, 281, 452-455.

63. Rubin, H., Fanshier, C., Cornelius, A., & Hughes, W. F. Tolerance and immunity in chickens after congenital and contact infection with avian leukosis virus. Virology, 1962, 17, 143-156.

64. Rübsamen, H., Ziemiecki, A., Friis, R. R., & Bauer, H. The expression of pp60 src and its associated protein kinase activity in cells infected with different trans-formation-defective temperature-sensitive mutants of Rous sarcoma virus. Virology, 1980, 102, 453-457.

65. Scher, C. D., Scolnick, E. M., & Siegler, R. Induction of erythroid leukemia by Harvey and Kirsten sarcoma virus. Nature, 1975, 256, 225-226.

66. Scolnick, E. M., Rands, E., Williams, D., & Parks, W. P. Studies on the nucleic acid sequences of Kirsten sarcoma virus: A model for the formation of a mammalian RNA-containing, sarcoma virus. J. Virol., 1973, 12, 456-463.

67. Scolnick, E. M., Goldberg, R. J., & Siegler, R. A bio-chemical and genetic analysis of mammalian RNA-containing sarcoma viruses. Cold Spring Harbor. Symp. Quant. Biol., 1975, 39, 885-895.

68. Scolnick, E. M., Vass, W. C., Howk, R. S., & Duesberg, P. H. Defective retrovirus-like 30S RNA species of rat and mouse cells are infectious if packaged by Type C helper virus. J. Virol., 1979, 29, 964-972.

69. Sheiness, D., & Bishop, J. M. DNA and RNA from uninfected vertebrate cells contain nucleotide sequences related to the putative transforming gene of avian myelocytomatosis virus. J. Virol., 1979, 31, 514-521.

70. Shields, A., Goff, S., Paskind, M., Otto, G., & Baltimore, D. Structure of the Abelson murine leukemia virus genome. Cell, 1979, 18, 955-962.

71. Souza, L. M., Strommer, J. N., Hillgard, R. L., Komaromy, M. C., & Baluda, M. A. Cellular sequences are present in the presumptive avian myeloblastosis virus genome. Proc. Nat. Acad. Sci., 1980, in press.

72. Spector, D. H., Varmus, H. E., & Bishop, J. M. Nucleotide sequences related to the transforming genes of avian sar-coma virus are present in DNA of uninfected vertebrates. Proc. Nat. Acad. Sci., 1978 a, 75, 4102-4106.

73. Spector, D. H., Baker, B., Varmus, H. E., & Bishop, J. M. Characteristics of cellular RNA related to the transforming gene of avian sarcoma viruses. Cell, 1978 b, 13, 381-386.
74. Stehelin, D., Guntaka, R., Varmus, H. E., & Bishop, J. M. Purification of DNA complementary to nucleotide sequences required for neoplastic transformation of fibroblasts by avian sarcoma viruses. J. Mol. Biol. 1976 a, 101, 349-365.
75. Stehelin, D., Varmus, H. E., Bishop, J. M., & Vogt, P. K. DNA related to the transforming gene(s) of avian sarcoma viruses is present in normal avian DNA. Nature, 1976 b, 260, 170-173.
76. Stephenson, J. R., Khan, A. S., Van de Ven, W. J. M., & Reynolds, F. H., Jr. Type C retroviruses as vectors for cloning cellular genes with probable transforming function. J. Nat. Cancer Inst., 1979, 63, 1111-1119.
77. Tooze, J. The molecular biology of tumour viruses. Cold Spring Harbor, New York: Cold Spring Harbor Press, 1973.
78. Tsichlis, P. N., & Coffin, J. M. Role of the c-region in relative growth rates of endogenous and exogenous avian oncoviruses. Cold Spring Harbor Symp. Quant. Biol., 1980, 44, 1123-1132.
79. Tsuchida, N., Gilden, R. V., & Hatanaka, M. Sarcoma virus-related RNA sequences in normal rat cells. Proc. Nat. Acad. Sci., 1974, 71, 4503-4507.
80. Van de Ven, W. J. M., Reynolds, F. H., Nalewaik, R. P., & Stephenson, J. R. Characterization of a 170,000 dalton polyprotein encoded by the McDonough strain of feline sarcoma virus. J. Virol., 1980, 35, 165-175.
81. Wang, L.-H., Duesberg, P. H., Beemon, K., & Vogt, P. K. Mapping RNase T1-resistant oligonucleotides of avian tumor virus RNAs: Sarcoma specific oligonucleotides are near the poly(A) end and oligonucleotides common to sarcoma and transformation-defective viruses are at the poly(A) end. J. Virol., 1975, 16, 1051-1070.
82. Wang, L.-H., Duesberg, P. H., Mellon, P., & Vogt, P. K. Distribution of envelope-specific and sarcoma-specific nucleotide sequences from different parents in the RNAs of avian tumor virus recombinants. Proc. Nat. Acad. Sci., 1976, 73, 1073-1077.
83. Wang, L.-H. The gene order of avian RNA tumor viruses derived from biochemical analyses of deletion mutants and viral recombinants. Annu. Rev. Microbiol., 1978, 32, 561-593.

84. Wang, S. Y., Hayward, W. S., & Hanafusa, H. Genetic variation in the RNA transcripts of endogenous virus genes in uninfected chicken cells. J. Virol., 1977, 24, 64-73.
85. Weyl, K. S., & Dougherty, R. M. Contact transmission of avian leukosis virus. J. Nat. Cancer Inst., 1977, 58, 1019-1025.
86. Witte, O. N., Dasgupta, A., & Baltimore, D. Abelson murine leukemia virus protein is phosphorylated in vitro to form phosphotyrosine. Nature, 1980, 283, 826-831.

Feline Leukemia and Sarcoma Viruses

M. ESSEX

Professor of Virology

Department of Microbiology
Harvard University School of Public Health
Boston, Massachusetts 02115

The role of RNA tumor viruses in the etiology of leukemia,
lymphoma and other tumors of cats provides firm evidence that
viruses can cause cancer under natural circumstances in higher
mammals. Although we now have a fairly clear understanding
about the epidemiology and natural history of feline leukemia
virus (FeLV) in the domestic cat population we still know
relatively little about how this agent causes neoplasia in the
individual cat. Conversely, although we know relatively
little about the origin and distribution of feline sarcoma
virus (FeSV) in the domestic cat population, we know more
about how this agent may exert an oncogenic effect.

NATURAL HISTORY

   Most domestic cats that roam freely in the average
suburban environment become exposed to FeLV during their
lifetime. This conclusion is based primarily on the observation that 40-80% of the stray cats from various cities have
antibodies to the feline oncornavirus-associated cell membrane
antigen (FOCMA) (4,26). A smaller proportion, perhaps 20-40%,
have antibodies to the virus structural proteins.
   Following exposure to FeLV, most cats avoid persistent
infection by mounting a virus neutralizing antibody response.
The major route for virus excretion is saliva (12) and
although the route of entry into the animal is not known, it
appears likely to be the oral cavity. Cats frequently "groom"
both themselves and each other with their tongues and virus
present in saliva will remain viable for reasonable time

periods (11). The eipthelial cells in the buccal cavity are sensitive to infection, and the buccal cavity, the tonsillar area, and/or the respiratory epithelium presumably represent the initial site of replication.

A significant proportion of the cats that become infected at the local site become viremic (16). Most experience only transient viremia, but a small proportion, perhaps 2%, become persistently viremic (10). Those that become persistently viremic have a dramatic increase in relative risk for the development of both neoplastic diseases and various non-neoplastic diseases. Almost all (eg. greater than 95%) of the cats that become persistently viremic will die because of some related disease process within 3-5 years after the time they become persistently viremic (13). Only about 20-40% will die of leukemia or lymphoma, while the rest will die from various non-neoplastic infecious diseases such as septicemia, peritonitis, and glomerulonephritis (6,13).

Cats viremic with FeLV presumably have an increased risk for the development of diseases such as septicemia and peritonitis because of the immunosuppressive effects exerted by the oncogenic agent. Healthy cats that become persistently infected with FeLV were found to have reduced levels of circulating lymphoid cells (6) and one of the virus structural proteins was shown to possess immunosuppressive activity in vitro (21). This immunosuppressive activity may also play an important role in allowing the development of leukemia or lymphoma by diminishing the immunosurveillance response directed to FOCMA (8). In fact, cats that were vaccinated with inactivated FeLV sometimes had an enhanced rate of lymphoma development if challenged with live FeLV rapidly thereafter (23). The incubation period for the development of diseases such as septicemia and peritonitis is short so that cats that become infected with these agents would die before the onset of clinical leukemia or lymphoma had a chance to occur. The incubation period for membranous glomerulo-nephritis is considerably longer, but this disease may occur as a result of the immune complexes formed by the renewable FOCMA and/or FeLV antigens in the circulation.

Since both healthy cats and sick cats that are persistently viremic continually excrete FeLV, and most viremic cats remain healthy for 1-2 years before developing disease, the healthy viremic cat is the major focus for distribution of FeLV in the environment (10). In fact, it appears that healthy cats may even excrete higher titers of infectious virus (10).

When cats are confined into densely populated conditions the distribution pattern of infection changes. A much larger proportion of the cats develop persistent viremia and thus a larger proportion also develop leukemia, lymphoma and other diseases (7,8). Under such conditions, "clusters" of leukemia or lymphoma may occur (2,8). Several factors probably contribute to this increase in disease incidence. First, most cats become infected with larger doses of virus and become exposed more frequently. Second, many cats become exposed to FeLV at younger ages, often while they are still nursing. Unless in highly concentrated conditions of confinement, nursing kittens would not be exposed to adults other than the mother until after weaning. Under laboratory conditions, when cats are inoculated with FeLV by parenteral routes, those inoculated at the youngest ages are most likely to develop tumors (18). Finally, under crowded conditions most infectious agents are more prevalent and chronic infections with other non-oncogenic cytopathic viruses and bacteria might also depress resistance to FeLV.

The most common neoplastic disease syndrome that occurs in cats that are persistently infected with FeLV is a T cell lymphoma (9,17). This frequently presents with the mediastinal cavity as the primary site for development but may also originate in lymph nodes or various other sites. Lymphomas also occur that are not T-cell in origin, many originating in the wall of the gastrointestinal tract. Several forms of true leukemias also occur in FeLV-infected cats. These include acute lymphoblastic leukemia, which is most often a T-cell disease, and erythroid and myeloid forms. Certain strains of FeLV also cause aplastic anemias (20). Whether the different forms of lymphomas and leukemias are caused by the same strains and subgroups or different strains is not known. Several strains and subgroups have been distinguished by interference (30), serum neutralization (29), host cell infectivity spectrum (31), and T1 oligonucleotide fingerprinting (27). It has been reported that infection with one subgroup may enhance transmission and infection with the others (19). All field isolates of subgroup B and C are found in cats that are also infected with A. The reason for this is unclear, since B and C can grow efficiently in the absence of A in cultured cells.

VIRAL GENOMES AND PROTEINS

FeLV and FeSV are similar in structure to comparable retroviruses of mice, chickens, and other species (5). The FeLV genomic RNA contains three genes that are essential for replication. These genes are positioned between ends that are terminally redundant, an apparent requirement for

circularization and integration of the DNA provirus. The
gene closest to the 5' end, designated "gag" for "group
specific antigen", encodes for a protein of about 75,000
daltons which subsequently undergoes post-translational
cleavage to release 4 peptides that compose the structure of
the virion cores. Designated from the 5' end of the RNA by
relative molecular weight, these peptides are designated p15,
p12, p30, and p10. All are immunogenic in infected cats (5),
but since they occupy an internal position in the virus
particles the immune response cannot lyse mature infectious
FeLV. However, these peptides are distributed on the cell
surfaces of both FeLV-producer normal cells and tumor cells.
It is conceivable that in this site they could serve as
targets for the lysis of infected cells as a means to control
replication.

The gene in the middle of the genome, designated pol
codes for the RNA dependent DNA polymerase or reverse
transcriptase. It also is immunogenic and many cats possess
antibodies to this protein but it is not clear that such
antibodies play any role in controlling infections and it is
hard to imagine how this might occur.

The third gene, env, codes for the virion envelope polyprotein, a complex of about 90,000 daltons which also undergoes postranslational cleavage to produce the gp70, a
glycoprotein that becomes the knobs at the surface of the
virus particles, and p15e, a hydrophobic peptide that serves
as the backbone of the virion envelope in which the gp70
molecules are inserted. Both the gp70 and p15e are also
present at the membranes of infected cells and can presumably
serve as targets for lysis by the immune system.

FeLV's that have been isolated from infected cats
replicate efficiently in various cells. However, the possibility that "replication-defective" forms of FeLV might exist
and play a role in leukemogenesis has not been ruled out.
Because of our knowledge about the structure of FeSV and how
this agent transforms cells (see below) it seems possible
that comparable forms of FeLV might exist as replication
defective recombinants that contain a newly added "luk" gene.
In fact, up to one-third of the cases of naturally occurring
feline leukemia and lymphoma occur in "FeLV-negative" cats (9).
However, such cats with "virus-negative" cases of leukemia
contain incomplete copies of representative DNA proviral
sequences in both tumor cells and normal cells (as do many
healthy cats). A portion of the cats with "virus-negative"
tumors also have low levels of selected viral proteins in
the circulation (32). All the major pathologic forms of
leukemia and lymphoma occasionally occur in "virus-negative"

cats although cats with "virus-negative" cases of neoplastic disease tend to be older at the time of presentation (15). Perhaps most importantly, cats known to be exposed to infectious FeLV have an increase in relative risk for development of "virus-negative" lymphoma that is just as high as the increase in risk for development of "virus-positive" lymphoma following known exposure to FeLV. In fact, we recently proposed an immunoselection hypothesis to postulate how cases of "virus-negative" feline leukemia and lymphoma might actually be caused by FeLV (5).

All strains of FeSV are defective for replication. They contain a genome that is only about 4.5 kilobase pairs in length as compared to about 8.5 kilobase pairs for the replication-competent FeLV's (33). As shown by restriction mapping and heteroduplexing, the redundant regions at the external ends of the FeSV are identical to those on the FeLV genome. Additionally, the regions in from the terminal repeats, up to about 1 kilobase pairs from each end are also similar if not identical to the appropriate helper FeLV. In the middle of the FeSV genome is a new and distinct sequence of about 1-5 kilobase pairs. Comparable sequences have been identified in other replication defective sarcoma and leukemia viruses of both birds and mammals. In the murine and avian viruses such sequences are believed to have originated from control genes present in host cells and limited evidence is available to support this position for FeSV (14).

Only one class of protein has been identified as being encoded by FeSV. This is a polyprotein composed of the 5' end of the gag gene product linked to a distinct peptide of 60,000-100,000 daltons usually designated "x" (34,37). The gag related portion contains FeLV p15, FeLV p12, and part but not all of FeLV p30. The size of the "gag-x" protein varies with the strain of FeSV. It is about 85,000 daltons for the ST strain, about 110 daltons for the GA strain, and about 150,000 daltons for the SM strain (24,38).

TRANSFORMATION AND TUMOR INDUCTION

The events that lead to the development of leukemia or lymphoma within the host are not well understood. Although we might suspect that such tumors are monoclonal because comparable tumors are in other species, no direct evidence is available to support that position. The shortest incubation period that ever occurs following inoculation of the virus is 15-25 weeks (18). During this period the thymus atrophies and it is subsequently replaced by the malignant cells. Lymphoid tumor cells are not unusual in appearance, but they contain FOCMA, the FeLV and FeSV-associated tumor

specific antigen. All lymphoid tumor cells express FOCMA,
irregardless of whether they are T or non-T cells, and
whether they are virus producer or non-producer (5). FOCMA
is not expressed on normal lymphoid cells; even, normal lymphoid cells that replicate FeLV. FOCMA is, however, expressed on FeSV-transformed fibroblasts, whether or not they
replicate helper FeLV or exist as "nonproducer" clones.
FOCMA is seen on both cat cells and non-feline cells (eg.
mink, rat) that were transformed with FeSV (35, 37).

The biochemical nature of FOCMA is still unclear. Molecules in the range of 65,000 daltons to 70,000 daltons have
been detected in both cultured lymphoma cells and FeSV-transformed nonproducer mink cells (36, 39). Rabbit antiserum
made to a p65 separated from membranes of FeSV-transformed
mink cells will cross-react with an antigen of 68,000 daltons
found on the membranes of lymphoma cells. Both molecules
will also react with typical FOCMA antiserum of cat origin.

Typical FOCMA antiserum of cat origin can also be used
to immunoprecipitate the "gag-x" proteins found by the metabolic labelling of FeSV-transformed mink cells (1). Cats
immunologically respond to both the gag and the "x" portions
of the molecule. The gag-x protein that is encoded by the
ST-FeSV is serologically closely related to the gag-x protein
found in GA-FeSV transformed mink cells even though the relative sizes of the molecules are different. The "x" portion
of the gag-x protein encoded for by the SM strain of FeSV
appears to be quite different.

The gag-x proteins are expressed in feline cells transformed by FeSV as well as mink and rat cells, and they are
expressed in superinfected FeLV-producer cells as well as
nonproducer cells (1). Although not always the case with
mutant strains of FeSV (3), the gag-x proteins are usually
expressed concordinately with phenotypic transformation.
Transfection of mouse cells with FeSV proviral DNA in the
absence of FeLV DNA induces transformation as well as the
appropriate gag-x protein (28).

The gag-x proteins are also expressed in cells freshly
biopsied from FeSV-induced tumors (1). The proteins in the
biopsied tumor cells are characteristic of the strain of FeSV
that induced the tumor, and indistinguishable from the analogous proteins that are expressed in fibroblasts transformed
by the same virus.

At least one strain of FeSV (GA) has also been used to
induce melanomas, a tumor that is very different from the
characteristic fibrosarcomas in that it arises from neuro-
ectodermal germ cells (22). The melanomas are preferentially
induced if FeSV is inoculated either intradermally or intra-

ocularly. In either case the virus apparently becomes exposed to many melanin containing cells. Cells from FeSV-
induced melanomas also contain the same gag-x proteins as
fibrosarcoma cells, indicating that such proteins are expressed concordinately with the malignant phenotype even across
germ-line barriers, if in fact the same strain of FeSV was
used to induce both tumors (1). This suggests that if the
gag-x proteins do play an important role in transformation,
these proteins must have a pleiotropic effect that can function in different cell types. Both FeSV-induced melanoma
cells and FeSV-induced fibrosarcoma cells are also positive
for FOCMA by membrane immunofluorescence.

Various feline tumor cell lines representative of spontaneous tumors not known to be associated with FeLV or FeSV
were also tested for both gag-x proteins of the ST-GA type,
and FOCMA. The tumors analyzed included chondrosarcomas,
osteosarcomas, mammary carcinomas and neurofibrosarcomas (1).
All were negative for both antigens, suggesting that these
activities are somehow specific to the feline retraviruses.
Cultured normal cat fibroblasts that were transformed with
dimethylbenanthracene were also checked and found to be negative (25).

SUMMARY

FeLV is a ubiquitous agent in the domestic cat population. Most cats become exposed to the virus but resist persistent viremia due to their immune response. Of the small
proportion that become persistently viremic a minority develop other non-neoplastic diseases, presumably because of
the immunosuppressive activity of the virus. The induction
period for leukemia development is 1-2 years. Of the cats
that develop spontaneous leukemia or lymphoma about one-third
do not contain replicating infectious FeLV, but most of these
animals also have a history of exposure to FeLV.

The mechanism by which FeLV causes neoplasia is not well
understood. Most lymphomas are T cell tumors and they express FOCMA, a tumor-specific cell membrane antigen. Extensive type or strain variation occurs among the FeLV's and the
possibility that replication defective variants occur has
not been excluded. FeSV is a replication-defective relative
of FeLV that causes morphologic tranformation of fibroblasts
in vitro and multicentric fibrosarcomas in vivo. FeSV-transformed cells, including non-producer clones, express both
FOCMA and "gag-x", a polyprotein which contains a portion of
the FeLV core proteins and a unique new protein which is
believed to be involved in transformation. The "gag-x" pro-

tein is characteristic of the strain of FeSV that causes the
pathology, and it is expressed in the same manner in both
transformed fibroblasts and tumor cells. In fact, the same
protein is expressed in both FeSV-induced fibrosarcomas and
FeSV-induced melanomas, suggesting that this protein may
function in a pleiotropic manner.

REFERENCES

1. Chen, AP, Essex, M, Mikami, T et al: The expression of
   transformation-related proteins in cat cells. In:
   Feline Leukemia and Sarcoma Viruses, Elsevier/North
   Holland Press, New York, 1980, in press.
2. Cotter, SM, Essex, M, Hardy, WD, Jr: Serological studies
   of normal and leukemic cats in a multiple-case leukemia
   cluster. Cancer Res 34:1061-1069, 1974.
3. Donner, L, Turek, LP, Ruscetti, SK et al: Transformation
   defective mutants of feline sarcoma virus which express a
   product of the viral src gene. J Virol 35:129-140, 1980.
4. Essex, M: Horizontally and vertically transmitted oncornaviruses of cats. Adv Cancer Res 21:175-248, 1975.
5. Essex, M: Feline leukemia and sarcoma viruses. In:
   Viral Oncology, Raven Press, New York, 1980, pp 205-229.
6. Essex, M, Hardy, WD, Jr, Cotter, SM et al: Naturally
   occurring persistent feline oncornavirus infections in
   the absence of disease. Infect Immun 11:470-475, 1975.
7. Essex, M, Jakowski, RM, Hardy, WD Jr et al: Feline oncornavirus associated cell membrane antigen. III Antibody
   titers in cats from leukemia cluster households. J Natl
   Cancer Inst 54:637-641, 1975.
8. Essex, M, Sliski, A, Cotter, SM et al: Immunosurveillance of naturally occurring feline leukemia. Science
   190:790-792, 1975.
9. Francis, DP, Cotter, SM, Hardy, WD, Jr et al: Feline
   leukemia and lymphoma: Comparison of virus positive and
   virus negative cases. Cancer Res 39:3866-3870, 1979.
10. Francis, DP, Essex, M, Cotter, SM et al: Feline leukemia
    virus infections: The significance of chronic viremia.
    Leukemia Res 3:435-441, 1979.
11. Francis, DP, Essex, M, Gayzagian, D: Feline leukemia
    virus: Survival under home and laboratory conditions.
    J Clin Microbiol 9:154-156, 1979.
12. Francis, DP, Essex, M, Hardy, WD, Jr: Excretion of feline
    leukemia virus by naturally infected pet cats. Nature
    269:252-254, 1977.
13. Francis, DP, Essex, M, Jakowski, RM et al: Feline lym-
    phoma: Descriptive epidemiology of a virally-induced
    malignancy in a closed cat population. Amer J Epidemiol
    111:337-346, 1980.

14. Frankel, A,E, Gilbert, JH, Porzig, EM et al: Nature and distribution of feline sarcoma virus nucleotide sequences. J Virol 30:821-827, 1979.
15. Gardner, MB, Rasheed, S, Rongey, RW et al: Natural expression of feline type C virus genomes. Prevalence of detectable FeLV and RD-114 gs antigens, type C particles and infectious virus in postnatal and fetal cats. Int J Cancer 14:97-105, 1974.
16. Grant, CK, Essex, M, Gardner, MB et al: Natural feline leukemia virus infection and the immune response of cats of different ages. Cancer Res 40:825-829, 1980.
17. Hardy, WD, Jr, Zuckerman, EE, MacEwen et al: A feline leukemia and sarcoma virus induced tumor virus specific antigen. Nature 270:249-251, 1977.
18. Hoover, EA, Olsen, RG, Hardy, WD, Jr et al: Feline leukemia virus infection: Age-related variation in susceptibility of cats to experimental infection. J Natl Cancer Inst 58:365-369, 1976.
19. Jarrett, O, Russell, PH: Differential growth and transmission in cats of feline leukemia viruses of sub-groups A and B. Int J Cancer 21:466-472, 1978.
20. Mackey, LJ, Jarrett, W, Jarrett, O et al: Anemia asso-iated with feline leukemia virus infection in cats. J Natl Cancer Inst 54:209-218, 1975.
21. Mathes, LE, Olsen, RG, Hebebrand, LC et al: Immuno-suppressive properties of a virion polypeptide, a 15,000-dalton protein, from feline leukemia virus. Cancer Res 39:950-955, 1979.
22. McCullough, B, Schaller, J, Shadduck, JA et al: Induction of malignant melanomas associated with fibrosarcoma in gnotobiotic cat inoculated with Gardner feline fibro-sarcoma virus. J Natl Cancer Inst 48:1893-1896, 1972.
23. Olsen, RG, Hoover, EA, Schaller, JP et al: Abrogation of resistance to feline oncornavirus disease by immunization with killed feline leukemia virus. Cancer Res 37:2082-2085, 1977.
24. Porzig, KJ, Barbacid, M, Aaronson, SA: Biological properties and translational products of three independent isolates of feline sarcoma virus. Virology 92:91-107, 1979.
25. Rhim, J, Nelson-Rees, WA, Essex, M: Transformation of feline embryo cells in culture by a chemical carcinogen. Int J Cancer 24:336-340, 1979.
26. Rogerson, P, Jarrett, W, Mackey, L: Epidemiological studies on feline leukemia virus infection. I. A serological survey in urban cats. Int J Cancer 15:781-785, 1975.

27. Rosenberg, ZF, Pedersen, FS, Haseltine, WA: Comparative analysis of the genomes of feline leukemia viruses. J Virol 35:542-546, 1980.
28. Rosenberg, ZF, Sahagan, BG, Snyder, HW,Jr: Biochemical characterization of cells transformed via transfection by feline sarcoma virus proviral DNA. Submitted for publication.
29. Russell, PH, Jarrett, O: The specificity of neutralizing antibodies to feline leukemia viruses. Int J Cancer 21:768-778, 1978.
30. Sarma, PS, Log T: Subgroup classification of feline leukemia and sarcoma viruses by viral interference and neutralization tests. Virology 54:160-170, 1973.
31. Sarma, PS, Log, T, Damine, J et al: Differential host range of viruses of feline leukemia-sarcoma complex. Virology 64:438-446.
32. Saxinger, C, Essex, M, Hardy, W et al: Detection of antigen related to feline leukemia virus in sera of "virus-negative" cats. In: Feline Leukemia and Sarcoma Viruses, Elsevier/North Holland Press, New York, 1980, in press.
33. Sherr, CJ, Fedele, LA, Donner, L et al: Restriction endonuclease mapping of unintegrated proviral DNA of Snyder-Theilen feline sarcoma virus: location of sarcoma specific sequences. J Virol 32:860-875, 1979.
34. Sherr, CJ, Sen, A, Todaro, GJ et al: Feline sarcoma virus codes for a phosphorylated polyprotein containing FOCMA, p15 and p12 antigens. Proc Natl Acad Sci USA 75:1505-1509, 1978.
35. Sliski, AH, Essex, M, Meyer, C et al: Feline oncornavirus-associated cell membrane antigen (FOCMA): Expression on feline sarcoma virus transformed nonproducer mink cells. Science 196:1336-1339, 1977.
36. Snyder, HW, Jr, Hardy, WD, Jr, Zuckerman, EE et al: Characterization of a tumour-specific antigen on the surface of feline lymphosarcoma cells. Nature 275:656-657, 1978.
37. Stephenson, JR, Khan, AS, Sliski, AH et al: Feline oncornavirus-associated cell membrane antigen (FOCMA): Identification of an immunologically cross-reactive feline sarcoma virus coded protein. Proc Natl Acad Sci USA 74:5608-5612, 1977.
38. Van de Ven, WJM, Khan, AS, Reynolds, FH, Jr et al: Translational products encoded by newly acquired sequences of independently derived feline sarcoma virus isolates are structurally related. J Virol 33:1034-1045, 1980.

39. Worley, M, Essex, M: Identification of membrane proteins associated with transformation-related antigens shared by feline lymphoma cells and feline sarcoma virus transformed fibroblasts. In: Feline Leukemia and Sarcoma Viruses, Elsevier/North Holland Press, New York, 1980, in press.

The Epstein-Barr virus;
its relation to Burkitt's lymphoma
and nasopharyngeal carcinoma

WERNER HENLE

GERTRUDE HENLE

Professors of Virology in Pediatrics
University of Pennsylvania School of Medicine
The Joseph Stokes, Jr., Research Institute
of The Children's Hospital of Philadelphia
Philadelphia, Pennsylvania 19104.

Among human cancers of possibly viral etiology Burkitt's
lymphoma (BL), the most frequent malignancy of African
children, appeared to be outstanding because several aspects
of its epidemiology were compatible with an infectious origin
(cf.[2]). In 1964, Epstein and his associates detected a
herpes type virus by electronmicroscopy in a small percentage
of cultured BL cells[3] which was relegated by most virologists
to a harmless passenger role in the tumor however because no
member of this group of DNA viruses had as yet been shown to
be oncogenic under natural or experimental conditions. When
the virus was proven by indirect immunofluorescence tests to
be unrelated to any known herpes virus[4] it was named the
Epstein-Barr virus (EBV) after the EB-1 culture of BL cells
in which it was first observed. EBV was found subsequently
also in lymphoblast cultures derived from peripheral lymphocytes of healthy donors or patients with various diseases
(cf.[23]).

Using the indirect immunofluorescence test in seroepidemiologic surveys (cf.[8]), antibodies to EBV were detected in
sera from all African BL patients but also in many sera from
African control children. Indeed, antibodies were found

anywhere in the world, even in the remotest areas, showing
that almost nobody escapes infection by EBV. BL patients
however had substantially higher titers of antibodies than
healthy controls, but similarly high titers were found also
in sera from patients with nasopharyngeal carcinoma (NPC),
used initially in immunodiffusion tests as controls for BL
sera[21]. This poorly or undifferentiated carcinoma, known
also as lymphoepithelioma because of abundant lymphocytic
infiltration, is especially common among Southern Chinese,
East and North Africans, and Alaskan natives but occurs at
low frequency anywhere in the world (cf.[16]). The ubiquity
of EBV suggested that it might cause primarily a common
benign disease and, indeed, it was shown to be the cause of
infectious mononucleosis (IM) (cf.[6]). A seronegative tech-
nician in our laboratory provided the initial clue when she
developed antibodies to EBV in the course of IM[7]. This self-
limited lymphoproliferative disease is unknown in those parts
of the world where primary EBV infections occur early in life
when they usually remain silent. In highly developed Western
Countries primary EBV infections are often postponed to
adolescence or later when they frequently induce IM.

The serologic approach has established EBV as the cause of
IM but in order to relate the virus etiologically to BL and
NPC it was necessary to provide additional evidence by four
approaches based on studies of animal tumor virus models: (1)
detection of fingerprints of EBV (nucleic acids, antigens) in
BL and NPC biopsies; (2) malignant transformation of normal
human cells by EBV in vitro; (3) induction of tumors by EBV
in non-human primates; and (4) detection of broader spectra
and higher titers of antibodies to EBV-specific antigens in
tumor patients as compared to controls and relation of changes
in the antibody patterns to the prognosis of the patients.

DETECTION OF VIRAL NUCLEIC ACIDS AND ANTIGENS

This approach has been highly successful (cf.[26]).
Productively EBV-infected cells are not found in tumor tissue
because they become targets of immune defenses and are
rapidly destroyed as soon as viral antigens are inserted into
their membranes. They appear spontaneously within a day
however among BL cells when placed in culture and in cultured
NPC biopsy cells after chemical induction. Over 97% of
African BL biopsies contain EBV DNA in amounts equivalent to
multiple viral genomes per cell and the lymphoma cells
express the EBV-associated nuclear antigen (EBNA)[17]. EBV DNA
or EBNA-positive cells have not been found in other types of

lymphomas, except among B cell lymphomas arising at enhanced frequency in immunologically compromised patients.

EBV DNA corresponding to multiple viral genomes per cell is regularly demonstrable in NPC biopsies[1]. It is present in the carcinoma cells and not in the lymphoid elements of the tumor[24]. The carcinoma cells thus express EBNA which is readily demonstrable in touch preparations of biopsies[13]. This test is of diagnostic value in cases of lymph node metastases in which the primary tumor has not been found. EBNA-positive carcinoma cells in the lymph node biopsy identify the postnasal space as the site of the primary tumor because carcinomas at other sites of head and neck or elsewhere have uniformly been free of EBV DNA or EBNA-positive carcinoma cells[1,14].

TRANSFORMATION OF NORMAL CELLS BY EBV IN VITRO

There are two types of EBV populations; one induces abortive cycles of viral replication in non-producer cultures; and the other transforms bone marrow-derived (B) but not thymus-derived (T) lymphocytes of man and other primate species in vitro into permanently growing lymphoblasts which carry EBV genomes and express EBNA (cf.[23]). The transformed lymphocytes do not conform in all aspects to BL cells (cf.[20]). While these too have B cell characteristics they are monoclonal in origin; i.e., each tumor arises from a single, malignantly transformed cell; they develop into lymphomas when injected subcutaneously into athymic (nude) mice; and they show a reciprocal translocation between the long arms of one of the #8 and 14 chromosomes. In vitro transformed B lymphocytes or lymphoblasts cultured from IM patients or viral carriers are polyclonal, do not grow in nude mice except when injected into immunologically privileged sites (the central nervous system) or into immunologically immature newborn animals and they do not show the 8;14 translocation. Thus, B lymphocytes transformed by EBV are not yet fully malignant although they are endowed with a permanent growth potential which is an attribute of cancer cells.

No epithelial cells have been infected or transformed by EBV. Because NPC cells survive only a few weeks in culture it is unlikely that their normal progenitors, even if infected and transformed by EBV, will grow indefinitely in vitro. However, during the short life span in culture NPC cells can be induced by certain antimetabolites to synthesize EA, VCA and infectious virus particles, proving that they contain complete viral genomes (cf.[16]).

INDUCTION OF TUMORS IN NON-HUMAN PRIMATES

This approach, like the preceding one, has been only
partly successful (cf.[19]). Injection of transforming EBV
into marmosets and two other primate species induces a
similar range of responses as seen in man; i.e., silent sero-
conversion in some, self-limited lymphoproliferation in
other, and fatal disseminated lymphomas in the remaining
animals. The lymphomas arising in marmosets are not
comparable to BL in at least two aspects. They arise at a
considerable frequency and within a few weeks, whereas BL is
rare and years elapse between the primary EBV infection under
the age of 3 years and the emergence of the tumor with a peak
incidence at the age of 6 years. Nevertheless these observations emphasize the oncogenic potential of the virus.
     No carcinomas have been induced to date in marmosets or
other primates by injection of EBV. Conceivably, topical
application of the virus is required, perhaps in conjunction
with one or more of the co-factors considered presently to
contribute to the development of NPC; i.e., chemical
carcinogens, respiratory viruses, etc., as will be discussed
later.

THE SPECTRUM OF EBV-SPECIFIC ANTIBODIES IN BL AND NPC

     In due course, a number of distinct EBV-determined antigens
have been differentiated by immunofluorescence techniques and
tests for the corresponding antibodies, including their
immunoglobulin (Ig) class, have been developed (cf.[10]). Most
useful for the serodiagnosis, prognosis and seroepidemiology
of EBV-associated diseases are the viral capsid antigen (VCA),
the D (diffuse) and R (restricted) components of the early
antigen (EA) complex, and the EB viral nuclear antigen (EBNA),
whereas the EBV-induced early and late cell membrane antigens
(MA) have played a lesser role because techniques for determination of antibodies to MA are too complex for routine use.
The tests have permitted to delineate antibody spectra
characteristic for each of the EBV-associated diseases which,
as shown in figure 1, differ from each other and from the
patterns observed in healthy individuals after long past
primary EBV infections (cf.[12]).
     In acute IM, high titers of IgM and IgG antibodies to VCA
are seen, a transient anti-D response, and absence as yet of
antibodies to EBNA which arise only in late convalescence.
The majority of IM patients also show transiently antibodies
to heterophil antigen of the Paul-Bunnell type which are

EBV-SPECIFIC ANTIBODY PATTERNS

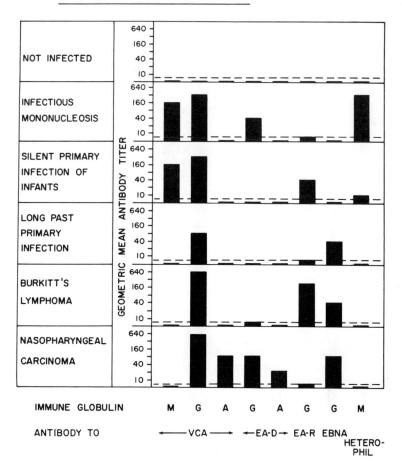

Figure 1. Antibody spectra and titers characteristic of EBV-associated diseases.

highly specific for the disease. In silent primary EBV infections under the age of 2 years, and possibly also later, the responses are similar to those seen in IM, except that antibodies to the EA complex are directed against R rather than D, and that heterophil antibodies do not arise or become at most barely detectable. The persistent viral carrier state which ensues regularly in the lymphoreticular system is responsible for life-long maintenance of IgG antibodies to VCA and EBNA. Antibodies to R, rarely to D, are detected at only low levels among those viral carriers who maintain relatively high anti-VCA titers. In African BL, high titers of IgG antibodies to R, which may even exceed those of VCA-specific antibodies, are characteristic, whereas in NPC high titers of IgG antibodies to D and especially IgA antibodies to VCA and D are outstanding features[5].

The antibody spectrum and titers in BL increase to some extent with the tumor burden and reflect to a considerable degree the prognosis of the patients[9]. Following therapy, continuing absence of antibodies to R or a steady, slow decline of anti-R titers indicate a good prognosis because most patients with these patterns have survived, after at most one or two early relapses, for more than 5 to 10 years without evidence of disease. In contrast, persistence or development of high anti-R titers during remissions denote that the patients face multiple, ultimately fatal relapses, even after disease-free periods of as long as 6 years (Biggar et al., submitted).

Only about 20% of American patients with a diagnosis of BL conform serologically to their African counterpart and they tend to be older[25]. Even a cluster of four young adult patients with EBV-associated BL has been observed in Pennsylvania[15]. Biopsies from such cases contain EBV DNA and EBNA-positive tumor cells. The other 80% of American patients have either no antibodies to EBV or show antibody patterns comparable to those of healthy individuals after long past primary EBV infections. Their tumors are free of viral DNA and EBNA-positive cells. Cultured cells derived from EBV-associated and EBV-free tumors apparently differ from each other in several aspects[18], suggesting that the two types of tumors may be distinct entities.

In NPC, the spectrum and titers of EBV-specific antibodies increase substantially with the total tumor burden; i.e., from stage I (tumor limited to the postnasal space) to stage II and III (cervical lymph node invasion at increasing distance from primary site) to the final stage IV (metastases spread to various organs)[11]. The incidence of IgG antibodies to D increases with advance of the disease from 60 to 97%, of IgA antibodies to VCA from about 80 to 95% and of IgA antibodies to D from 30 to 75%. Correspondingly, the geometric mean titers of these as well as of VCA-specific IgG antibodies increase up to 10-fold. After therapeutic reduction or eradication of the tumor, the antibody spectra and titers slowly decrease. In a 5 year follow-up study of over 100 NPC patients in Hong Kong[11] about half of the cases showed a steady, gradual decline in antibody titers to lower (IgG anti-VCA) or even non-detectable levels (VCA- and D-specific IgA antibodies). These patients remained free of disease throughout the observation period. About one third of the patients showed, after an initial satisfactory response to therapy, increases in the spectrum and titers of some or all of the antibodies. These increases often became evident months before clinical detection of relapses at the primary or metastatic sites. About 15% of the patients showed a combination of the two patterns discussed; i.e., an initial decline in antibody titers, foreboding a good prognosis, followed by a reversal of the trend toward broadening of the antibody spectrum and increases in titers. The reversal became evident months before clinical recognition of renewed tumor activity. In the remaining small number of patients, the tumor invaded the central nervous system by direct extension from the postnasal space without metastasizing to cervical lymph nodes. The antibody pattern of these cases was not characteristic of NPC because the tumor burden remained small until shortly before death.

The EBV-specific serology has practical aspects in NPC: (a) it serves to monitor patients during remissions because increases in antibody spectrum and titers alert to imminent relapses. They should lead to an intensified search for the site(s) of renewed tumor activity and, if found, to early resumption of therapy; (b) screening of populations at high risk of NPC for IgA antibodies to VCA may identify tumor-bearing individuals before they are sufficiently affected or disturbed to seek medical attention. This has been convincingly demonstrated in large-scale surveys in the People's Republic of China, involving nearly 160,000 individuals over 30 years of age. Among the over 1,000 persons with IgA antibodies to VCA, 48 cases of NPC were found on subsequent clinical examination (presented at the International Conference on Herpesviruses, Atlanta, Georgia, March 17-21, 1980). Since the patients so discovered were in stages ranging from I to IV they in part must have shown clinical symptoms of the disease but had chosen to disregard them; and (c), evidence has been presented that the titers of antibodies reactive in EBV-specific antibody-dependent cellular cytotoxicity also reflect the prognosis of NPC patients; high titers are favorable whereas low titers are not (cf.[22]).

CONCLUDING REMARKS

It is difficult to reconcile the available evidence with a mere passenger role of EBV in BL or NPC. The conclusion

seems inescapable that EBV plays an active role in the
development of both tumors but its exact nature remains to
be elucidated. It is generally thought that cancers do not
arise in a single step but that at least two, and possibly
more events precede their emergence. As to BL, EBV is now
considered to be the initiator, establishing in the course of
primary infections a persistent subpopulation of B lymphocytes which carries viral genomes, has a permanent growth
potential, but remains under control of the host's immune
defenses. If primary EBV infections occur in early infancy,
as observed in Africa, immature lymphocytes may be transformed possibly giving rise to clones of immature EBV-
carrying cells. Only one of these "preneoplastic" cells
needs to be converted by a second event into a fully autonomous, fully malignant cell to give rise to a monoclonal,
EBNA-positive Burkitt's lymphoma. Whatever induces the 8;14
chromosomal translocation might well be the second factor
which seems to affect preferentially, but not exclusively
EBV-transformed lymphoid cells. An unusually extensive
persistent viral infection or holoendemic malaria might have
such a mutagenic effect. Other factors of an immunologic,
genetic, hormonal, nutritional or other nature might singly
or in combinations facilitate the rare final emergence of
the tumor.

Regarding NPC, even more questions remain unresolved. It
is not yet known how the EBV genomes become associated with
the carcinoma cells. While no normal epithelial cells have
been found infectible or transformable by EBV in vitro, the
appropriate type of cells have perhaps not yet been cultured.
Another possibility would be that enveloped virus particles
or viral DNA-containing lymphoid cells, intermittently
present in nasopharyngeal secretions, become fused with
epithelial cells of the postnasal space during infections by
parainfluenza or other viruses known to cause fusion of cells.
Whatever the answer, other factors must play contributing
roles, such as a genetic predisposition among Southern
Chinese, ingestion or inhalation of nitrosamines or other
chemical carcinogens, nutritional deficiencies or a decline
in immunologic surveillance.

It is easy to suggest the use of an EBV vaccine for eradication of BL and NPC but development of a vaccine from a
potentially oncogenic virus faces numerous, difficult
problems. They concern among others, a non-malignant cellular
source of the virus, the assessment of safety and potency of
the vaccine, the duration and degree of protection against
primary infection and establishment of a persistent viral
carrier state, and the logistics of its administration after

the loss of maternal antibodies and <u>before</u> natural infection under the field conditions existing in regions where BL or NPC are most prevalent. Because of the many hurdles to be mastered, progress will not be fast but work toward a satisfactory vaccine should procede with due caution if for nothing else but the prevention of IM in adolescents and young adults because this disease can be extremely severe, very prolonged and occasionally fatal.

REFERENCES

1. Andersson-Anvret M, Forsby N, Klein G, Henle W: Studies on the occurrence of Epstein-Barr virus-DNA in nasopharyngeal carcinomas, in comparison with tumors of other head and neck regions. Int J Cancer 20:486-494, 1977.
2. Epstein MA, Achong BG: The relationship of the virus to Burkitt's lymphoma, in Epstein MA and Achong BG (eds): The Epstein-Barr virus. Berlin, Heidelberg, New York, Springer Verlag, 1979, pp 322-337
3. Epstein MA, Achong BG, Barr YM: Virus particles in cultured lymphoblasts from Burkitt's lymphoma. Lancet 1:702-703, 1964.
4. Henle G, Henle W: Immunofluorescence in cells derived from Burkitt's lymphoma. J Bact 91:1248-1256, 1966.
5. Henle G, Henle W: Epstein-Barr virus-specific IgA serum antibodies as an outstanding feature of nasopharyngeal carcinoma. Int J Cancer 17:1-7, 1976.
6. Henle G, Henle W: The virus as the etiologic agent of infectious mononucleosis, in Epstein MA and Achong BG (eds): The Epstein-Barr virus. Berlin, Heidelberg, New York, Springer Verlag, 1979, pp 297-300
7. Henle G, Henle W, Diehl V: Relation of Burkitt tumor associated herpes-type virus to infectious mononucleosis. Proc Natl Acad Sci (USA)59:94-101, 1968.
8. Henle W, Henle G: Seroepidemiology of the virus, in Epstein MA and Achong BG (eds): The Epstein-Barr virus. Berlin, Heidelberg, New York, Springer Verlag, 1979, pp 61-78
9. Henle W, Henle,G, Gunven P, et al.: Patterns of antibodies to Epstein-Barr virus-induced early antigens in Burkitt's lymphoma. Comparison of dying patients with long-term survivors. J Nat Cancer Inst 50:1163-1173,1973.
10. Henle W, Henle G, Horwitz CA: Epstein-Barr virus-specific diagnostic tests in infectious mononucleosis. Human Pathology 5:551-565, 1974.

11. Henle W, Ho HC, Henle G, et al.:Nasopharyngeal carcinoma: Significance of changes in Epstein-Barr virus-related antibody patterns following therapy. Int J Cancer 20:663-672, 1977.
12. Henle W, Henle G, Lennette ET: The Epstein-Barr Virus. Scientific American 241(1):48-59, 1979.
13. Huang DP, Ho JHC, Henle W, Henle G: Demonstration of EBV-associated nuclear antigens in NPC cells from fresh biopsies. Int J Cancer 14:580-588, 1974.
14. Huang DP, Ho HC, Henle W, et al.: Presence of EBNA in nasopharyngeal carcinoma and control patient tissues related to EBV serology. Int J Cancer 22:266-274, 1978.
15. Judson SC, Henle W, Henle G: A cluster of Epstein-Barr virus-associated American Burkitt's lymphoma. New Engl J Med 297:464-468, 1977.
16. Klein G: The relationship of the virus to nasopharyngeal carcinoma, in Epstein MA and Achong BG (eds): The Epstein-Barr virus. Berlin, Heidelberg, New York, Springer Verlag, 1979, pp 340-350
17. Lindahl T, Klein G, Reedman BM, et al.: Relationship between Epstein-Barr virus (EBV) DNA and the EBV-determined nuclear antigen (EBNA) in Burkitt lymphoma biopsies and other lymphoproliferative malignancies. Int J Cancer 13:764-772, 1974
18. Magrath IT, Pizzo PA, Whang-Peng J, et al.: Characterization of lymphoma-derived cell lines: Comparison of cell lines positive and negative for Epstein-Barr virus nuclear antigen. I. Physical, cytogenetic, and growth characteristics. J Nat Cancer Inst 64:465-476, 1980.
19. Miller G: Experimental carcinogenicity by the virus in vivo, in Epstein MA and Achong BG (eds): The Epstein-Barr virus. Berlin, Heidelberg, New York, Springer Verlag, 1979, pp 352-372
20. Nilsson K: The nature of lymphoid cell lines and their relationship to the virus, in Epstein MA and Achong BG (eds): The Epstein-Barr virus. Berlin, Heidelberg, New York, Springer Verlag, 1979, pp 227-281
21. Old LJ, Boyse EA, Oettgen HF, et al.: Precipitating antibody in human sera to an antigen present in cultured Burkitt's lymphoma cells. Proc Natl Acad Sci (USA)56:1699-1704, 1966.
22. Pearson GR: In vitro and in vivo investigations on antibody-dependent cellular cytotoxicity. Curr Top Microbiol Immunol 80:65-96, 1978.
23. Pope JH: Transformation by the virus in vitro, in Epstein MA and Achong BG (eds): The Epstein-Barr virus. Berlin, Heidelberg, New York, Springer Verlag, 1979, pp 205-223

24. Wolf H, zur Hausen H, Klein G, et al.: Attempts to detect virus-specific DNA sequences in human tumors. III. Epstein-Barr viral DNA in non-lymphoid nasopharyngeal carcinoma cells. Med Microbiol Immunol 161:15-21, 1975.
25. Ziegler JL, Andersson M, Klein G, Henle W: Detection of Epstein-Barr virus DNA in American Burkitt's lymphoma. Int J Cancer 17:701-706, 1976.
26. zur Hausen H: Oncogenic herpesviruses. Biochem Biophys Acta 417:25-53, 1975.

Hepatitis B virus and
primary hepatocellular carcinoma

W. THOMAS LONDON
Senior Research Physician

BARUCH S. BLUMBERG
Associate Director for Clinical Research
The Institute for Cancer Research
The Fox Chase Cancer Center
Philadelphia, Pennsylvania 19111

In the 1950's workers in West and East Africa proposed the
hypothesis that primary hepatocellular carcinoma (PHC) (which
was and is extremely common in large parts of Africa, Asia,
Oceania and elsewhere) followed infection with the agent of
viral hepatitis. It was not possible to test this view at
that time, since the virus could not be detected; but after
the discovery of Australia antigen and its identification
with a hepatitis virus (later designated hepatitis B virus,
HBV) in 1967, it could be directly studied. (See Table 1 for
nomenclature of HBV components and associated antibodies.)
When sensitive tests for the surface antigen of the hepatitis
B virus (HBsAg) were developed, a series of studies in Asia
and Africa consistently showed a much higher frequency of
infection with HBV in patients with PHC than in what appeared
to be appropriate controls. Encouraged by those findings, we
and others in Africa, Asia, Europe and America proceeded to
test the hypothesis that persistent infection with HBV is
necessary for the development of PHC. A substantial body of
data has now been collected, employing a variety of
techniques and disciplines which support this hyothesis, and
these will be reviewed below. (Additional references and

This work was supported by USPHS grants CA-06551, RR-05539
and CA-06927 from the National Institutes of Health and by an
appropriation from the Commonwealth of Pennsylvania.
Address reprint requests to:
Baruch S. Blumberg, M.D.
Institute for Cancer Research
7701 Burholme Avenue
Philadelphia, PA 19111

TABLE 1
Nomenclature of hepatitis B virus components and serology

HBsAg - hepatitis B surface antigen, the major antigenic
           determinant on the surface of the virion of HBV
HBcAg - hepatitis B core antigen, the major antigenic
           determinant on the core of HBV
HBeAg - hepatitis B e antigen, probably a soluble component
           of the core of HBV
anti-HBs - antibody to HBsAg
anti-HBc - antibody to HBcAg
anti-HBe - antibody to HBeAg

HBV-DNA - the core of the virus contains a double stranded,
     circular DNA ($\sim$ 3000 bp) with a single stranded region of
     variable length.
DNA polymerase - the core also contains a DNA polymerase
     capable, _in vitro_, of incorporating nucleotide triphos-
     phate into the DNA genome and filling in the single
     stranded gap.

information will be found in two recent papers[3,12]).
Although some of the crucial studies are not yet completed
and/or published, the evidence is now sufficiently impressive
to conclude that the hypothesis is much more likely to be
supported than rejected; and actions consequent on its
validity, we believe, are warranted. If the hypothesis is
correct, then it would be appropriate to test a consequent
hypothesis; prevention of infection with hepatitis B virus
will, in due course, decrease the incidence of PHC. In 1970
Millman and Blumberg[18] introduced a novel method for the
preparation of a vaccine against hepatitis B virus produced
by extraction of HBsAg from the peripheral blood of hepatitis
carriers. Vaccines prepared on this general principle have
been tested in animals and humans. The results so far are
encouraging, and more extensive field tests of the vaccine
are now in progress. There is also a large body of data on
how HBV is transmitted. Hence, it is now possible to conduct
research on public health strategies for the prevention of
HBV infection; and such studies are in progress. Methods of
transmission will be briefly reviewed later in this paper.
     If the hypothesis (that persistent infection with HBV is
necessary for the development of most cases of PHC) is valid,
then a model is necessary to explain the role of the virus in
the development of PHC. The traditional model for the relation of DNA viruses to cancers holds that portions of the DNA

of the virus enter the DNA of a host cell and transform it to
a cancerous cell. This explains the initiation of a cancer
but does not deal with some of the clinical and epidemiologic
observations on the HBV-PHC relation. We have proposed a
model with novel features that explains the known characteristics of the HBV-PHC relation and that also generates
specific experiments and studies. It is important to stress
that this model has recently been formulated and new studies
are now being devised and executed in an effort to reject it;
that is, it is a model that has not yet been effectively
tested.

By 1970 it had become apparent that HBV had characteristics which were different from other viruses. As a
heuristic device, we suggested a group term, "Icron," to
designate HBV and other infectious agents which might be
found in the future with sufficiently similar characteristics
to be grouped with HBV[4]. The word Icron was derived as an
acronym on the name of the Institute for Cancer Research in
Philadelphia (where our studies had been done) with a neuter
Greek ending.

We predicted that other agents would be found with
characteristics similar to HBV, and later, when the intimate
relation of HBV to PHC became apparent, that Icrons would
also be related to preventable cancers. The molecular
biologists have now described fundamental characteristics of
HBV which allow the definition of these agents in specific
chemical and immunologic terms. The prediction has been
fulfilled in that four "Icron" agents are now known and at
least two of these are related to cancer. These will be
discussed in the final portion of the paper.

EVIDENCE TO SUPPORT THE HYPOTHESIS THAT PERSISTENT INFECTION
WITH HBV IS REQUIRED FOR THE DEVELOPMENT OF MOST CASES
OF PRIMARY HEPATOCELLULAR CARCINOMA (PHC)

1. PHC occurs commonly in the regions of the world where
chronic carriers of HBV are prevalent and much less frequently
in areas where carriers are found at low prevalence. We have
completed several extensive studies in West Africa (Mali,
Senegal), Asia (Korea) and the United States (Philadelphia),
the results of which are consistent with this statement[3].

2. Case-control studies have shown that up to 80% of
patients with PHC living in endemic areas are HBsAg(+) and up
to 87% are anti-HBc(+) (Tables 1 and 2). In the same areas,
controls have much lower frequencies of HBsAg and anti-HBc.

Table 2

		PHC		CONTROLS	
		Hepatitis B surface antigen			
Country	No. tested	% Positive		No. tested	% Positive
Greece	189	55.0		106	4.7
Spain	31	19.3		101	2.0
U.S.A.	34	14.7		56	0
Senegal	291	51.9		100	12.0
Mozambique	29	62.1		35	14.3
Uganda	47	47.0		50	6.0
Zambia	19	63.1		40	7.5
S. Africa	138	59.5		200	9.0
Taiwan	84	54.8		278	12.2
Singapore	156	35.3		1516	4.1
Japan	260	37.3		4387	2.6
Vietnam	61	80.3		94	24.5
		Antibody to hepatitis B core antigen			
Greece	80	70.0		160	31.9
Spain	31	87.0		101	14.8
U.S.A.	33	48.5		56	0
Senegal	291	87.3		100	26.0
S. Africa	76	86.0		103	31.7
Hong Kong	37	70.3		58	36.2

Frequency of hepatitis B surface antigen (HBsAg) and antibody against hepatitis B core (anti-HBc) in patients with PHC and controls. Only studies using radioimmunoassay or a test of equivalent sensitivity for HBsAg and in which controls were included are used. These data have not been corrected for age. (Adapted from Szmuness[29] and Yarrish et al.[34].)

Even in the U.S., patients with PHC have significantly higher frequencies of HBsAg and especially anti-HBc in their blood than controls. That is, serological evidence of persistent infection with HBV is significantly more common in the cases of PHC than in the controls.

3. Most cases (~80%) of PHC arise in a liver already affected with cirrhosis and/or chronic active hepatitis. If chronic hepatitis and cirrhosis are steps on the way to the development of liver cancer, then case-control studies of these two diseases should also show higher prevalences of chronic infection with HBV in the cases compared with appropriate controls. Studies in Africa and Korea have demonstrated that most of the patients with these chronic liver diseases are or have been persistently infected with HBV (HBsAg(+) and/or anti-HBc(+)) (See, for example, Reference 9).

4. Since PHC is a cancer of the liver, one would expect to find signs of HBV infection in the hepatic tissues of patients with the disease. HBV proteins can nearly always be demonstrated in such tissues by histochemical stains or immunological techniques[20]. HBsAg and HBcAg are either not detected or found in small quantities in the tumor cells, themselves, but are found in the non-malignant cells adjacent to the expanding tumor and elsewhere in the liver. These antigens are not found in the livers of uninfected individuals or in persons with anti-HBs in their serum.

5. If persistent HBV infection "causes" PHC, such infection should precede the occurrence of PHC. To test this hypothesis, it is necessary to identify "healthy" chronic carriers of HBV and controls who are not carriers and follow the individuals in such groups over a period of several years for the development of PHC. Two studies of this prospective design are currently in progress; one in Japan directed by Sakuma and his colleagues[25] and a second in Taiwan conducted by Beasley and Lin[1]. In the study in Japan, all employees of the Japan National Railway in the Tokyo district between the ages of 40 and 60 had a blood sample drawn as part of their annual physical examinations. The workers found to have HBsAg in their blood were tested again six months later. If they were still positive, they were designated chronic carriers. Three hundred and forty-one such individuals were identified compared with 17,843 HBsAg(-) non-carriers. Over the succeeding six months to three and one-half years, three cases of PHC occurred among the carriers, whereas none was observed among the non-carriers.

Beasley's study in Taiwan was conducted on male civil servants, also between the ages of 40 and 60. Three thousand carriers were identified in a fashion similar to that used in

Table 3

	No. of Patients	Developed PHC
HBsAg(+)	30	7 (23.3%)
HBsAg(-)	85	5 (5.9%)
Total	115	12 (10.4%)

Development of PHC in Japanese patients with cirrhosis of the liver followed for one to four and a half years. Nearly a quarter of the patients in whom the cirrhosis was associated with HBV but only six percent of those presumably due to other causes developed PHC[22].

Japan. The controls were 3000 HBsAg(-) individuals matched by age, sex, and place of origin in mainland China or Taiwan and an additional 18,000 HBsAg(-) males between the ages of 40 and 60 not matched for place of origin. The subjects have been followed for more than four years. Forty-three cases of PHC have occurred during the follow-up, and all but one of the cases have developed in the chronic carriers. The relative risk of developing PHC was more than 200x greater for carriers than non-carriers (personal communication, Beasley). These two studies provide very strong support for the hypothesis that chronic infection with HBV is etiologically related to PHC.

6. As stated previously (point 3), PHC usually develops in a liver affected by cirrhosis and/or chronic hepatitis. Some investigators have argued that any hepatotoxic agent (e.g. alcohol, liver parasites such as Schistosoma mansoni) that causes cirrhosis is associated with an increased risk of developing PHC and that hepatitis B virus is "just" one more hepatotoxic agent. Therefore, a particularly rigorous test of the hypothesis that chronic infection with hepatitis B virus imparts an increased risk of PHC beyond its role in the production of cirrhosis is to compare the incidence of PHC in patients with cirrhosis who are or are not chronic carriers of HBV. Such a study is being carried out in Japan by Obata and colleagues[22]. Beginning in April 1973, patients with cirrhosis were categorized as HBsAg(+) or (-), carefully evaluated to be sure that they did not have PHC on admission to the study and then followed for the development of PHC. As shown in Table 3, the patients who were HBsAg(+) were at about four times the risk, during a three- to four-year follow-up period, of developing PHC as the HBsAg(-) patients.

7. In populations where HBV is endemic (i.e. sub-Saharan Africa, Asia, Oceania), there is good evidence that many of the chronic carriers arise as a result of infection transmitted from their mothers early in life (at the time of delivery, in the period after birth when the mother and child have considerable close contact, or, perhaps, prenatally). That is, the mothers themselves are chronic carriers and offspring born at times when the mothers are infectious are likely to become chronic carriers[2]. The potential infectiousness of the mothers appears to be associated with the presence of intact hepatitis B virions, DNA polymerase and HBeAg in their peripheral blood. Among members of a population, individuals infected at birth or within the first few months of life will have been chronic carriers of HBV longer than chronic carriers of similar age infected later in life. Therefore, if the duration of being a chronic carrier

is related to the likelihood of developing PHC, one could predict that the mothers of patients with PHC would be more likely to be chronic carriers than the mothers of control individuals of similar age who do not have PHC. We conducted such a study in Dakar, the capital of Senegal in West Africa, and found that about 70 per cent of the mothers of patients with PHC were HBsAg(+) compared with only 14 per cent of the mothers of controls. Even when mothers of PHC patients were compared with mothers of HBsAg(+) carriers without cancer, the mothers of the cancer patients were significantly more likely to be HBsAg(+)[10]. In collaboration with Chung Yong Kim of the National University Hospital and our colleague Hie-Won Hann, we have carried out similar studies in Seoul, South Korea, and the findings are consistent with the African studies[9] (Table 4).

    8. Most studies of the relationship of viruses to cancer have been done in experimental animals or tissue culture systems. It is thought that the genomes of such viruses or DNA transcripts of RNA viruses become integrated into the genomes of host cells and the product of a viral gene is required to produce malignant transformation of the cell.

    Jesse Summers of this Institute, and his collaborators have tested this hypothesis. He isolated HBV DNA and, with the use of DNA polymerase from E. coli, made radioactive copies of the HBV DNA which, in turn, could be used as probes to see whether viral DNA was present in PHC tissue, i.e. would hybridize with DNA in the liver tumor cells. His studies demonstrated viral DNA in the liver cells of patients with PHC who showed evidence of HBV infection in their blood. The viral DNA, however, was located within protein cores and did not appear to be integrated into the genome of the tumor cells. Because it is not certain that a given block of tissue removed at autopsy is free of non-tumor cells and blood, it is difficult to know whether the viral DNA was extracted from malignant or non-malignant hepatocytes. In any event, Summers was unable to demonstrate integration of the HBV genome into any hepatocyte genomes.

    Recently, Marion and Robinson[16] studied a unique tissue culture preparation originally developed by Alexander of South Africa from the liver of an African patient who had died of PHC. They found that part of the genome of HBV was integrated in three places into the DNA of the chromosomes of the Alexander liver cells. Brechot et al.[5] have reported integration of HBV DNA into the tumor cells of a single patient with PHC. It is not clear at present how common such integration is, and future studies will be required to understand the role of this phenomenon.

Table 4

| | SENEGAL | | | | KOREA | | | |
| | Mothers of PHC | | Mothers of CONTROLS | | Mothers of PHC | | Mothers of CONTROLS | |
	No. tested	% Pos	No. tested	% Pos	No. tested	% Pos	No. tested	% Pos
HBsAg	28	72	28	14	9	44	114	4
anti-HBc	28	72	28	14	9	100	46	52
anti-HBs	28	11	28	54	9	44	114	45

Frequency of HBsAg, anti-HBc and anti-HBs in mothers of PHC patients compared to controls. (For Senegal, the controls were mothers of individuals who did not have PHC, but who were usually carriers of HBsAg. For Korea, the controls were other women in the same population[10,9].)

9. The existence of primary carcinoma of the liver, associated with a virus similar to HBV, in Marmota monax is an additional piece of evidence supporting the hypothesis.

Robert Snyder has trapped in the wild and maintained at the Philadelphia Zoological Garden for the past 18 years a colony of Pennsylvania woodchucks (Marmota monax). During this period, he performed postmortem examinations on 102 woodchucks; 23 of these had primary liver cancer, and three had chronic active hepatitis. He further noted that, as in humans with PHC, the tumors in the animals were usually associated with chronic hepatitis and, sometimes, cirrhosis.

Several years ago we had examined the sera of some of these animals for the presence of the surface marker of the hepatitis B virus, HBsAg, but did not detect it. Summers studied these sera again, this time with more rewarding results[28]. He based his investigation on the hypothesis that viruses of the same class as HBV would have a similar nucleic acid structure and similar DNA polymerase. That is, they would contain a circular, double stranded DNA genome with a single stranded region and a DNA polymerase capable of filling in the single stranded region to make a fully double stranded circular DNA. He assayed serum samples from the woodchucks for particles containing a DNA polymerase with this activity; about 15 per cent of the serum samples had such particles. He and his colleagues went on to study three animals in detail: two that had died of liver cancer and one of a myocardial infarction. They found that the two animals with liver tumors had particles in their sera very much like the three types of particles associated with HBV; the animal without tumor did not have such particles. The viral DNA was, as predicted, very similar to HBV in size and structure.

Recently, Werner, from our laboratory, and her colleagues at ICR[33] found cross reactivity between the surface (WHsAg) and core (WHcAg) antigens of the woodchuck hepatitis virus (WHV) and the comparable antigens on human HBV. Antisera against HBcAg precipitates the cores of WHV, and antisera against WHV cores (anti-WHc) precipitates HBcAg. There is also cross reactivity of the surface antigens but it is less than for the core antigens. Antibody against HBsAg (anti-HBs) will not precipitate WHsAg or vice versa, but antibody to WHsAg (anti-WHs) will agglutinate red blood cells coated with HBsAg, and anti-HBs antibodies will agglutinate erythrocytes coated with WHsAg.

A carrier state for WHV in Marmota monax which appears to be analogous to the HBsAg carriers in humans has been found. The frequency of carriers among Pennsylvania and New Jersey woodchuck populations is 10-20%, similar to that found for HBV in several human populations.

Liver cancer in the woodchuck is not what is generally thought of as a laboratory model of a human disease, that is, it was not designed or "created" by an investigator for his purposes; rather it is a naturally occurring disease related to a naturally occurring virus, both of which have remarkable features in common with their human counterparts.

Taken together, these nine bodies of evidence strongly support the hypothesis that persistent infection with HBV is required for the development of most cases of PHC, and we will now proceed to discuss the consequences of accepting the validity of this statement.

PREVENTION OF INFECTION WITH HEPATITIS B VIRUS

The study of the epidemiology and transmission of HBV has been considerably advanced by the availability of several sensitive methods of detecting responses to infection. These include the surface antigen of the virus (HBsAg), antibody against the surface (anti-HBs) and core (anti-HBc) antigens, various subtypes of the surface antigen, an antigen apparently on or in the core (HBeAg) and antibody to this antigen (anti-HBe), and the specific DNA polymerase present in the serum (see Table 1).

There are several methods by which HBV can be transmitted. Blood transfusion has been a major method of transmission, and this has been controlled to a large extent by the testing of donor blood. Contaminated blood can also be transmitted from one individual to another by other means, i.e. injection of drugs (particularly illicit drugs) using contaminated equipment, tatooing, ritual circumcision, shared razors, etc. There is also indirect and direct evidence that there are several insect vectors. Field infection rates of about 1 in 200 have been found for several species of mosquitoes in Africa and mosquito carriage has also been reported elsewhere. African bedbugs (Cimex hemipterus) collected from beds whose main occupants are hepatitis carriers have a high frequency (more than 50%) of HBV carriage and may represent a means of transmission from one to another occupant of the same bed, perhaps through the medium of contaminated bedbug feces. This may be particularly important in mother-child transmission since they often both occupy the same bed when the child is young. The virus has been identified in saliva and it can possibly be spread by the respiratory route[12].

In many communities family transmission appears to be a common form of spread and maternal transmission is particularly important. In completed or nearly completed families there is a much higher frequency of HBV carriers among the offspring of carrier mothers than in the offspring of mothers who are not carriers. However, in our African studies, we have found that children rarely acquire the carrier state until after 4-5 months of age, after which the offspring of the carrier mothers may commonly be infected. The time of maternal transmission may be different in Asia and elsewhere. Among siblings, particularly brothers of carriers, we have found particularly high prevalences (30-50%) of persistent infection.

Although it is generally assumed that HBV is not transmitted by the fecal-oral route, it is possible that the virus may be transmitted in this manner. Small quantities of blood (up to 30 ml/24 hrs) are always excreted from the intestinal tract and in the presence of intestinal parasites or peptic ulcer, larger quantities (>100 ml/24 hrs) may be passed in the feces. HBsAg has not been detected in feces of infected individuals. However, there are constituents of the human intestine, including certain bacteria, which are known to affect the surface antigen in a manner to make it undetect-able by techniques using specific antibodies against surface antigen. It is particularly important to study the problem of fecal transmission in places such as China, where large amounts of human waste are used as agricultural fertilizers.

If the vaccine described in the introduction proves to be both safe and effective, then it can have a major role in prevention programs. Since, at least in Africa, children do not appear to be infected immediately after birth, it may be possible to vaccinate them at 4-6 months of age and provide protection against infection later in their childhood. A variety of conventional public health measures based on the knowledge of viral transmission and used in conjnction with the vaccine could result in effective control measures; and studies on these are planned and are in progress.

In the regions of the world where PHC is common, acute and particularly chronic liver disease due to HBV are major causes of mortality and morbidity. Hence, it is likely that prevention programs could be justified on this basis alone and the effect on prevention of PHC, it if occurs, would be an additional benefit. This situation is different from the proposals for a "cancer vaccine" for cancers which are rare in relation to other causes of mortality and morbidity. In the case of rare cancers, it might be considered unwise to vaccinate a large number of people to protect a very small number of potential victims.

A MODEL FOR THE RELATION OF HEPATITIS B VIRUS
TO PRIMARY HEPATOCELLULAR CARCINOMA

The generally accepted model for how viruses cause cancer
is that DNA from the virus or a DNA transcript of the genome
of a retrovirus is integrated into the genome of the host
cell. A product of an integrated viral gene produces
"malignant transformation" of a cell and all of the progeny
of that cell are cancer cells. There is now evidence from
avian virus-tumor systems that the product of the transforming gene is a protein kinase[6],[11] which preferentially
phosphorylates tyrosine[7]. Robinson's recent observations
that part of the HBV genome is integrated into the DNA of the
Alexander hepatocellular carcinoma cell line and that the
core of HBV contains a protein kinase are consistent with
this model[24]. Although this is an attractive hypothesis, it
does not account for many of the epidemiologic and clinical
characteristics of PHC in humans and woodchucks; for example,
the long interval from the time of infection to the development of clinical cancer (30 to 50 years in humans, 23 to 100
months in woodchucks), the background of chronic liver
disease, the marked male predominance, and several histopathological features. We have proposed another model which does
not deal directly with the transformation event but attempts
to account for the clinical and epidemiological observations.
In the livers of patients with PHC, the tumor cells
contain little or no viral protein (HBsAg or HBcAg), whereas
the non-malignant cells, particularly those adjacent to the
tumor, frequently contain HBsAg in their cytoplasm and cell
membrane and less commonly HBcAg in their nuclei[19],[31]. In
those instances in which HBsAg has been demonstrated in tumor
cells, the antigen was found in only a small percentage of
the total PHC cases studied and only in a few foci within
those tumors. In the serum of PHC patients, HBsAg is often
observed at low levels, lower than the concentrations seen in
chronic carriers and patients with chronic active hepatitis
or cirrhosis[21]. An explanation for this phenomenon is that
as the tumor grows, non-malignant cells which produce HBsAg
are replaced by malignant ones which produce little or no
HBsAg. There is also serological evidence that patients with
PHC are not actively replicating HBV. Even when HBsAg is
present in their blood, they generally lack HBeAg and have
detectable anti-HBe[32].
We propose that in the liver of humans (or animals which
can be infected with related viruses), there are two
populations of cells. The first, and initially much larger
population, readily becomes infected with HBV (or in the

case of woodchucks, WHV), actively synthesizes viral
proteins, and probably replicates infectious virus.
Hereafter, we will refer to these as S (susceptible) cells.
The second population, which may initially be very small, is
relatively resistant to HBV infection. We shall call these R
(resistant) cells. If these cells become infected, they do
not actively replicate virus and they synthesize little or no
viral proteins. In individuals who are chronically infected
with HBV or WHV, S cells have a shortened survival either (or
both) as a result of an immune response (albeit inadequate)
to viral and cellular antigens expressed on the surface of
virus-infected hepatocytes or because cells which are
actively replicating virus, even if they are not lysed by
this process, are metabolically compromised and ultimately
have a shortened life span. In the liver, the stimulus for
cells to divide is death or removal of hepatocytes. Thus, in
individuals with persistent HBV or WHV infection, there would
be continuous cell death and continuous cell regeneration.
These are recognized clinically as chronic hepatitis and
cirrhosis. During this process, the second or resistant cell
population, because of the selective pressure described,
would gradually expand relative to the first. As a result of
random mutation, exposure to environmental carcinogens (e.g.
aflatoxin) or integration of HBV or WHV DNA, or other
"transforming" phenomenon, the dividing liver cells would
give rise to mutant hepatocytes, some of which could be
malignant ("transformed"). The malignant clones with the
best chance of survival would be those that arose from the
resistant cell population. That is, hepatocytes that lacked
receptors for HBV or, once infected, lacked the ability to
express HBV antigens would escape damage from immune
responses to antigens on virus infected cells and metabolic
damage from active viral replication.

In considering this model, the first question that arises
is, What is the origin of the two cell populations? A
simple explanation consistent with cell biology is that R
cells represent an earlier stage in the differentiation of
hepatocytes and S cells a later or fully differentiated
stage. That is, R cells can divide and differentiate into S
cells, but S cells cannot give rise to R cells. Therefore, a
given R cell may divide into two R cells, one R cell and one
S cell, or two S cells. S cells (if they can divide) can
only give rise to other S cells (Figure 1). Since the
selective pressure of persistent HBV infection is applied
only to S cells, R cells will gradually accumulate.
Transformation of an R cell ensures that that R cell will
give rise to other R cells, thereby greatly increasing the

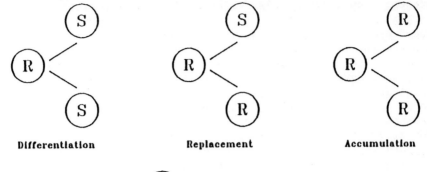

Differentiation   Replacement   Accumulation

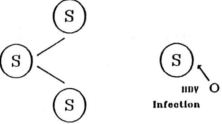

HBV

Infection

Replacement

Figure 1 — Accumulation of resistant (R) cells

S cells are differentiated hepatocytes which are susceptible
to infection with HBV. This compromises their survival and
ability to replicate. R cells are (relatively) resistant to
infection with HBV; they divide in response to the death of
S cells and replace S cells with a probability less than 1.
Therefore, R cells will gradually accumulate in the presence
of persistant HBV (or WHV) infection.

rate of accumulation of a particular clone of R cells. This
process eventually results in a clinically significant
cancer. Even assuming that the transformation event can
occur either in R or S cells, HBV infection would limit the
replication of a transformed S cell and this would not lead
to a clinical cancer (Figure 2).

In humans, newborn infants and fetuses probably do not
replicate HBV. Although umbilical cord bloods of babies born
to HBsAg(+) mothers are sometimes HBsAg(+), blood withdrawn
from these infants in the first few days of life is always
HBsAg(-)[23,26,27]. According to our model, the fetal and
newborn liver is composed of R cells. After birth there is
further cell division and differentiation giving rise to S
cells which can replicate virus. Six weeks of age is about
the earliest that HBsAg has been detected in an infant.

HBV infection in infancy (first six months of life) is
associated with a high probability of persistent infection[23,27], whereas infection later in childhood or in adult
life usually (> 90% of the cases) results in a transient
infection[13]. This would be consistent with the explanation
that early in life there are mostly R cells and few S cells.
After exposure to HBV, the few S cells become infected,
replicate virus, and eventually die. The infection is taking
place, however, at a time when the S population is increasing
and the R population is decreasing in size as a result of
cell division and differentiation. Thus, new susceptible
cells are continuously available to maintain the infection.
Later in life the reverse is true; most cells in the liver
are S and few are R. Infection results in the death of large
numbers of S cells (acute hepatitis) and an insufficient
number of S cells are generated from R cells or uninfected S
cells in the time required to maintain the infection.

A further consequence of this model is that the selective
pressure of HBV infection against S cells must be sustained
in order to maintain the stimulus for regeneration of the
liver and the accumulation of R cells. If the infection
ceases, the selective pressure is removed, R cells will stop
accumulating and the risk of developing a tumor falls
sharply. In humans, males are much more likely to develop
PHC than females, even though male and female babies are
equally exposed to HBV carrier mothers (or siblings)[29,9].
There is evidence that HBV infection is less persistent in
females than males. This has been demonstrated in adults
with chronic renal disease by London and Drew[13] and Szmuness
et al.[30], and there is support for this in free living
populations (Mazzur, S. - unpublished data).

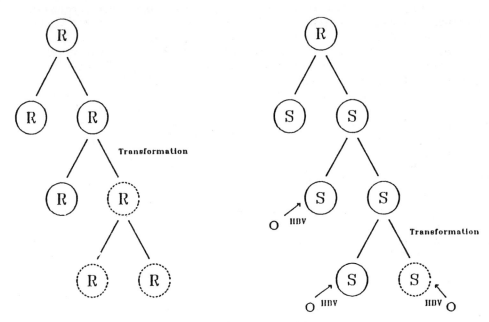

Figure 2 – Development of cancer

The death of S cells stimulates liver regeneration, R cells can give rise to R cells or S cells, but S cells can only divide into other S cells. As a result of a transformation event (integration of a viral genome, spontaneous mutation, or chemical carcinogen induced mutation) either an R cell or an S cell could become malignant. Neoplastic S cells would be selected against by the persistant viral infection whereas transformed R cells would be stimulated to divide by the cell death caused by the viral infection.

This model has some features in common with that proposed
by Emmanuel Farber for chemical carcinogenesis in liver[8]. He
suggested that the initiating event by a carcinogen is to
make a population of cells resistant to the cytotoxicity of
other chemicals (promoters). When exposed to proliferative
stimuli (death of non-initiated cells, partial hepatectomy),
foci of initiated cells would expand and ultimately give rise
to cancers which kill the host animal. If the promoters are
applied for a short time and removed, the foci of initiated
cells gradually disappear and the liver returns to a normal
state.

This proposed cellular model was created to account for
the observed epidemiologic, clinical and pathogenetic
characteristics of the HBV-PHC relation. It can now be used
to generate a series of hypotheses and predictions to test
the validity of the model and its assumptions. It should be
emphasized that the validity of this model does not affect
the conclusions reached in the previous two sections of this
paper.

OTHER VIRUSES RELATED TO HBV WITH A SIMILAR
RELATION TO CANCER (ICRONS)

There are few things that are entirely unique in nature.
As discussed in the introduction, we postulated that there
would be other viruses similar to hepatitis B virus. This
implies that there are other cancers and chronic diseases
that might be preventable in the same manner that we have
proposed for the prevention of chronic liver disease and PHC.
The prediction that there are other Icrons has been fulfilled
by the discovery of three other viruses, woodchuck hepatitis
virus (WHV, described in detail above)[28]; ground squirrel
hepatitis virus (GSHV)[15] and duck hepatitis B virus (DHBV)[17],
all of which have many virological and epidemiologic similarities to HBV. WHV is associated with cancer of the liver, and
DHBV has been localized in the liver. Cancer of the liver is
common in domestic ducks from several regions of China.

Characteristics of these viruses are shown in Table 5
where they are compared to the "type specimen," that is, HBV.
The characteristics listed in the tables can be used in the
search for other viruses that might fall in this group. An
important feature of Icrons and one of the earliest known
characteristics of "Australia antigen" is the presence of
large amounts of surface and other antigens in the peripheral
blood of individuals who are carriers. Carriers may be very
common in some (but not all) populations of the species in

Table 5. Characeristics of Icrons

	VIRUS			
Particles	HBV	WHV	GSHV	DHBV
Present in large quantities in blood	+	+	+	+
Virion structure double shell	+	+	+	+
Virion diameter, nm	40–45	40–45	47	40
Surface antigen particle, nm	20–25	20–25	15–25	35–60
Elongated surface antigen, length in nm	>500	>500	>750	not seen
Core, nm	27	27	∿ 27	27

DNA

	HBV	WHV	GSHV	DHBV
Circular	+	+	+	+
Double and single stranded	+	+	+	+
DNA polymerase	+	+	+	+
Nucleotides (number)	3182	3300	3200	3000
Homology with HBV, %	100	3–5	?	?

Antigens

	HBV	WHV	GSHV	DHBV
Surface (HBV, cross-reacting %)	HBsAg	WHsAg (0.1–1)	?	DHBsAg
Core (HBV, cross-reacting %)	HBcAg	WHcAg (5–10)	?	DHBcAg
e	+	?	?	?
surface subtypes	yes	?	?	?

Responses to infection

	HBV	WHV	GSHV	DHBV
Carrier state, % in populations	0.1– 20	0–20	0–50	7–18
anti-surface antigen, % in population	anti-HBs 0–50	anti-WHs 25	?	?
anti-core antigen, % in population	anti-HBc 0–60	anti-WHc	?	?
anti-e antigen	+	?	?	?

Clinical conditions

	HBV	WHV	GSHV	DHBV
acute hepatitis	+	?	?	?
chronic hepatitis	+	+	?	?
cirrhosis	+	?	?	?
PHC	+	+	?	?

Male-female ratios

	HBV	WHV	GSHV	DHBV
Carriers	M>F	M∿F	M∿F	?
Acute hepatitis	M>F	?	?	?
Chronic hepatitis	M>F	?	?	?
PHC	M≫F	?	?	?

Hepatitis B virus (HBV) is compared to woodchuck hepatitis virus (WHV), ground squirrel hepatitis virus (GSHV) and duck hepatitis B virus (DHBV). The viruses are found respectively in humans (Homo sapiens) eastern woodchucks (Marmota monax), Beechey ground squirrel (Spermophilus beecheyi) and domestic ducks of various breeds. The symbol ∿ indicates approximately, and ? that information is not available.

which the virus is found. For example, up to 50% of certain Beechey ground squirrel population samples studied were infected with GSHV. Many of the individuals who are not carriers will have antibody against surface antigen, and others may have antibody against the core antigen. In human populations residing in high incidence areas, more than 70% of individuals will eventually develop anti-HBs. This means that normal individuals may be screened to find a virus (or an antibody against it) that causes serious disease in some of those infected with the virus. Since the frequency of infected individuals is very high in many of the populations of the species, this could facilitate the discovery of viruses. Suscepted sera can be screened for particulate DNA polymerase or for the antigens or antibodies found in one or more of the viruses (e.g. HBsAg, WHsAg, HBcAg, WHcAg, DHBsAg, etc. or antibodies against these).

The objective of this research, then, would be the discovery of additional Icron-class viruses and their disease associations. A clue to the disease association could be obtained by determining which organ or organs harbor the virus in the normal study subjects.

REFERENCES

1. Beasley RP, Lin CC: Hepatoma risk among HBsAg carriers. Am J Epidemiol 108:247, 1978.
2. Blumberg BS: Australia antigen. A review with comments on maternal effect. Bull Acad Med Toronto 45:45-51, 1972.
3. Blumberg BS, London WT: Hepatitis B virus and primary hepatocellular carcinoma: The relation of "Icrons" to cancer. Seventh Cold Spring Harbor Conference on Cell Proliferation, September 4-9, 1979 (in press).
4. Blumberg BS, Millman I, Sutnick AI, London WT: The nature of Australia antigen and its relation to antigen-antibody complex formation. J Exp Med 134:320-329, 1971.
5. Brechot C, Pourcel C, Louise A, Rain B, Tiollais P: Presence of integrated hepatitis B virus DNA sequences in cellular DNA of human hepatocellular carcinoma. Nature, 1980 (in press).
6. Collett MS, Erikson RL: Protein kinase activity associated with the avian sarcoma virus s r c gene product. Proc Natl Acad Sci USA 75:2021-2024, 1978.

7. Eckhart W, Hutchinson MA, Hunter T: An activity phosphorylating tyrosine in polyoma T antigen immunoprecipitates. Cell 18:925-933, 1979.

8. Farber E: Experimental liver carcinogenesis: a perspective, in Remmer H, Bolt HM, Banasch P, Popper H (eds): Primary Liver Tumors. Lancaster, U.K., MTP Press Ltd., 1978, pp. 357-375.

9. Hann HL, London WT, Whitford P, Kim CY, Blumberg BS: Hepatitis B virus and primary hepatocellular carcinoma: Family studies in Korea. Proc Am Soc Clin Oncol 20: C-588, 1979. Abstract.

10. Larouze B, London WT, Saimot G, et al.: Host responses to hepatitis B infection in patients with primary hepatic carcinoma and their families. A case/control study in Senegal, West Africa. Lancet 2:534-538, 1976.

11. Levinson AD, Oppermann H, Levintow L, et al.: Evidence that the transforming gene of avian sarcoma virus encodes a protein kinase associated with a phosphoprotein. Cell 15:561-572, 1978.

12. London WT, Blumberg BS: A strategy for cancer prevention: Hepatitis B virus and primary cancer of the liver. Scientific American, 1980 (in press).

13. London WT, Drew JS: Sex differences in response to hepatitis B infection among patients receiving chronic dialysis treatment. Proc Natl Acad Sci USA 74:2561-2563, 1977.

14. London WT, Sutnick AI, Blumberg BS: Australia antigen and acute viral hepatitis. Ann Intern Med 70:55-59, 1969.

15. Marion PL, Oshiro LS, Regnery DC, et al.: A virus in Beechey ground squirrels which is related to hepatitis B virus in man. Proc Natl Acad Sci USA 77:2941-2945, 1980.

16. Marion PL, Robinson WS: Hepatitis B virus in a human hepatocellular carcinoma liver. Seventh Cold Spring Harbor Symposium on Cell Proliferation, September 4-9, 1979 (in press).

17. Mason WS, Seal G, Summers J: A virus of Pekin ducks with structural and biological relatedness to human hepatitis B virus. J Virol 1980 (in press).

18. Millman I, Blumberg BS: Perspectives de la vaccination contre le virus de l'hepatite B. Rev Prat 28:1943-1951, 1978.

19. Nayak NC, Dhark A, Sachdeva R, et al.: Association of human hepatocellular carcinoma and cirrhosis with hepatitis B virus surface and core antigens in the liver. Int J Cancer 20:643-654, 1977.

20. Nayak NC, Sachdeva R: Localization of hepatitis B
    surface antigen in conventional paraffin sections of the
    liver: Comparison of immunofluorescence, immunoperoxi-
    dase, and orcein staining methods with regard to their
    specificity. Am J Path 81:479-492, 1975.
21. Nishioka K, Mayumi M, Okochi K, et al.: Natural history
    of Australia antigen and hepatocellular carcinoma, in
    Nakahara W, Hirayama T, Nishioka K, Sugano H (eds):
    Analytic and Experimental Epidemiology of Cancer. Tokyo,
    University of Tokyo, 1973, pp. 137-146.
22. Obata H, Hayashi N, Motoike Y, et al.: A prospective
    study on the development of hepatocellular carcinoma from
    liver cirrhosis with persistent hepatitis B virus
    infection. Int J Cancer 25:741-747, 1980.
23. Okada K, Yamada T, Miyakawa Y, Mayumi M: Hepatitis B
    surface antigen in the serum of infants after delivery
    from asymptomatic carrier mothers. J Pediat 87:360-363,
    1975.
24. Robinson W: The HBcAg/anti-HBc system and DNA
    polymerase, in Proceedings of the Vth International
    Congress of Liver Diseases. Basel, Switzerland,
    October 5-7, 1979 (in press).
25. Sakuma K, Ohtake H, Okada K, Mayumi M: Studies in Japan
    on railroad workers. Personal communication. (Hepatitis
    Scientific Memorandum.)
26. Schweitzer IL: Vertical transmission of the hepatitis B
    surface antigen. Am J Med Sci 270:287-291, 1975.
27. Stevens CE, Beasley RP, Tsui J, Lee W: Vertical
    transmission of hepatitis B antigen in Taiwan. N Engl J
    Med 292:771-774, 1975.
28. Summers J, Smolec JM, Snyder R: A virus similar to human
    hepatitis B virus associated with hepatitis and hepatoma
    in woodchucks. Proc Natl Acad Sci USA 75:4533-4537,
    1978.
29. Szmuness W: Hepatocellular carcinoma and hepatitis B
    virus: Evidence for a causal association. Prog Med
    Virol 24:40-69, 1978.
30. Szmuness W, Harley EJ, Ikram H, Stevens C: Socio-
    demographic aspects of the epidemiology of hepatitis B,
    in Vyas GN, Cohen SN, Schmid R (eds): Philadelphia,
    Franklin Institute Press, 1978, pp. 297-320.
31. Thung SN, Gerber MA, Sarno E, Popper H. Distribution of
    five antigens in hepatocellular carcinoma. Lab
    Invest 41:101-105, 1979.
32. Werner BG, Murphy BL, Maynard JE, Larouze B: Anti-e in
    primary hepatic carcinoma. Lancet 1:696, 1976.

33. Werner BG, Smolec JM, Snyder R, Summers J: Serological relationship of woodchuck hepatitis virus to human hepatitis B virus. J Virol 32:314–322, 1979.
34. Yarrish RL, Werner BG, Blumberg BS: Association of hepatitis B virus infection with hepatocellular carcinoma in American patients. 1979 (in preparation).

Radiation Hazards

Radiation Hazards

ARTHUR C. UPTON

Director and Chairman
Institute of Environmental Medicine
New York University Medical Center
New York, New York

INTRODUCTION

It is almost 80 years since the carcinogenic effects of ionizing radiation were first recorded. In the interim, such effects have been documented extensively in human and animal populations, under widely differing conditions of exposure. The types of growths induced, their distribution in time, their relation to the dose received, and the influence of age, sex, and other physiological factors on their occurrence have been characterized to a greater degree than with cancers caused by any other environmental agent. our experience with radiation-induced neoplasia leads to conclusions that have far-reaching implications for cancer in general.

No attempt will be made in this report to review radiation carcinogenesis comprehensively or in detail, especially since certain aspects of the subject are to be dealt with in a later session during this conference. Instead, this survey is intended merely to provide a broad overview of the carcinogenic risks of low-level radiation and to highlight salient questions remaining to be resolved.

HISTORICAL HIGHLIGHTS

Within a decade after Roentgen's discovery of the X-ray, in 1895, the first cancer attributed to radiation was reported to arise on the hand of a radiologist as a complication of radiation dermatitis. Within the next few years dozens of similar cases were described. Other early examples of radiation-

This manuscript was prepared under support by Grant #ES00260 from the National Institutes of Environmental Health Sciences and Grant #CA13343 from the National Cancer Institute.

induced cancer include osteosarcomas and cranial sinus carcinomas associated with radium poisoning in luminous dial paint-
ers, lung cancers in pitchblende and uranium miners, and
leukemia in pioneer American radiologists (see reviews by
Furth and Lorenz, 1954; Upton, 1975).

Confirming and extending these findings in human beings
were early experiments on the carcinogenic effects of radiation in laboratory animals. By 1935, a variety of tumors had
been reported in rats, mice, rabbits and guinea pigs following
their exposure to X-rays or radium (Upton, 1975).

While it became evident in the early part of this century
that large, tissue-destructive amounts of ionizing radiation
were carcinogenic, the possibility that smaller amounts might
also increase the risk of cancer was not given serious credence until 50 years later, when analysis of the leukemia
incidence in atomic-bomb survivors, radiologists, and certain
groups of irradiated patients led E. B. Lewis (1957) to postulate that the frequency of the disease varied as a linear,
nonthreshold function of the radiation dose. Moreover, by
extrapolating the postulated dose-incidence curve down to zero
dose, Lewis inferred that 10-20 per cent of "spontaneous"
leukemias in the general population might be attributable to
natural background radiation.

In suggesting that carcinogenic effects could result from
natural background irradiation, Lewis contradicted the prevailing views of the day, which envisioned genetic effects to
be the only significant hazard of low-level irradiation. Because Lewis's hypothesis was sobering as well as iconoclastic,
it provoked sharp debate on the dose-incidence relation, which
has continued up to the present time. The salient data now
available are summarized briefly below.

HUMAN DOSE-INCIDENCE DATA

Cancers of a growing variety of types are known to be increased in incidence in irradiated populations (Table 1). The
magnitude of the increase varies with the type of cancer, the
conditions of irradiation, the age and sex of the exposed population, and the time after exposure. The data come predominantly from observations at moderate-to-high doses of radiation and in few instances are available over a wide enough
range of doses to allow any inferences about the shape of the
dose-incidence curve. Hence, the carcinogenic risks of low-
level radiation can be estimated only by extrapolation from
observations at higher doses and dose rates, based on unproven
assumptions about the nature of the dose-incidence relation
and the mechanisms of carcinogenesis.

TABLE 1

Cancers Linked to Radiation in Particular Populations[+]

Type of Cancer	Atom bomb radiation			Medical radiation											Occupational radiation			
	Japanese atom bomb survivors	Marshall Islanders	Nuclear test participants	Ankylosing spondylitis (x-ray)	Ankylosing spondylitis (radium)	Benign pelvic disease	Benign breast disease	Multiple chest fluoroscopy	Tinea capitis (children)	Enlarged thymus (infants)	Thorotrast	Thyroid cancer (I-131)	In utero x-ray	Diagnostic x-ray	Radium dial painters	Radiologists	Uranium & other miners	Nuclear workers
Leukemia	***		*	***	*	**					***		***	*		***		*
Thyroid	***	**							**	**		*						
Female breast	***						***	***		*								*
Lung	***			***													***	
Bone	**			*	***										***			
Stomach	**			**														
Esophagus				**														
Bladder	**																	
Lymphoma (incl. mult. myeloma)	**			**							**					**		*
Brain									*			*				**		
Uterus					*													
Cervix	*																	
Liver	*										***					***		
Skin	*								**	**						**	**	
Salivary gland									**	**	*							
Kidney				*														
Pancreas	*																	*
Colon						**												
Small intestine						**									*			
Rectum																		

+ Strong associations are indicated by ***, meaningful but less striking associations by **, and suggestive but unconfirmed associations by *

From Interagency Task Force, 1979

Leukemia

All types of leukemia except chronic lymphatic leukemia
have been observed to be increased in incidence in irradiated
populations. The relative frequencies of the different types
and their distributions in time after irradiation vary, depending on sex, age at irradiation, dose, quality of radiation, and other exposure factors (NAS/BEIR, 1972, 1980; UN,
1977). In acutely irradiated populations, the overall excess
of leukemia appears within 25 years and subsides 10-20 years
after exposure.

In the most heavily irradiated atomic-bomb survivors the
cumulative incidence during the first 28 years after irradiation is 10-20 times higher than normal, with the largest excess in those who were either children or elderly adults at
the time of exposure. The excess rises more steeply with the
dose at Hiroshima than at Nagasaki and the curve for Hiroshima
appears linear while that for Nagasaki is compatible with
either a linear or a curvilinear regression (Figure 1). Since
the radiations at Hiroshima included a large component of fast
neutrons, while those at Nagasaki were composed almost entirely of gamma rays, the differences between the leukemia rates
in the two cities have been inferred to reflect a high relative biological effectiveness (RBE) of fast neutrons for
leukemia induction, such as has been observed in experimental
animals (Upton *et al.* 1970; NAS/BEIR, 1980). The data for
both cities are consistent with a linear-quadratic function of
the form:

$$I_D = C + aD_g + bD_g^2 + cD_n$$

where I is the annual incidence at dose D, C is the incidence
at zero dose, D_g is the gama ray component of dose D, D_n is
the neutron component of dose D, and a, b, and c are constants,
with the values: a = 0.99, b = 0.0085, and c = 27.5 (NAS/BEIR,
1980).

The excess of leukemia in irradiated spondylitics compares
closely with that in atomic-bomb survivors, with 29.15 excess
leukemia deaths in 112,970 person-years of followup. The
excess, related to an estimated mean marrow dose of about 214
rads, corresponds to an absolute risk of 1.2 leukemia deaths
per 10^6 person-years per rad (NAS/BEIR, 1980).

A comparable excess of leukemia per unit dose has been observed in other irradiated populations, with the exception of
those exposed to diagnostic radiation *in utero*. In the latter,
the data point to an excess of approximately 25 fatal leukemias
per million children per year per rad, from birth to age 12;

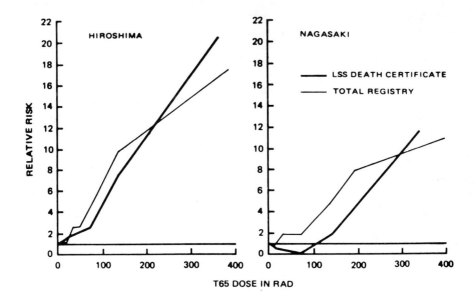

Figure 1.   Dose response for leukemia mortality in atomic-
             bomb survivors of Hiroshima and Nagasaki. Data
             based on LSS sample and death certificates,
             1950-1974, are compared with those based on
             atomic-bomb survivors' survey and total leukemia
             registry, 1946-1974. (Reprinted with permission
             from Beebe et al., 1978.)

however, the contribution of factors other than radiation to
the causation of the disease in these children remains to be
excluded (NAS/BEIR, 1980).

Cancer of the Breast

    Although its high sensitivity was unsuspected until about
15 years ago, the female breast now appears to be more susceptible to radiation carcinogenesis than any other tissue in
the adult, if judged on the basis of absolute, as opposed to
relative, risks. The excess carcinomas of the breast in
atomic-bomb survivors, women receiving radiation therapy to
the breast for acute postpartum mastitis or other benign diseases, and women subjected to repeated fluoroscopic examination of the chest during treatment of pulmonary tuberculosis
with artificial pneumothorax approximate 3-10 cases per million person-years per rad, depending on age at irradiation

(NAS/BEIR, 1980). In general, sensitivity appears to decrease
with increasing age at exposure. The minimum latent period
also appears to be age-dependent: the excess cancer in women
irradiated during their teens took longer to appear than that
in women irradiated after middle age, such that the radiation-
induced breast cancers resemble other breast cancers in age
distribution (NAS/BEIR, 1980).

The dose-incidence relationship appears virtually the same
in a-bomb survivors as in irradiated mastitis patients and
multiply fluoroscoped women, in spite of marked differences
between the groups in duration of exposure (Boice *et al*. 1979).
This fact, coupled with the shapes of the dose-incidence
curves in the low-to-intermediate dose range, supports the interpretation that the incidence of this form of cancer varies
as a linear, nonthreshold function of the dose (NAS/BEIR,
1980).

Carcinoma of the Thyroid Gland

An increased incidence of thyroid neoplasm has been observed in atomic-bomb survivors, Marshall Islanders accidentally
exposed to nuclear fallout from a weapons test, and persons
treated with X-rays to the head and neck region for various
non-neoplastic conditions (Table 1). The lesions include benign adenomas as well as papillary and follicular adenocarcinomas, but no significant numbers of more malignant forms of
thyroid cancer. Hence, mortality from the disease has been
minimal to date (UN, 1977; NAS/BEIR, 1980).

The increase in incidence appears within 10-15 years after
exposure and persists in one study for the full 35 years of
follow-up (Hempelmann, 1977). The excess is evident at doses
in the 6-20 rad range and increases with dose up to 1500 rads,
in keeping with a linear, nonthreshold regression corresponding to about 4 carcinomas and 12 adenomas per million person-
years per rad (NAS/BEIR, 1980). In women the excess is about
three times as large as in men (NAS/BEIR, 1980). On the basis
of relative risk, as opposed to absolute risk, the thyroid
appears more susceptible to radiation carcinogenesis than any
other organ, except the bone marrow (NAS/BEIR, 1980).

Other Neoplasms

In addition to the above types of cancer, other neoplasms
have occurred at increased rates in atomic-bomb survivors and
other irradiated populations (Table 1). Because the induction
period for solid tumors is substantially longer, in general,
than that for leukemias, the ratio of such tumors to leukemias
increases with time after irradiation, as does the diversity

of tumor types. On the basis of findings in the atomic-bomb
survivors, irradiated spondylitics, and American radiologists,
the cumulative numbers of excess deaths in these populations
from all cancers other than leukemia are expected ultimately
to exceed the numbers of deaths from leukemia by a factor of
3-6 (UN, 1977; NAS/BEIR, 1980). From comparison of the relative frequencies of the various cancers, expressed in terms of
the excess of each type of cancer per unit dose, it is evident
that different tissues and organs vary markedly in their susceptibility to radiation carcinogenesis, for reasons yet to be
determined (Table 2).

TABLE 2
Lifetime Cancer Risks of Low-Level Radiation[a]

Site	Risk per million person-rems	
	Fatal Cancers	Incident Cancers
Bone marrow(leukemia)	15-40	20-60
Thyroid	10	20-150
Breast(women only)	50	50-200
Lung	25-50	25-100
Brain Stomach Liver Colon Salivary glands	10-15 (each)	15-25
Bone Esophagus Small Intestine Urinary bladder Pancreas Lymphatic tissue	2-5 (each)	5-10
Skin	1	15-20
Total(both sexes)	100-250	300-400

[a]From NAS (1972, 1980), UN (1977), Jablon and Bailar (1980).

EXPERIMENTAL DOSE-INCIDENCE DATA

Carcinogenesis in Laboratory Animals

A wide variety of neoplasms has been induced by irradiation
in experimental animals, comprising growths of virtually all

histologic types (UN, 1977). Among the different neoplasms, the dose-incidence relationships vary widely in shape and in slope, owing in part to differences in the mechanisms of carcinogenesis. In the induction of some neoplasms, for example-- such as ovarian tumors and thymic lymphomas in the mouse, hair follicle adenomas in the rat, and osteosarcomas in the dog-- the killing of certain types of cells seems to play a key role in promoting neoplasia, whereas the killing of cells may inhibit tumorigenesis in other instances (UN, 1977). As yet, too little is known about the relevant mechanisms of carcinogenesis to explain fully the diversity of observed dose-incidence patterns.

In few instances has the dose-incidence relation been determined over a wide range of doses, extending down into the region below 50 rads, or has the influence of dose rate and radiation quality been well characterized. In the absence of further information, therefore, the effects of low-level irradiation on the incidence of most experimentally induced neoplasms will remain highly uncertain.

On the basis of the limited evidence that is available, the following generalizations can be made: 1) high-LET radiations (alpha particles, protons, fast neutrons) are more carcinogenic per unit dose than low-LET radiations (X-rays, gamma rays, beta-radiations), at least in the low-to-intermediate dose range; 2) the excess of most types of neoplasms per unit dose decreases with decreasing dose and dose rate of low-LET radiations, but decreases less, if at all, (or may even increase) with decreasing dose and dose rate of high-LET radiations; 3) at high dose rates, the dose-incidence curve for most neoplasms passes through a maximum at intermediate-to-high doses and decreases with further increase in the dose; 4) although radiation is carcinogenic in essentially all mammals, susceptibility to radiation carcinogenesis varies widely among species, strains, organs, tissues, and cells, for reasons which are poorly known; 5) the induction of neoplasms may be enhanced or inhibited after irradiation by hormonal, immunological, or other factors modifying the expression of radiation-induced carcinogenic changes; 6) the neoplasms induced by irradiation are indistinguishable from those arising through other causes (U.N., 1977).

The mechanisms of radiation carcinogenesis at high dose levels involve such a diversity of interacting effects that no single dose-incidence function can be expected to apply to all types of neoplasms. However, if the carcinogenic effects of low-level radiation in a given organ are postulated to result primarily from the neoplastic transformation of one of its cells by damage to the genes or chromosomes of the affected cell, then a function of the following form can be predicated on radiobiological grounds:

$$I_D + (C + aD + bD^2)e^{-(pD + qD^2)}$$

where I_D is the incidence of neoplasms at dose D, and a, b, p, and q are constants (Upton, 1977). The values of the coefficients a and b are such for low-LET radiation that the linear term (aD) predominates at low doses and low dose rates, and the quadratic term (bD^2) at high doses and high dose rates. With high-LET radiation, on the other hand, the values are such that the linear term predominates at all doses and dose rates. The values of the coefficients p and q are such as to account for the saturation of the dose-incidence curve at high doses. Although the above expression must be assumed to be a gross over-simplification of the dose-incidence relationship, for the reasons stated, it conforms surprisingly well to some experimental dose-incidence data (eg., Robinson and Upton, 1978).

Cell transformation *In Vitro*

The transforming effects of ionizing radiation on cells *in vitro*, which can be elicited in human as well as animal cells (Borek, 1980), are consistent with its carcinogenic effects *in vivo*. Although studies of radiation-induced neoplastic transformation *in vitro* are still limited in number and scope, they represent a promising approach for quantifying effects on cells in the low-to-intermediate dose range, for exploring interactions between radiation and other factors influencing neoplasia, and for investigating mechanisms of carcinogenesis at the cellular level. To the extent that cells transformed *in vitro* acquire the capacity to proliferate indefinitely and to produce progressively growing tumors on innoculation into appropriate test animals, neoplastic transformation *in vitro* may be considered analagous in certain respects to carcinogenesis *in vivo*.

Studies on the dose-effect relationship for transformation *in vitro* are few in number as yet, and their methodology is still in early stages of development. Nevertheless, several important conclusions already emerge from relevant experiments with Syrian hamster embryo (Borek, 1979a) and C3H 10T½ mouse embryo (Little *et al* 1979; Elkind and Han, 1979; Lloyd, *et al* 1979) fibroblasts: 1) the percentage of cells transformed increases with increasing dose, reaching a plateau in the region of 150-400 rads of x-rays; 2) the transforming effectiveness of high-LET radiation is greater than that of low-LET radiation; 3) depending on the cell system used, transforming

effects are detectable with doses as low as 0.1 rad of fast
neutrons or 1 rad of x-rays; 4) the rate of transformation
varies, depending on the cell system, radiation dose, and culture conditions used; 5) the rate of transformation may be
modified by agents that promote or inhibit carcinogenesis *in
vivo*; 6) a dose of 50-300 rads of x-rays divided into two
fractions separated by an interval of five hours can cause a
higher rate of transformation than the same dose delivered in
a single exposure (Borek, 1979b; Elkind and Han, 1979).

Although research to date has not succeeded in defining the
subcellular lesions involved in transformation, it has laid
the foundation for incisive and analytical studies which
should advance our knowledge significantly in the not-too-
distant future. The information available thus far points
strongly to DNA damage as the initiating event in radiation-
induced cell transformation, in keeping with data on the
transforming effects of chemical carcinogens (Miller, 1979).

Assessment of the Risks of Low-Level Radiation

Existing evidence is insufficient to define unambigously
the dose-incidence relationship for low-level radiation carcinogenesis, or to exclude the possible existence of a threshold at low dose levels. Nevertheless, the growing body of
information from observations on irradiated human populations,
experimental animals, and cultured cells argues increasingly
against the existence of a threshold. In this respect, the
observations on carcinogenesis are consistent with findings
on dose-incidence relationships for radiation-induced mutagenesis, chromosome damage, and cell killing (U.N., 1977;
Furcinitti and Todd, 1979).

Although present knowledge may not justify the assumption
of a threshold for radiation carcinogenesis, the biological
effectiveness of low-LET radiation generally decreases with
decreasing dose and dose rate for carcinogenic effects in laboratory animals, as for most other biological effects, including the induction of mutations and chromosome aberrations
(U.N., 1977). Hence, in the absence of evidence to the contrary, a linear-quadratic model may be more appropriate than a
linear model for use in estimating risks of low-LET radiation
at low doses by extrapolation from observations at higher
doses (Brown, 1977; Upton, 1977; U.N., 1977; NAS/BEIR, 1980).

With human breast cancer, the data are more consistent with
a linear model than with a linear-quadratic model; however,
the data for most other types of human cancer are indetermin-
ate. In view of uncertainties about the appropriate model to
use in estimating the overall cancer risks at low doses, the
members of the NAS/BEIR Committee were divided in their

opinions, as is reflected in the wide range of estimates presented in their 1980 report (NAS/BEIR, 1980).

The estimates shown in Table 2, which represent values intermediate between extremes of the ranges reported by the U.N. (1977) and NAS/BEIR (1980) Committees, may be used as an interim basis for assessing the cancer risks associated with various types of radiation exposure. Such estimates have been useful in evaluating the risk-benefit relationship in mass mammographic screening for early detection of breast cancer (Upton, *et al* 1977; Shore, 1979) and in assessing the adequacy of existing radiation exposure limits for radiation workers and the public (IRCP, 1977). According to such estimates, it has been calculated that exposure of the general population to natural background radiation and radiation from man-made sources may account for about 2-3 percent of the existing cancer burden (Table 3). Such a small contribution is not measurable with existing epidemiological techniques.

TABLE 3
Estimates of Contribution of Radiation Exposure to Burden of Fatal Cancer in the U.S. Population[a]

Source of Radiation	Annual Dose (person-rems)	Lifetime Cancer Mortality Commitment (Number of Fatal Cancers)
Natural background	20,000,000	5,000
Healing arts (diagnostic X-rays)	17,000,000 (14,800,000)	4,250 (3,670)
Nuclear weapons fallout	1,300,000	375
Technologically enhanced natural radiation (mining + milling, etc.)	1,000,000	250
Nuclear energy	30,000	9
Consumer products	6,000	1.5
Total	39,345,000	<10,000[b]

[a] From Jablon and Bailar, 1980.

[b] Value = 2.5% of total natural cancer mortality per year (400,000).

   While some observers have critized the above estimates as
being too low, on the basis of what they have interpreted to
be disproportionately heightened cancer rates in certain
groups of radiation workers (Mancuso et al 1970; Najarian and
Colton, 1978; Gofman, 1979), children exposed to nuclear fallout from Nevada weapons tests (Lyon et al 1979), and patients
exposed to diagnostic irradiation (Bross and Natarajan, 1972,
1977), their contentions have been judged to deserve little
credence without further evidence (NAS/BEIR, 1980). Their
claims have, nevertheless, aroused public concern about the
adequacy of existing radiation protection policies, and safety
measures (Interagency Task Force, 1979).
   There is thus clearly need for continuing research on the
carcinogenic hazards of low-level radiation, both through
follow-up of irradiated human populations and through investigation of appropriate experimental models. It is entirely
conceivable that, because of cell killing and other forms of
radiation injury at high doses and high dose rates, the risks
of carcinogenic effects at low doses may be larger than those
predicted on the basis of existing extrapolations (Table 2),
especially if some of the effects at low doses occur selectively in subpopulations of unusually high sensitivity.
These and other issues cannot be resolved without further
study of the relevant mechanisms of carcinogenesis, as well
as the relevant dose-effect relationships (Land, C.E., 1980).

                              REFERENCES

Beebe, G.W., H. Kato, and C.E. Land. Studies of mortality of
   the A-bomb survivors. 6. Mortality and radiation dose,
   1950-1974. Radiat. Res. 75:138-201, 1978.
Boice, J.D., Jr., C.E. Land, R.E. Shore, J.E. Norman, and M.
   Tokunaga. Risk of breast cancer following low-dose exposure. Radiology 131:589-597, 1979.
Borek, C. Malignant transformation in vitro: criteria,
   biological markers, and application to environmental
   screenings of carcinogens. Radiat. Res. 70:209-232, 1979a.
Borek, C. Neoplastic transformation following split doses of
   X-rays. Br. J. Radiol. 50:845-846, 1979b.
Borek, C. X-ray-induced in vitro neoplastic transformation of
   human diploid cells. Nature 283:776-778, 1980.
Bross, I.D.J., and N. Natarajan. Leukemia from low-level
   radiation. Identification of susceptible children. N. Engl.
   J. Med. 287:107-110, 1972.
Bross, I.D.J., and N. Natarajan. Genetic damage from diag-
   nostic radiation. J. Amer. Med. Assoc. 237:2399-2401, 1977.

Elkind, M.M., and A. Han. Neoplastic transformation and dose fractionation: Does repair of damage play a role? Radiat. Res. 79:233-240, 1979.

Furth, J. and E. Lorenz. Carcinogenesis by ionizing radiations. IN: Radiation Biology, Vol. 1., edited by A. Hollaender, McGraw-Hill, New York, 1954, pp. 1145-1201.

Furcinitti, P.S. and P. Todd. Gamma rays: further evidence for lack of a threshold dose for lethality to human cells. Science 206:475-476, 1979.

Gofman, J.W. The question of radiation causation of cancer in Hanford workers. Health Physics 37:617-639, 1979.

Hempelmann, L.H. Thyroid neoplasms following irradiation in infancy, IN: L.J. DeGroot, L.A. Frohman, E.L. Kaplan, and S. Refetoff, Eds. Radiation-Associated Thyroid Carcinoma. New York: Grune & Stratton, 1977, pp. 221-229.

Interagency Task Force on the Health Effects of Ionizing Radiation. Report of the Work Group on Science. U.S. Dept. of Health, Education, and Welfare, Washington, D.C. 1979.

Jablon, S. and J. Bailar. The contribution of ionizing radiation to cancer mortality in the United States. Prev. Med. 9:219-226, 1980.

Land, C.E. Estimating cancer risks from low doses of ionizing radiation. Science 209:1197-1203, 1980.

Lewis, E.B. Leukemia and ionizing radiation. Science 125: 965-975, 1957.

Little, J.B., H. Nagasawa, and A.R. Kennedy. DNA repair and malignant transformation: Effect of X-irradiation, 12-0-tetradecanoyl-phorbol-13-acetate, and protease inhibitors on transformation and sister-chromatid exchanges in mouse 10T1/2 cells. Radiat. Res. 79:241-255, 1979.

Lloyd, E.L., M.A. Gemmell, C.B. Henning, D.S. Gemmell, and B.J. Zabransky. Transformation of mammalian cells by alpha particles. Int'l. J. Radiat. Biol. 36:467-478, 1979.

Lyon, J.L., M.R. Klauber, J.W. Gardner, and K.S. Udall. Childhood leukemias associated with fallout from nuclear testing. New Eng. J. Med. 300:397-402, 1979.

Mancuso, T.F., A. Stewart, and G. Kneale. Radiation exposures of Hanford workers dying from cancer and other causes. Health Physics 33:369-385, 1977.

Miller, J.A. Concluding remarks on chemicals and chemical carcinogenesis. IN: Carcinogens: Identification and Mechanisms of Action, edited by Griffin, A.C. and Shaw, C.R., Raven Press, New York, 1979, pp. 455-469.

Najarian, T., and T. Colton. Mortality from leukemia and cancer in shipyard nuclear workers. Lancet 1:1018-1020, 1978.

National Academy of Sciences Advisory Committee on the Biological Effects of Ionizing Radiation (BEIR), The effects

on populations of exposure to low levels of ionizing
radiation. National Academy of Sciences. National
Research Council, Washington, 1972, 1980.

Robinson, C.V. and A.C. Upton. Competing-risk analysis of
leukemia and non-leukemia mortality in X-irradiated male
RF mice. J. Natl. Cancer Inst. 60:995-1007, 1978.

Shore, R.E. Application of epidemiologic studies of radia-
tion-induced breast cancer to mammographic screening
guidelines. IN: Radiation Research (Proc. 6th Int'l.
Congress of Radiat. Res., 1979, Tokyo), edited by Okada,
S., Imamura, M., Terashima, T., and Yamaguchi, H. Japanese
Assoc. Radiat. Res., Tokyo, 1979, pp. 973-979.

United Nations Scientific Committee on the Effects of Atomic
Radiation. Sources and Effects of Ionizing Radiation.
Report to the General Assembly, with Annexes, United
Nations, New York, 1977.

Upton, A.C. Physical carcinogenesis: radiation - history and
sources. IN: Cancer, A comprehensive treatise, edited by
Becker, F.F., Plenum, New York, 1975, pp. 387-403.

Upton, A.C. Radiobiological effects of low doses: implications
for radiological protection. Radiation Res. 71:51-74, 1977.

Upton, A.C., G.W. Beebe, J.M. Brown, C.J. Shellabarger, and
E. Quimby. Report of NCI ad hoc working group on the risks
associated with mammography in mass screening for the detection of breast cancer. J. Natl. Cancer Inst. 59:481-493,
1977.

Upton, A.C., M.L. Randolph and J.W. Conklin. Late effects of
fast neutrons and gamma-rays in mice as influenced by the
dose rate of irradiation induction of neoplasia. Radiat.
Res. 41:467-491, 1970.

Risk of Thyroid Cancer
After Irradiation in Childhood

ELIZABETH D. WOODARD, M.D., M.P.H.

*Asst. Professor of Oncology in
Preventive Medicine and in Radiology
University of Rochester Medical Center
Rochester, New York*

INTRODUCTION

In 1950, Duffy and Fitzgerald suggested that there might be an association between prior[4] x-ray treatment for thymic enlargement and thyroid cancer. Two papers published in 1955 substantiated this association. One was a retrospective study by Clark of 15 patients with thyroid cancer,[1] all of whom had a history of x-ray treatment in infancy. The other was a retrospective study by Simpson, Fuller and Hempelmann of 1,700 subjects treated in Rochester, New York, with x-rays in infancy for thymic[14] enlargement, and their 1,800 non-irradiated siblings. The irradiated individuals had a higher incidence of leukemia, and of benign and malignant thyroid neoplasms than their sibling controls.

Since those early reports, it has become evident that irradiation of other sites in the head and neck also incurs a risk of thyroid cancer. In a report of a worldwide survey of thyroid cancer in childhood, Winship and Rosvoll reported that 76% of cases were associated with a history of prior[16] irradiation of various structures in the head and neck. The findings of Hazen, Hempelmann, et al in 1966 in a retrospective study of 971 persons treated with x-rays in childhood for lymphoid hyperplasia of the nasopharynx suggested that the thyroid glands of children between age 5 and 15 were as sensitive to the oncogenic action of radiation as those of infants.[6] The greater propensity in children for the development of benign thyroid nodularities has been demonstrated in the studies[2] of the Marshallese islanders exposed to radioiodine, and for the development of thyroid carcinoma in the Japanese atomic bomb survivors exposed to total body,

high energy ionizing radiation.[9] The latter study has also
identified an increased risk of radiation-induced thyroid
cancer up to 50 years of age at the time of radiation exposure. Reports of patients treated for adolescent acne have
similarly demonstrated that the radiosensitive period extends
beyond early childhood and the period of risk into adulthood.[3,5,7,12] Studies involving children treated with x-rays
for tinea capitis have corroborated these findings and, in
addition, have demonstrated a risk at a thyroid dose as low
as 6 to 9 rads.[11,13]

THYMUS-IRRADIATED SERIES

With these preliminary remarks, having identified only
a few of the significant studies ongoing in the field of
radiation-induced thyroid cancer, I would like to turn to the
study of thymus-irradiated children initiated by Dr. Louis
Hempelmann at the University of Rochester nearly thirty years
ago. This series, as shown in Table 1, is now based on 2,872
subjects treated with x-rays in infancy during the period
1926 to 1957 in Monroe County in Upstate New York. The
health of these individuals and their 5,055 non-irradiated
siblings has been followed by mailed health questionnaires
since 1953. Because the treatments were given in ten facilities over a 31 year period with different diagnostic
criteria and standards of practice, the population represents
a selected group, but not a homogeneous one. Approximately
90% of the children were less than six months of age when
treated. Most received one or two treatments. If more than
one treatment was given, the interval was usually less than

TABLE 1
Characteristics of Thymus-Irradiated Series

	Treated Subjects		Untreated Siblings	
	All	Subgroup C	All	Subgroup C
Number	2,872	261	5,055	349
Mean Age (1979)	33	41	32	37
% Males	58	64	51	51
% Jewish	8	48	5	38
Mean Thyroid Dose (rads)	119	399		

one week. The radiation dose to the thyroid gland ranged
from 5 to 1000 rads with a mean dose of 119 rads.

One subgroup (C), treated by a private radiologist using
large doses and large ports (resulting in the inclusion of
the thyroid gland in the primary x-ray beam and a mean thyroid dose of 399 rads), was identified early in the study
as being at an exceptionally high risk of thyroid neoplasia.
These 261 individuals were informed of their risk of nodular
disease and offered limited screening in 1964-65 including
physical examination of the thyroid gland and P.B.I. deter-
minations. The results of screening 105 individuals
projected to the entire subgroup gave a prevalence of nodular
thyroid disease of 28% and a prevalence of thyroid cancer of
5%.[10] No other clinical screening has been conducted in this
study.

The results of the fourth mail survey completed in 1971
were published in 1975.[7] The irradiated population was shown
to have a high risk of several types of neoplasms, the
highest being the risk of thyroid neoplasia. Extrathyroid
neoplasms did not occur in sufficient numbers to permit
statistical analysis for the effects of sex, age, and dose
on incidence.

Recently, with the assistance of Dr. Roy Shore at New York
University the data from the 1971 survey have been reanalyzed
using more powerful statistical methods.[12] The risk factors
evaluated are summarized in Table 2. In that analysis, it
was demonstrated that the dose response for thyroid cancer
exhibited both a linear and dose-squared component. No dose-
squared component was evident for thyroid adenomas. This

TABLE 2
Risk Factors for Thyroid Cancer

Thyroid Dose
  Risk proportional to dose with linear and dose-squared
    component.
  Risk estimate 3.8 cancers/10^6 persons/year/rad.
  Fractionation decreases risk.
Latency
  Incidence increasing with time.
  No evidence of inverse relationship with dose.
Jewish Factor
  Relative risk 3.5.
Sex Factor
  Females: absolute risk estimate 5.2 cancers/10^6 persons
  /year/rad; Relative risk = 29.
  Males: absolute risk estimate 1.8 cancers/10^6 persons
  /year/rad; Relative risk = 60.

finding for thyroid cancer is consistent with current radiobiological theory for low-LET radiation which suggests the
yield of tumors will be proportional to dose for small dose
and/or fractionated or protracted radiation exposure; the
dose-squared component will be negligible. The overall risk
estimates were 3.8 thyroid cancers/10^6 persons/year/rad and
4.5 thyroid adenomas/10^6 persons/year/rad. Linear extrapolation from high dose data appeared to overestimate the risk
of thyroid cancer at low doses by a factor of 2 to 3.
Although it could be shown for thyroid adenomas, there was
no evidence relative to thyroid cancer of diminished radiation effect at the highest doses. This is probably explained
by dose fractionation. Few received more than 300 rads per
treatment, and treatments were separated by days or weeks.
At lower total doses (less than 400 rads) there was a suggestion that dose fractionation diminished the thyroid cancer
response, but a similar effect was not seen for thyroid
adenomas. On the contrary, fractionation appeared to increase
the yield of thyroid adenomas.

   Although the earliest thyroid cancer was observed at 6
years post-irradiation, the increased risk of thyroid neoplasia was evident to 40 years post-irradiation, the maximum
length of observation. The excess incidence of thyroid
cancer appeared to be increasing with time. Similarly the
risk of adenomas, first evident at 12 years post-irradiation,
showed no decline with time. The analysis reaffirmed that
there was no evidence for an inverse relationship between
thyroid radiation dose and thyroid cancer latency. Inasmuch
as the latency for cancer was less than that for adenomas,
this study does not substantiate the hypothesis that adenomas
progress to cancer.

   In the reanalysis of variations in susceptibility by sex
and ethnicity, the significance of the Jewish effect was
again demonstrated (RR = 3.5). Synergism between sex and
ethnicity for thyroid cancer could not be shown. Females had
a significantly higher absolute risk estimate but a lower
relative risk estimate than males. Neither a multiplicative
model nor an additive model fit the sex-difference data
adequately for radiogenic cancer in this study.

   The fifth questionnaire survey of this population has been
recently completed. Although analysis of the data is not
complete, there are a few observations that can be made based
on the crude data. Six new thyroid cancers have occurred
in the irradiated series bringing the total to 30 cancers.
The first thyroid cancer in the control group has developed
in a 48 year old female. Thirty-three new thyroid adenomas
have been surgically removed in the irradiated group and

twelve in the control group, making a total of 85 adenomas in
the irradiated group and 18 in the controls. Not included
in the totals are eleven cases of second nodules, all benign,
in the irradiated group (four in thyroid cancer patients) and
two benign recurrences in the controls. The cumulative incidence of surgically removed thyroid nodules (benign and malignant) to date in the irradiated group is 4% (115/2872) and
of thyroid cancer is 1% (30/2872). In the sibling control
group of comparable age, the cumulative incidence of total
thyroid nodularity is 0.4% (19/5055), one-tenth that of the
irradiated group, and of thyroid cancer is 0.02% (1/5055), a
fifty-fold difference.

OTHER SERIES

   In contrast to the Rochester study, the Michael Reese
group demonstrated in their clinical screening program
involving 1,056 irradiated subjects a prevalence of palpable
nodular thyroid disease of 16.5%.[5] Thyroid imaging detected
an additional 10.7% for a prevalence of total nodularity of
27.2%. Of those operated, one third proved to have malignant
lesions. As was previously noted, with the exception of the
limited program in 1964 involving 105 persons, clinical
screening for thyroid disease has not been part of the
Rochester program. In the 1964 program, it was demonstrated
that the ratio of surgically removed lesions to clinically
palpable lesions was one to three; that is, the questionnaire
survey asking about surgically excised lesions appeared to
underestimate the actual number of clinically palpable
nodules by a factor of three.[10] Just as our program may
underestimate risk, screening programs, such as that at
Michael Reese, may overestimate risk by detecting occult
thyroid lesions of uncertain clinical significance. It is
interesting to note, however, that the risk estimate for the
tonsil-nasopharynx treated subjects in the Michael Reese
study as shown in Table 3 is comparable to that of the thymus
series.
   For comparison purposes, risk estimates for thyroid nodularity are listed for five studies in Table 3. The most
recently reported estimate of risk of thyroid cancer in the
Israeli study of persons irradiated for tinea capitis is
somewhat higher, $8.3/10^6$ persons/year/rad.[11] It should be
noted that this study relates to irradiated Jewish children
who, as the Rochester study has shown, may be at increased
risk of radiation-induced thyroid carcinogenesis. In addition, as suggested in the recent report, the younger children,

TABLE 3
Thyroid Nodularity in Irradiated Populations

Population studied	Absolute Risk[a]	
	Malignant	Benign
Rochester thymus-irradiated[12]	3.8+0.3	4.5+0.4
Michael Reese tonsil-adenoid[5]	4.5	n.a.
Israeli tinea capitis[11]	8.3	n.a.
Marshallese islanders[2]	3.5[b] 10.5[c]	29[b] 14[c]
Japanese atomic bomb survivors[15]	1.4	n.a.

[a] Cases/10^6 persons/year/rad

[b] Persons <age 10 at exposure

[c] Persons >age 10 at exposure

less than 6 years of age, may actually have received a higher thyroid dose than has been estimated or perhaps because of an age effect have a higher risk than older children.

Risk estimates from the study of Marshallese islanders exposed to radioactive fallout suggest a lower risk for thyroid cancer but a two-fold increased risk for benign thyroid lesions in children less than ten as compared to those over ten at exposure.[131] Although clinical experience suggested that ^{131}I would be less effective in producing thyroid tumors, the higher energy of the short-lived isotopes ([132]I, [133]I, and [135]I) probably caused the increase above that expected from similar doses of ^{131}I alone. The lower incidence of thyroid cancer in children on Rongelap in the Marshall Islands was probably due to the high thyroid dose causing cell destruction. These data and that on thyrotoxic patients given ^{131}I therapy suggest that children are two to three times more susceptible to radiation-induced benign thyroid nodules than adults.[8]

In the studies of atomic bomb survivors, Parker indicated an apparent dependence of thyroid cancer incidence on age at exposure.[9] For clinically diagnosed cancers, the mean rate of detection for those less than ten at the time of the bomb was nearly 4 times that for those age 20 or over at the bomb.[15]

PATHOLOGY

In all of the studies, the thyroid cancers have been well differentiated lesions which have a good prognosis. Few fatalities have been reported relative to radiation-induced thyroid cancer. The 1977 UNSCEAR report indicated a 3% case fatality. In the Rochester series of 30 cancers, 12 are papillary, 8 follicular, 9 mixed papillary-follicular, and 1 anaplastic carcinoma. With the exception of the anaplastic carcinoma, this distribution is typical of other series of radiation-induced thyroid cancer. Two of the six new cases in the thymus-irradiated series have proven fatal. One case, a footnote in the 1975 paper[7] and now confirmed, developed in a 37 year old woman who had received 2,931R to the chest (531R for thymic enlargement and 2,400R one year later for Hodgkin's Disease). She developed an anaplastic thyroid carcinoma and died of widespread metastases. The second fatality involved a 43 year old male who had received 412 rads to the thyroid gland and subsequently developed a mixed papillary-follicular carcinoma of the thyroid gland first presenting at age 40 and 41 as undifferentiated metastases to the cervical lymph nodes and lung respectively. These two fatal cases in addition to a new case in a 37 year old female are the oldest irradiated subjects to develop thyroid cancer in our series.

SUMMARY

In summary, the risk of induction of thyroid cancer following irradiation in childhood appears to be of the order 3.5 to 8.3 cancers/10^6 persons/year/rad within about 30 years of irradiation.[13] A risk of neoplasia is evident at a thyroid dose of 6 rads. Dose-response data for the Rochester thymus-irradiated series indicate a linear and a dose-squared component for thyroid cancer. At lower total doses (<400 rads), the Rochester data suggest that dose fractionation diminishes the thyroid cancer response. Thyroid cancer has appeared earlier than adenomas; the minimum reported latency[2] being 4 years for thyroid cancer[11] and 9 years for adenomas. The Rochester data indicate the excess incidence of thyroid neoplasia persists to 40 years, the maximum period of follow-up. For thyroid cancer, there is no evidence of an inverse relationship between dose and latency in the Rochester series. Such a relationship was suggested for thyroid adenomas. A higher absolute risk of thyroid neoplasia has been demonstrated in all series for females and in the Rochester series for Jewish subjects as well. Whether age at exposure influences incidence of thyroid cancer and/or latency is not yet clear. Despite the increased incidence of thyroid cancer, mortality from the well-differentiated malignant lesions is low.

REFERENCES

1. Clark, D: Association of irradiation with cancer of the thyroid in children and adolescents. JAMA 159:1007-1009, 1955.
2. Conard, R: Summary of thyroid findings in Marshallese 22 years after exposure to radioactive fallout, in DeGroot, L (ed): Radiation-Associated Thyroid Carcinoma. New York, Grune & Stratton, 1977, pp 241-257.
3. DeGroot, L, Paloyan, E: Thyroid carcinoma and radiation: A Chicago endemic. JAMA 225:487-491, 1973.
4. Duffy, B, Fitzgerald, P: Thyroid cancer in childhood and adolescence. A report on 28 cases. Cancer 3:1018-1032, 1950.
5. Favus, M, Schneider, A, Stachura, M, et al: Thyroid cancer occurring as a late consequence of head-and-neck irradiation. N Eng J Med 294:1019-1025, 1976.
6. Hazen, R, Pifer, J, Toyooka, E, et al: Neoplasms following irradiation of the head. Cancer Res 26:305-311, 1966.
7. Hempelmann, L, Hall, W, Phillips, M, et al: Neoplasms in persons treated with x-rays in infancy: Fourth survey in 20 years. JNCI 55:519-530, 1975.
8. Maxon, H, Thomas, S, Saenger, E, et al: Ionizing radiation and the induction of clinically significant disease in the human thyroid gland. Amer J Med 63:967-978, 1977.
9. Parker, L, Belsky, J, Yamamoto, T, et al: Thyroid carcinoma after exposure to atomic radiation. Ann Int Med 80:600-604, 1974.
10. Pincus, R, Reichlin, S, Hempelmann, L: Thyroid abnormalities after radiation exposure in infancy. Ann Int Med 66:1154-1164, 1967.
11. Ron, E, Modan, B: Benign and malignant thyroid neoplasms after childhood irradiation for tinea captitis. JNCI 65:7-11, 1980.
12. Shore, R, Woodard, E, Pasternack, B, Hempelmann, L: Radiation and host factors in human thyroid tumors following thymus irradiation. Health Phys 38:451-465, 1980.

13. Shore, R, Albert, R, Pasternack, B: Follow-up study of patients treated by x-ray epilation for tinea capitis. Arch Environ Health 31:17-24, 1976.

14. Simpson, C, Hempelmann, L, Fuller, L: Neoplasia in children treated with x-rays in infancy for thymic enlargement. Radiology 64:840-845, 1955.

15. United Nations Scientific Committee on the Effects of Atomic Radiation: Sources and Effects of Ionizing Radiation. New York, United Nations, 1977, pp 384-385.

16. Winship, T, Rosvoll, R: Thyroid carcinoma in childhood: Final report on a 20 year study. Clin Proc Child Hosp 26:327-348, 1970.

Radiogenic Breast Cancer: Age Effects and
Implications for Models of Human Carcinogenesis

John D. Boice and Robert N. Hoover

Environmental Epidemiology Branch
National Cancer Institute
Bethesda, Maryland 20205

Introduction. Studies of populations exposed to ionizing radiation have led to the identification of a preventable cause of cancer in our society. Over the years preventive measures have been taken to reduce population exposure, including more conservative use of medical radiation, reduction of patient exposure from medical x-ray equipment and stringent environmental and occupational radiation protection guidelines. These measures undoubtably reduce the cancer burden in society. For example, children are no longer irradiated for enlarged thymus glands, tuberculosis patients no longer receive fluoroscopic screening, thorotrast is no longer used as a radiographic contrast medium, mammography exposures have been reduced by an order of magnitude during the last decade, and uranium miners, radiologists and luminescent watch makers are no longer exposed to high levels of radiation. Radiation studies, however, have also provided insights into mechanisms of cancer, and observations made from human studies are now being incorporated into theories of carcinogenesis.

Radiation Studies. The increased risk of human breast cancer following irradiation has been more thoroughly studied than any other radiogenic tumor, with the possible exception of leukemia.[5,8,17] Large-scale studies have found dose-dependent increases in breast cancer incidence in women with pulmonary tuberculosis whose artificial pneumothorax treatment was monitored by fluoroscopic chest examination,[3,18,23] in Japanese women exposed to the atomic bomb,[20,32,34] and in women treated therapeutically with x ray for acute[21,27] and chronic[1] breast conditions. These studies indicate:[5,8,17]

(1) that the underlying relationship between radiation dose and breast cancer incidence is most consistent with linearity, even at doses under 50 rad,
(2) that fractionation does not appear to diminish risk,
(3) that radiogenic cancers do not begin to be apparent until perhaps 10 years or more post-irradiation,
(4) that risk continues throughout life or at least for 40 years,

(5) that the patterns of age-specific incidence of breast
    cancer are the same for exposed and nonexposed women,
    differing only in magnitude,

(6) and that age at exposure is the most important factor
    influencing subsequent risk.

Of these major findings, the association with age, and risk
factors associated with age, have formed a basis for the
development of several models of hormonal carcinogenesis.[16,22]
These observations are discussed in detail below.

Age at exposure. Apart from the radiation dose, the major
determinant of subsequent breast cancer risk is the age at
exposure. The three major studies to date provide strong
evidence for cancer induction in females exposed at ages
10-39, with girls 10-19 years of age having the greatest risk
(Table 1).[5,8,17]

Table 1
Age-specific risk estimates,[8] excess cancer($\pm$1s.d.)/10^6WY-rad

Age at exposure	Atomic Bomb Survivors[17]	Massachusetts TB-Fluoroscopy[3]	Rochester Mastitis[27]
0-9	0.0	$\cdots$	$\cdots$
10-19	9.2$\pm$2.2	8.7$\pm$3.1	a
20-29	2.9$\pm$0.88	3.8$\pm$3.1	6.3$\pm$2.0
30-39	4.9$\pm$2.5	(6.9$\pm$4.5)[a,b]	9.4$\pm$3.4
40-49	-1.0$\pm$0.45	a,b	(52.1$\pm$21.0)[a]
50+	3.3$\pm$2.2	$\cdots$	$\cdots$
All ages	3.6	6.2	8.3

[a]Estimate based on small numbers and may be misleading.
[b]Observed cancers not in excess of population expectation.

Given the variation in the nature of the exposures, as well
as the substantial differences in the populations exposed,
the similarity of age-specific risk estimates is remarkable,
particularly in the younger ages where the numbers are large
enough to provide stable estimates. It is interesting that
American women who are at high natural risk of breast cancer,[19] are at comparable risk of radiogenic cancer with
Japanese women who are at low natural risk. Crude estimates
of radiation risk suggest that Japanese women are at lower
risk of radiogenic cancer, but this is because the Japanese
population had higher proportions of very young and very old
women who thus far seem to be at much lower risk. The best
estimate of risk among American women exposed after age 20 is
6.6 excess cancers per million women per year per rad
(6.6/10^6WY-rad) after a latent period of about 10 years.[5,8]

To date, there is little evidence that radiation exposures before the age of 10 carry any future risk of radiogenic breast cancer. Among atomic bomb survivors, no excess breast cancers (only 5 total) have occurred among 9,300 women who were under age 10 at exposure and followed to age 30-39.[17,32] These women may not yet be old enough for a risk to have been detected. This seems unlikely, however, since: (1) among 4,200 women exposed at ages 5-9 and followed to age 30-39, only 3 breast cancers occurred, whereas for 5,100 women exposed at ages 10-14 and followed to the same age (30-39 yr), 13 breast cancers had occurred;[17] (2) a recent followup, adding 4 more years of mortality observation, i.e., to age 34-43, has failed to demonstrate an excess risk in those aged 0-9 at exposure;[14] and (3) in a study of 1,200 women exposed as infants to high dose irradiation for enlarged thymus glands, no breast cancers have been reported despite follow-up periods up to 40 years,[11] although the radiation fields may not have completely included the breasts in all cases. Further observations of the A-bomb survivors should provide a definitive answer to whether the immature breast is in fact relatively resistant to radiation damage. If it is, it may be that radiation damage is repaired before the proliferation of breast tissue during menarche, that there are few breast cells at risk for transformation, or that for other reasons breast tissue may not be susceptible to carcinogens before breast budding.

Adolescence, including menarche, appears to be the period of greatest risk for the induction of subsequent breast cancers.[3,23,32] Exposures at ages 10-19 carried the greatest risk for atomic bomb survivors ($9.0/10^6$WY-rad) and TB-fluoroscopy patients ($8.7/10^6$WY-rad).[5] Studies of atomic bomb survivors indicate that women exposed at ages 10-14, around the time of menarche (ave=14.5yr), had the greatest increased incidence of breast cancer.[20,32] The Massachusetts survey of TB-fluoroscopy patients also reported the highest risk for women exposed just before or during their first menses, although the numbers of breast cancers were quite small (3 observed vs 0.28 expected).[4] Possibly, exposures that occur just before menarche, during the period of breast budding and hormonal changes, are especially damaging.[4]

All studies, with the exception of the mastitis series,[27] indicate that radiogenic risk falls with increasing age at exposure from menarche to menopause. This is particularly apparent for the TB-fluoroscopy series[3] where no excess breast cancers were found in women exposed after age 30, and in a Swedish study[1] of women irradiated for benign breast conditions.

Data on women exposed after age 50 are sparse, e.g., only 3 breast cancers occurred in such women in the A-bomb survivors[17] exposed to greater than 100 rad, but the risk associated with such exposure appears to be quite low.

Menopause. Exposures occurring around the time of menopause also appear to carry little or no risk. The atomic bomb survivor study showed no excess risk in more than 2,000 women exposed during their forties.[32] In fact, a significant negative dose-response was reported, i.e., increased dose resulted in decreased breast cancer incidence. This anomalous negative dose-response for Japanese women may be associated with these women receiving total-body exposure, including ovarian irradiation. A study in Hiroshima indicated that amenorrhea occurred in over half of the women aged 40-49 at the time of the bombing.[25] Amenorrhea was permanent for most of these women, whereas it was transient for all women exposed under age 35. Possibly, the disruption of ovarian function for those aged 40-49 at exposure may have decreased subsequent breast cancer risk.

Women undergoing radiation castration have shown significant decreases in death due to breast cancer.[30] Similarly, studies of cervical cancer patients who received large therapeutic doses to the pelvis and ovaries have also shown a decreased risk of developing breast cancer as a second tumor.[15] Particularly provocative findings from these studies are: (1) the decrease in risk of breast cancer appears to be greater than that experienced by women having undergone surgical castration at similar ages; and (2) the protective effect of ovarian irradiation applies also to exposures incurred after the ages of natural menopause, when surgical intervention has no effect.[33] One possible explanation for these findings is that irradiation might produce selective killing of cells in the ovary. Perhaps the estrogen-producing cells are more sensitive to cell killing by irradiation than androgen-producing cells. Irradiation coupled with pituitary hormonal stimulation to the ovary might produce a relatively higher androgen/estrogen ratio in peri- and post-menopausal women that could possibly retard the manifestation of an already induced breast cancer (S. Korenman, personnal communication). At least one other study has reported a low breast cancer risk among women with relatively high levels of endogenous androgens as measured a relatively short time prior to diagnosis.[6] In any event, the effect of ovarian irradiation on subsequent breast cancer risk appears to be an important area for further evaluation.

<u>Pregnancy, Parity, and Lactation</u>. Full-term pregnancies have a profound effect on subsequent breast cancer risk with risk rising with increasing age at first birth, and nulliparous women being at greatest risk unless first pregnancy occurs after about age 35.[19] The TB-fluoroscopy study[4] indicated that nulliparous women (8.7 cancers/10^6WY-rad) were at increased excess risk of radiogenic cancer when contrasted with women exposed before (0.9/10^6WY-rad) or after (0.4/10^6WY-rad) their first pregnancy, but at less risk than women exposed at the time of pregnancy (17.1/10^6WY-rad). The numbers, however, were small and require confirmation. It is noteworthy that a full-term pregnancy after irradiation appeared to lower the risk of radiogenic breast cancer, i.e., exposed nulliparous women who years later became pregnant were at lower risk than exposed nulliparous women who remained nulliparous.[4] Interestingly, a study of dogs that received whole-body irradiation also found an increased risk of death due to mammary tumors in nulliparous but not parous beagles.[7]

The women irradiated for postpartum mastitis[27] had all just given birth, and experienced the largest age-specific risks.[5,17] In contrast to all other experiences, the radiation risk appeared to rise slightly with increasing age at exposure, and was high among those aged 30-44 at exposure. A recent animal experiment[13] has found high excess cancers in rats when exposure occurred during pregnancy or lactation; and it is conceivable that the inflamed and lactating breasts at the time of exposure may have influenced risk in the mastitis patients. In the mastitis series it was also noted that exposure just after a late first pregnancy, i.e. after age 29, carried a greater risk than exposures after earlier first pregnancies, and it was recommended that intense screening of so called high risk women by mammography for early detection of breast cancer be done cautiously for women who were nulliparous or over age 30 at the time of their first delivery.[28]

It has been suggested that reproductive history influences the latent interval between exposure and clinical diagnosis of breast cancer,[35] supposedly through an acceleration of tumor growth by a pregnancy in a small number of women. If this were a widespread phenomenon, however, it might be expected that the average latent period would be longer for nulliparous women than for women irradiated prior to pregnancy, but this was not the case in the Massachusetts TB-fluoroscopy study. The average latent period was 23.4 yr for nulliparous women and 28.8 yr for parous women; the average ages at exposure were 26.4 yr and 21.1 yr, and the average ages at diagnosis for breast cancer were 49.8 yr and 49.9 yr, respectively (J.Boice, unpublished data). The hypothesis, however, deserves to be tested in a larger series.

Sex. Radiation-induced breast cancer appears predominantly in women. Males, of course, do have breasts, although minimal ductal tissue. The fact that male breasts do not experience periodic endocrine stimulation may be related to the small incidence of natural and radiogenic breast cancer. To date, no male breast cancers have been reported in followup studies of atomic bomb survivors,[2] TB-fluoroscopy patients,[23] or thymic irradiated children.[11]

Summary of Human Studies. The following generalizations, based on relatively substantial data, are consistent with the human studies on radiation-induced breast cancer:

(1) adolescent exposures carry the greatest risk, especially exposures around menarche;
(2) risk appears to fall with increasing age at exposure from menarche up to the time of menopause;
(3) latency is inversely related to age at exposure;
(4) the age-specific incidence patterns of breast cancer are the same for exposed and nonexposed women, differing only in magnitude; and
(5) and risk continues thoughout life or at least for 40 years.

The following tentative generalizations are based on less substantial data:

(1) the immature breast, and perhaps also the post-menopausal breast, may be relatively radioresistant;
(2) exposures during and immediately after pregnancy may be particularly hazardous;
(3) nulliparous women appear to be at greater radiation risk than parous women;
(4) exposed women who remain nulliparous may be at greater risk of radiogenic breast cancer than nulliparous women who later become parous;
(5) and ovarian irradiation may reduce risk beyond the effect of castration.

Many of these conclusions are receiving further evaluation in ongoing followup and case-control studies.

Hypotheses on Breast Carcinogenesis.

The observations made in human studies of radiation-induced breast cancer can be or have been incorporated into general models of breast carcinogenesis.

1. Previous Hypothesis. Prior to many of the observations reported in this paper, MacMahon, Cole and Brown[19] described in clear detail how the epidemiology of human breast cancer indicates that a woman's lifetime risk of breast cancer appears to be determined to a substantial extent during the early years of reproductive life. Their interpretation of this pattern was that some aspect of estrogen metabolism in the years after menarche may be linked to breast cancer risk throughout life. A number of observations from the studies of radiogenic breast cancer outlined above support the importance of early reproductive life in the etiology of breast cancer. For example: (1) radiation exposure around the time of menarche appears to incur the greatest risk; (2) irradiation before menarche seems to carry little or no risk; (3) risk of exposure after menarche appears to fall with increasing age at exposure; (4) the age-specific incidence patterns of breast cancer are similar for exposed and nonexposed women, differing only in magnitude; i.e., although exposures may have occurred as early as adolescence, the clinical presentation of breast cancer did not occur until the ages normally associated with increased incidence, implying that non-radiogenic cancers may also have been initiated during a similar period in early reproductive life.

2. Recent Hypotheses.
(a) Two-stage model. Moolgavkar, Day and Stevens[22] have recently elaborated upon a two-stage model for breast carcinogenesis. The model assumes that two discrete and irreversible events are required for cell transformation. Since each event must occur during cell division, tissue growth and rapid cell turnover would influence susceptibility. Observations made in atomic bomb[32] and TB-fluoroscopy studies[4,5] were incorporated into this model, under the assumption that radiation affects breast tissue by transforming a proportion of susceptible normal cells into intermediate cells. It is the interpretation of these authors that: (1) The absence of a radiation effect in women exposed under age 10 is because few cells are dividing before the period of breast development, i.e., there are few susceptible cells at risk; (2) the reported decreased radiation risk in parous women compared to nulliparous women[4] is consistent with the first full-term pregnancy reducing the number of susceptible cells in parous women, perhaps from the enhancement of breast cell differentiation by a pregnancy; and (3) the fact that radiation-associated risk is highest at puberty and falls with increasing age at irradiation is consistent with a proliferative advantage of intermediate cells, in which one of the two irreversible events has already occurred, a proliferative advantage that would be greatly reduced at menopause when a decrease in the turnover rate of breast epithelium is accompanied by involu-

tion and dysfunction.   In other words, the longer the period
between irradiation of susceptible cells and menopause the
longer the time for radiation-induced intermediate cells to
proliferate and the greater the risk.

(b) Estrogen window.   Korenman[16] has recently modified two
earlier hypotheses concerned with the protective effect of
progesterone[9,26] into an estrogen window hypothesis that
assumes that endocrine status influences susceptibility to
environmental carcinogens.   The actions of estrogen and
prolactin, unopposed by the action of progesterone, are
assumed to increase susceptibility of the mammary epithelium
to environmental carcinogens.   Two main induction periods, or
"windows" are proposed.   These are the periods in a woman's
life characterized by increased estrogen and diminished
progesterone secretion.   The first window opens with the
onset of ovarian activity before menarche and closes at the
onset of regular ovulatory menstrual cycles.   The second
window opens in the peri-menopausal period with the appearance
of irregular, prolonged follicular phase, and anovulatory
cycles, and closes with the cessation of ovarian function.
The hypothesis assumes that breast tissue is particularly
susceptible to environmental carcinogens when these endocrine
windows are open, and is relatively refractory to carcinogenesis at all other times.   Several observations from radiation studies were noted by the author as being consistent
with this model.   (1) The lack of a breast cancer excess in
atomic bomb survivors exposed under age 10 is consistent with
this being prior to the opening of the first endocrine window.
(2) The increased susceptibility of the breast to exposures
just before and around menarche[3,32] was considered compatible
with this being the time when the first window is open.   (3)
The absence of a significant excess risk among atomic bomb
survivors and TB-fluoroscopy patients exposed at ages 30-49
is consistent with this being after the first window was
closed and prior to the opening of the second.   (4) The nonsta-
tistically significant risk reported for atomic bomb survivors
exposed after age 50 was considered possibly consistent with
the opening of the second window.   (5) The concordance of the
patterns of age-specific incidence curves between exposed and
nonexposed Japanese women, differing only in magnitude, was
considered consistent with the hypothesis that a long latent
period applies to both radiogenic and non-radiogenic cancers.

As can be seen, the credibility of models for the hormonal
carcinogenesis of human breast cancer can be tested and new
models developed by relying on observations from epidemiologic
studies of radiogenic breast cancer.   The fact that several
models are consistent with the same set of observations is
not surprising, given the similarity these models have to

each other. We anticipate, however, that these models could
be meaningfully tested and appropriately altered by incorpo-
rating a number of other observations concerning radiation-
induced breast cancer. With respect to current observations,
it would be most interesting to learn how the following
observations would fit into or alter existing models: (1)
the very high risks possibly associated with exposures occurring during pregnancy in TB-fluoroscopy patients,[4] and those
definitely associated with exposures just after pregnancy in
postpartum mastitis patients;[27] (2) the apparent increase, or
at least absence of a decrease, in risk with age at exposure
in patients irradiated for postpartum mastitis;[27] (3) the
possible increased risk associated with exposures after a
late first pregnancy contrasted with exposures after earlier
pregnancies;[28] (4) the protection afforded by a pregnancy
following exposure in nulliparous women;[4] and (5) the absence
of a radiation effect of exposures during the peri-menopausal
period in atomic bomb survivors.[32]

Although radiation-induced breast cancer is relatively well
studied, a number of associations are not as yet adequately
investigated and might very well contribute to the refinement
of existing models. Included are evaluations of the relationship between radiation and other breast cancer risk factors.
For example, is the effect of radiation influenced if the
exposed woman has a relative who developed breast cancer, has
a personal history of breast cancer, is obese or has had
prior benign breast disease? It would also be useful to
evaluate further the effect of ovarian irradiation, the
effect of breast irradiation during and just after pregnancy,
and the effect of radiation on the immature and the post-
menopausal breast.

Models of carcinogenesis for other tumors. Radiation studies
are perhaps more readily interpretable than studies of some
other environmental carcinogens because exposure generally
occurred during a short period of time, can be identified and
quantified, and latent period, age susceptibility and period
of life-time risk can be evaluated readily. If intensive
evaluation of these observations have already been profitably
incorporated into models of breast carcinogenesis, perhaps
equally important will be similarly intensive studies of
radiation-induced cancer of other sites. Such studies could
lead to the alteration of a variety of existing models, or
assist in the development of new models of human carcinogenesis. Studies of tumors that react to radiation in a similar
fashion as the breast, e.g., the thyroid, or in an opposite
fashion, e.g., bone marrow-leukemia, might be particularly
instructive.

Both breast and thyroid cancers are under hormonal control, occur at higher rates in females in both exposed and non-exposed populations, and occur in subcutaneous organs. For both, radiogenic risk appears to fall with increasing age at exposure, and both are associated with linear or near-linear dose-response relationships.[5,10,11,17,29] The risk of radio-genic thyroid cancer appears greatest if exposure occurs during childhood and this has been interpreted as indicating that rapidly proliferating cells injured by radiation could be more likely to develop abnormally than cells irradiated in later life.[10] As noted, this analogy holds for the breast as well.[4] Finally the excess risk of thyroid cancers induced in infancy emerges with an abrupt rise in incidence during adolescence, suggesting the possible influence of thyroid-stimulating hormone as a promoting factor.

If the epidemiology of radiation-induced thryoid and breast cancers are similar, there are major differences between aspects of breast cancer and of leukemia as reported in atomic bomb survivors[12] and patients irradiated for ankylosing spondylitis.[31] Specifically, (1) for the breast linearity appears to be a reasonable representation of dose response, while leukemia appears to be curvilinear.[8] (2) The Relative Biological Effectiveness (RBE) for neutron exposure and breast cancer is consistent with 1.0,[17] while for leukemia and all other radiogenic cancers it has much larger values.[8] (3) The human breast appears to be the only site for which fractionation or splitting of dose does not diminish risk,[3] while for leukemia fractionation reduces risk in practically all experimental situations.[24] (4) In contrast to the wave-like temporal pattern shown for radiation-induced leuke-mia,[12,31] there is no evidence that breast cancer risk decreases with time after reaching some maximum value.[3] (5) Finally, the relationship between age at exposure and risk differs dramatically for breast cancer compared with leukemia: on an absolute scale, radiogenic breast cancer risk appears to decrease with increasing age at exposure from menarche to menopause, whereas the risk for leukemia increases.[2,31] Pre-puberty exposures also appear to carry little or no radiogenic breast cancer risk, whereas for leukemia the greatest relative risk occurs at this time.[12] Elucidation of the reasons behind these differences may provide insights into the environmental and host determinants of cancer as well as suggest fresh ideas for future research.

Epidemiologic studies of radiation-induced cancer have led directly to cancer prevention through the setting of radia-tion protection guidelines for occupational, medical and public exposures. However, in the long run, perhaps the most important contributions will be the insights into basic mechanisms of human carcinogenesis gained through such studies. The intensive epidemiologic evaluations of radiogenic cancer, while thus far few, have been productive of leads to such insights, and should be a major area of emphasis in cancer research in the immediate future.

REFERENCES

1. Baral E, Larsson LE, Mattsson B: Breast cancer following irradiation of the breast. Cancer 40:2905-2910,1977.
2. Beebe GW, Kato H, Land CE: Studies of the mortality of A-bomb survivors. 6. Mortality and radiation dose, 1950-1974. Radiat Res 75:138-201,1978.
3. Boice JD Jr, Monson RR: Breast cancer in women after repeated fluoroscopic examinations of the chest. J Natl Cancer Inst 59:823-832,1977.
4. Boice JD Jr, Stone BJ: Interaction between radiation and other breast cancer risk factors. In: Late Biological Effects of Ionizing Radiation, Vol 1. Vienna, International Atomic Energy Agency, 1978, pp 231-249.
5. Boice JD Jr, Land CE, Shore RE, et al: Risk of breast cancer following low-dose radiation exposure. Radiology 131:589-597,1979.
6. Bulbrook RD, Hayward JL, Spicer CC: Relation between urinary androgen and corticoid excretion and subsequent breast cancer. Lancet 2:395-398,1971.
7. Chrisp CE, Phemister RD, Anderson AC, et al: Pathology in a lifespan study of x-irradiated adult female beagles. In: Biomedical Environmental Research ERDA Research and Development Program, UC-48. Springfield, VA, Natl Tech Inf Serv, 1976, pp 28
8. Committee on the Biological Effects of Ionizing Radiation (BEIR III). The Effects on Populations of Exposure to Low Levels of Ionizing Radiation. National Academy of Sciences, Washington, D.C., 1980.
9. Grattarola R: The premenstrual endometrial pattern of women with breast cancer. Cancer 17:1119-1122,1964.
10. Hempelmann LH: Risk of thyroid neoplasms after irradiation in childhood. Science 160:159-163,1968.
11. Hempelmann LH, Hall WJ, Phillips M, et al: Neoplasms in persons treated with x-rays in infancy: Fourth survey in 20 years. J Natl Cancer Inst 55:519-530,1975.
12. Ichimaru M, Ishimaru T, Belsky JL: Incidence of leukemia in atomic bomb survivors belonging to a fixed cohort in Hiroshima and Nagasaki, 1950-71. Radiation dose, years after exposure, age at exposure, and type of leukemia. Jpn J Radiat Res 19:262-282, 1978.

13. Jacrot M, Mouriquand J, Mouriquand C, Saez S: Mammary carcinogenesis in Sprague-Dawley rats following 3 repeated exposures to 14.8 MeV neutrons and steroid receptor content of these tumor types. Cancer Letters 8:147-153,1979.
14. Kato H, Schull WJ: Mortality experience of atomic bomb survivors, 1950-78. Presented to the 6th International Congress of Radiation Research, Tokyo, Japan, May 1978.
15. Kleinerman R, Boice J, Curtis R, Flannery J: Second cancers following radiation for cervical cancer. Am J Epidemiol 112(abs):442,1980.
16. Korenman SG: Oestrogen window hypothesis of the aetiology of breast cancer. Lancet 1:700-701,1980.
17. Land CE, Boice JD Jr, Shore RE et al: Breast cancer risk from low-dose exposures to ionizing radiation: Results of parallel analysis of three exposed populations of women. JNCI 65:353-376,1980.
18. MacKenzie I: Breast cancer following multiple fluoroscopies. Br J Cancer 19:1-8,1965.
19. MacMahon B, Cole P, Brown J: Etiology of human breast cancer: A review. J Natl Cancer Inst 50:21-42,1973.
20. McGregor DH, Land CE, Choi K, et al: Breast cancer incidence among atomic bomb survivors, Hiroshima and Nagasaki, 1950-1974. J Natl Cancer Inst 59:799-811,1977.
21. Mettler FA Jr, Hempelmann LH, Dutton AM, et al: Breast neoplasms in women treated with x rays for acute postpartum mastitis. A pilot study. J Natl Cancer Inst 43:803-811,1969.
22. Moolgavkar SH, Day NE, Stevens RG: Two-stage model for carcinogenesis: Epidemiology of breast cancer in females. JNCI 65:559-569,1980.
23. Myrden JA, Hiltz JE: Breast cancer following multiple fluoroscopies during artiticial pneumothorax treatment of pulmonary tuberculosis. Can Med Assoc J 100:1032-1034, 1969.
24. National Council on Radiation Protection and Measurements, NCRP Report No.64. Influence of dose and its distribution in time on dose-response relationships for low-LET radiations. Washington, D.C.,1980.
25. Sawada H: Sexual function in female atomic bomb survivors 1949-57: Hiroshima. Hiroshima, Atomic Bomb Casualty Commission TR 34-59,1959.
26. Sherman BM, Korenman SG: Inadequate corpus luteum function: A patho-physiological interpretation of human cancer epidemiology. Cancer 33:1306-1311,1974.
27. Shore RE, Hempelmann LH, Kowaluk E, et al: Breast neoplasms in women treated with x-rays for acute postpartum mastitis. J Natl Cancer Inst 59:813-822,1977.

28. Shore RE: Application of human studies of radiation-induced breast cancer to mammographic screening guidelines. In: Radiation Research: Proceedings of the Sixth International Congress of Radiation Research (Okada S, et al, eds). Tokyo, Japanese Association of Radiation Research, 1979, pp 973-979.
29. Shore RE, Woodard ED, Pasternack BS, Hempelmann LH: Radiation and host factors in human thyroid tumors following thymus irradiation. Health Phys 38:451-465,1980.
30. Smith PG, Doll R: Late effects of x irradiation in patients treated for metropathia haemorrhagica. Br J Radiol 49:224-232,1976.
31. Smith PG, Doll R: Age- and time-dependent changes in the rates of radiation-induced cancers in patients with ankylosing spondylitis following a single course of x-ray treatment. In: Late Biological Effects of Ionizing Radiation, Vol 1. Vienna, International Atomic Energy Agency, 1978, pp 205-218.
32. Tokunaga M, Norman JE Jr, Asano M, et al: Malignant breast tumors among atomic bomb survivors, Hiroshima and Nagasaki, 1950-74. J Natl Cancer Inst 62:1347-1359,1979.
33. Trichopoulos D, MacMahon B, Cole P: The menopause and breast cancer risk. J Natl Cancer Inst 48:605-613,1972.
34. Wanebo CK, Johnson KG, Sato K, Thorslund TW: Breast cancer after exposure to the atomic bombings of Hiroshima and Nagasaki. N Engl J Med 279:667-671,1968.
35. Woods KL, Smith SR, Morrison JM: Parity and breast cancer: evidence of a dual effect. Br Med J 281:419-421,1980.

Childhood Cancer and Prenatal
Irradiation

BRIAN MACMAHON

Professor
Department of Epidemiology
Harvard School of Public Health
Boston, Massachusetts

The question of whether in utero exposure to diagnostic
x-rays increases the risk of childhood cancer does not have
the clinical urgency that it had when it was first raised in
1956. The first reports that an association existed led to
a dramatic reduction in the use of x-ray for obstetrical
diagnosis. With the development of alternative diagnostic
methods, there is now virtually no obstetric indication for
x-raying a living fetus, although non-obstetric exposures
continue to occur - wittingly and unwittingly. The issue
nevertheless remains an important one, not only because of
the continuing exposures but also from the standpoint of
basic radiobiology. If the human fetus is substantially
more susceptible to radiation carcinogenesis than is the
post-nate - as some interpret the data - this has broad
implications to the setting of exposure limits in non-
medical as well as medical settings, and it would suggest
that, once again, man is different from other species in
ways that it would be useful for us to know about.
  The recent report of the Third Committee on the Biological Effects of Ionizing Radiations[2] (BEIR III) makes the
task of reviewing the information available on this question
somewhat less burdensome. It does little to resolve the
difficulties that have prevailed during the past quarter
century in drawing convincing conclusions from it. The BEIR
committee is thorough in its review of this topic, succinct
in its statements and appears reasonably unanimous in its
conclusions and uncertainties - at least in this section of
its report. I could probably do no better than try to
recount these for you.

223

An association exists. It seems beyond reasonable doubt
that there is a statistical association between exposure to
diagnostic x-rays while in utero and probability of developing malignancy in the first ten years of life. There are
some studies in which no association has been found, but none
are of sufficient size to be incompatible, in statistical
terms, with chance deviation from the estimates of risk derived from the larger, positive studies. The estimates of
relative risk associated with prenatal exposure (all forms
combined) are generally in the range of 1.4-1.5, indicating
a 40-50 per cent increase in risk for exposed fetuses.

The association is clearly confounded by a host of social,
medical and methodologic variables. Extensive efforts have
been made to take such confounding into account, but, while
relative risk estimates can be modified substantially by
stratification, no single variable or combination of
variables has been identified whose use reduces the relative
risk estimates below 1.4.

The association appears to exist for leukemia and for each
of the categories of solid tumor that occurs in sufficient
numbers to be examined.

Is the association causal? Here one senses one of the
committee's principal uncertainties. The evidence that
infants exposed to x-rays in utero differed from those not
exposed in ways that affected their overall mortality rates -
as well as their cancer-specific rates - is clear. It
suggests strongly the possibility that there was some characteristic of the mothers of exposed infants, or of their pregnancies, that was associated with - or perhaps an indication
for - an x-ray examination, and which was also associated
with the probability of the infant developing malignancy.
On the other hand, no such factor has been identified in
spite of careful evaluation of a wide range of maternal and
gestational characteristics[5,6] and, indeed, one cannot offer
a likely candidate that has not been evaluated.

One observation which the BEIR committee considered persuasive evidence in favor of the association being causal
was that of Mole[7], who pointed out that the increased risk
following exposure was at least as great for infants born
of dizygotic twin pregnancies as for births in singleton
pregnancies. The frequency of x-ray exposure in the
dizygotic twin pregnancies was 55 per cent, in contrast to
10 per cent in singleton pregnancies. Since the higher
level of exposure in twin pregnancy is attributable to the
twinning itself, and since dizygotic twins do not have a
higher cancer rate than singletons, this suggests that at
least the excess cancers in the x-rayed twins cannot be

attributed to confounding introduced by any of the variety
of medical and obstetric indications for which the singletons
were x-rayed. The committee's reservation that Mole's
findings were based on "a reinterpretation of published data
with which the author did not claim direct familiarity" does
not seem particularly cogent.

On the other hand, at least two sets of observations weigh
against the association being causal. First, experimental
data do not indicate that the fetus of other species is any
more susceptible to carcinogenesis by irradiation than are
infant or adult animals. In fact, there are notable observations to the contrary[1,8,10] - that is, of <u>lower</u> susceptibility of the fetal animal. Second, Jablon and Kato[4] found
no significant excess of deaths from cancer in children who
had been <u>in utero</u> at the time of the atomic bombings of
Hiroshima and Nagasaki. There was one death among some 1200
individuals (of whom approximately 250 were exposed to fetal
doses above 20 rads - many substantially above), whereas
0.75 would have been expected at Japanese national rates.
On the basis of available dose estimates, Jablon and Kato
considered this experience to be statistically incompatible
with the dose-response relationship derived from diagnostic
x-ray data[9]. Pointing to the uncertainties in the dose
estimates in both sets of data, Mole[7] noted that the upper
limit of the risk estimate from the atomic bomb data <u>might</u>
be compatible with the estimates from diagnostic radiography
"but only if all the assumptions in the calculations are
chosen with that intent". Hardly a ringing rebuttal of the
conclusion of Jablon and Kato.

Finally, while it is not inconceivable that fetal doses
in the 1 to 2 rad range would increase cancer risk by 40 or
50 per cent, one must acknowledge that biologic plausibility
argues against it. As Jablon and Kato remark[4]: "It seems,
to say the least, a puzzle why x-ray doses of the order of
1-5 rad to third-trimester fetuses should cause cancers
within ten years whereas (largely) gamma-ray doses exceeding
100 rad to children below ten years should produce cancers
only after a latent period of thirteen years or more".

Personally, I find the constancy of the relative risks
over all the major categories of malignancy the most difficult feature of the relationship to accept. It is true that
this feature was not found in the largest prospective study
of the question, in which the association was found for
leukemia but not for other malignancies[3]. However, this
study provided some of the clearest evidence there is of the
social and medical differences between exposed and unexposed
infants. In light of these differences - which were

reflected in differences in overall, as well as leukemia-
specific, mortality - it is difficult to put a great deal
of weight on the findings. By far the largest body of data
on the whole matter is that of the Oxford survey, and here
the same relative risk is seen for other tumors as for
leukemia. The same was observed in New England[6]. If the
existence of the association for solid tumors is in question,
then the principal bases for the existence of the association for leukemia (the Oxford and New England studies) are
also in jeopardy. We must accept this constancy of relative
risk over tumor types as a feature of the association as
presently understood. It is true that radiation carcinogenesis has been observed in a wide range of tissues in
children and adults, but the dose-response relationships, the
relative risks associated with given doses and the latent
periods are remarkable in their variety. Whey, then, should
fetal tissue respond in a way that appears to be constant -
not, it may be noted, in terms of tumor incidence per rad,
but in proportion to the incidence of tumors in the same
tissue when not exposed?

Other characteristics of the association. The data of
the Oxford survey have been explored intensively to charac-
terize the radiation-cancer relationship in terms of dose-
response, trimester of pregnancy at exposure and other
features. Stewart and Kneale[9] claim that a linear dose-
response relationship can be demonstrated in the Oxford data,
and a suggestion of some dose-response association was
evident in New England[4,6]. In the Oxford study the highest
relative risk was seen for infants exposed in the first
trimester. In the New England study, x-rays early in
pregnancy were under-ascertained, and this issue could not
be examined. The BEIR committee comments on these observations and the numerous interpretations and re-interpretations
that have been made of them over the years. The statistical
sophistication applied to the data by many writers is awe-
inspiring, but the discussion can have only a feathery substance when the analyses and re-analyses are essentially
limited to one set of data. Further, interest in these
refinements can follow only an acceptance of the causal
nature of the association. In this acceptance, I seem to
lean more towards the negative than did the BEIR committee.

What next? As indicated at the beginning of this presentation, I (with others) regard the question of whether
diagnostic x-rays increase the cancer risk to a fetus as an
important one. I expect to have conveyed the impression that

I (with others) do not regard the question as answered. How can we get, or at least approach, an answer? The difficulties include the facts that: (1) exposures are now too infrequent to provide the basis for a substantial study, (2) mothers' memories cannot credibly provide unbiased ascertainment of exposure, and (3) records of exposure are, at best, difficult to access and, at worst, missing in ways that are not free of bias. With these constraints, it is difficult to believe that a better data set than that of the Oxford survey - or even a set of comparable size and quality - will be forthcoming. The BEIR committee felt that further studies of irradiated twins are warranted. I suggest that studies of particular populations of twins would be informative, regardless of whether their radiation status is known. There was a time when a radiograph was to a twin pregnancy as a birth certificate is to a birth. Can it be true that only 55 per cent of twin pregnancies were x-rayed? Even if it were, and the relative risk associated with x-ray were 1.4, twins should still have a cancer rate 20 per cent higher than that of singletons. Yet currently available evidence suggests that their rate is lower - or at least not higher. If the latter were confirmed, it would be difficult to maintain that the association of fetal x-ray exposure with cancer risk was causal. While a study of twins would have to be a large one, it is worth noting that, while the records of x-ray exposure are ephemeral, the fact of being a twin is not. The problems of determining the cancer rate of infants born of twin pregnancies should be only mechanical. Short of some such indirect evaluation, it seems likely that the question of the association between fetal irradiation and childhood cancer will fade into medical history - unresolved and the source of more confusion than understanding.

REFERENCES

1. Cahill DF, Wright JF, Godbold JH, et al: Neoplastic and life-span effects of chronic exposure to tritium. II. Rats exposed in utero. J Natl Cancer Inst 55:1165-1169, 1975
2. Committee on the Biological Effects of Ionizing Radiations, Division of Medical Sciences, Assembly of Life Sciences, National Research Council: The Effects on Populations of Exposure to Low Levels of Ionizing Radiation. Washington, D.C., National Academy of Sciences, 1980.

3. Diamond EL, Schmerler H, Lilienfeld AM: The relationship of intra-uterine radiation to subsequent mortality and development of leukemia in children. A prospective study. Amer J Epidemiol 97:283-313, 1973

4. Jablon S, Kato H: Childhood cancer in relation to prenatal exposure to atomic-bomb radiation. Lancet ii:1000-1003, 1970

5. Kneale GW, Stewart AM: Mantel-Haenszel analysis of Oxford data. 1. Independent effects of several birth factors including fetal irradiation. J Natl Cancer Inst 56:879-883, 1976

6. MacMahon B: Prenatal x-ray exposure and childhood cancer. J Natl Cancer Inst 28:1178-1191, 1962

7. Mole RH: Antenatal irradiation and childhood cancer: causation or coincidence? Br J Cancer 30:199-208, 1974

8. Reincke U, Stutz E, Wegner G. Tumoren nach einmaliger Rontgenbestrahlung weisser Ratten in verschiedenem Lebensalter. Zeits f Krebsforsch 66:165-186, 1964.

9. Stewart A, Kneale GW: Radiation dose effects in relation to obstetric x-rays and childhood cancers. Lancet i: 1185-1188, 1970

10. Upton AC, Odell TT Jr., Sniffen EP: Influence of age at time of irradiation on induction of leukemia and ovarian tumors in RF mice. Proc Soc Exp Biol Med 104:769-772, 1960

Overall Risks of Cancer in A-Bomb

Survivors and Patients Irradiated

for Ankylosing Spondylitis

GILBERT W. BEEBE

Clinical Epidemiology Branch
National Cancer Institute
National Institutes of Health
Bethesda, Maryland

Ionizing radiation is an effective tool in experimental carcinogenesis, and the existence of large bodies of quantitative
data on man should in time constitute a major resource for
exploring ideas about carcinogenesis in man. Historically,
the bulk of the human data on radiation carcinogenesis has
come from the British ankylosing spondylitis patients and from
the Japanese A-bomb survivors. These studies have provided
the basis for the risk estimates of the International Commission on Radiological Protection, the Medical Research Council
(MRC), the National Academy of Sciences (NAS), and the United
Nations Scientific Committee on the Effects of Atomic Radiation, on which radiation protection procedures have come to
depend. The greater value of the two series, however, may
ultimately lie in their quantitative data on the variation in
risk of radiogenic cancer associated with characteristics of
host and of exposure situation, data that may be used to test
theories of carcinogenesis. Both series remain under observation and have just begun to provide the larger numbers
essential for statistical stability.

Although the risk estimates derived from the two series are
by no means definitive, and their implications for low-dose
effects are subject to debate, many of their findings are
quite solid and may well have implications for theories of
carcinogenesis in man.

ANKYLOSING SPONDYLITIS PATIENTS

The British ankylosing spondylitis series, about 14,000
mostly male patients treated by x-ray in British clinics from
1935-1954, was developed by Court Brown and Doll at the request
of the MRC in 1955.[10] The reports on the ankylosing spondylitis patients are notable for their quantitative emphasis
and for their consideration of many factors that influence
risk estimates in addition to size of dose: age at exposure,
sex, time after exposure, dose-fractionation, cell-type,
possible existence of a threshold dose, and form of dose-
response curve. The major publication is the 1957 MRC monograph on leukemia[4] in which Court Brown and Doll, with only
about 35 excess cases to work with, demonstrated that the
risk attributable to radiation increases with increasing
dose and with age at exposure, that the latent period can be
as short as 2-3 years, and that excess leukemia by type is
not proportional to its natural occurrence, chronic lymphocytic leukemia (CLL) not having been observed. In addition,
the authors interpreted their findings as suggesting that
there may be no threshold dose below which radiation is
without leukemogenic effect, and that the dose-response
function may be linear. Their views evidently provided much
of the force behind the shift from the previously dominant
concept of the "safe" dose to the present "no threshold"
hypothesis favored by most radiation biologists. With duration of follow-up ranging up to 20 years, but averaging only
5.5 years, the linear estimate of absolute risk was about
0.5 excess cases per million persons per year per rad to the
spinal marrow.
Subsequent reports on the series[5,15] extending follow-up
to 1970, show that the leukemogenic effect peaked about 3-8
years after irradiation and was substantially complete 20
years after exposure. These later reports also show that
excess solid tumors of heavily exposed sites, e.g., lung and
stomach, began to occur about 6-8 years after treatment
and at a lower level of relative risk, but in much greater
numbers than excess leukemias, and continued to appear even
20 years after irradiation. Excess tumor mortality in the
lightly irradiated sites is not statistically significant.
The most recent report[15] reveals an increase in risk of both
leukemia and solid tumors with increasing age at irradiation,
an increase that is roughly proportional to natural mortality.
Only for leukemia have dose-specific estimates been published
by Doll and his colleagues, but a considerable effort at
dose reconstruction has been under way for some time and
there is every reason to expect that dose-specific information
will soon become available for the solid tumors as well.[14]
Meanwhile, the 1980 BEIR III report[11] from the NAS gives

tentative organ dose estimates prepared by Fabrikant and
Lyman that are used there to derive linear risk estimates
for major sites.

The observational nature of the study of the British series
of ankylosing spondylitis patients invites reservations and
criticisms of the findings and their interpretation as evidence of an association between ionizing radiation and the
risk of leukemia and of solid tumors of heavily irradiated
sites. Patients with ankylosing spondylitis are known to be
at higher risk for certain diseases and therapeutic modalities
other than x-ray, especially drugs, might be thought to
increase their risk of cancer. Court Brown and Doll anticipated these criticisms in their 1957 report on leukemia,[4]
pointing out that the distribution of the excess by cell-type
differed from that found among the untreated cases, citing a
smaller study of ankylosing spondylitis patients who did not
receive x-ray treatment and among whom no excess leukemia was
found, noting that the excess leukemia risk increased with x-
ray dose, and discounting the likelihood that other forms of
therapy might be responsible for the association seen between
radiation dose and leukemia. A recent follow-up of ankylosing
spondylitis patients not treated by x-ray[16] has lent further
support to their position on leukemia and provided no reason
to believe that such patients have a higher risk of solid
tumors except possibly for cancer of the colon which may be
associated with ankylosing spondylitis through its connection
with ulcerative colitis. In 1980 perhaps the most compelling
evidence of the validity of the findings and of their interpretation by Doll and his colleagues is their consistency with
those from other studies.[11,19]

A-BOMB SURVIVORS

Three major samples are used in cancer studies at the Radiation Effects Research Foundation, formerly the Atomic Bomb
Casualty Commission: (1) The Life Span Study (LSS) sample of
82,000 survivors and 27,000 subjects not in the city (NIC) at
the time of the bomb, for whom mortality follow-up through the
Japanese family registration system is 100 percent complete
and supplemented by cancer registries in both cities; (2) the
Adult Health Study sample, a subsample of the LSS sample,
consisting of 15,000 survivors and 5,000 NIC subjects seen in
ABCC/RERF clinics at two-year intervals; and (3) the In Utero
Mortality sample of 1,800 exposed in utero and 900 controls.
The last published analysis of the experience of the LSS
sample was for the period 1950-1974 and covered 1.7 million
person years of follow-up for the 82,000 exposed to the
bombs.[2] Their average external dose is 27 rads. From 1950-

1974 there were 19,646 deaths among them, 4,031 attributed to neoplasms; by 1978 cancer deaths exceeded 5,000.[6]

With two-thirds exposed to less than 10 rads, the large LSS sample is predominantly a low-dose sample, but the two cities differ markedly, Nagasaki having many fewer in the low-dose range. Although neutrons formed only about 1 percent of the total dose in Nagasaki, they contributed 23 percent of the dose in Hiroshima. These differences set the stage for remarkable differences in the dose-reponse characteristics of radiation carcinogenesis in the two cities.

Sites and Types of Cancer

In addition to leukemia, by 1975 solid tumors of the thyroid, breast, lung, stomach, and esophagus had been linked with radiation dose in the A-bomb survivors. Suspicion had also fallen on the bladder, salivary gland, liver, large bowel, and pancreas. An excess of deaths from cancer of lymphatic and hematopoietic tissues other than leukemia was also seen in the 1950-1974 analysis. In their preliminary report on the 1950-1978 analysis given at the Radiation Research Congress in Tokyo last year, Kato and Schull indicated that there is now definite evidence of excess mortality from cancer of the large bowel (except rectum) and from multiple myeloma.[6] The list of affected sites has been increasing slowly since 1962,[17] when evidence of excess thyroid cancer became definite, and it can only be supposed that still other sites may be added to the list. Two organs known to be sensitive to the carcinogenic action of ionizing radiaticn, namely, skin and bone, have thus far provided no evidence of involvement. Even more important, no new variety of cancer peculiar to radiation has been detected.

Despite a vigorous pathology program, only very limited information on cell types has been provided, largely because the number of excess deaths from radiogenic cancer in the LSS sample is not large. For 1950-1974 it was estimated that only 90 leukemia deaths and 103 deaths from other cancers could be attributed to the radiation exposure.[2] For leukemia, however, the sample is large enough to conclude definitely that CLL is not increased by atomic radiation. There is also a suggestive city difference in excess chronic granulocytic leukemia (CGL), Hiroshima subjects having a marked excess, Nagasaki subjects much less. Finally, although the more malignant forms of thyroid cancer (anaplastic and medullary) have not been linked with atomic radiation, the thyroid sample is small and these forms are not among the most prevalent cell-types in naturally occurring thyroid cancer.[12]

Tissue sensitivity to the carcinogenic effect of ionizing

radiation can be measured in terms of relative risk or absolute risk, with somewhat different results. Relative risk
puts leukemia in a class by itself, cancer of breast or thyroid next, and cancer of lung, stomach, or esophagus at a
distinctly lower level. Absolute risk permits little distinction among leukemia, breast cancer, and thyroid cancer in
the category of greatest sensitivity, with lung cancer, etc.,
in a distinctly lower risk group. Again, the relative paucity
of excess cases, other than leukemia and breast cancer, makes
closer comparisons unreliable. But certainly cancer of skin
or bone can be put in the lowest category at the present time.

Distribution of Excess Cases over Time

Remarkable differences in temporal distribution of excess
cases are seen between leukemia and solid tumors, and by age
at exposure. The leukemogenic effect begins 2-4 years after
exposure, reaches a maximum at 6-7 years post-exposure, and
has essentially disappeared 30 years after exposure. The
solid tumor excess cannot be pinpointed so accurately, since
relative risks are lower and excess cases, except for breast
cancer, fewer. But it is plain that radiogenic solid tumors
are slower to appear initially, and continue much longer, than
radiogenic leukemias.

Evidence that high doses shorten the time of appearance of
excess tumors is seen only for leukemia.[9]

Age at exposure plays an important role in determining
length of minimal latent period for solid tumors, but apparently not for leukemia. For leukemia, excess cases appear
soon in all age groups at exposure, cease early in the
youngest age groups, and are most sustained in intermediate
age groups. For breast cancer, no excess has appeared among
those under age 10 in 1945; in the remaining age groups the
minimal latent period is longer the younger the age in 1945.
For lung cancer, by 1974 no effect could be seen in those
under age 35 in 1945 but by 1978 Kato and Schull observed
excess lung cancer in all but those under 10 in 1945, and the
minimal latent period was again longer the younger the age in
1945.[6] These age differences have been interpreted as evidence that solid tumors of radiogenic origin appear at the
ages of natural incidence, and as being generally supportive
of a relative risk model with respect to time and narrowly
applied to a particular tumor in a particular population.

Host Factors

Not all of the influence of age in 1945 is seen in the
temporal distribution of excess cases, for there are important
differences among age groups in magnitude of carcinogenic

response. This is most clearly seen in leukemia, for which
the experience is now complete. Those under age 10 in 1945,
and those 50 or older, suffered excess cases at rates much
higher than those of intermediate age groups. Similarly,
women aged 10-19 in 1945 have, thus far, the greatest excess
risk of breast cancer of any age group. But the breast cancer
experience is still incomplete.

Dose-Response Functions and Their Derivatives

Currently the A-bomb survivor data fuel the controversy
over the choice of dose-response models, the relative biological effectiveness (RBE) of neutrons, and the size of low-dose
effects. The observations on leukemia incidence, breast
cancer incidence, and mortality from all forms of cancer
except leukemia, are extensive enough to be exploited in this
fashion,[11] but definitive results may be forthcoming only for
breast cancer if present trends continue.[18]

Leukemia

Through 1974 there were only 34 deaths from leukemia among
survivors in the Nagasaki LSS sample; with only two of these
in the range of 10-99 rads (external dose), the dose-response
plot is decidedly curvilinear, although linearity is not
rejected by statistical test. In the larger Hiroshima sample
there were 110 deaths, 25 in the 10-99 rad range, and the plot
is quite linear. Whether the curvilinear appearance of the
Nagasaki plot reflects merely sampling variation, or the dose-
response function for leukemia resulting from low-LET radiation truly is curvilinear, remains uncertain and quite
controversial. Whatever the reason, the result is that estimates based on the LSS cohort inevitably show gamma radiation
to be a weak carcinogen in comparison with neutrons. Table 1

TABLE 1
Regression Analysis of Leukemia Incidence,
Hiroshima and Nagasaki, 1950-1971

| Analysis | Dose-Response Function | | |
	L - L	LQ - L	Q - L
Goodness of fit (P)	.49	.49	.42
Tests of coefficients (P)			
Gamma dose	< .01	NS	–
Gamma dose^2	–	NS	< .01
Neutron dose	< .01	<.01	< .01
Neutron RBE, 1 rad neutrons	11.3	23.2	47.1
Excess cases/10^6PY,* 5 rads**	11.2	5.2	0.35

* Persons per year ** Tissue dose, low-LET
Source: NAS BEIR III Report, 1980

summarizes the recent BEIR III analysis in which three dose-
response models were fitted to the LSS incidence data for
1950-1971. These models are all linear in neutron dose but
differ as to the gamma dose, being either linear (L-L),
"linear-quadratic" (LQ-L), or so-called "pure quadratic" (Q-
L). The data are not robust enough to discriminate among the
three models, and low-LET coefficients for the LQ-L model are
quite unstable. The RBE for neutrons is a constant 11.3 under
the L-L model, and $47.1/D_n^{1/2}$ under the pure quadratic model.
At one rad of neutrons, the three RBE estimates are, by model:
L-L, 11.3; LQ-L, 23; and Q-L, 47.1. For an acute dose of 5
rads of gamma radiation to the bone marrow the risk per
million persons per year varies under the three models as
follows: linear, 11.2; linear-quadratic, 5.2; and pure
quadratic, 0.35. Although I do not think we are justified in
taking such low-dose estimates too seriously, they are the
best we have. They suggest that there is no great difference
between linear and linear-quadratic models in the low-dose
region, and that the pure quadratic model generates estimates
lower by more than an order of magnitude. The BEIR III
Committee expressed guarded preference for the linear-
quadratic model for leukemia.

Breast Cancer

Breast cancer, is, of course, far more prevalent than
leukemia among female A-bomb survivors and excess cases have
already occurred in greater numbers.[18] The series is large
enough to provide strong support for the near-equivalence of
risk in the two cities and for linearity of dose-response.[18]
The most recent data analyzed in the BEIR III fashion by Land
et al.,[8] are summarized in Table 2. Notably, with all coefficients constrained to be positive, the LQ-L model reduces
to the L-L model, and although the Q-L model cannot formally
be rejected on the basis of the goodness of fit test, with

TABLE 2
Regression Analysis of Breast Cancer Incidence,
Hiroshima and Nagasaki, 1950-1974

Analysis	Dose-Response Function		
	L - L	LQ - L	Q - L
Goodness of fit (P)	.94	.91	.39
Tests of coefficients (P)			
Gamma dose	< .01	< .01	–
Gamma dose^2	–	(coeff=0)	.02
Neutron dose	NS	NS	NS
Neutron RBE, 1 rad neutrons	1.4	≤1.4	40.7
Excess cases/10^6PY,* 5 rads**	10.9	10.9	0.1

* Persons per year   ** Tissue dose, low-LET
Source: Land et al., JNCI, 1980

P=.39, it does not fit nearly as well as the linear model for
which P=.94, and the quadratic term does not significantly
improve the fit of the LQ-L model. The neutron coefficient
does not differ significantly from 0 under any model and the
RBE of neutrons under the linear model is only 1.4 $\pm$ 1.9.
Annual low-dose, low-LET estimates are subject to much less
uncertainty for breast cancer than for leukemia but appear to
be of about the same magnitude; they pertain to a longer
period of excess risk, however. Estimates of the effect of 5
rads of low-LET radiation to breast tissue are 10.9, 10.9, and
1.3 excess breast cancer cases per million persons per year
for the three models, linear, linear-quadratic, and quadratic,
respectively.

All Cancer Mortality except Leukemia
Since excess mortality attributable to forms of cancer
other than leukemia is not large enough to sustain analyses
by site, the NAS BEIR Committee chose to estimate the combined
mortality risk of all forms of cancer other than leukemia.
Its analysis, based on A-bomb survivor data for 1950-1974 with
the exclusion of an arbitrary latent period, 1945-1954, is
given in Table 3. All three models fit equally well.
Striking is the fact that none of the gamma risk coefficients
differs significantly from 0, which reflects the fact that
there is very little evidence of any association between dose
and cancer risk in the Nagasaki mortality data. The test for
a linear increase with dose returns a P of .10. Since the
association is quite significant for the Hiroshima data in the
same test (P <.001), substantially all of the carcinogenic
effect in Hiroshima is attributed to neutrons. Since we know
that thyroid cancer and breast cancer are both significantly
related to dose in Nagasaki, the analysis in Table 3 is really
unacceptable as an indication of the general carcinogenic risk

TABLE 3
Regression Analysis of Cancer Mortality
(Excluding Leukemia), Hiroshima and Nagasaki,
1955-1974

Analysis	Dose-Response Function		
	L - L	LQ - L	Q - L
Goodness of fit (P)	.30	.23	.28
Tests of coefficients (P)			
Gamma dose	NS	NS	-
Gamma dose^2	-	(coeff=0)	NS
Neutron dose	.01	.02	<.01
Neutron RBE, 1 rad neutrons	44.2	$\leq$ 44.2	120
Excess cases/10^6PY,* 5 rads**	7.0	7.0	0.1

* Persons per year   ** Tissue dose, low-LET
Source: NAS BEIR III Report, 1980

associated with low-LET radiation. The NAS BEIR Committee
circumvented this troublesome problem by making two quite
arbitrary assumptions: (1) that in the LQ-L model the ratio
of the linear to the quadratic coefficient is independent of
type of cancer, so that the empirically obtained ratio for
leukemia may be used; and (2) the RBE of neutrons relative to
gamma radiation is also independent of type of cancer, so that
the relationship obtained for leukemia may be used for other
forms of cancer. When this was done, the low-dose risk
estimates for an acute dose of 5 rads of low-LET radiation
were 17.4, 7.2, and 0.46 excess cancer deaths per million
persons per year, for the modified linear, linear-quadratic,
and quadratic models respectively.

Criticisms

No epidemiologic study is entirely adequate or free from
defects, and the study of the A-bomb survivors is no exception.
The Nagasaki sample is much too small in the low-dose range,
dosimetry is based on the recollections of survivors of their
location when the bombs fell, males of military age in the
sample were largely those who were unfit for military service,
and the ascertainment of cancer depends in large part on the
death certificate. In addition, its critics[7,13] argue that
(1) the dose estimates should not exclude fallout and
early entrants into Hiroshima after the bombing have had a
higher risk of leukemia than the study of those directly
exposed suggests; and (2) the cataclysmic effect of the
bombings selected for survival individuals whose normal expectation of cancer and other chronic disease is well below that
of the general population. Investigations by Japanese,
British, and U.S. physicists have shown that fallout probably
contributed only in a very minor way, except for a small
agricultural community outside of Nagasaki, and to a lesser
extent in several suburban communities west of Hiroshima. It
has not been possible, or thought necessary, to adjust the
dose of the survivors for fallout or induced radiation.[1]
Moreover, published estimates of the leukemia risk of early
entrants are internally inconsistent, and the regression
estimates of leukemia risk per person-year-rads would be
little changed by any upward adjustment of the doses for
presumed contributions from fallout. Whether the holocaust
selected for survival individuals with a less than average
expectation of mortality from cancer and other diseases is
highly speculative and without empirical foundation.[3]

SIGNIFICANCE OF FINDINGS FOR THEORIES OF CARCINOGENESIS

Which of the findings of the two major human series are

definite enough to provide some factual basis for testing
theories of human carcinogenesis? I would pick the following,
but without attempting to guess their relative importance:
(1) Ionizing radiation is a fairly general carcinogen affecting most, if not all, sites of cancer and generating no unique
type of its own.
(2) At least a few cell-types appear not to result from
ionizing radiation; certainly CLL is in this exceptional class
and there may be others.
(3) The strength of the carcinogenic effect of the same
amount of energy released in a given volume of tissue is not
proportional to natural incidence by site.
(4) With the notable exception of leukemia the incidence of
radiogenic cancer tends to follow the natural age-specific
incidence of each form of cancer; minimal latent periods are
correlated with the interval between age at exposure and the
age at which incidence normally becomes appreciable; high
doses do not appear to accelerate the appearance of radiogenic
tumors, except possibly for leukemia.
(5) For most, but not all, forms of cancer, high-LET radiation seems to produce more cancer per rad at a given site
than does low-LET radiation; the breast may be the outstanding
exception.
(6) Partial-body exposure differs little from whole-body
exposure in carcinogenic effect when comparisons are based on
tissue dose.
(7) For most tumors, there is no evident threshold dose; skin
and bone are, however, likely exceptions.
(8) The minimal latent period for leukemia is notably shorter
than that for solid tumors; the duration of the effect also
seems to be shorter.

REFERENCES

1. Arakawa ET: Radiation dosimetry in Hiroshima and Nagasaki
    atomic-bomb survivors. N Engl J Med 263:488-493, 1960.
2. Beebe GW, Kato H, Land CE: Studies of the mortality of A-
    bomb survivors. 6. Mortality and radiation dose, 1950-
    1974. Radiat Res 75:138-201, 1978.
3. Beebe GW, Land CE, Kato H: The hypothesis of radiation-
    accelerated aging and the mortality of Japanese A-bomb
    victims, in Late Biological Effects of Ionizing Radiation,
    vol 1. Vienna, International Atomic Energy Agency, 1978,
    pp. 3-27.
4. Court Brown WM, Doll R: Leukaemia and aplastic anaemia
    in patients irradiated for ankylosing spondylitis.

Medical Research Council Special Report Series No. 295.
London, Her Majesty's Stationery Office, 1957, p. 135.

5. Court Brown WM, Doll R: Mortality from cancer and other causes after radiotherapy for ankylosing spondylitis. Br Med J 2:1327–1332, 1965.

6. Kato H, Schull WJ: Mortality experience of atomic bomb survivors, 1950–1978. Presented at the Sixth International Congress of Radiation Research, Tokyo, 1979.

7. Kneale GW, Stewart AM: Pre-cancers and liability to other diseases. Br J Cancer 37:448–457, 1978.

8. Land CE, Boice JD Jr, Shore RE, et al.: Breast cancer risk from low-dose exposures to ionizing radiation: Results of parallel analysis of three exposed populations of women. JNCI 65:353–376, 1980.

9. Land CE, McGregor DH: Temporal distribution of risk after exposure, in Nieburgs HE (ed): Prevention and Detection of Cancer. Part 1: Prevention, Vol 1: Etiology. New York, Marcel Dekker, 1977, pp 831–843.

10. Medical Research Council: Hazards to Man of Nuclear and Allied Radiations. London, Her Majesty's Stationery Office, 1956, p 89.

11. National Academy of Sciences, Committee on the Biological Effects of Ionizing Radiations: The Effects on Populations of Exposure to Low Levels of Ionizing Radiation. Washington, D.C., National Academy of Sciences, 1980, Typescript ed, p 638.

12. Parker LN, Belsky JL, Yamamoto T, et al.: Thyroid Carcinoma Diagnosed Between 13 and 26 Years After Exposure to Atomic Radiation. A Study of the ABCC-JNIH Adult Health Study Population, Hiroshima and Nagasaki, 1958–71. Hiroshima, Atomic Bomb Casualty Commission TR 5-73, 1973, p 21.

13. Rotblat J: The puzzle of absent effects. New Sci 75:475–476, 1977.

14. Smith PG: Personal communication.

15. Smith PG, Doll R: Age- and time-dependent changes in the rates of radiation-induced cancers in patients with ankylosing spondylitis following a single course of x-ray treatment, in: Late Biological Effects of Ionizing Radiation, vol 1. Vienna, International Atomic Energy Agency, 1978, pp 205–214

16. Smith PG, Doll R, Radford EP: Cancer mortality among patients with ankylosing spondylitis not given x-ray therapy. Br J Radiol 50:728–734, 1977.

17. Socolow EL, Hashizume A, Neriishi S, Niitani R: Thyroid carcinoma in man after exposure to ionizing radiation: A summary of the findings in Hiroshima and Nagasaki. N Engl J Med 268:406–410, 1963.

18. Tokunaga M, Norman JE Jr, Asano M, et al.: Malignant breast tumors among atomic bomb survivors, Hiroshima and Nagasaki, 1950–74. JNCI 62:1347–1359, 1979.
19. United Nations Scientific Committee on the Effects of Atomic Radiation: Sources and Effects of Ionizing Radiation, Report to the General Assembly. New York, United Nations, 1977, p 725.

Risk of Cancer
Associated with
Occupational Exposure
in Radiologists and
Other Radiation Workers

GENEVIEVE M. MATANOSKI, M.D., DR. P.H.

Professor
Department of Epidemiology
The Johns Hopkins University
School of Hygiene and Public Health
Baltimore, Maryland

Increasing use of external radiation in industry has renewed previous concerns about the hazards associated with chronic exposure to low levels of ionizing radiation. Recent studies of workers in nuclear facilities have suggested that they have an increased risk of cancer, especially multiple myeloma and pancreatic cancer (1,2). Another occupational group which probably had low doses of gamma rays has been reported to have a high risk of leukemia (3). In contrast to these relatively recent uses of radioactive materials, professionals associated with medicine have been exposed to x-rays since the 19th century. This presentation will emphasize the changing effects seen in radiologists over 70 years in order to emphasize differences in their mortality experience from early periods of practice when exposure to radiation was high to the current era of medicine when procedures should require very low levels of radiation.

Occupational studies of exposure to external radiation have had many problems associated with both measurement of the radiation and exposure to other toxic materials. Studies of radiologists are no exception to these problems. However, studies of these professionals have major advantages over other working groups. The records of exposed populations

The study was supported by Grant #OH 00465 from the National Institute for Occupational Safety and Health.

241

exist for long periods of time so one can study the effect of chronic exposure over 60 to 80 years. Unlike other members of the workforce, radiologists as an occupational group remain within their same profession throughout their lifetime. There are groups of physicians who have exposures to the same confounding variables as radiologists such as drugs and infections but who have no or lower doses of radiation and, therefore, can be used for comparison. The follow-up of these specialists is virtually complete due to their professional visibility. Their high socioeconomic status and education assure accurate diagnosis of medical conditions.

The study population consists of five medical societies. The cohorts who entered the professional groups between 1900 and 1929 consist of radiologists from the American Roentgen Ray Society (ARRS) and a comparison population of pathologists in the American Association of Pathologists and Bacteriologists (AAPB). The recent members of the specialties who entered professional societies from 1920 through 1969 include radiologists in the Radiological Society of North America (RSNA), internists in the American College of Physicians (ACP) and specialists in the American Academy of Ophthalmology and Otolaryngology (AAOO). These are all professional groups which were originally studied in the fifties by Drs. Seltser and Sartwell (4,5) and which have been subsequently updated (6,7). Initially, it was hypothesized that the internists would be exposed to radiation but at lower levels than radiologists and members of the other societies would have little or no exposure. Recent records have indicated that otolaryngologists have radiation exposures in recent years and their data have been analyzed separately from ophthalmologists in the later cohorts.

The radiologists in these professional societies number about 6500 with over twice that number in the control groups. Their combined experience represents about 750,000 person years. In Table 1, the mortality experience of all radiologists is compared to that of other specialty societies using U.S. white male rates for indirect adjustment by age and time. The results suggest that radiologists have higher mortality from all causes, all cancers, cardiovascular disease and stroke. The only causes for which radiologists do not show a consistently higher mortality than those of other specialists are the group of external causes - suicides, homicides and accidents.

Has the risk of cancer mortality changed for radiologists as their expected level of radiation has been reduced? Previous data as well as more recent analyses indicate that age and

TABLE 1
Comparison of Mortality of Radiologists
and Other Specialists

Cause of Death	Ratio of SMR* RSNA ACP	RSNA AAOO
All Causes	1.22	1.31
Cancers	1.34	1.56
Diseases Nervous System	1.32	1.34
Diseases Circulatory System	1.20	1.29
External Causes	1.05	0.96
All Other	1.22	1.39

* SMR=ratios of mortality indirectly age and
time adjusted against U.S. white male rates.

time adjusted rates for all cancers are highest in
radiologists compared to other specialists from the youngest
ages in the earliest cohorts of entry, 1900 through 1939.
The only difference in the pattern of excess mortality which
occurs in the later cohorts is that radiologists appear to
have a preferential cancer mortality in the youngest age
groups since they experience lower death rates than in other
specialty groups. However, at later ages, their cancer
mortality becomes higher than that seen in other specialists.

The ranking of the societies by cancer mortality rates
suggests a gradient of mortality similar to that originally
hypothesized for radiation dose for all cohorts.
Radiologists have the highest rates, internists and
otolaryngologists have slightly lower rates and the lowest
cancer death rate is attributed to ophthalmologists.

At exactly what age does this excess risk seem to occur?
The cancer death rates for each of the newer societies from
1920 on have been standardized against U.S. white male rates
and the standardized mortality ratios have been compared
between societies. The data in Figure 1 indicate that the
risk for all causes is not higher until the age of about 50
years when the ratio jumps from .55 to .75 for radiologists.
This age is about 25 years after the usual age of graduation
from medical school. From that age on, the radiologists have
consistently higher ratios than other specialty groups.

Similar data for cancer mortality is shown in Figure 2.
The curve is more irregular but suggests that the excess
mortality risk also begins at age 50 and continues throughout
the remaining age groups. The curve is very similar to that
of all mortality.

How long after entry into the society do radiologists first
show an excess risk of all deaths and of cancer? Using the

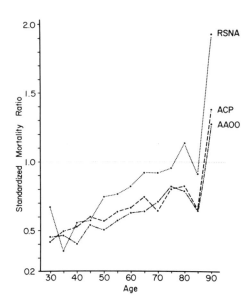

Figure 1. Standardized mortality ratios by age for all causes of death.

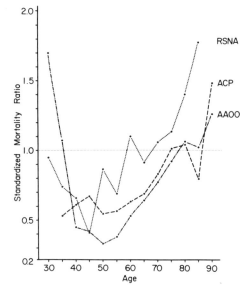

Figure 2. Standardized mortality ratios by age for all cancers.

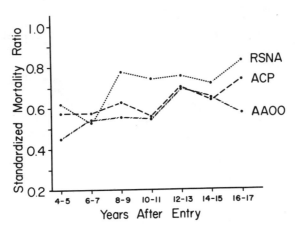

Figure 3.   Standardized mortality ratios by years after entry
            for all causes of death.

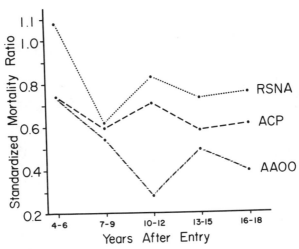

Figure 4.   Standardized mortality ratios by years after entry
            for all cancers.

combined cohorts in recent societies and the mortality ratios
standardized against U.S. white males as in the previous
analysis, it is apparent in Figure 3 that the risk of all
cause mortality begins to increase at about 8 or 9 years
after entry into the society. In Figure 4 similar ratios for
cancer mortality do not have as sharp a peak, perhaps because
of small numbers. However, the excess mortality seems to
occur about 10-12 years after entry into the specialty group,
a few years later than the increase described for all causes.
Entry into a specialty group occurs on the average 10 to 12
years after the physician's graduation from medical school
and at a point when he may already have had exposure to
radiation during his training and early period of practice.
   It is important to identify the specific sites of cancer
which are contributing to the excess cancer mortality and
to determine whether they are the same as those associated
with radiation exposure in other populations. For this
analysis, an internal comparison has been utilized since all
deaths within the specialty populations have been coded by
the same criteria. The standardized mortality ratios
represent adjustments for age and time using a log linear
regression model. A significant p-value for differences
between the societies is indicated by a double asterisk.
   The mortality ratios for selected cancer sites are
presented in Tables 2, 3 and 4. The sites selected represent

TABLE 2
Standardized Mortality Ratios (SMRs)
for ARRS and AAPB in Entry Period 1900-1929
All Cancer and Selected Cancers

Cause	SMR* ARRS	AAPB	
All Cancer	1.47	0.75	**
Oral cavity	1.32	0.80	
Stomach	1.55	0.74	
Colon	1.64	0.69	
Liver primary	0	1.67	**
Liver secondary	2.35	0	
Pancreas	1.56	0.69	
Lung	0.67	1.25	
Prostate	1.25	0.88	
Skin	2.55	0.27	**
Other-unspec. Ca	1.19	0.93	
Lymph. + Hemato.	1.87	0.54	**

* Adjusted for age and year of entry into study.
   Comparison based on total study population.
** p < .05

those which we think might be associated with an exposure to radiation either from other studies or from our own preliminary data. There are other sites which have high ratios in radiologists in several cohorts such as bladder, brain, and kidney and which are not included in the tables but, as with other sites, they are not associated with significant differences. In Table 2, the oldest society of radiologists with entrants from 1900-1929 is compared to the control society of pathologists and bacteriologists. There is an excess risk of all cancer, skin cancer, and lymphatic and hematopoietic cancers with ratios of 2.0, 9.5, and 3.5 respectively. The excess for primary liver cancer is associated with the group of pathologists rather than the radiologists. Although none of the mortality ratios for other cancer sites are significantly different, several sites are higher in radiologists than pathologists; these are oral cavity and pharynx, stomach, colon, pancreas, and prostate. In the 1920-1939 cohort of entry for the RSNA, ACP and AAOO (Table 3), we find that the total cancer mortality is high in radiologists and significantly different between societies. The sites with significant variation between groups and for which radiologists are highest include oral cavity, secondary liver, skin, lymphatic and hematopoietic tissue cancers, and unspecified cancers. It is noteworthy that few cancer sites appear to have an excess mortality in

TABLE 3
Standardized Mortality Ratios (SMRs)
for RSNA, ACP and AAOO in Entry Period 1920-1939
All Cancer and Selected Cancers

Cause	RSNA	ACP	AAOO	
All Cancer	1.38	0.94	0.85	**
Oral	2.17	0.52	0.95	**
Stomach	1.01	0.98	1.04	
Colon	1.25	0.98	0.87	
Liver primary	1.45	1.20	0.44	
Liver secondary	3.22	0.43	0.40	**
Pancreas	0.97	1.02	0.99	
Lung	0.96	1.13	0.85	
Prostate	1.24	1.03	0.81	
Skin	3.38	0.32	0.49	**
Other-unspec. Ca	1.69	1.07	0.48	**
Lymph. + Hemato.	1.64	0.81	0.87	**

* Adjusted for age and year of entry into study.
  Comparison based on total study population.
** p < .05

both time periods; exceptions are skin, oral cavity, hematopoietic system and total cancers. In Table 4, the mortality for these societies is presented for the 1940-1969 cohort of entry. The AAOO has been divided into two groups, the otolaryngologists and the ophthalmologists, because of the higher radiation exposure in the former group. Again we see an excess risk of total cancer mortality among radiologists which is about two times higher than it is in ophthalmologists. Only lung and colon cancers show significant differences between societies and this variation is not always associated with higher risks in radiologists. Skin cancer even in these later cohorts is associated with excess mortality in radiologists. Only oral and pharyngeal tumors have a high mortality ratio in radiologists consistently through all cohorts of entry. It is noteworthy in the final cohort that there is no excess of lymphatic and hematopoietic cancers in radiologists.

Tables 5, 6 and 7 present data on other specific diseases including subclasses of leukemia, multiple myeloma, lymphosarcoma, Hodgkin's, aplastic anemia and arteriosclerotic heart disease. In the earliest period, 1900-1929, radiologists have a significant 15-fold excess risk of leukemia which is associated with excesses of both

TABLE 4
Standardized Mortality Ratios (SMRs)
for RSNA, ACP and AAOO Ophthalmologists and
Otolaryngologists in Entry Period 1940-1969
All Cancer and Selected Cancers

Cause	SMR*			
	RSNA	ACP	AAOO otol	AAOO op
All cancer	1.15	1.08	1.01	0.59 **
Oral	2.88	0.31	2.00	0 **
Stomach	1.33	1.09	0.76	0.64
Colon	0.60	1.36	0.97	0.32 **
Liver primary	0.56	1.52	1.35	0
Liver secondary	0.70	1.13	1.66	0
Pancreas	0.72	1.13	1.41	0.46
Lung	1.22	1.15	0.97	0.33 **
Prostate	1.01	0.89	0.98	1.40
Skin	2.41	0.76	0.58	0.51
Other-unspec. Ca	0.75	1.16	0.94	0.80
Lymph. + Hemato.	1.07	1.04	1.08	0.75

* Adjusted for age and year of entry into study.
  Comparison based on total study population.
** p < .05

acute and myeloid leukemia (Table 5). They also have a
7.8-fold significant excess of aplastic anemia. The risk of
arteriosclerotic heart disease is about 20% higher than in
pathologists.

As seen in Table 6, the leukemias in the second cohort of
entry, 1920-1939, are still significantly higher in
radiologists than in the other societies and, again, this
excess is associated with the subtypes of acute and myeloid
leukemia that one might expect from exposure to radiation.
There is no excess of lymphatic leukemia. In this cohort a
significant excess of lymphosarcoma is demonstrated. This
cancer site was high for radiologists in the previous group
but the difference was not significant. Aplastic anemia
still occurs with significant excess mortality in radiologists
and the excess is almost identical to that in the previous
cohort. The 27% excess risk of arteriosclerotic heart
disease in radiologists as compared to members of the AAOO is
significantly different.

The final and most recent cohort of entrants into the
specialties are depicted in Table 7. The data are
impressive because of the complete absence of any excess risk
of leukemia among radiologists. There is some evidence of an
excess among otolaryngologists who, we suspect, may have had
a substantial exposure to radiation in recent years. For the

TABLE 5
Standardized Mortality Ratios (SMRs)
for ARRS and AAPB in Entry Period 1900-1929
Radiation-Related Diseases

Cause	SMR*		
	ARRS	AAPB	
Leukemia	2.41	0.16	**
Acute	2.68	0	**
Myeloid	2.74	0	**
Lymphatic	1.39	0.78	
Monocytic	2.78	0	
Other & Unspec.	2.13	0	
Multiple Myeloma	0	1.52	
Lymphosarcoma	1.82	0.60	
Hodgkin's Disease	2.98	0	
Other Lymphomas	0	1.42	
Aplastic Anemia	2.36	0.30	**
ASHD	1.12	0.94	

*   Adjusted for age and year of entry into
    study. Comparison based on total study
    population.
** p < .05

TABLE 6
Standardized Mortality Ratios (SMRs)
for RSNA, ACP and AAOO in Entry Period 1920-1939
Radiation-Related Diseases

Cause	SMRs* RSNA	ACP	AAOO	
Leukemia	2.01	0.79	0.62	**
Acute	2.23	0.78	0.55	**
Myeloid	2.39	0.71	0.43	**
Lymphatic	1.34	0.85	0.95	
Monocytic	0.78	1.01	1.15	
Other & Unspec.	2.90	0.63	0.41	
Multiple Myeloma	0.89	0.86	1.00	
Lymphosarcoma	2.73	0.40	0.80	**
Hodgkin's Disease	0.53	1.32	0.71	
Other Lymphomas	0.60	0.69	1.68	
Aplastic Anemia	2.70	0.59	0.37	**
ASHD	1.15	1.00	0.91	**

* Adjusted for age and year of entry into study.
  Comparison based on total study population.
** $p < .05$

TABLE 7
Standardized Mortality Ratios (SMRs)
for RSNA, ACP, AAOO Ophthalmologists and
Otolaryngologists in Entry Period 1940-1969
Radiation-Related Diseases

Cause	SMRs* RSNA	ACP	AAOO otol	AAOO op	
Leukemia	1.00	0.90	1.56	0.70	
Acute	1.17	0.67	2.60	0.40	
Myeloid	1.69	0.90	0	1.85	
Lmyphatic	0.63	1.22	1.12	0.65	
Monocytic	0	1.41	1.84	0	
Other & Unspec.	0	0	4.95	0	
Multiple Myeloma	2.05	0.81	1.48	0	**
Lymphosarcoma	0.41	1.49	0.80	0.63	
Hodgkin's Disease	1.14	1.04	0	1.50	
Other Lymphomas	1.07	0.83	0	2.26	
Aplastic Anemia	0	0	0	0	
ASHD	1.15	0.95	1.06	0.93	

* Adjusted for age and year of entry into study.
  Comparison based on total study population.
** $p < .05$

first time among the cohorts of entry we see a two-fold
excess risk of multiple myeloma in radiologists compared to
ophthalmologists and a lesser excess in otolaryngologists.
There is a similar relative risk of arteriosclerotic heart
disease as in previous cohorts and this difference is already
approaching significance with a p-value of .07.

The time at which leukemia appears in excess after entry
into a professional society is displayed in Figure 5. The
standardized mortality ratios for leukemia using U.S. white
male rates for standardization for the cohorts entering the
radiology society from 1920 through 1939 are graphed for the
time periods after entry. There is a peak at about 3 to 5
years after entry into the society and another peak 15 to
16 years after entry. The excess persists to termination of

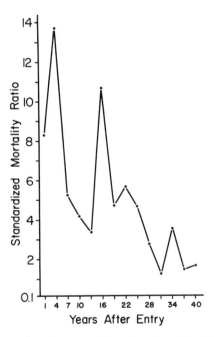

Figure 5. Standardized mortality ratios for leukemia by years
after entry into the Radiological Society of North
America. Entry 1920-1939.

the study. The observed excess is 14 times the rate in U.S.
white males at the first peak and 10 times the rate in the
second peak. We are investigating further the possible
reasons for the bimodality. It cannot be attributed to
changing rules for entry into the society. It is possible
that the peaks represent different types of leukemia. It may
be an artifact due to small numbers.
    From these data it is apparent that radiologists exposed to
continuous doses of radiation throughout 40 or more years of
practice experience an excess risk of cancer mortality which
is about 1.5 to 2 times higher than that of other
specialists. They have shown a smaller 20 percent increase
in other chronic diseases but no excess in deaths from
external causes. The risk of mortality for the specialists
in most cohorts follows the gradient that we would expect
based on their presumed exposure to radiation.
    The overall excess of cancer is not caused by a consistent
excess of lesions at any one site with the exception of oral
and skin cancers which are high throughout the 70 years of
follow-up. The all cancer ratios are significantly high in
radiologists because several cancer sites have high or the
highest mortality ratios in this specialty group compared to
others for each time period examined. The specific sites of
excesses change over time with stomach cancer having the
highest risk in one period, colon in another, and lung in the
third. The times of excess of stomach and lung cancer seem
to conform to the times when deaths from cancer at these sites
were excessive in the general population. Are the observed
excesses in radiologists related to an enhancement by
radiation of an underlying environment cancer risk? Selection
bias in choosing an occupation may also play a role.
    The U.S radiologists had a risk of acute and myeloid
leukemia and aplastic anemia in the earliest cohorts but
those excesses have disappeared for entrants into the
profession after 1940 and multiple myeloma has appeared to
be consistently high in cohorts of entry from 1930 on. We
propose that the excesses of leukemia and aplastic anemia
may have been due to high doses of radiation and these doses
have subsequently decreased with a resultant decline in these
diseases. It has been estimated that doses to the marrow of
radiologists in a lifetime of practice in early periods may
have been as high as 600 to 800 rads, a sizable dose. We may
now be seeing only excesses of cancer related to low dose
chronic exposure to radiation. These outcomes may be
specifically multiple myeloma and a general carcinogenic
effect at several sites. However, the overall excess of

cancer remains the same. It is true that the British
radiologists have not shown an excess risk of cancer in the
cohorts who entered the specialty after 1920 even though
there was a significant excess in earlier periods (8). The
early radiologists also had excess skin cancer, leukemia
and aplastic anemia although the numbers were small and the
authors placed relatively little importance on the findings.
They did not see an overall risk in mortality even when
using doctors as comparisons and this is not surprising since
specialists usually have a preferred mortality experience
compared even to general practitioners.

Could the effects we are now seeing be due to a selective
bias for entry into the radiology specialty? This is, of
course, a possibility. The fact that several causes as well
as cancer appear to be showing an excess risk would support
this supposition. However, many physicians choose their
specialty at graduation from medical school which is about 10
years before entering the society. It is difficult to see
how they are predicting their selectivity for disease this
far in advance. It is also difficult to explain the
consistency of the rise in the risk at a specific age, about
50 years, and at a specific time after entry into the society
on the basis of selection bias. The sudden increase in risk
suggests exposure to an environmental agent at a single point
in time. The excesses by society consistently occur with the
gradient one might expect if the variation in radiation
exposure between the groups is the major factor associated
with cancer and other diseases. It will be necessary to
examine more closely these risks in populations
occupationally exposed to low-doses of external radiation in
order to determine whether the subtle differences observed in
recent cohorts of radiologists actually exist.

REFERENCES

1 Mancuso T, Stewart A, Kneale G: Radiation Exposures of
  Hanford Workers Dying From Cancer and Other Causes. Health
  Physics 33: 369-384, 1977.
2 Marks S, Gilbert ES, Breitenstein BD: Cancer Mortality in
  Hanford Workers, in Late Biological Effects of Ionizing
  Radiation. Vol 1. Proceedings of a Symposium. Vienna,
  International Atomic Energy Agency, 1978, pp 369-386.
3 Najarian T, Colton T: Mortality from Leukemia and Cancer
  in Shipyard Nuclear Workers. Lancet 1: 1018-1020, 1978.

4 Seltser R, Sartwell PE: The Application of Cohort Analysis to the Study of Ionizing Radiation and Longevity in Physicians. Am J Public Health 49: 1610-1619, 1959.

5 Seltser R, Sartwell PE: The Influence of Occupational Exposure to Radiation on the Mortality of American Radiologists and Other Medical Specialists. Am J Epidemiol. 81: 2-22, 1965.

6 Matanoski GM, Seltser R, Sartwell PE, et al: The Current Mortality Rates of Radiologists and Other Physician Specialists: Deaths from All Causes and from Cancer. Am J Epidemiol 101: 188-198, 1975.

7 Matanoski GM, Seltser R, Sartwell PE, et al: The Current Mortality Rates of Radiologists and Other Physician Specialists: Specific Causes of Death. Am J Epidemiol 101: 199-210, 1975.

8 Court-Brown WM, Doll R: Expectation of Life and Mortality from Cancer Among British Radiologists. Br Med J 2: 181-187, 1958.

Industrial and Lifestyle Carcinogens

Industrial and Life-Style Carcinogens[1]

MICHAEL B. SHIMKIN

Professor of Community Medicine and Oncology
Department of Community Medicine
University of California, San Diego, School of Medicine
La Jolla, California 92093

HISTORICAL PRELUDE

Pott's description, in 1775, of scrotal cancer among chimney sweeps, is a milestone in our understanding of cancer. Here was a specific cancer in a specific occupation, evoked by a specific agent; prevention was as obvious as the cause.[16]

During the Nineteenth Century, some half-dozen other occupational environments were described in which long-term contact with oils and tars led to the appearance of skin cancers. In 1895, Rehn added the occurrence of urinary bladder cancers among workers in the dye industry. The responsible agent acted not at the site of contact, but required transport through the body in order to manifest a distant carcinogenic effect.

Oncology during the Nineteenth Century was preoccupied with histogenesis, and experimental cancer research had to await the introduction of transplantable tumors. Little attention was paid to industrial cancers, which were considered to be exotic occurrences without general relevance. Prevention of cancer was limited to early detection and prompt surgical treatment. Primary prevention, the prevention of occurrence, was seldom mentioned. As an example, primary prevention was not one of the goals at the founding in 1913 of the American Society for the Control of Cancer, the precursor of the American Cancer Society.

[1] Prepared with assistance of Contract NIH 263-78-C-0095 from the National Cancer Institute.

The discovery of experimental tar cancer made in 1915 by
Yamagiwa and Ichikawa, and the isolation of carcinogenic polycyclic hydrocarbons from tar, accomplished by Kennaway and his
group by 1930, opened the period of chemical carcinogenesis.[16]
The emphasis of laboratory research in cancer became biochemical, stimulated by the possibility of endogenous production of
carcinogens from cholesterol. And, indeed, the female sex
hormone was shown to be carcinogenic, the first clearly defined chemical carcinogen of endogenous origin.

Minimal research investment was made before World War II on
environmental sources of carcinogens. The pioneer endeavors
of William Hueper and of Leon Shabad in this direction were
recognized only many years later. However, during the 1950s
the causative relation of tobacco smoking to lung cancer was
demonstrated, essentially by epidemiologic methods. The discovery elevated cancer epidemiology and statistics to legiti-
mately recognized scientific pursuits, aroused predictable
commercial repercussions, and lay unexploited by the public.
A major environmental carcinogen had been identified. It was
not an industrial contaminant, but a habit of a large proportion of the population, a part of their life style.

Environmental concerns have been a prominent feature of our
society during the past several decades. Rachel Carson's
"Silent Spring," published in 1962, warned us of the consequences of saturating our environment with insecticides. Her
book remains a worthy symbol of the environmental period.

Cancer has shared in the environmentalist orientation.
Epidemiologists pointed out geographic differences in cancer
rates, their relationships to habits and occupations, and
their changes in migrant populations. Extrapolations from
such differences led to widely publicized pronouncements that
90 percent of all cancers were environmental, and thus potentially preventable. Further statistical elaborations assigned
20 percent of all cancers to occupations, and even a larger
proportion to nutrition. Symposia,[9] conferences,[8] and publications,[5] on environmental carcinogens and on cancer prevention proliferated. National and international groups of
experts periodically regrouped and re-analyzed data available
on man and on animals.[1] A shelf of muck-raking, alarmist
books appeared on the neglect of environmental carcinogens,
and interpreted the neglect as a conspiracy between science
and business. From an obscure specialty of a few public
health practitioners, environmental cancer became a topic of
public concern and governmental involvement.

The rise of interest in environmental carcinogens and
cancer prevention also coincided with public disappointment in
the achievements of cancer research. The solution of the
cancer problem has been a national commitment since 1937, and

expanded along managerial lines in 1971. Too much was prom-
ised, or was implied as a promise, from massive programs in
cancer chemotherapy and in viral oncology. No magic bullet
that cured all cancers emerged, and no virus causing all
cancers in man was identified. Public awareness of cancer and
of cancer research, carefully promoted by publicity, became
intense. It also became more sophisticated, although not
always correct.

One consequence of the stimulated acquaintance of the
public with cancer was to make cancer the main concern in
problems that had many more immediate and serious hazards.
The first cause of death and disability in industry is acci-
dental trauma, not neoplasms. The possibility of perishing
from ionizing radiation is much greater as a consequence of
a disputation between world powers over fossil fuel than it is
from the dangers of nuclear energy plants.

The public, as well as the scientific community, must be
kept appraised, and kept correctly and honestly appraised,
not only of our successes but also of our disappointments and
errors. Neither science nor the public are well served by
exaggerated, premature announcements and messianic exhorta-
tions. Such pronouncements support budget increases, but are
not convincingly hedged or retracted. Nor do numerical values
added to guesses convert guesses into facts.

What, then, are the facts about environmental carcinogens,
from industrial and from more general sources? What are the
dangers, and how are we to avoid them? Are we living in a sea
of carcinogens - or a miasma of fear?

CARCINOGENESIS

Attempts to answer the questions posed above require con-
ceptualization of the process of carcinogenesis. Figure 1 is
a diagrammatic guide for this discussion.

Cancer is a chronic pathological endpoint of a prolonged,
complex process. It is a result of exogenous or endogenous
stimuli interacting with cells of a genetically susceptible
host. The interaction is influenced by a myriad of factors
that either enhance or retard the reaction. Among the factors
related to the stimulus are the dose, concentration, schedule,
vehicle, and route. Among the factors related to the host
are age, sex, nutritional and immunological status, other
diseases, and undoubtedly the complex of psychological influences. The balance between the stimulus and the host
determines the proportion of neoplasms evoked and the rate
at which they appear.

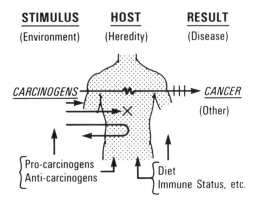

Figure 1. A Scheme of Carcinogenesis.

Responses to stimuli leading to cancer are, as other processes, dose-dependent. The greater or more prolonged the
stimulation, the more cancers will arise, and the earlier will
be the appearance of the cancers. The range over which this
relationship exists is limited and is not necessarily linear.
At higher doses, toxic effects may inhibit the neoplastic reaction. At lower doses, the reaction may be obscured by the
background noise of the spontaneous rate of neoplasia for the
population. Nevertheless, as Paracelsus said five centuries
ago, "the poison is in the dose."

The no-threshold concept for carcinogens has been of theoretical importance, but empirically and practically its value
is dubious. As a basis of legislation, such as the Delaney
Clause, which prohibits the addition of any amount of carcinogens to food, it has the clarity of the Ten Commandments.
However, it requires human interpretation and a definition of
what is a carcinogen. Are carcinogens a group of compounds
distinct from all other chemicals? It seems more logical not
to separate them from the universe of chemical substances, and
not to demand safety standards that are absolute. For one
thing, there may be more risk in trying to reach absolute
safety than the risk that is avoided.[3]

The activity of a carcinogen can be modified by other
chemicals in the environment and in the host. The earliest
example of co-carcinogenesis was adduced from the demonstration that the amount of the active carcinogen in tar, benzo(a)-
pyrene, was insufficient to account for the numbers of cancers
induced, and that other chemicals in the mixture were acting
as co-carcinogens or promoters without themselves being carcinogens. A more recent interest has been on agents that reduce or retard carcinogenesis, such as antioxidants or

selenium. This research field now bears the attractive name
of chemoprevention. Enhancement or inhibition of carcinogenesis can also occur through metabolic changes of the host.
Perhaps the clearest demonstration of this are the studies of
Albert Tannenbaum,[17] showing that limitations in nutrition reduced spontaneous and induced tumors of several types in mice.

Some carcinogens seem to exert their activity only at the
point of contact; the best example is ultraviolet radiation.
Other carcinogens require carriers for impingement or penetration; hematite particles for polycyclic hydrocarbons delivered
to the lung are an example. Carcinogens that enter the body
undergo complex chemical conversions that may include detoxification and excretion, or produce more active carcinogens.
The best examples of the latter are afforded by the classical
investigations of James and Elizabeth Miller,[11] using primarily aromatic amines.

In addition to the pharmacodynamics of dose and concentration, and to metabolic conversions, carcinogens have specificity of action in regard to the end-organ in which the
neoplastic reaction is evoked. When a rat is injected with
7,12-dimethylbenz(a)anthracene, DMBA, a potent carcinogen,
practically all of its tissues soon fluoresce, indicating the
wide distribution of the chemical. Yet tumors, arising many
weeks later, are restricted to but a few end-organs such as
the breast. There must be neoreceptors[14] involved in the induction of neoplasia, similar to the estrogen-receptor model.
These neoreceptors are not static structural entities, but
reactive states modified by a variety of conditions, such as
the age and sex of the host.

It is commonly accepted that carcinogenesis is not a sudden
event, but that it goes through stages of initiation, promotion, and growth, which in turn may consist of multiple
stages. The original stimulus may be a pulse dose, such as
exposure to radiation, but the reactions that occur until the
overt neoplasm is evident are multiple.

It is also commonly accepted that the ultimate cellular
reaction that manifests itself as cancer involves the DNA of
the nucleus, producing a permanent, genetically transmissible
change. As Berenblum[4] has written, not all neoplastic situations fit neatly into this scheme, and consideration of the
exceptions may be more informative than the rule. The most
intriguing alternate hypotheses include the possible role of
viruses integrated into the genome, and the role of differentiation.

There is an element of circular thinking in the definition
of carcinogens. Active, obvious carcinogens pose little problems. These are agents that produce histologically and bio-

logically malignant killing neoplasms of several types in several species of animals. Usually small doses of such chemicals are sufficient to demonstrate carcinogenic effects. The
problems, of course, are with agents that are given in maximum tolerated amounts over the lifetime of animals, and at
terminal autopsy are found to be associated with a greater
proportion of some type of tumors than the untreated controls.
Should these chemicals be labeled as carcinogens, and designated as such in comparing other procedures for testing carcinogenic activity? At what point should such data be considered to define potential hazard to man, and therefore come
under the purview of regulatory actions?

Lists of chemicals, viruses and physical agents that have
been called carcinogenic in animals now include literally
thousands of entities, although many are analogues of parent
compounds. Obviously, agents carcinogenic in animals should
be suspected of having carcinogenic import for man. Yet extrapolations from animal data to man require caution, especially since data on animals are usually obtained under conditions not encountered in man. Few indeed are chemicals ingested by man at maximum tolerated doses over the whole lifetime.

Adding fuel to the discussions and arguments regarding extrapolation of animal data to man are even more disparate information sources on *in vitro* systems.[2] The fact that many
established carcinogens are also mutagens has bracketed these
two biological responses in the minds of many, extending the
lists of potential human hazards. As an example,[10] studies on
drinking water report the presence, in minute amounts, of 23
carcinogens and suspected carcinogens and 30 mutagens and suspected mutagens. Tests for mutagenicity on bacteria involve
not only life-term exposure to the agent tested, but exposure
over several generations of unicellular organisms that lack
the homeostatic mechanisms which multicellular organisms have
evolved.

Data on mutagenesis and teratogenesis, of course, are valuable and must not be ignored. In my opinion, however, none
should be extrapolated to indicating hazard for man until
there is more knowledge than is available at present. The
first need often is to replicate the *in vivo* findings. Secondly, there should be more dose-response information so that
quantitation can be gauged over several orders of magnitude.
Thirdly, the nature of the cellular masses should be tested by
transplantation, to assure that these are biological as well
as morphological cancers. The non-metastasizing invasive lesions of the bladder seen in old male rats fed large doses of
saccharin are not the pathological entity that killed Hubert
Humphrey.

HUMAN CARCINOGENS

Environmental agents that have induced cancer in man, on
evidence acceptable to qualified committees, are listed in
Table 1. The exact number can be increased by specifying
closely related agents - such as alkylating agents used in the
treatment of cancer - or decreased by grouping. The important
category of polycyclic aromatic hydrocarbons, for example,
includes many mixtures and chemicals.

One traditional presentation of carcinogens has been to
array the agents by the situational exposure: occupational,
medicinal, or general. There is obvious overlap between such
categories. Industrial exposures do not stop conveniently at
the gates of the plant, and industrial effluents become contaminants of the regional water supply. Another division that
can be made is by the route of entry: skin contact, ingestion,
or inhalation. These also overlap, as inhaled agents are also

TABLE I
Human Carcinogens

Agent	Site
Aflatoxin	Liver
Alkylating agents	Marrow
Androgens	Liver
Aromatic amines	Urinary bladder
Arsenic	Skin, lung
Asbestos	Lung, serosa
Benzene	Marrow
Benzidine	Urinary bladder
Chloromethyl ether	Lung
Chromium	Lung
Estrogens	Uterus, vagina
Immunosuppressants	Lymphatic
Isopropyl oil	Nasal sinus
Mustard gas	Lung
Nickel	Nasal sinus
Phenacetin	Kidney
Polycyclic aromatic hydrocarbons	Skin, lung
Radiation, ionizing	Skin, marrow, etc.
Radiation, ultraviolet	Skin
Schistosoma haematobium	Urinary bladder
Vinyl chloride	Liver
Viruses	Lymphatic

Modified from Althouse et al.[1]

ingested and also come in contact with body surfaces. Chemical structure can be used as a framework, but human populations are usually exposed to complex mixtures rather than to
single chemicals. An alphabetical listing is as informative
as any, but should serve as a simple check list rather than
implying other meanings.

In terms of the populations exposed and the carcinogenic
effects elicited, a half-dozen of the agents stand out as of
primary importance. These include the polycyclic aromatic
hydrocarbons, the active constituents of the ubiquitous
products of incompletely burned vegetable material, the oils,
shales, tars of industry, and the condensates of smoke of
tobacco and of engines powered by fossil fuel. The aromatic
amines, and their role in dye, rubber and many other industrial processes, are perhaps the second more important class
of carcinogens. Asbestos, silicates of many physical and
chemical forms, have gained special recent recognition as
potentiators of exposure to other agents, especially the inhalation of tobacco fumes. Although asbestos is a carcinogen
for serosal surfaces, perhaps as an example of "solid state"
carcinogenesis, its main role appears to be to promote impingement and penetration of other carcinogens. The female
sex hormones, as replacements of lost youth, represent perhaps
the best recent example of medicinal, iatrogenic carcinogenesis, but may already be a chapter of the past. Certainly
the use of diethylstilbestrol as a useless aid in the preservation of pregnancy is now of historical and litigious
interest only. Aflatoxin and *Schistosoma haematobium*, prominent in the African and Asian tropics, are of little or no
consequence in Europe and the United States.

Viruses are now included in the list of human carcinogens.[6]
Certainly the Epstein-Barr virus is etiologically related to
the African childhood lymphoma and to nasopharyngeal carcinoma, and herpes hominis 2 and hepatitis B viruses may be related to genital and hepatic neoplasms.

A prominent omission from Table 1 is nitrosamine, because
no role has been as yet demonstrated for it in human carcinogenesis. Yet the activity of this class of compounds,
and their autosynthesis from nitrites and amines, make them
obvious candidates for our search of endogenous carcinogens.

The list includes several metals, and vinyl chloride, as
more typical examples of agents to which industrial groups
are exposed. The import of these agents to the general
population is unknown, but must be very small.

If there is anything clear about carcinogenesis, it is that
the exposure is almost always intense and prolonged. The
process takes 7 to 20 years to eventuate in cancer. During
such a length of time, alterations occur in the host,

nutritionally, hormonally and immunologically. All such
alterations influence the development and the growth of the
neoplasm.

The first question of a putative carcinogen for man should
be whether man indeed is exposed to it at all. In California
we plant oleanders along the highways. Oleanders are poison-
ous plants, but we do not use them in salads and consider that
their beauty is of no danger to us. The second question
should be, how much of the chemical does indeed get on or into
man. The third should be what happens metabolically to the
chemical. This is undoubtedly the most important area for
future research on carcinogenesis, to define the enzymatic and
other metabolic mechanisms devised by our body to guard
against the perils of the environment. In fact, the definition of such measures and their effectiveness will lead to
the understanding of individual susceptibility, probably the
next large step to be achieved in the clinical sciences.[9]

IMPORTANCE OF HUMAN CARCINOGENS

Having defined certain chemicals and other agents that
induce cancer in man, the next question is how important, in
the total occurrence of cancer, are these agents.

One line of evidence has been adduced from rates of incidence and mortality from cancer during the past thirty years.
During this time chemical industrial production has increased
and, if related to cancer, should have increased the occurrence of cancer.

When adjusted for age, no remarkable increases are observed
during the past four decades.[7,13] In fact, there has been a
decline in mortality rates under 45 in the United States,
interpreted by some as being due to therapeutic improvements,
especially chemotherapy. Increased mortality among men has
been attributed to the pandemic of lung cancer due to cigarette smoking, and the male rates show no increase when lung
cancer is removed from the calculations.

These data leave much to be desired. Cancer is a conglom-
erate of many disparate neoplastic diseases, some of which
have gone up (such as pancreatic as well as pulmonary cancer),
and others which have gone down (such as cancer of the stomach
and uterine cervix). The balance remains fairly constant, for
reasons that may evoke the disquieting thought that the population rate for cancer remains even and that changes occur
primarily as shifts between various entities.

Another factor to be considered is that the occurrence of
cancer today reflects exposures of a decade or more before.
Also important is that the study of total cancer may obscure

minor, specific neoplastic epidemics such as the estrogenic
cancers of the vagina and of the endometrium. Such occurrences are revealed by clinical suspicions and astute special
studies. The resources of the NCI SEER program are becoming
of increasing importance in detecting neoplastic rises in
defined populations. Employees in industries that could be
followed through mortality among the retirees, via social
security rosters, would be another valuable and frugal resource that would yield valuable information.

In any case, studies on the incidence and mortality in
human populations do not support an important role for industrial carcinogens in the total cancer occurrence. By far
the most important single carcinogen is our old enemy, tobacco
smoking.

As a general pattern, cancer favors more technological,
supposedly more advanced and advantaged populations. Many of
the correlations of nutrition and cancer drawn between populations are no more prominent than correlations made to the
gross national product. A recent study of Finland,[18] for
example, concludes that ". . . the general environment and way
of life which has been called urban or developed puts the
individual under an increased risk of most types of cancer.
The specific factors involved remain to be defined." Unknown
factors are also involved in the low incidence of cancer
among religious groups that practice abstinence from tobacco,
alcohol, follow a frugal semi-vegeterian diet, and have many
other selective factors that remain to be defined.[12]

In regard to specific neoplasms, it is one matter to discover that ionizing radiation produces acute myelocytic
leukemia, or carcinoma of the thyroid, and another matter to
assign what proportion of these neoplasms are indeed caused or
related to this factor. In our society, every citizen has the
right to claim that his leukemia is the result of an atomic
bomb test or a defoliant exposure. The measure of the actual
risk, and the translation of this risk to individual situations, however, is a legal rather than a scientific evaluation.

At an important conference held in 1979 at the American
Health Foundation, with Ernest Wynder[19] in the chair, experts
were asked to make estimates of the role of various risk
factors in cancer. Their conclusions are extracted and summarized in Table 2.

It is difficult to relate these estimates to some of the
assertions about the importance of known environmental carcinogens and the possibilities of cancer prevention. Tobacco
smoking is a primary controllable environmental factor, with
alcohol as an enhancing factor, perhaps through solubilizing
other carcinogens. All cancers must involve nutritional and

TABLE 2

Factors in Cancer, as Summarized at the Conference on the Primary Promotion of Cancer, New York, 1979.

	Men	Women
	Percent of Cancers Involving Factors	
Smoking	25–35	5–10
Alcohol	7	2
Occupation	6	2
Nutrition	30	30–50
Food contaminants	0	0
Drugs	<1	<1
Air pollution	0	0
Ionizing radiation	<3	<3
Ultraviolet radiation	(skin 50)*	(skin 50)*
Heredity	10–25	10–25
Viruses	<1	<1
Immunodeficiency	<1	<1

*Excluded from total cancers.
Derived from Wynder[19]

genetic factors, but these factors require further definition if they are to be useful in preventive measures. As far as more specific factors are concerned, the estimates of their role in human carcinogenesis varies from zero to 3 percent.

Cancer is a multifactorial disease, and the numbers in Table 2 must *not* be added to yield a neat 100 percent, or any other simple summation.

PREVENTION OF CANCER

An important reason for being interested in causation and risk factors is to have the knowledge upon which preventive measures can be devised and practiced. The present climate abroad in the land favors prevention as the approach against cancer. At least we talk about it more than we used to.

I am devoted to preventive medicine, but its limitations are only too obvious. Redemption of sins is closer to the human condition than a blameless life. Redemption is quick and visible; a blameless life, alas, only promissory. So is prevention as apposed to treatment.

But it is an error to compare or to appose treatment and prevention. Both are necessary and desirable. The choice between the two depends upon their relative ease and effectiveness rather than upon any cosmic considerations. If we had a chemical that would cure cancer by a few intravenous injections and leave no serious sequelae, there would be less need for prevention. If such a miracle drug existed for cancer of the uterine cervix, for example, there would be less need for community Pap smear programs, not to mention cancer warnings about early coitus and multiple sex partners.

When measures of primary prevention of cancer available to us at present are analyzed, it soon becomes obvious that the recommendations are not limited to cancer, but represent measures of general health protection. This is summarized in Table 3, which points out the same facts about primary prevention of industrial carcinogenesis. Cancer prevention is health protection, and should not be separated from it. Such separation is encouraged by health agencies bearing the label of cancer. They jealously guard their budgets and their turf, and are careful not to impinge upon the turf of other categorical prerogatives. It is high time they got together.

Preventive oncology is but a part of preventive medicine,[15] which in turn is but a part of medicine, a part of society. Control of cancer will be achieved by new knowledge acquired through research on causes and on cures. Special units propounding and applying the limited knowledge available to us at present are useful as an interim device.

The final goal of *all* cancer research is cancer control. And in this we are not doing badly, unless we overpromise and raise anticipations beyond realistic levels. Thus, progress in cancer chemotherapy is real and obvious, albeit it is limited to a few categories of neoplasia. It has not made a serious impress upon the big cancer killers, of the breast, lung, prostate, and large intestine, which account for over 50 percent of all cancer deaths. Viral oncology has not uncovered a cancer virus inducing all human cancers. But here

TABLE 3
Primary Prevention of Cancer

A. General
1. Do not smoke tobacco or substitutes
2. Do not drink alcohol
3. Eat sparingly a "prudent" diet
4. Avoid unnecessary x-rays
5. Avoid excessive sun exposure
6. Avoid inappropriate drug intake
B. Industrial
1. Avoid or minimize contact with irritants
2. Avoid or minimize ingestion of foreign materials
3. Avoid or minimize inhalation of foreign materials
4. Use appropriate protective measures and devices

progress also is real and important, with one viral entity being involved in two types of human cancer, and two other viruses threatening to make the list also. Perhaps some day we may have truly preventive vaccines against some cancers.

We must encourage research and application of the findings to cancer prevention. But such applications should not be at the expense of research on treatment, on virology, and on many other approaches. At the same time, cancer prevention should be in the vanguard of reuniting preventive medicine of all diseases as an integral part of the health protection of all people.

We are going forward. Let us continue.

SUMMARY

It is established that a significant proportion of cancer in man is man-made. Some occupational groups provide the clearest examples, but social habits also are associated with cancer risk. Cancer occurrence is related to population density, to the industrial-economic activity of the area, and, as other diseases, favors the poor. Hygienic measures in the working places, and hygienic habits of life reduce cancer rates.

Primary prevention of cancer, neglected for too long, is a wise social and individual goal. Application and exploitation of available knowledge might produce 30 to 40 percent reduction in cancer. The elimination of tobacco use alone, if not replaced by similar vices, would prevent a 100,000 cases a year in the United States alone. But the prevention of cancer awaits research findings to be made in the future.

REFERENCES

[1] Althouse, R., Huff, J., Tomatis, L. et al. An evaluation of chemicals and industrial processes associated with cancer in humans based on human and animal data: IARC Monographs, vols. 1-20. *Cancer Research* 40:1-12, 1980.

[2] Ames, B.N. Identifying environmental chemicals causing mutations and cancer. *Science* 204:587-93, 1979.

[3] Ashby, E. *Reconciling Man With the Environment*. Palo Alto: Stanford University Press, 1978.

[4] Berenblum, I. Established principles and unresolved problems in Carcinogenesis. *J. Natl. Cancer Inst. 60:723-26, 1978.*

[5] Dayan, A.D. and Brimblecombe, R.W. (eds.). *Carcinogenicity Testing: Principles and Problems*. Baltimore: University Park Press, 1978.

[6]DeThé, G. Viruses as causes of some human tumors? Results and prospectives of the epidemiologic approach. In *Origins of Human Cancer*, H.H. Hiatt, J.D. Watson and J.A. Winsten (eds.) pp. 1113-31. Coldsprings Harbor Lab. 1977.

[7]Devesa, S.S. and Silverman, D.T. Cancer incidence and mortality trends in the United States: 1935-74. *J. Natl. Cancer Inst.* 60:545-71, 1978.

[8]Griffin, A.C. and Shaw, C.R. (eds.). *Carcinogens: Identification and Mechanisms of Action*, p. 487. New York: Raven Press, 1979.

[9]Harris, C.C. (moderator). Individual differences in cancer susceptibility. *Ann. Int. Med.* 92:809-25, 1980.

[10]Kraybill, H.F. Evaluation of public health aspects of carcinogenic/mutagenic biorefractories in drinking water. *Preventive Med.* 9:212-18, 1980.

[11]Miller, E. Some current prospectives on chemical carcino-genesis in humans and experimental animals. *Cancer Research* 38:1479-96, 1978.

[12]Phillips, R.L. Role of life-style and dietary habits in risk of cancer among Seventh-Day Adventists. *Cancer Research* 35:3513-22, 1975.

[13]Pollack, E.S. and Horn, J.W. Trends in cancer incidence and mortality in the United States: 1969-76. *J. Natl. Cancer Inst.* 64:1091-1103, 1980.

[14]Shimkin, M.B. Carcinogenesis: frontiers in inner space. *Ann. N.Y. Acad. Sci.* 163:2:1026-29, 1969.

[15]Shimkin, M.B. Overview: Preventive Oncology. In *Persons at High Risk to Cancer*, J.F. Fraumeni, Jr. (ed.). pp. 435-48. New York: Academic Press, 1975.

[16]Shimkin, M.B. *Contrary to Nature*. Washington: Government Printing Office, 1977.

[17]Tannenbaum, A. and Silverstone, H. Nutrition in relation to cancer. *Advances in Cancer Research* 1:451-501, 1953.

[18]Teppo, L., Pukkala, E., Hakama, M. et al. Way of life and cancer incidence in Finland. *Scand. J. Social Med.*, Suppl. 19, 1980.

[19]Wynder, E.L. (chmn.). Conference on the Primary Prevention of Cancer: Assessment of Risk Factors and Future Directions. *Preventive Med.*, 9:163-332, 1980.

The Metabolic Activation of
Chemical Carcinogens

ELIZABETH C. MILLER

WARF Professor of Oncology
McArdle Laboratory for Cancer Research
University of Wisconsin Medical School
Madison, Wisconsin 53706

It has been evident for several decades that chemical carcinogens with a variety of structures can cause tumors to develop
in experimental animals and in the human. Many of the carcinogens belong to one of several groups of chemicals, e.g. polycyclic aromatic hydrocarbons, aromatic amines and amides, N-
nitroso amines and amides, alkylating agents, and halogenated
hydrocarbons. Within each of these groups there are a number
of chemicals that possess carcinogenic activity and others
that possess little or no carcinogenic activity.

METABOLISM OF CARCINOGENS IN RELATION
TO INITIATION AND PROMOTION

Carcinogenesis is now generally recognized as a multistage process (Berenblum 1974; Slaga et al, 1978). The first
stage is known as initiation. It occurs rapidly and is
essentially irreversible. The initiated cells appear not
to be tumor cells, and they can not be recognized directly.
They are known to exist by the fact that the application
of another chemical, known as a promoter, causes them to
develop into tumor cells that replicate to yield gross tumors.
The second step, promotion, requires a much longer time than
the initiation stage, and promotion appears to be reversible
in the early phases. It has been possible to dissect these
stages because some chemicals have essentially only initiating
activity and others act primarily as promoters. However, most
of the chemicals involved in the induction of cancer appear

269

to be complete carcinogens, i.e., to possess both initiating
and promoting activities. The relative amounts of initiating
and promoting activity for different complete carcinogens may
differ greatly.

Furthermore, most chemical carcinogens are not active
in the forms administered and require metabolism to ultimate
carcinogens (E. C. Miller & Miller, 1976; J. A. Miller
& Miller, 1979). This activating metabolism may occur in
one step, or it may involve the intermediate formation of
proximate carcinogens. In addition, metabolism to inactive
derivatives occurs. Thus, one factor that determines the
carcinogenicity of a chemical under a given set of conditions
is the relative proportions of its metabolism that leads to
carcinogenically active products and to inactive metabolites.

The metabolites that are active in the initiation of
carcinogenesis have the special property of being strong
electrophilic reactants (E. C. Miller and Miller, 1976;
J. A. Miller and Miller, 1979). Electrophilic reactants
are positive or uncharged molecules with electron-deficient
atoms that react by sharing electron-pairs of electron-
rich atoms such as S, O, and N. These reactants are typified
by the alkylating agents. Broadly speaking, free radicals,
i.e., reactive species with unpaired electrons, are also
electrophilic and can abstract hydrogen atoms from other
molecules. Although their initial reactions are hit-and-
run attacks, free radicals generated in nucleic acids or
proteins can react with other free radicals to yield macro-
molecule-bound carcinogen residues (Cavalieri, 1976; Kriek,
1979; Ts'o et al., 1974).

Reaction of electrophiles with DNA can result in mutations,
and the predominant view is that the initiation step of
carcinogenesis is usually, if not always, a mutagenic event.
In that case DNA would be the critical target of the electrophilic reactants for initiation. However, there are no
compelling data that specify mutation as the only possible
basis of initiation (see E. Miller, 1978; Rubin, 1980;
Weinstein et al., 1978).

On the other hand, the available evidence strongly indicates that the promotion stage of carcinogenesis does not
depend on alteration of DNA. In the case of complete carcinogens, i.e., those that possess both initiating and promoting
activity, electrophilic metabolites initiate the carcinogenic
process and non-electrophilic metabolites (or the parent compound) may promote the initiated cells. In addition, electrophilic reactants may also function as promoting agents.
Studies with the skin tumor promoter tetradecanoyl phorbol
acetate suggest that the cell membrane is a critical target
for promotion (Weinstein et al., 1978). On the other hand,

the reactions of electrophilic compounds in promotion may
not always be specific; those reactions that result in cell
death may have indirect promoting activity through the
stimulus of cell death on reparative hyperplasia.

GENERAL ASPECTS OF CARCINOGEN METABOLISM

Although the capacity of the liver for the metabolism of
chemical carcinogens is generally greater than that of other
tissues, sensitive methods have shown that metabolism of
carcinogens, at least at low levels, can occur in a wide
variety of tissues.

Furthermore, metabolism may occur at a number of sites on
most carcinogens, and more than one type of metabolism may be
possible for a given functional group. Although one or more
of the metabolic products are electrophilic and essential
for carcinogenic activity, the major share of the metabolism
ultimately yields non-electrophilic metabolites which have
no known function in the carcinogenic process. However, the
possible roles of the non-electrophilic metabolites in
tumor promotion have generally not been examined.

The enzymes that metabolize carcinogens are generally
localized in the cytosol or the endoplasmic reticulum. However, some cytochrome P-450 monooxygenases, originally considered to be associated only with the endoplasmic reticulum,
also occur in the nuclear envelope (Kasper, 1976). Although
only a few per cent of the total cellular cytochrome P-
450 monooxygenase is in the nuclear envelope, the proximity
of the products formed there to the DNA may make these
reactions more important, at least for initiation, than the
quantitative aspects suggest. On the other hand, continuity
of the endoplasmic reticulum with the outer leaflet of the
nuclear envelope may facilitate the transfer of electrophilic
reactants formed within the endoplasmic reticulum to the
nucleus. Specific cytosolic proteins for transport of some
electrophilic products to the nucleus have also been suggested (Ketterer, 1980; Mainigi and Sorof, 1977).

ELECTROPHILIC METABOLITES OF REPRESENTATIVE CARCINOGENS

The best studied of the carcinogens with regard to their
metabolic activation and reactivity are the potential donors
of simple alkyl groups (Magee et al., 1976; O'Connor et al.,
1979). The four potential methylating agents in Figure 1
are each relatively potent carcinogens and, except for
cycasin, are representative of classes of carcinogens with

POTENTIAL ALKYLATING AGENTS

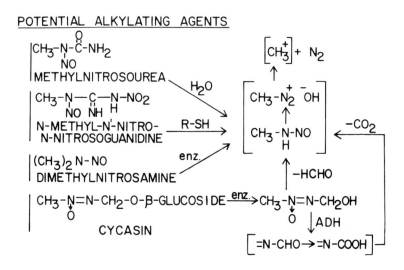

Figure 1. The metabolic activation of potential methylating
           agents.

relatively broad species and tissue susceptibilities. In
each case metabolism leads to the formation of a methyl
diazonium ion, which gives rise to the methylating species.
The formation of alkyl diazonium ions from $\underline{N}$-alkyl-$\underline{N}$-nitros-
amides and $\underline{N}$-alkyl-$\underline{N}$-nitrosimides occurs non-enzymatically
on reaction with water or sulfhydryl groups, respectively,
under physiological conditions. Activation of dimethylnitrosamine occurs through oxidation of one methyl group by a
cytochrome P-450 monooxygenase in the endoplasmic reticulum;
the unstable monomethylnitrosamine rearranges rapidly to the
methyl diazonium ion. In the case of cycasin the first step
is hydrolysis of the β-glucosidic bond; β-glucosidase is
found in animals primarily in the bacteria of the intestinal tract. Further activation can apparently occur either
by loss of formaldehyde or by oxidation with alcohol dehydrogenase to the aldehyde, subsequent oxidation to the acid,
and loss of carbon dioxide (Fiala et al., 1978; Grab & Zedeck,
1977). 3,3-Dimethyl-1-phenyltriazene yields a methylating
species through oxidation by a cytochrome P-450 monooxygenase,
rearrangement of the monomethylalkylaryltriazene, and addition
of a proton (Preussmann et al., 1969) (Figure 2).
     The toxic pyrrolizidine alkaloids, which are constituents
of plants from a number of genera and are hepatocarcinogenic
in rodents, each contain a nuclear double bond alpha to an
esterified carbinol (Culvenor & Jago, 1980; E. C. Miller

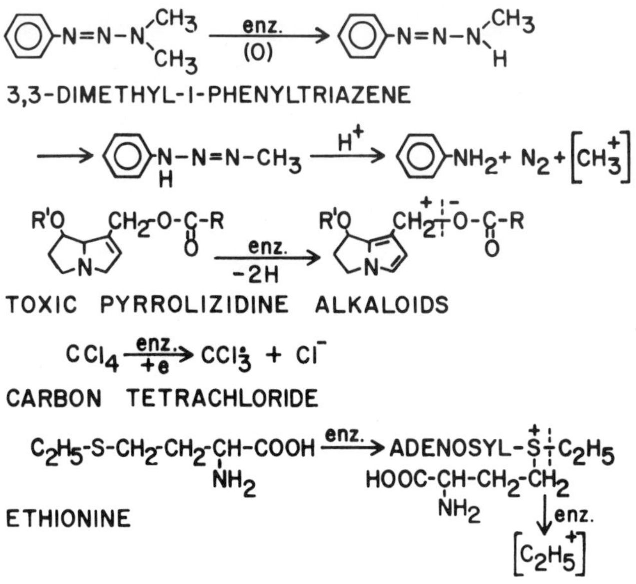

3,3-DIMETHYL-1-PHENYLTRIAZENE

TOXIC PYRROLIZIDINE ALKALOIDS

$$CCl_4 \xrightarrow[+e]{enz.} CCl_3^{\cdot} + Cl^-$$

CARBON TETRACHLORIDE

$$C_2H_5\text{-}S\text{-}CH_2\text{-}CH_2\text{-}CH\text{-}COOH \xrightarrow{enz.} ADENOSYL\text{-}\overset{+}{S}\text{-}C_2H_5$$

ETHIONINE

Figure 2.   The metabolic activation of some potential alkylating agents.

& Miller, 1979). This structure is dehydrogenated by a cytochrome P-450-dependent enzyme to a pyrrolic ester. Carbon
tetrachloride, another hepatocarcinogen, is enzymatically
reduced in the endoplasmic reticulum, apparently by a cytochrome P-450-dependent enzyme, to a CCl_3 free radical. The
hepatocarcinogen ethionine is converted to its S-adenosyl
derivative by a cytosolic transferase, which can then ethyl-
ate nucleic acids (E. C. Miller & Miller, 1979).
    2-Acetylaminofluorene (Figure 3) is one of the more com-
plex carcinogens for which the metabolic activation has been
worked out in some detail for one target tissue, the liver
(E. C. Miller & Miller, 1976; Kriek, 1979). The first step
is N-hydroxylation by a cytochrome P-450 monooxygenase in
the endoplasmic reticulum. A cytosolic hepatic sulfotransferase converts the proximate carcinogen N-hydroxy-2-acetyl-
aminofluorene to N-sulfonoxy-2-acetylaminofluorene, which
is a strong electrophilic reactant and which appears to be
a major ultimate carcinogen in rat liver. N-Hydroxy-2-
acetylaminofluorene is also converted to a nitroxide free
radical by one-electron oxidants, such as peroxidases, and
this free radical dismutates to yield the reactive ester
N-acetoxy-2-acetylaminofluorene. These esters react with

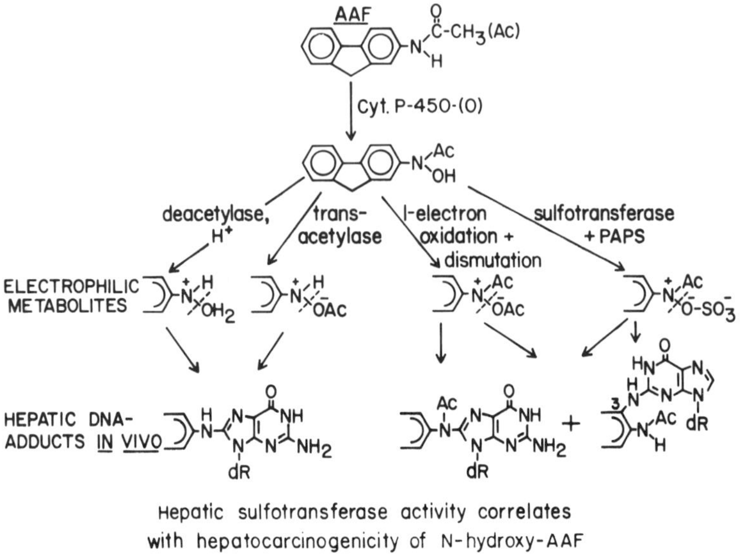

AAF

Cyt. P-450·(O)

deacetylase,   trans-   l-electron   sulfotransferase
H⁺   acetylase   oxidation +   + PAPS
dismutation

ELECTROPHILIC
METABOLITES

HEPATIC DNA-
ADDUCTS IN VIVO

Hepatic sulfotransferase activity correlates
with hepatocarcinogenicity of N-hydroxy-AAF

Figure 3.   The metabolic activation of 2-acetylaminofluorene
in rat liver.

nucleic acids to yield guanine adducts in which the N-acetyl
group is retained. N-Hydroxy-2-acetylaminofluorene is also
a substrate for a cytosolic transacetylase which converts
it to N-acetoxy-2-aminofluorene. Both this electrophilic
ester and the protonated hydroxylamine, formed by deacetyla-
tion of N-hydroxy-2-acetylaminofluorene in the endoplasmic
reticulum, react to yield non-acetylated products. The hepatic DNA and RNA from rats given N-hydroxy-2-acetylamino-
fluorene contain both acetylated and non-acetylated adducts.
Although metabolic attack occurs at many sites on the
hydrocarbons, in the past few years great attention has been
focussed on the so-called diolepoxides of the hydrocarbons as
the principal ultimate carcinogenic metabolites (Gelboin and
Ts'o, 1978; Sims, 1980). These products are formed in a
three-step reaction as exemplified in Figure 4 for benzo(a)-
pyrene. Epoxidation catalyzed by a cytochrome P-450 monooxygenase occurs at the 7,8-position and this epoxide is hydrolyzed by epoxide hydrase. The resulting trans-7,8-dihydrodiol
is then epoxidized at the 9,10-position in a stereoselective
manner. Other studies indicate that the formation of similar

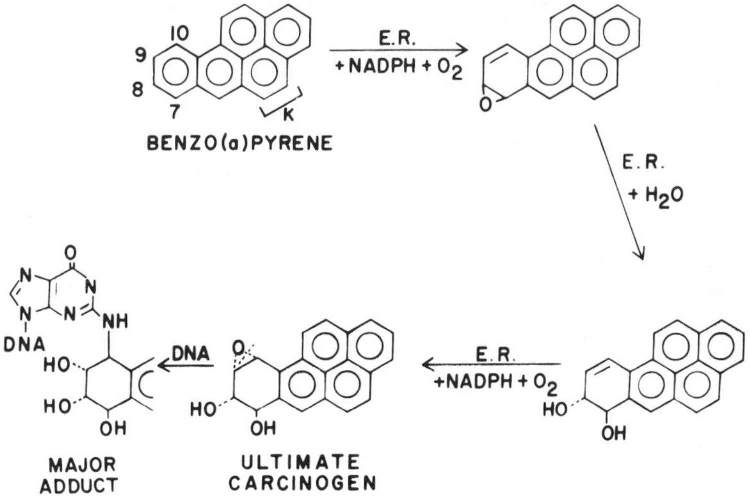

Figure 4. The metabolic conversion of benzo[a]pyrene to
           a reactive diolepoxide.

diolepoxides in which the substituents are all on adjacent
carbon atoms on one ring and in which the epoxide is in the
"bay region" formed by the angular rings may be a general
mechanism for the enzymatic activation of the polycyclic
aromatic hydrocarbons in carcinogenesis (Wood et al., 1979).

APPROACHES TO CANCER PREVENTION BASED ON KNOWLEDGE OF
THE METABOLISM OF CHEMICAL CARCINOGENS

Even though our knowledge on the metabolism of chemical
carcinogens and on the mechanisms of chemical carcinogenesis
is still far from complete, the available data and concepts
provide opportunities that can and have been exploited
toward the prevention of human cancer. The generalization
that strong electrophilic reactivity is a basic requirement
for the initiation of carcinogenesis and knowledge of the
metabolic activation and deactivation of many chemicals
are providing useful approaches toward the reduction of
exposure. For instance, some predictions with regard to
electrophilic reactivity and possible carcinogenicity can
be made from inspection of chemical structures (e.g., those
proposed for use as drugs, industrial intermediates, etc.)

for substituents with electrophilic reactivity under physiological conditions and for potential metabolism to derivatives containing such functional groups. Further, mutation
systems, frequently fortified with tissue preparations for
metabolic activation, are now being widely used to screen
for chemicals with potential electrophilic activity (McCann
et al., 1975; Purchase et al., 1978; Rinkus and Legator,
1979). Malignant transformation of mammalian cells in
culture, sometimes supplemented with tissue preparations
for metabolism of the chemicals, provide useful assay systems
in which the formation of cancer cells is the endpoint
(Pienta et al., 1977; Purchase et al., 1978). The use of
human tissues is beginning to provide information on the
metabolic similarities of human and animal cells with respect
to their abilities to activate and deactivate carcinogens.

Despite the usefulness and importance of these and other
short-term tests, for the present the results from such
assays can only be used as prescreens for potential carcinogenic activity. The abilities of chemicals to induce cancer
in whole animals still provide the only approach that we
have for the evaluation of their potentials for actually
causing cancer. Even then, the metabolic differences between
the experimental animals and any human population make the
extrapolation of animal carcinogenicity data to the estimation of human risks very difficult. Furthermore, humans
are exposed to a wide variety of chemicals in all parts of
their environments, including their food and the products of
the microorganisms in their gastrointestinal tracts. These
environmental chemicals possess a wide range of biological
activities, and some may be expected to have initiating
activity, promoting activity, or complete carcinogenicity.
In addition, a wide variety of foreign chemicals, including
some that occur naturally in foods (Wattenberg, 1979),
induce increased synthesis and increased tissue levels of
certain enzymes such as the monooxygenases, epoxide hydrase,
and glutathione-$\underline{S}$-transferase. Altered levels of one or more
enzymes can change the metabolic balance between competing
reactions, and this alteration may profoundly affect the
dispositions of a broad range of chemical carcinogens.

It is apparent that the quantitative aspects of the
metabolism of chemical carcinogens in humans, as well as
in experimental animals, will differ as a function of the
genetic make-up of the individual, nutritional conditions,
hormonal balance, and exposures to other chemicals. Furthermore, conditions that reduce or increase the metabolism of
a given chemical to carcinogenically active products could
increase, reduce, or have no effect on the metabolism of
other chemical carcinogens or toxins to their active and

inactive metabolites. It is evident that much more study
on these metabolic relationships will be needed before
purposeful alterations of the levels of carcinogen-metabo-
lizing enzymes can be used as practical approaches for
cancer prevention in human populations.

REFERENCES

Berenblum, I. Carcinogenesis as a Biological Problem.
Amsterdam/Oxford: North-Holland, 1974.

Cavalieri, E., Roth, R., & Rogan, E. C. Metabolic activation
of aromatic hydrocarbons by one-electron oxidation in
relation to the mechanisms of tumor intiation. In R.
I. Freuendenthal and P. W. Jones (Ed.), Carcinogenesis,
Vol. I, Polynuclear Hydrocarbons; Chemistry, Metabolism,
and Carcinogenesis. New York: Raven Press, 1979, 181-
190.

Culvenor, C. C. J., & Jago, M. V. Carcinogenic plant products
and DNA. In P. L. Grover (Ed.), Chemical Carcinogens
and DNA. Boca Raton, Fla.: CRC Press, 1979, 161-186.

Fiala, E. S., Kulakis, C., Christiansen, G., & Weisburger,
J. H. Inhibition of the metabolism of the colon carcinogen,
azoxymethane, by pyrazole. Cancer Res., 1978, 38, 4515-
4521.

Gelboin, H. V., & Ts'o, P. O. P. (Ed.) Polycyclic Hydrocarbons
and Cancer: Molecular and Cell Biology. New York:
Academic Press, 1978.

Grab, D. J., & Zedeck, M. S. Organ-specific effects of the
carcinogen methylazoxymethanol related to metabolism by
nicotinamide adenine dinucleotide-dependent dehydrogenases.
Cancer Res., 1977, 37, 4182-4189.

Kasper, C. B. Chemical and enzymic composition of the
nuclear envelope. In P. L. Altman and D. D. Katz (Ed.),
Cell Biology. Bethesda, Md.: Federation of American
Societies for Experimental Biology, 1976, 395-400.

Ketterer, B. Interactions between carcinogens and proteins.
Brit. Med. Bull., 1980, 36, 71-89.

Kriek, E. Aromatic amines and related compounds as carcinogenic hazards to man. In P. Emmelot and E. Kriek (Ed.),
Environmental Carcinogenesis: Occurrence, Risk Evaluation,
and Mechanisms. Amsterdam/New York/Oxford: Elsevier/North-
Holland, 1979, pp. 143-164.

Magee, P. N., Montesano, R., & Preussmann, R. N-Nitroso
compounds and related carcinogens. In C. E. Searle (Ed.),
Chemical Carcinogens, ACS Monograph 173. Washington:
American Chemical Society, 1976, 491-625.

Mainigi, K. D., & Sorof, S. Evidence for a receptor protein

of activated carcinogen. Proc. Natl. Acad. Sci., U.S.A.,
1977, 74, 2293-2296.

McCann, J., Choi, E., Yamasaki, E., & Ames, B. N. The
detection of carcinogens as mutagens in the Salmonella
microsome test: Assay of 300 chemicals. Proc. Natl. Acad.
Sci., U.S.A., 1975, 72, 5135-5139.

Miller, E. C. Some current perspectives on chemical carcinogenesis in humans and experimental animals: Presidential
address. Cancer Res., 1978, 38, 1479-1496.

Miller, E. C., & Miller, J. A. The metabolism of chemical
carcinogens to reactive electrophiles and their possible
mechanisms of action in carcinogenesis. In C. E. Searle
(Ed.), Chemical Carcinogens. American Chemical Society
Monograph No. 173, Washington: American Chemical Society,
1976, 737-762.

Miller, E. C., & Miller, J. A. Naturally occurring chemical
carcinogens that may be present in foods. In: A. Neuberger
and T. H. Jukes (Ed.), International Review of Biochemistry,
Biochemistry of Nutrition 1A, Vol. 27. Baltimore: University Park Press, 1979, 123-165.

Miller, J. A., & Miller, E. C. Perspectives on the metabolism
of chemical carcinogens. In P. Emmelot and E. Kriek
(Ed.), Environmental Carcinogenesis. Amsterdam: Elsevier/
North-Holland Biomedical Press, 1979, 25-50.

O'Connor, P. J., Saffhill, R., & Margison, G. P. N-Nitroso
compounds: Biochemical mechanisms of action. In P.
Emmelot and E. Kriek (Ed.), Environmental Carcinogenesis.
Amsterdam: Elsevier/North-Holland, 1979, 73-96.

Pienta, R. J., Poiley, J. A., & Lebherz, W. B., III. Morphological transformation of early passage golden Syrian
hamster embryo cells derived from cryopreserved primary
cultures as a reliable in vitro bioassay for identifying
diverse carcinogens. Int. J. Cancer, 1978, 19, 642-655.

Preussmann, R., Druckrey, H., Ivankovic, S. & von Hodenberg,
A. Chemical structure and carcinogenicity of aliphatic
hydrazo, azo, and azoxy compounds and of triazenes, potential in vivo alkylating agents. Ann. N. Y. Acad. Sci.,
1969, 163, 697-714.

Purchase, I. F. H., Longstaff, E., Ashby, J., Styles, J. A.,
Anderson, D., Lefevre, P. A., & Westwood, F. R. An evaluation of 6 short-term tests for detecting organic chemical
carcinogens. Brit. J. Cancer, 1978, 37, 873-959.

Rinkus, S. J., & Legator, M. S., Chemical characterization
of 465 known or suspected carcinogens and their correlation
with mutagenic activity in the Salmonella typhimurium
system. Cancer Res., 1979, 39, 3289-3318.

Rubin, H. Is somatic mutation the major mechanism of malignant transformation? J. Natl. Cancer Inst., 1980, 64,

995-1000.

Sims, P. The metabolic activation of chemical carcinogens. Brit. Med. Bull., 1980, 36, 11-18.

Slaga, T. J., Sivak, A., & Boutwell, R. K. Mechanisms of Tumor Promotion and Cocarcinogenesis, 588 pp. New York: Raven Pres, 1978.

Ts'o, P. O. P., Caspary, W. J., Cohen, B. I., Leavitt, J. C., Lesko, S. A., Jr., Lorentzen, R. J., & Schechtman, L. M. Basic mechanisms in polycyclic hydrocarbon carcinogenesis. In P. O. P. Ts'o, and J. A. DiPaolo (Ed.), Chemi-cal Carcinogenesis, Part A. New York: Marcel Dekker, 1974, 113-147.

Wattenberg, L. W. Inhibitors of chemical carcinogenesis. In P. Emmelot, and E. Kriek (Ed.), Environmental Carcinogenesis. Amsterdam/New York/Oxford: Elsevier/North-Holland, 1979, 241-263.

Weinstein, I. B., Yamasaki, H., Wigler, M., Lee, L.-S., Fisher, P. B., Jeffrey, A., & Grunberger, D. Molecular and cellular events associated with the action of initiating carcinogens and tumor promoters. In A. C. Griffin and C. R. Shaw (Ed.), Carcinogens, Identification and Mechanisms of Action. New York: Raven Press, 1978, 399-418.

Wood, A. W., Levin, W., Chang, R. L., Yagi, H., Thakker, D. R., Lehr, R. E., Jerina, D. M., & Conney, A. H. Bay-region activation of carcinogenic polycyclic hydrocarbons. In P. W. Jones and P. Leber (Ed.), Polynuclear Aromatic Hydrocarbons. Ann Arbor, Mich.: Ann Arbor Science, 1979, 531-551.

Detection of Carcinogens

JEFFREY C. THEISS

Associate Professor of Environmental Sciences
University of Texas Health Science Center at Houston
School of Public Health
Houston, Texas   77025

The first long-term carcinogenicity test was carried out in 1915 when it was demonstrated that tumors developed when rabbit ears were painted with coal tar. Since this time some 7,000 chemicals have been tested for carcinogenicity in long-term animal bioassays. While the utility of long-term animal bioassays in assessing the carcinogenicity of chemicals is accepted by many, these bioassays are very expensive ($500,000 or more per chemical) and very time consuming (3.5 years per chemical). It is thus not realistic to use this approach alone in attempting to determine how many of the approximately 70,000 chemicals which are in commercial use in the U.S. possess carcinogenic activity.

Many different and imaginative approaches to carcinogen bioassay are presently under development which will help to determine which of the great variety of chemicals present in the environment may pose a carcinogenic hazard to man. These assay systems are relatively inexpensive and rapid and thus provide the potential for testing a large number of chemicals in a reasonable amount of time. In this paper various approaches to carcinogen bioassay will be described; the current utility of these short-term tests in the regulatory process will be indicated; and future areas of effort in short-term testing will be suggested.

CONCEPTUAL OUTLINE OF THE CARCINOGENIC PROCESS

To understand the various approaches to carcinogen bioassay it is first necessary to have a grasp of the currently accepted view of the mechanisms involved in the carcinogenic process. These mechanisms are outlined in Figure 1.

It is currently accepted that the great majority of carcinogens are electrophilic compounds or are chemicals which can be metabolized to become electrophiles. These ultimate carcinogens then interact with the DNA of the cell, causing DNA damage. This damage under certain conditions is detect-

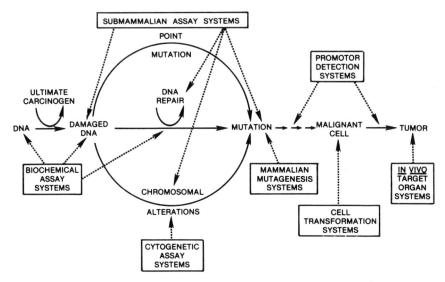

Figure 1. Conceptual Outline of the Approaches to Carcinogen Bioassay.

able microscopically as chromosomal alterations. The cell possesses enzymes which repair the damaged DNA and when a mistake in this repair process occurs a mutation may develop which will increase the neoplastic potential of that cell. When one or more of these mutations occurs within the cell it will lose the ability to function in a controlled fashion and will become neoplastic. Under proper conditions within the host, this neoplastic cell will divide repeatedly to form a tumor.

When this process runs to completion as the result of exposure to a single chemical that chemical is considered a complete carcinogen. When exposure to a chemical results in a mutation which increases the neoplastic potential of the cell but does not produce a neoplastic cell which will go on to form a tumor that chemical is considered an initiator. Complete carcinogens often function as initiators at low doses. When exposure to an initiator is followed by exposure to a promotor the carcinogenic process will run to completion. In this case the promoting substance is an integral part of the carcinogenic process and the process is called sequential carcinogenesis. Several substances have also been found to facilitate the carcinogenic process by enhancing the response of the host to a complete carcinogen. The ways this enhancement may occur include: increased metabolism of carcinogens to their ultimate electrophilic form or decreased metabolism of these ultimate carcinogens to non-toxic substances; increased sensitivity of the DNA to carcinogen induced damage; alterations in DNA repair leading to increased mutagenic events; and alterations in the immune or hormonal status of the host which facilitate the growth of neoplastic cells to form a tumor. Substances which enhance the carcinogenic process in this fashion are termed permissive promotors. Thus, in determining the potential carcinogenic hazard of a chemical to man we should ideally assess the ability of this chemical to act as an initiator, promotor and permissive promotor in addition to determining the complete carcinogenic activity of the chemical

APPROACHES TO CARCINOGEN BIOASSAY

The various short-term tests which are under development utilize end-points for assessing the carcinogenicity of chemicals which are predicated on the underlying mechanisms for carcinogenesis depicted in Figure 2. Each of these approaches to carcinogen bioassay is briefly summarized below.

Biochemical Assay Systems

There are five end-points used in biochemical assay systems. Unscheduled DNA synthesis in cells or tissues exposed to a chemical is assessed by measuring the incorporation of a radioactively labelled nucleoside into DNA when normal replicative DNA synthesis has been inhibited. Unscheduled DNA synthesis is taken as a measure of the amount of DNA repair induced by the interaction of the chemical with DNA and resulting damage. DNA fragmentation is examined by labelling DNA with radioactivity, exposing the target cells or tissue to the chemical under test and determining the amount of radioactive label eluted from the DNA as fragments. Single strand DNA breaks may be detected by a decrease in sedimentation velocity or an increase in fluorescence of DNA extracted from cells exposed to a chemical. DNA binding is most often assessed by using radioactively labelled test chemicals. A delayed rebound of DNA synthesis after DNA synthesis inhibition resulting from exposure to a chemical has also been associated with the mutagenic activity of several chemicals. All of these systems are rapid, inexpensive, sensitive and can use a variety of target cells and tissues, including human cells. The end-points of these assays, however, are very distant from the induction of a tumor in an experimental animal and thus the specificity of these tests in assessing for carcinogenic activity may be questioned.

Submammalian Assay Systems

A variety of submammalian organisms have been utilized in testing chemicals for carcinogenic activity. These organisms include prokaryotic microorganisms (bacterial), eukaryotic microorganisms (fungi), insects and plants. A great variety of end-points are used in these bioassay systems.

In prokaryotic microorganisms, the induction of both reverse mutations, measured by the reversion of auxotrophic mutants to prototrophic organisms, and forward mutations, measured by the induction of resistance to certain cytotoxic agents, is taken as evidence of the mutagenicity of test chemicals. The ability of chemicals to induce prophage residing within bacteria to lyse these bacteria is taken as evidence of the occurrence of DNA damage because single strand breaks in DNA triggers the induction of prophage. The hypersensitivity of DNA repair deficient mutants to chemicals also provides evidence for the occurrence of DNA damage because these deficient mutants would be less able to repair this damage. The bacteria which are most often used in these bioassay systems are *Salmonella typhimurium*, *Escherichia coli* and *Bacillus subtilis*. These bioassays are often carried out *in vitro*. They may be used, however, in a host-mediated assay in which the test organisms are inoculated into a mammalian host followed by exposure of the host to the test chemical, retrieval of the test organisms and assessment of chemically induced alterations in those organisms. *In vitro* tests using prokaryotic microorganisms may also be utilized to assess the mutagenic activity present in body fluids (urine, bile, etc.). These fluids may be derived either from test animals exposed to a chemical, in which case the animal serves as an activating system for the chemical, or these fluids may be derived from humans, in which case the bacterial test system serves as a system for monitoring the exposure of humans to mutagenic substances.

These prokaryotic test systems are very useful because they are well defined, inexpensive, rapid and technically easy to perform. However, while positive results in these test systems generally correlate well with carcinogenic activity, there are notable exceptions (metals, chlorinated hydrocarbons, non-mutagenic promoting substances) which indicate that these prokaryotic test systems alone are not sufficient for determining the carcinogenic activity of all chemicals.

The major eukaryotic microorganisms which are used in chemical testing are *Saccharomyces cerevisiae*, *Neurospora crassa and Aspergillus nidulans*. Since these organisms possess chromosomes, they utilize several end-points which reflect chromosomal effects of chemicals in addition to assessing the ability of chemicals to induce point mutations. The advantage of these systems is that they are the simplest available for investigating chemically induced chromosomal alterations. The chief limitation of these systems is their

relative inefficiency in detecting carcinogens requiring metabolic activation.

Among the insects, *Drosophila melanogaster* are very suitable for assessing mutagenic activity of chemicals because
they contain many carcinogen activating enzymes; they possess
well defined genetic markers which are easily scored; and a
variety of genetic effects such as the induction of sex-
linked recessive lethal mutations, dominant lethal mutations,
sex-chromosome losses, partial chromosome losses and translocations can be tested. The main limitation of the *Drosophila* test systems is that quantitative dose-response curves
are difficult to generate.

Several plants such as tradescantia, corn, soybean, barley
and ferns have also been utilized to assess the mutagenic activity of chemicals. Laboratory tests for determining the
mutagenic activity of chemicals are usually carried out on
plant seeds. Plants are also used for *in situ* monitoring for
the presence of mutagens in the environment by positioning
plants in areas where the presence of mutagens is suspected
and determining the development of mutations in these plants.

Mammalian Mutagenesis Systems

Several mammalian systems have also been developed to test
chemicals for mutagenic activity. *In vitro* test systems utilize primary rodent cell cultures, rodent cell lines or primary human cell cultures. In these systems mutagenicity is
assessed by exposing cells to the chemical under test and
then incubating these cells with a cytotoxic agent to determine the number of mutants in the cell population which are
resistant to the toxic effect of the selective agent. The
major genetic loci which are used in these systems are the
thymidine kinase locus, the hypoxanthine-guanine phosphorib-
osyl transferase locus and the ouabain resistant locus. The
majority of *in vivo* mammalian germinal mutation systems are
not very useful as short-term tests for carcinogenic activity
because they require large numbers of animals and a long period of time to complete. However, the mouse dominant lethal
test, which measures the effect of chemicals on fetal resorp-
tion in female mice mated to male mice exposed to the test
chemicals, and the mouse sperm abnormality test, which asses-
ses the occurrence of atypical sperm in chemically exposed
mice, are two *in vivo* germinal mutation systems which may
have utility in testing chemicals for carcinogenicity. Two
in vivo mammalian somatic mutation systems which show promise
are the spot test and the eye test, both of which utilize the
induction of mutation in melanocytes as a measure of carcinogenic potential. In the spot test these mutations are expressed phenotypically as localized changes in coat color and

in the eye test mutations produce areas of dark pigmented
cells in the pink retina of treated mice. An advantage of
mammalian mutagenesis tests is that these tests use mammalian
cells as targets and, in the *in vivo* systems, test chemicals
are subjected to the pharmacological factors which come into
play when humans are exposed to these chemicals. A limitation of these tests is that they examine mutagenic effects
at only a few select loci within the genome and, in the *in
vivo* systems, mutagenic effects are only assessed in a few
specific tissues of the chemically exposed animals.

Cytogenetic Assay Systems

   Cytogenetic assay systems utilize a variety of mammalian
cells and tissues, ranging from cultured rodent cells to somatic human tissues. One major end-point for these assay
systems is the microscopic detection of chromosomal aberrations. Staining techniques which enable the sister chroma-
tids of a chromosome to be differentiated have allowed the
use of a more subtle chromosomal alteration, called sister-
chromatid exchange, as an end-point in cytogenetic assay systems. Another end-point utilized in these assay systems is
the relatively easily detected micronucleus formation, which
results from chromosomal breakage fragments or lagging chromosomes which remain in the cytoplasm after completion of
mitosis. These cytogenetic assay systems in general are useful in testing for carcinogenicity because there is an extremely good qualitative correlation between the ability of
chemicals to induce chromosomal alterations and their ability
to induce specific locus mutations. Cytogenetic tests which
utilize human tissues are particularly important because they
can be used in monitoring humans for exposure to mutagenic
chemicals. The major problem with these cytogenetic bioassay
systems is thàt agents which are potent inducers of mutations are often poor inducers of chromosomal alterations and
vice versa. Thus, these test systems are not particularly
useful in quantifying the potential carcinogenic potency of
chemicals.

Cell Transformation Systems

   Cell transformation systems which utilize primarily rodent
fibroblastic cell cultures, are very useful in assessing
chemicals for carcinogenic activity because transformed cells
resulting from chemical exposure will develop into tumors
when injected into rodents. These test systems are thus utilizing a more direct measure of carcinogenic activity as
their end-point. In addition to acquiring the ability to
form tumors *in vivo*, transformed cells are altered in several
other ways. Transformed cells are released from contact

inhibition and can thus pile up to form multilayered foci of
cells. They also lose anchorage dependence and can thus form
colonies when suspended in soft agar. Individual transformed
cells also are often morphologically altered and grow in a
disordered fashion, producing colonies of cells which are
morphologically altered. When one or more of these alterations is accompanied by acquisition of the ability to produce
tumors *in vivo*, these alterations may be used as *in vitro*
criteria for neoplastic transformation. Three popular criteria are: the development of transformed foci of piled up
cells on monolayers of normal cells; the development of colonies of transformed cells at low population density; and the
development of cell colonies in soft agar. One of the major
short-comings of cell transformation systems is that they
utilize fibroblastic cells while the major human cancers
arise from epithelial cells. Efforts are underway, however,
to develop and validate transformation systems which use epithelial cells as well as systems which use human cells.

In Vivo Target Organ Systems

In vivo target organ systems utilize the occurrence of
tumors in a specific organ or tissue of animals exposed to a
chemical as an end-point for carcinogenicity. One approach
along these lines is to assess the development of tumors at
the site of application (skin painting, subcutaneous injection, intramuscular injection). The advantage to this approach is that the development of tumors in living animals
can be detected by palpation and thus both the time for tumor
development and the total incidence of tumors which develop
in response to a carcinogen can be assessed. Problems with
this approach include rapid diffusion from the injection
site, systemic activation of test chemicals, and non-
specificity of the tumor response to some substances (solid
state carcinogenesis). Another *in vivo* target organ approach
involves the use of a variety of organ specific tumor models
which serve as models for specific human cancers (hamster
lung, mouse colon, rat colon, rat bladder, rat mammary gland).
These tumor models are not particularly useful as a tool in
screening for carcinogenicity because chemicals may produce
tumors in organs other than the one under observation. These
systems are potentially useful, however, in characterizing
those carcinogens for which organ specificity is known,
either from other animal studies or from human epidemiological studies. One target organ system which has been used extensively in the screening of chemicals for carcinogenicity
and appears to be responsive to a great variety of carcinogens, regardless of their organ specificity, is the mouse
pulmonary adenoma bioassay. The target cell for this bioassay is the type 2 cell which resides in the alveoli of the

lung and the end-point for determining carcinogenicity is the
appearance of pulmonary adenomas (pearly-white, raised nodules) on the lung surface. This system is an excellent
screening tool because it is quantitative, rapid (6 months),
inexpensive ($10,000 per chemical), and it is technically
easy to determine the carcinogenic response to chemicals
(adenomas on the lung surface). The problems with this system include the high spontaneous incidence of pulmonary adenomas in older mice, the questionable malignancy of these
adenomas and the possibility that chemicals which require
more than 6 months of exposure to elicit a carcinogenic response will not be detected in this system

Promotor Detection Systems

The development of promotor detection systems is a recent
undertaking but substantial progress has already been made.
In vitro systems for detecting promoting activity utilize
end-points such as the induction of plasminogen activator and
the inhibition of metabolic cooperation between cells which
have been associated with the biological activity of known
promoting substances. Enhancement of cell transformation induced by an initiating dose of carcinogen is another end-
point used in these *in vitro* bioassays. These systems are
useful in detecting promotors which are an integral part of
the carcinogenic process but they will not detect permissive
promotors which affect the carcinogenic process indirectly
through alterations induced in the host. The most well established *in vivo* system for detection of promoting activity
is the mouse skin system, which served as the model for de-
delopment of the sequential carcinogenesis scheme. Recently
however, many *in vivo* promotor detection systems which utilize tumors that arise systemically within the host have been
developed (rat liver, rat colon, rat bladder, mouse lung).
These systems will be particularly useful in assessing chemicals for permissive promoting activity.

Metabolic Activation

One important common feature of all of the *in vitro* approaches to carcinogen bioassay which have been described
above is the incorporation of a system for activating carcinogens into these bioassays. The standard system for activating carcinogens in *in vitro* tests is a homogenate of rat
liver called the S-9 fraction. A recent comparison of carcinogen activation by liver homogenates, intact cellular systems, and rodent tissues *in vivo* indicated many important
differences in metabolic activation. The standard S-9 metabolic activation system may thus not reflect *in vivo* activation of the chemicals under test and results obtained in *in
vitro* systems which utilize an S-9 fraction should thus be

viewed with caution.

Conclusions

In reviewing the various approaches to carcinogen bioassay, certain conclusions can be formed. It is obvious that a tremendous variety of test systems are under development. Each test system has certain problems associated with it but a battery of such test systems may effectively predict carcinogenicity. In the course of testing using such a battery, much valuable information may be obtained in addition to determining qualitatively the carcinogenicity of the chemical under test. This information may eventually help in quantifying the carcinogenic risk of a particular chemical to exposed human populations.

CURRENT UTILITY OF SHORT-TERM TESTS IN THE REGULATORY PROCESS

The Interagency Regulatory Liaison Group (composed of the Environmental Protection Agency, the Food and Drug Administration, the Occupational Safety and Health Administration and the Consumer Product Safety Commission) recently issued a report dealing with the scientific bases for identification of potential carcinogens and estimation of risks. In this report experimental evidence from long-term animal bioassays is considered definitive evidence that a particular substance poses a potential carcinogenic hazard to exposed human populations. In the opinion of these governmental agencies evidence from short-term tests presently do not alone constitute definitive evidence for or against carcinogenicity. Short-term tests may, however, be used to confirm positive results obtained from long-term animal studies and to select chemicals that require further long-term investigations.

In setting forth policies for the identification, classification and regulation of potential occupational carcinogens, the Occupational Safety and Health Administration has adopted the same view of the utility of short-term tests as the Interagency Regulatory Liaison roup. OSHA considers five short-term test approaches to be sufficiently validated for use in regulatory decisions. These tests include: the induction of DNA damage and/or repair; mutagenesis in submammalian species; mutagenesis in mammalian somatic cells; mutagenesis in mammalian germinal cells; and neoplastic transformation of mammalian cells in culture. Positive results in two of these validated short-term tests are taken by OSHA as confirmatory evidence for the carcinogenicity of a substance which gave positive results in a single long-term animal bioassay. Thus, at their current state of development, short-term tests do not play a central role in decisions regarding the carcinogenicity of chemicals.

FUTURE EFFORTS IN SHORT-TERM TESTING

In view of the great potential utility of short-term tests in assessing the carcinogenicity of chemicals, we should continue to develop and validate these test systems so that test batteries may be developed which will provide definitive evidence of carcinogenicity. By closely integrating these experimental systems with epidemiological studies conducted in human populations we may better be able to obtain a true assessment of the carcinogenic hazard particular chemicals pose to man.

REFERENCES

Bigger, G.A.H., Tomaszewski, J.E., Dipple, A., Lake, R.S. Limitations of metabolic activation systems used with *in vitro* tests for carcinogens. Science 209:503-505, 1980.

Griffin, A.C., Shaw, C.R. (Eds.), Carcinogens: Identification and Mechanisms of Action. New York: Raven Press, 1979.

Hollaender, A., and de Serres, F.J. (Eds.), Chemical Mutagens -Principles and Methods for Their Detection. Volume 5. New York: Plenum Press, 1978.

Hollstein, M., McCann, J., Angelosanto, F.A. and Nichols, W.W. Short-term tests for carcinogens and mutagens. Mutation Res. 65:133-226, 1979.

Interagency Regulatory Liaison Group. Scientific bases for identification of potential carcinogens and estimation of risks. J. Natl. Cancer Inst. 63:244-268, 1979.

Kilbey, B.J., Legator, M., Nichols, W., Ramel, C. (Eds.), Handbook of Mutagenicity Test Procedures. New York: Elsevier, 1977.

Occupational Safety and Health Administration. Identification, classification and regulation of potential occupational carcinogen. Fed. Reg. 45:5001-5296, 1980.

Saffiotti, U. Identifying and defining chemical carcinogens. In H.H. Hiatt, J.D. Watson, and S.A. Winsten (Eds.), Origins of Human Cancer. Cold Spring Harbor Laboratory, 1977, 1311-1326.

Shimkin, M.B., and Stoner, G.D. Lung tumors in mice: Application to carcinogenesis bioassay. Adv. Cancer Res. 21: 1-58, 1975.

Slaga, T.J., Sivak, A., and Boutwell, R.K. (Eds.), Carcinogenesis - A Comprehensive Survey. Volume 2. Mechanisms of Tumor Promotion and Cocarcinogenesis. New York: Raven Press, 1978.

Yotti, L.P., Chang, C.C., and Trosko, J.E. Elimination of metabolic cooperation in Chinese hamster cells by a tumor promotor. Science 206:1089-1091, 1979.

Population-based Tumor Registries
in the Identification of
Occupational Carcinogens

DONALD F. AUSTIN

Chief, Resource for Cancer Epidemiology Section
California State Department of Health Services
1450 Broadway
Oakland, California 94612

There are three approaches to the identification of environmental carcinogens:

1. By accident (historical)
2. Substance testing (Ames test, etc.)
3. Population monitoring

The first is how it has usually been done in the past. From the time of Sir Percival Potts until now, nearly every carcinogen having a detectable effect in humans has been discovered long after the fact and not as a result of any systematic approach to identification, e.g., asbestos, vinyl cloride, radium, aniline dyes, etc. We can no longer rely on haphazard means of identifying carcinogens. Two systematic approaches are now possible, basically those of biologic screening and epidemiology. Each has its particular strengths and weaknesses.

Substance testing is relatively simple, fast and cheap. It allows us to make sensible decisions regarding substances before seeing an effect in humans. It can not test for all possible combinations or metabolites of chemicals and may have no direct relationship to actual human cancer being experienced.

Population monitoring is slower and more expensive but has a direct application to cancer being experienced by a population. In other words, it is directed towards identifying those carcinogen exposures not prevented through other approaches.

The National Cancer Institute's SEER Program, (Surveillance, Epidemiology and End Results) covers over 10 percent of the population of the U.S. with a population-based cancer reporting system, although receiving only 1 percent of the annual NCI budget. The Resource for Cancer Epidemiology (RCE), a section of the California Department of Health Services, operates one of the field offices of this program in the San Francisco Bay Area. We are now beginning to recognize this program as a major resource in identifying occupational carcinogens. I'd like to present to you the points which led us to this recognition.

In 1976, we reported a dramatic increase in the incidence of endometrial cancer.[5] The increase was almost exclusively among white women over the age of 50.[1,2] Although there was a small incidence increase among women 45-49 years, every 5-year age group over 50 had an increase approximately double that of ten years earlier (Fig 1). Case-control studies done by others indicated that this increase was due to the widespread use of exogenous estrogens among post-menopausal women.[3,4,6.]

An unquestionable incidence increase for all women was detected in spite of the fact that:

- only menopausal and post-menopausal women were exposed to the causative agent,
- not all menopausal or post-menopausal women were taking estrogens, and
- about one-third of women over 50 had had a hysterectomy and therefore couldn't contribute to uterine cancer incidence.

An effect was detected because the etiologic agent was sufficiently widespread to affect the incidence for an entire population group and also because the high risk group could be characterized by demographic factors available from population census data; namely age, race and sex. If the high risk group had been a small percent of the general population, expecially if it had been persons of both sexes, all ages and races who worked at a particular trade or in a specific factory, it never would have been detected.

POINT ONE: IF WE ARE TO MONITOR CANCER IN THE POPULATION CHARACTERIZED BY OTHER THAN AGE, RACE AND SEX, WE MUST MONITOR SPECIFIC SMALL POPULATION GROUPS.

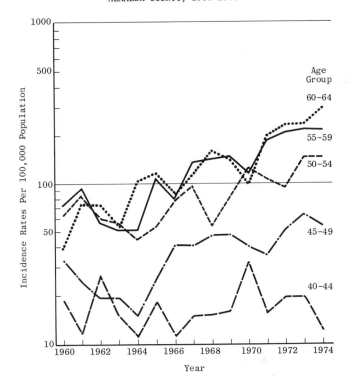

INVASIVE CARCINOMA OF THE CORPUS UTERI
INCIDENCE RATES FOR WHITE FEMALES, BY FIVE YEAR AGE GROUP
ALAMEDA COUNTY, 1960-1975

The experience with uterine cancer illustrated something
else. 1976 was the first year in over a decade in which there
was a decrease in the incidence of endometrial cancer. In
subsequent years the rate continued to decline as rapidly as
it rose reaching, in 1979, the approximate rate for 1972.
This rise, and subsequent decline, paralleled the patterns of
estrogen sales in western United States. This does not fit
the traditional model of a carcinogen with a long latent
effect, although the incidence increase among women 50-54
years also indicates that these women could not have been exposed to estrogen for very long. This represents a different
biologic model than that represented by asbestos and mesothelioma, or cigarette smoking and lung cancer. Estrogen and
endometrial cancer fit the model for a promoter, rather than
a true carcinogen.

At least three models exist now for the effects of environmental agents on cancer risk. The first is that of asbestos
and mesothelioma (Fig 2). Here the exposed have a risk
nearly undetectable from the non-exposed risk (both near zero)

Donald F. Austin

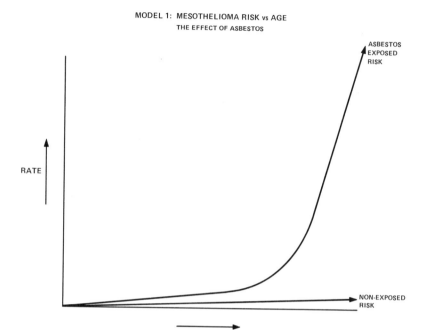

MODEL 1: MESOTHELIOMA RISK vs AGE
THE EFFECT OF ASBESTOS

until a period of latency has passed, i.e., 15-30 years.
Then the rate for mesothelioma increases to several thousand
times the rate of the unexposed, and this dramatic increase
cannot be altered. In this case, eliminating exposures benefits primarily by preventing others from becoming initially
exposed. The already exposed are on an unchangeable risk path.

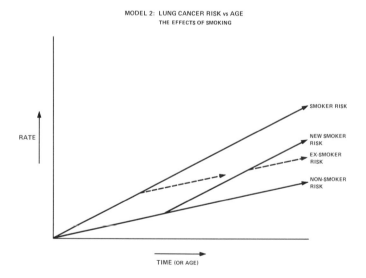

MODEL 2: LUNG CANCER RISK vs AGE
THE EFFECTS OF SMOKING

The second model is cigarette smoking and lung cancer (Fig 3). Here the exposed person's risk rises more rapidly with age than the non-exposed, but when the exposure ceases, the subsequent rate of increase is on a gentler slope, comparable to that of the non-smoker. Ending the exposure cannot undo the progression of risk to date but it can prevent further progression at the accelerated rate.

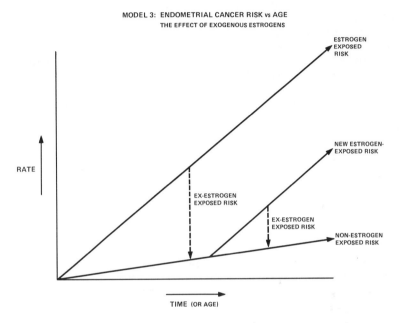

MODEL 3: ENDOMETRIAL CANCER RISK vs AGE
THE EFFECT OF EXOGENOUS ESTROGENS

The third model is that of estrogen and endometrial cancer (Fig 4). Here the exposed person's risk also increases at a much higher rate than the non-exposed. However, when exposure ceases, the risk soon returns to the risk of the non-exposed. Preventing further exposures to these agents contributes immediate rewards, especially to those already exposed.

POINT TWO: AN ENVIRONMENTAL AGENT CAN HAVE A POTENT EFFECT ON CANCER INCIDENCE YET WHEN IT IS REMOVED, THE RISK AMONG THE EXPOSED CAN RETURN TO THE PRE-EXPOSURE RISK. THE CONCEPT THAT THE CANCERS OF TODAY ARE THE RESULT OF EXPOSURES 20 to 30 YEARS AGO IS NOT INVARIABLY TRUE. THEY MAY BE DUE TO EXPOSURES OF SEVERAL MONTHS AGO.

We began to establish specific cohorts within our cancer incidence area on the basic premise that if we had the name of every member of a group (e.g., plumbers) residing within our area, we could establish the cancer incidence within the group, since every resident case of cancer in our area is recorded by name. Searching for occupational carcinogens by population monitoring must proceed in two steps. The first is to identify a group at high risk for some particular cancer; the second is to identify the specific exposure responsible for the elevated risk. We attempted to determine the sensitivity of our approach to the first step. Sources of potential error are: 1) incomplete registration of cancer cases, 2) inaccurate listing of name or address of occupational cohort members, and 3) failure of the linkage. To assess these potential errors we tested a cohort known to be at high risk, which had been followed for mortality through the traditional follow-up methods. We chose the local asbestos worker's union, a group of 235 members, for which we established annual membership rosters for 1972-1977. These rosters we linked to the registry files for the same years. Our results, 13 cancer diagnoses in 12 individuals were rewarding (Table 1). In an overnight computer run, we found every case found by the traditional death search method, plus eight cases not yet entered in the mortality files.

POINT THREE: THIS METHOD IS EXTREMELY SENSITIVE.

TABLE 1

Results of the Match of a Cohort of 235 Members of the Asbestos Workers Union Against the Annual Cancer Incidence Files, 1972-1977. California Tumor Registry

Site of Cancer	Number
Lung	4*
Pleura**	2
Peritoneum**	2
Colon	2
Rectum	1
Prostate	1
Brain	1
All Cancer	13

 * One from each category is the same individual
** Mesotheliomas

We next applied the methodology to several cohorts not known to be at high risk. The first roster, all employees of the Lawrence Livermore Laboratory, was provided to us by the

management of that nuclear research facility. We analyzed
the occurrence of malignant melanoma in that group because of
rumors among employees of excessive numbers of this malignancy.
We established that this cohort, for the years 1972-77, had
experienced malignant melanoma at three to four times the expected rate (Table 2). We are now carrying out the step necessary to identify the probable cause.

TABLE 2

Comparison of Observed and Expected Numbers of
Malignant Melanoma Among White Employees of the
Lawrence Livermore Laboratory Resident in Alameda
and Contra Costa Counties, by stage and sex. 1972-1977

Melanoma	Observed	Method A[1] Expected	O/E	Method B[2] Expected	O/E
Males	17	5.59	3.04	3.87	4.40*
In Situ	3	0.83	3.61	0.13	23.08
Invasive	14	4.76	2.94	3.74	3.74*
Females	2	0.80	2.50	0.73	2.74
In Situ	0	0.14	–	0.13	–
Invasive	2	0.66	3.03	0.60	3.33
Total	19	6.39	2.97	4.60	4.13*
In Situ	3	0.96	3.13	0.26	11.54
Invasive	16	5.43	2.95	4.34	3.69*

*$p < .0001$

1. Method A has the LLL employees included in the numerator
   and denominator of the reference population.
2. Method B has the LLL employees removed from the numerator
   and denominator of the reference population.

The excess melanoma risk was identified in 1980. Its cause
may not be identified until 1981. The risk was apparently
operative in 1972 and, had the analysis been done, the excess
risk for the period 1972-74 would have been apparent five
years ago. In other words, an excess risk operative for nearly a decade could have been detected at least five years
earlier, had we looked. How many other potential cohorts are
there at elevated risk, perhaps contributing only a dozen excess cases to a county and therefore masked when looking at
general population data?

POINT FOUR: NUMEROUS SMALL EPIDEMICS OF OCCUPATIONAL
CANCER MAY CURRENTLY EXIST, WHICH WILL REMAIN UNDETECTED AND
UNCORRECTED WITHOUT MONITORING SPECIFIC OCCUPATIONAL COHORTS.

Probably many instances exist of risks elevated severalfold,
which will only be evident when looking at the appropriate
small cohort. The means of monitoring these small cohorts
now exists in a significant proportion of this country. In
addition to the population-based cancer reporting systems
sponsored by the SEER Program, large systems exist in New York
State, Los Angeles, and a number of smaller areas. At little
cost, labor and industry can enter into a partnership with
population-based reporting systems to form industrial cancer
registries for the rapid identification and subsequent control
of occupational carcinogens.

REFERENCES

1. Austin, DF, Roe, K. An Increase in Cancer of the Uterine
    Corpus in the San Francisco-Oakland SMSA, 1960-1975.
    JNCI 62:13-16, 1979.
2. Austin, DF, Roe, K. Uterine Cancer Incidence, San Fran-
    cisco Bay Area, 1960-1975, State of California, Department
    of Health. Monograph, Vol. 5, #1, 1978.
3. Mack TM, Pike MC, Henderson BE, et al. Estrogens and
    endometrial cancer in a retirement community. N Engl J
    Med. 1976; 294:1262-7.
4. Smith DC, Prentice R, Thompson DJ, Hermann WL. Associa-
    tion of exogenous estrogen and endometrial carcinoma.
    N Engl J Med. 1975; 293:1164-7.
5. Weiss NS, Szekely DR, Austin DF. Increasing incidence of
    endometrial cancer in the United States. N Engl J Med.
    1976; 294:1259-62.
6. Ziel HK, Finkle WD. Increased risk of endometrial carci-
    noma among users of conjugated estrogens. N Engl J Med.
    1975; 293:1167-70.

Partially supported by SEER Contract No. N01-CP-81018

Three Decades of Environmental Concern

DAVID P. RALL, M.D., PH.D.

Director
National Institute of Environmental Health Sciences
Research Triangle Park, North Carolina

Thank you for inviting me to speak today. It is a pleasure to
talk to you about the emerging field of environmental health
science.

The American historian, Frederick Jackson Turner, proposed
the theory that in order to understand the American consciousness,
one must first realize the importance the idea of the frontier
played in the development of that consciousness.

We are by and large a Nation of immigrants, people who left
the crowded cities of Europe and later, other parts of the
world, and settled first on a thin band along the coast.
Later, as more people arrived, the settlers pushed inward into
the Ohio and Tennessee Valleys. In the 19th century, Horace
Greeley would proclaim, "Go West, Young Man, Go West."
Opportunity was to be found in developing new areas of the
country.

With the possible exception of Alaska--the development of
which is now a topic of hot Congressional debate--America has
reached the limits of its frontiers.

We've discovered that while in the past we used to be able to
escape from our problems by moving on, we now find there's nowhere else to go. We've reached the frontier. I suggest that
this represents a drastic change not only in the way that we
live, but also in the way that we conceptualize.

This realization has had a profound impact on our society.

Just two decades ago in November 1960, a Presidential Commission on National Goals issued a report describing areas expected
to be of national concern in the coming decade. Among the fifteen goals cited, not one concerned environmental pollution.
But by the end of the decade, we had witnessed an extraordinary
revolution in popular thinking. People were beginning to talk

299

about there being possible limits to growth. An international economist, Barbara Ward, described our planet as "Space Ship Earth." Suburbanites were organizing to recycle their trash.

All of these changes, both profound and less profound, are the result of recognition that Earth is not an endlessly open system, but rather a living, breathing, essentially closed system. Whereas we used to be able to pick up and move on, now the country is settled. What I do is going to affect the next guy. There is no escape.

What does this have to do with environmental cancer and its control?

I suggest that the recognition that this Earth is a self-contained living system makes a world of difference in how we will be able to live on it.

During the last three decades we have begun to see and be able to measure the effects of actions which followed from the belief that we live in a world without limits. Now we must face the consequences of the mistakes which flow from that assumption: air and water pollution, nuclear and chemical waste dumps, ozone depletion and other problems of scarcity. A limited world simply cannot continue to absorb the byproducts of an increasingly dirty industrial society. The Earth is a living system and it can tolerate a certain amount of abuse. Like the body, it, too, has a threshold. And when that threshold is breached, mankind is in trouble.

Let's take a look at air pollution, for example. Until the industrial revolution, coal--which was discovered by Marco Polo to be in use in more advanced civilizations of Asia--was regarded by Europeans as an "unnatural" product. Its sulfurous emissions were associated with anti-clerical forces. King Richard the Third of England, who reigned from 1377 to 1399, and Henry the Fifth, who ruled from 1413 to 1422, took steps to regulate strictly the use of coal. Yet eventually coal was to become the fuel for the industrial revolution. As early as 1661, long before England became the world's first superpower, London had an air pollution problem. This was recognized by John Evelyn, a founding member of the Royal Society, who in that year wrote a paper entitled, "Fumigum: or the Inconvenience of the Aer and Smoke of London Dissapated; Together with Some Remedies Humbly Proposed." Unfortunately, the problem did not become serious enough to force action until 300 years later.

In the United States, we had one of our first experiences with the limits of growth--or perhaps more accurately, the results of uncontrolled growth--in the town of Donora, Pennsylvania, population at the time, 14,000. The town, which sits in the Monongahela River Valley, thought it was blessed with the riches of employment brought by its smelters, open hearths and its sulfuric acid plant. That was, until Saturday, October 30, 1948, when its first citizen dropped dead as a result of an unusual weather condition that suffocated the town in its own pollution.

By the time the episode was over, 20 people were dead, most due to asthma or chronic heart disease, and 6,000 had been seriously ill.

Similar problems were occurring in Los Angeles. In the 1940s and 1950s people began to notice the lack of visibility and the burning in their eyes and say it was caused by something they called "smog." Like Donora, Los Angeles is vulnerable to suffocating atmospheric inversions--in Los Angeles, for as much as 260 days a year. So in 1947, recognizing that air pollution crosses political boundaries and thus cannot be controlled on a city-by-city basis, the California Legislature passed our first Air Pollution Control Act.

As we entered the 1950s and citizens in other cities became concerned about the quality of their air as well, Congress became involved. The first national air pollution law was passed in 1955 but did little more than provide for some research and demonstration grants. In 1963, the Congress passed the Clean Air Act but left enforcement to the states--a fatal flaw since, unfortunately, air pollution is an interstate problem. In 1965, it passed the Motor Vehicle Air Pollution Control Act and the Department of Health, Education, and Welfare set emissions control regulations.

In response to the need for better control of air pollution, Congress has over the years made the legislation increasingly stringent and it appears increasingly difficult to administer. Next year, the legislation comes up for amendment once more and we can expect to see another battle over how much control is needed and how much it will cost to do the job.

I used air pollution as a specific example of how we've come to recognize a serious environmental health problem and how we've begun to respond.

Within the last three decades we have witnessed the passage of a plethora of other new laws responding to other environmental problems: The Federal Insecticide, Fungicide and Rodenticide Act in 1947; The Federal Water Pollution Control Act in 1948; The National Environmental Policy Act in 1969, which required for the first time an assessment of the environmental impact of major Federal projects before approval; Occupational Safety and Health Act in 1970, giving workers the right to a safe and healthful workplace; and Safe Drinking Water Act in 1974. And in 1976, two landmark bills passed, the Toxic Substances Control Act, which requires that information on chemicals be collected and requires determining the risk of new and existing chemicals before marketing, and the Resource Conservation and Recovery Act, which requires that waste chemicals be safely disposed of or eliminated.

If these laws work as intended, the Nation will have most of the requisite tools to protect the public from exposures to hazardous and carcinogenic chemicals in a variety of media, both in the general environment and the workplace.

There is one problem which remains unresolved by legislation which we hear much about today. The magnitude of that problem was illustrated vividly in 1978 when the inhabitants of a little community in Niagara Falls, New York, called the Love Canal became victims of a chemical disaster, one which will be remembered as vividly as air pollution in Donora. There is still a great debate about the actual effects of that environment on the human population; the residents complained of unusual sickness, dermatologic problems, miscarriages, birth defects and neurological disorders. And, we really cannot predict the long-term health effects of their exposure.

Buried in the long-abandoned canal near the elementary school is a repository of highly suspect chemicals many of which cause cancer in animals--dioxin, C-56, benzene, PCBs, and a host of other wastes, buried by the Hooker Chemical Company before there was a Federal law regulating such disposal. Hundreds of families had to be evacuated and hundreds of others are waiting. Before Love Canal became headline material, few realized that all the wastes we had so carelessly seen buried somewhere would come back to haunt us.

Congress is now struggling to decide who will pay to clean up the estimated 30,000 sites where toxic chemicals have been dumped in the past. These chemicals are not only a potential hazard to those in the immediate area, but they present the very real possibility of contaminating for a very long time the vital water supply sources upon which hundreds of thousands of Americans depend. Once this legislation is passed, we will have the legal tools needed to control environmental health hazards.

But will we have the knowledge we need to address these problems? And if we don't have all the answers--even if we are working diligently to get them--will an increasingly worried public understand? Here we face another frontier, a frontier of research and of education. Prior to the 1960s, the public understood disease as a simple cause and effect mechanism. If you caught a bug and your body couldn't fight it, you got sick. Scientists were viewed favorably because they could often find these bugs and develop miracle vaccines. Thus, during the 1950s, Jonas Salk became a folk hero--and rightly so--for developing a vaccine for polio, a terrible disease that harms our children in a horrible way.

The 1960s brought troubling knowledge of new kinds of diseases about which there was, and remains, little knowledge. Rachel Carson's book, The Silent Spring, published in 1962, raised public and scientific awareness of environmentally-induced diseases. She focused on pesticides, substances which like other organic compounds created de novo in the post-war period are persistent both in the environment and the human body.

The environmental diseases which some of these chemicals can cause are, in a sense, a more difficult problem for science than viral or bacterial diseases. Unlike infectious agents, these substances are not acutely toxic at the levels at which we normally experience them. Their effects may only appear 20 or 40 years later as cancer or in succeeding generations as birth defects. And, unlike the infectious diseases which we have conquered, these agents do not leave readily discoverable biological markers to tell us what we are looking for. And, for those such as PBBs and Agent Orange, for which some symptoms may be evident immediately after exposure, the symptomology is not yet well understood. Unlike the more familiar infectious diseases, many of the agents have some particularly nasty habits: they bioaccumulate in the ecologic system, thereby increasing the risk of exposure; they can interact with one another--and here I am thinking of the synergy between smoking and exposure to asbestos, for instance--and they can bioaccumulate in our fat tissue to be mobilized and cause problems long after exposure.

Before I discuss how we, as scientists, should approach the problem of dealing with these new initiators of disease, I want to discuss the public perception of the problem.

The public has become increasingly alarmed about environmental problems, PBBs in Michigan, asbestos disease among shipyard workers, Agent Orange exposure among Vietnam veterans, toxic waste dumps in the neighborhood, and countless other incidents of polluted air and contaminated water that make the environment a front page or evening news concern. In cases where people feel directly threatened--as at Love Canal--there are fear and anger. In other cases, as with the saccharin controversy, there is confusion. And, unfortunately, science can become a joking matter for Johnny Carson and even David Brinkley.

What is a concerned public to make of the headlines that appeared in connection with the saccharin controversy?

CANCER RATE SEEN HIGHER IN SACCHARIN TESTED OFFSPRING (3/77)
STUDY FINDS SACCHARIN DOES NOT CAUSE CANCER (5/77)
SACCHARIN AND HUMAN BLADDER CANCER ARE DIRECTLY LINKED IN CANADIAN STUDY (6/77)

EXPERTS WARN OF CANCER DANGER TO CHILDREN DRINKING DIET SODA (5/79)
SWEETENERS CALLED WEAK CARCINOGEN (2/80)

Or take the case of NTA:

U.S. REPORT LINKING NTA, BIRTH DEFECTS IN RATS SEEN KILLING ROLE IN DETERGENTS (12/70)
CHEMICAL IS CLEARED FOR DETERGENT USE--U.S. SAYS ANIMAL CARCINOGEN HAS SMALL RISK FOR HUMANS: OTHER EXPERTS DISAGREE (6/80)
EPA ALLOWS USE OF POSSIBLE CARCINOGEN AS PHOSPHATE SUBSTITUTE IN DETERGENTS (6/80)

Both of these substances are weak carcinogens. In both cases, animal tests provided the first indication of concern. The subsequent controversy has been one of public policy, not science. But one wonders how well the science involved--both what is known, and more importantly, what is not known--is being communicated to the public and the policy makers. Certainly in the case of saccharin, the debate has tended to misinterpret the extent of scientific consensus on the use of animal tests to predict human carcinogenicity.

In the case of saccharin, the Congress passed an exemption to the Delaney Amendment to the Food, Drug and Cosmetic Act which thereby allows saccharin to continue to be marketed. The Delaney Amendment says simply that no substance which causes cancer in animals can be used as a deliberate food additive. The fact that Congress has exempted saccharin from the requirement does not negate the positive animal studies nor the National Cancer Institute epidemiological study, nor the Canadian epidemiological study. What it does indicate is that Congress felt that the risk of using saccharin was acceptable for the Nation's public health and that individuals should make their own choices.

This is an appropriate division of labor. Scientists must inform society of the scientific facts as best we can and society's elected representatives must make the tough decisions about what ought to be done.

But, while this is an appropriate division of labor, it is definitely not an easy one. Scientists are reluctant to go beyond what they believe they can say with certainty and, as a result, it often looks to others as if we have very little definitive to say. Having received our contribution, however meager it may seem, legislators must then act on the basis of factors that are certainly difficult to quantify in a scientific sense. Often their actions give the illusion that, presto, the problem is solved when actually only a framework for problem-solving may have been created.

In the case of NTA, the preliminary positive animal studies a decade ago suggested the possible hazard. The Public Health Service recommended against using NTA at the time. Subsequent review of these data has found the risk to be lower than that for many carcinogens. Thus EPA, again making a policy decision, decided it did not want to allocate its limited resources to such a low risk substance when far greater hazards remain to be controlled.

There are a lot of difficult questions to answer when you get to decision time. In any given decision, these questions involve costs and benefits, and this includes the questions of costs to whom and benefits for whom. These are not simple equations because the burdens of the decisions are not found equally throughout society.

In these circumstances, it is the scientist's job to try to quantify, insofar as possible, the risk. And it is up to legislators--and their surrogates in the executive branch--to decide how to treat substances like NTA and saccharin within the framework of our scientific knowledge and legal traditions. The question is not whether we will live with risk, but how much of a risk we are willing to tolerate and how risk will be distributed among us. Many of these regulatory decisions involve different risk factors for, among others: workers, children, the elderly and consumers of particular products (dietary and lifestyle patterns), and those who are genetically susceptible. Concepts of fairness and justice need to be applied. All we can do to help assure that these decisions are properly made is to raise significant questions and where possible to point out the particular impacts of various decisions on different people.

Our first job as scientists becomes identifying those substances which pose a threat to human health. We live in a chemical universe. Since 1943, the production of synthetic organic chemicals has increased from 32 billion pounds to a level of 321 billion pounds, a ten-fold increase. It is estimated that there are some 30,000 different chemicals in production, very few of which have been adequately tested. It is the job of the scientific community to identify those prime candidates for testing, those chemicals for which we can assume there is a significant exposure and for which we suspect a possible hazard.

Once we have selected chemicals for testing, we use a mix of human data and laboratory findings.

Epidemiological studies are useful in themselves and in supporting what has been found in animal studies. Populations which have previously been exposed to a substance in an amount sufficient to cause a discernible effect and which can be related to exposure can be studied. Risk can then be predicted on the basis of this retrospective experience. However, epidemiology cannot anticipate hazards for substances which have not yet been introduced into commerce or have only relatively recently been introduced, such as saccharin.

The standard scientific tool used to identify toxic chemicals in the laboratory is the two-sex, two-species lifetime study of experimental animals. This type test determines if a chemical causes cancer and/or damages certain organ systems such as the liver, lung, kidney, or endocrine system. The test is weak at predicting reproductive, developmental, neurobehavioral and mutagenic effects.

The study of even a single compound is expensive and time consuming. It can take up to four years to complete, requiring hundreds of hours of scarce professional time. These limitations have stimulated the development and validation of new in vitro test methods that will allow us to determine more quickly and less expensively the toxicological potential of a compound.

The use of such laboratory tests for assessing potential human toxicity is essential. It is particularly so for those cases in which there is a new product, or a greatly increased exposure to an old product for which no human data are readily available; and also for those situations in which human data are either of low quality or extremely difficult to obtain or interpret.

I believe that the results of animal tests can and do predict for toxicity in man with an acceptable degree of certainty. When supplemented by epidemiological results which demonstrate a relation between a chemical and human disease, the argument for control of that particular substance is strong. In addition, I anticipate that the quantitative value of laboratory tests for risk estimation will increase as these testing methods are developed and improved.

The next task is to analyze the data and develop an estimation of risk.

The process of estimating human response from laboratory animal data involves several steps and a multitude of problems and assumptions. The toxic response observed in experimental animals should relate qualitatively to a corresponding human health effect. For instance, it is generally assumed that induced carcinogenesis in laboratory rodents implies a carcinogenic response in humans, although not necessarily of the same site and type. With mutagenesis the relation is less clear. For example, we do not know if elevated mutation rates in the mouse necessarily relate directly to human disease.

The next step involves inferences of dose-response relationships for humans from an appropriate animal model. Because of sample size limitations the experimental dose rates used in the animal models are generally at much higher levels than the environmental levels of concern. In order to estimate the response at lower environmental levels mathematical models for development of dose-response relationships are required. The estimated low-dose responses will depend greatly upon the model utilized; therefore, the model chosen should have a sound biologic basis.

Extrapolation of the estimated low-dose results obtained from the animal data to humans is the next phase. In the past this procedure has generally assumed the "median" man response is equivalent to that of the "median" mouse, with little attention given to the heterogeneity of the human population and susceptible subgroups. Another constraint is that few quantitative toxicity studies have been made over a wide range of species. To improve understanding of various toxicities and classes of agents, a better understanding of intra- and inter-species variability is needed. Species comparisons on a metabolic and pharmacokinetic basis would significantly improve the quality of the existing extrapolation methods.

The extrapolation procedure so far described is performed typically on a compound-by-compound basis. However, this type approach does have some problems. When a wide range of compounds is considered this way, the totality of the individual risk estimates is often ignored. Exposure to multiple substances, each with a similar toxicity, perhaps with the same target organ, could collectively produce an effect more harmful than the sum of their individual toxicities; or a substance which is individually innocuous may interact with other substances in such a way that exposure to them in combination is harmful and combination toxicity will be the challenge of the 1980s.

These are some of the complicating factors which should be taken into account in estimating risk. Another important consideration is that of disease latency particularly in cancer. Not only do we need to discover what level and type of exposure precipitated disease, but also the extent to which intervening exposures may have aggravated the disease.

Those are the principles and procedures that should guide we scientists as we develop the knowledge policy makers need to protect the public from environmental disease.

I spoke earlier about the wide-ranging array of rather complex but vital number of environmental laws passed in the last three decades. The enforcement of these laws--the Clean Air Act, the Safe Drinking Water Act, the Toxic Substances Control Act, the Resource Conservation and Recovery Act, the Pesticide Act-- will require rather massive infusion of environmental health

manpower if they are to be effective. There may be 1,000
trained toxicologists in this country right now and that's only
half as many as we need. I expect that within five years we
will only have 500 more--still far fewer than will be needed
as we face the challenge of protecting the public health.

Toxic chemicals are adding to the disease burden of the
United States in a significant, although as yet unquantifiable
way. Moreover, I believe this problem will become more acute
in the years to come. It is likely that the magnitude of the
public health risk associated with toxic chemicals is increasing
and will continue to do so until the hazardous agents are identified and brought under control. And even then, due to the long
latency period associated with their effects, the Nation will
continue to pay the price of the past haphazard proliferation
and disposal of toxic chemicals.

In our history, it is not unusual for mankind to have to pay
such a heavy price for his ignorance. In the field of infectious disease, if man had known just a little about what are
now considered elementary sanitary practices, millions would
not have died because of repeated plagues. One can only hope
that we do a better job in anticipating the possible effects
of toxic chemicals than mankind did with these earlier diseases.

Scientists have always played an important role in our Nation's
progress. I am sure we will do as well in the future.

Thank you.

REFERENCES

*Carson, R. Silent Spring. New York: Houghton Mifflin Co., 1962.

Host Defense against Cancer

Host Defense Against Cancer

HERBERT F. OETTGEN

Memorial Sloan-Kettering Cancer Center
New York, New York

The past two decades have seen a great resurgence of interest
in approaches to cancer based on immunology. Such approaches
have been based on the belief that there is something unique
about a cancer cell that distinguishes it from normal cells,
that this difference can be recognized by the host's immune
system, and that immunological recognition triggers host defense. It is my purpose to set down some of the principles of
cancer immunology as they have been developed over the years
and to describe current directions and questions. While our
goal is the understanding and control of cancer in man, the
object of the most intensive and precise study in this field
has been the mouse, and so I will refer often to results obtained with this experimental animal. With the rapid growth
of interest in cancer immunology, the field has become widely
diversified, the only obvious link between different approaches being the application of immunological techniques.
Nevertheless, a number of major topics have emerged over the
years.
In the area of immunogenetics, the coupling of serology and
genetic analysis has contributed much to answering some basic
questions about cancer, such as the identification of genes
involved in cancer susceptibility, expression of cancer antigens and immunity to cancer. The early discovery that genes
in the major histocompatibility complex influence susceptibility to leukemia in the mouse has led to continuing efforts
to find a comparable association between major histocompatibility antigens and cancer susceptibility in humans. It was
later realized that H-2 genes also control the immune response
to antigens, and there is now much interest in defining the
role of H-2 linked genes in immune reactions to cancer antigens. In the study of oncogenic viruses, immunological techniques have always played an important role. Advances have
depended to a large extent on the serological reagents that

permitted identification of structural and non-structural
components of RNA and DNA tumor viruses. Serological reagents have also been indispensable for the monitoring of immunochemical procedures aimed at isolating and characterizing
cancer antigens.

Progress in cancer immunology has of course been much influenced by recent advances in fundamental aspects of general
immunobiology. As our knowledge of the intricate regulatory
network that governs the immune response has grown, with the
findings of helper cells, suppressor cells, antigen presentation by macrophages, soluble regulatory factors, H-2 restriction and idiotype - anti-idiotype networks, we can expect
that similar influences regulate the immune response to tumors. Understanding immune regulation, and how to manipulate
it in favor of tumor rejection, has become a major focus of
interest. A question which continues to be asked is why tumors commonly continue to progress despite readily demonstrable immune responses by their hosts. It should be noted
that it is equally uncertain how grafts of heart or kidney,
or parasites, survive quite successfully in the face of demonstrable immune recognition. As the various escape mechanisms are better understood, more rational approaches can be
developed to increase the effectiveness of natural and synthetic immunoregulatory agents, and of active immunization
with tumor antigens.

With these general comments about the major issues facing
the field, I want to turn to some topics that have been of
particular interest to my colleagues and myself for many
years. The fundamental question is, of course, do tumor specific antigens in fact exist? In tracing the history of attempts to answer this question, it was the development of the
inbred mouse and the resulting understanding of the genetics
of transplantation immunity that provided the foundations on
which the field was to grow. The first milestone in the
search for tumor-specific antigens was reached in 1943 when
it was discovered that inbred mice could be immunized against
a tumor that developed in a mouse of the same inbred strain
(13). This work received little notice at the time, and 10
years passed before further evidence for tumor specific antigens was provided in a series of mouse tumors (11). Figure 1
illustrates the important features of these experiments. The
original tumor in the primary host is excised and passed into
a number of genetically uniform mice of the same inbred
strain by subcutaneous implantation. When the grafts have
reached a diameter of approximately 1 cm, they are removed
from some of the mice - Group A in Figure 1. Meanwhile, the
tumors in Group B are allowed to grow further in order to
maintain the tumor in serial passage. At a later date these

transplants of the tumor are used to challenge Group A, and these mice are found to resist this second implant of the tumor.

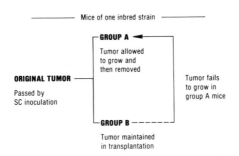

Figure 1. Demonstration of tumor-specific cell surface antigens by transplantation experiments.

Yet even these results were not universally accepted because the possibility continued to be raised that there were residual undetected genetic differences among members of the same inbred strains. This criticism was met when it was shown that even a mouse in which the tumor was originally induced could be immunized against cells from its own tumor, eliminating any doubt that tumor resistance might be due to transplantation antigens alone (22). These initial findings have been confirmed by many laboratories around the world; they represent the cornerstone of the field of tumor immunology. A consistent and remarkable feature of chemically induced tumors in this type of experiment is that each tumor elicits immunity to itself but not to any other tumor. Even when two tumors are induced with the same carcinogen in the same animal, they can be shown to have distinct antigens. By contrast, transplantation studies with tumors induced by oncogenic viruses such as polyoma virus, SV40 or adenoviruses, have shown that all tumors induced by the same virus have the same virus-specified cell surface antigen; immunization with any one tumor confers resistance to any other.

Tumors caused by any one agent, chemical or viral, vary greatly in their immunizing capacity. Naturally occurring tumors in mice have generally been found to be only weakly antigenic, and in certain cases they do not appear to be antigenic at all in transplantation experiments (14). These findings have been used by some as an argument to question the whole basis of immunological approaches to cancer. There are at least two reasons, however, to disagree with these conclusions. First, the value of immunological approaches to cancer does not depend on the validity of the immunosurveillance theory. The basic tenet in the field is that cancer cells are antigenically distinguishable from their normal progenitors, whether this leads to immune recognition or not. Secondly, there is no reason to believe that all cancer antigens will be recognized as transplantation antigens capable of eliciting rejection. In fact, with the several known escape routes available to tumor cells, it is surprising that cancer antigens were demonstrable at all by tests for transplantation resistance. It is simply not known whether tumor specific antigens are characteristic of all cancers without exception, or whether cells can be cancerous without gaining these distinctive markers. On the basis of current evidence it would be premature to form an opinion on this question.

Although transplantation techniques provided the first evidence for tumor-specific cell surface antigens, serological techniques, have a far greater potential for analyzing the surface composition of tumor cells. As advances are made in methods that demonstrate cellular immune reactions in vitro, these are likely to take their place with serological techniques in the analysis of cell surface antigens of tumors in the future. Present knowledge of these antigens, however, has come almost exclusively from the application of serological techniques. Mouse leukemia cells have been a favorite for study, because they can be easily obtained in free suspension. The great majority of mouse leukemias are T cells of thymic origin, and this has allowed the serologist to study the leukemia cell side by side with its normal counterpart, the thymocyte. As a consequence of this advantage, more is known about the surface antigens of normal and malignant T cells than almost any other cell population.

Three major categories of surface antigens in addition to the antigens of the major histocompatibility complex, H-2, have now been recognized on thymocytes and leukemia cells of the mouse. The first can be illustrated by a family of antigens, called Lyt antigens, that mark all cells undergoing T cell differentiation but are not expressed by any other cell. These antigens have been termed differentiation antigens because the genes controlling their expression are activated only in cells following a particular pathway of differentiation. Two systems of Lyt antigens have been defined. Lyt-1 antigen, coded for by a locus on chromosome 19, and Lyt-2 and -3 antigens, coded for by a single locus or closely linked loci on chromosome 6 (1,17). Great interest in Lyt antigens was generated by the finding that T cells with different functional activities could be distinguished on the basis of their

Lyt phenotypes (20,41). Cytotoxic T cells were found to express Lyt-2 and -3 antigens, whereas helper T cells did not.

The second category of mouse leukemia cell surface antigens is the TL system, called because the only types of cells on which it is found are normal mouse thymocytes and leukemia cells (31). Normal mouse strains can be classified as TL-positive and TL-negative on the basis of typing the thymus for TL antigen. TL is inherited as a Mendelian dominant trait, and genetic analysis has placed the TL locus, designated Tla, on chromosome 17 in close proximity to H-2 (3). The unusual feature of TL is that when leukemias arise in mice that lack TL on their thymocytes, the leukemia cells may express it. This has been interpreted to indicate that all mice have the genetic information for TL but that other genes control whether or not it will be expressed on normal thymocytes. Leukemogenesis disturbs this genetic repression, resulting in the anomalous appearance of TL on the surface of the leukemia cell. The appearance of TL antigens on the leukemia cells of TL-negative mice is the clearest example of a qualitative change in gene expression associated with malignancy.

Another remarkable feature of TL antigens is their disappearance from leukemia cells when they are exposed to antibody. This phenomenon, termed antigenic modulation, was discovered when TL-positive leukemia cells were found to grow as well in TL-immunized mice with high levels of TL antibody as in non-immunized mice (2). It was found that the leukemia cells growing in TL-immunized mice had lost the TL antigen. When these leukemia cells were transplanted into mice lacking antibody, however, the antigen reappeared on the cell surface. Antigenic modulation of the TL antigen is now known to be one example of the phenomenon that cell surface molecules can undergo conformational and positional changes as a consequence of antibody attachment leading to patching, capping, and in some cases temporary disappearance from the cell surface. Two important lessons have been learned from the study of TL antigens. One is that tumor antigens can be normal differentiation antigens or tumor-specific antigens, depending on the genetic background of the tumor-bearing host. The other is that not all tumor antigens can be detected as transplantation antigens. The existence of TL would have been missed had transplantation tests been the only method used for their detection.

The third and last category of leukemia antigens I would like to discuss briefly are antigens related to the murine leukemia virus or MuLV. Much that we know about the biology of this virus and the leukemias it causes was learned through the application of serological techniques for detecting viral antigens. A range of MuLV antigens have now been identified.

They include structural components of the virus particle,
viral antigens that become incorporated into the cell surface
and soluble antigens that are shed by MuLV infected cells into the body fluids.   The gp[70]-related systems that have been
defined provide markers for each of the MuLV classes, with
G(IX) distinguishing two types of ectropic MuLV, G(ERLD)
identifying all xenotropic MuLV and G(AKSL2) being a marker
for dualtropic MuLV (33). Aside from their value in typing
viral isolates, analysis of these antigens has revealed the
striking influence that genetic host factors have one viral
gene expression. We know that the genetic information MuLV is
ubiquitous in mice as an integral part of the genome, and that
these viral genes are transmitted from generation to generation along with the rest of the mouse genes (39). Whether or
not MuLV genes are fully expressed, is determined by other
genes that differ from one inbred mouse strain to the next.
Complete, partial or no expression of gp[70] determinants on the
surface of thymocytes has been found in different mouse
strains, and low or high expression of MuLV determinants parallels low or high incidence of leukemia in these strains (32).
  With the range of surface markers that have been identified
on T cells of the mouse, the surface phenotype of normal thymocytes and leukemias of thymic origin is becoming well characterized. A comparison of the surface antigens of three
leukemias that have been extensively studied with the corresponding normal thymocyte population is shown in Table 1.

TABLE 1

Cell Surface Phenotype of Normal
Thymocytes and Leukemia Cells

		H-2	Thy-1	Lyt	TL	MuLV				
						GCSA	G$_{IX}$	G$_{(RADA 1)}$	G$_{(ERLD)}$	G$_{(AKSL 2)}$
AKR	Thymocytes	+	+	+	−	+	+	+	+	+
	Spontaneous leukemia AKSL 2	+	+	−	−	+	+	+	+	+
A strain	Thymocytes	+	+	+	+	−	+	−	+	−
	X-ray-induced leukemia RADA 1	+	+	−	+	−	+	+⃞	+	−
C57BL/6	Thymocytes	+	+	+	−	−	−	−	+	−
	X-ray-induced leukemia ERLD	+	+	+	+⃞	−	−	−	+	−

⃞ Represent leukemia-specific antigens in the strain of origin

With regard to TL and MuLV-related antigens, the surface phenotype of the first leukemia, AKSL2, does not differ from normal thymocytes. By contrast, the two other leukemias express antigens not found on the corresponding thymocytes, G(RADAl) in the case of leukemia RADAl, in the G(RADAl) negative A strain, and TL in the case of leukemia ERLD in the TL negative strain C57BL/6 (33). The recognition that cell surface antigens such as TL and G(RADAl) may be leukemia-specific in some strains, yet be normally expressed as differentiation antigens in other strains, has been an important contribution of basic immunogenetics to tumor immunology. Antigens that are leukemia-specific in the strictest sense, that is, antigens restricted to leukemia cells and never expressed by any normal cell, have not yet been found.

Although a good start has been made, we still have only a superficial understanding of the enormous variety of surface antigens on normal and malignant cells in the mouse. Other antigens have been identified, but they have not been analyzed sufficiently to be placed in one category or another. Of course, the ultimate aim of this research is not simply to compile an inventory of cell surface antigens but to use these antigenic markers to understand how the cell surface is constructed, how malignancy changes that structure and how the immune system responds to such changes.

A major challenge remains the serological definition of the individually distinct transplantation antigens that were first detected on chemically induced sarcomas but are now known to exist on other tumors as well. Although this class of tumor antigens was recognized over 25 years ago, our knowledge of these antigens has advanced very little because it has not been possible to develop serological reagents for their detection and characterization. Recently, two antigens with an exceedingly restricted distribution have been defined on methylcholanthrene-induced sarcomas with antibody derived from hyperimmunized mice (8,9). The detection of these antigens provides the first serological probes to investigate the nature of these highly restricted cellular antigens. Questions to be answered are whether these antigens are related to the individually-distinct transplantation antigens, whether they are products of a single locus or multiple loci, whether they are causally related to malignant transformation or preexist before transformation as a polymorphic family of molecules distinguishing normal cells, and whether they are coded for by transfecting DNA. These and other questions can be addressed now that the first antigens of this type are accessible to serological analysis.

Let us now consider what is known about human cancer antigens. Despite the enormous volume of literature addressing

the question of tumor-specific surface antigens of human cancers, the existence of such antigens must still be considered
speculative. The general impression by many tumor immunologists as well as others that tumor-specific antigens have
been demonstrated in many types of human cancer is simply not
justified. The critical issue is specificity, and defining
the specificity of a serologic or cell-mediated immune reaction is much easier in the mouse than in man. In laboratory
animals, the availability of inbred strains permitted the
transplantation studies that established the existence of distinctive cell surface antigens in tumors. The serologic definition of these antigens in the mouse has also depended on inbred populations to provide the necessary reagents.

     In the absence of these advantages, the human cancer serolo-
gist is still attempting to evolve approaches that can cope
with the issue of specificity. Antisera prepared against
human cancer cells in foreign species, while at first appearing tumor-specific, have in every instance turned out to be
directed against normal cellular products that are either
present in higher concentration in tumor cells or are found in
restricted normal cell populations. Surveys of human sera for
reactivity with cell surface antigens of allogeneic tumor
cells, usually cell lines considered representative of one
type of cancer, form the basis for many reports in the literature. They are rarely, if ever, interpretable as tumor-specific reactions, however, because unknown participation of alloantibodies in the reactions observed is extremely difficult to
exclude.

     What I want to illustrate here is how our group has ap-
proached this issue and where we are in our attempts to answer
the two key questions of the field: do human cancer antigens
exist and, if so, do they elicit an immune response in humans?
Our initial decision to stress serological approaches to these
questions had nothing to do with prejudices about the relative
importance of humoral vs. cellular immune reactions against
cancer. It was simply based on the fact that defining the
specificity of a serological reaction is far easier than doing
so for reactions involving lymphoid cells. In the evolution
of our serological study, we have attempted to develop as
rigorous and comprehensive an approach as possible to the
analysis of cell surface antigens of human cancer and the
issue of cancer specificity.

     The serological method that we used initially is referred to
as autologous typing. It has several essential features. We
use tissue culture lines as target cells because only continuously available target cells permit the frequently repeated
serological testing that ensures reproducibility. The initial
tests are restricted to autologous combinations of serum and

tumor cells to eliminate the contribution of alloantibodies
and to detect antigens of the individually-distinct category.
We use several serological techniques to reduce the possibility that antibody of a particular immunoglobulin class might be
missed, and we determine specificity by extensive use of absorption analysis, which includes the testing of various cultured autologous normal cells. As cultured target cells are
required, the studies have been restricted to malignant melanoma (6,42,43), astrocytoma (35) and renal cancer (44), tumors
that can be cultured more easily than other tumors.

Over the past several years, sera from more than 100 patients with these tumor types have been analyzed by autologous
typing. The result of these studies has been that three classes of cell surface antigens can be defined by autologous
antibody. Class 1 antigens are individually distinct, restricted to autologous tumor, and cannot be found on autologous normal cells or any other normal or malignant cell. Class
2 antigens are shared tumor antigens, expressed not only by
autologous tumors but also by allogeneic tumors of similar
and in some cases dissimilar origin. In contrast, Class 3
antigens are not restricted but widely distributed on normal
and malignant cells, autologous, allogeneic and xenogeneic.
The largest number of reactions detected by autologous typing
are due to antibodies directed against Class 3 antigens, and
such antibodies in addition to alloantibodies undoubtedly
account for the majority of positive reactions recorded in
past serological studies of human cancer and for many mistaken
claims of tumor specificity.

Let me briefly review our findings with malignant melanoma.
One hundred twenty melanoma cell lines have been established
in our laboratory, a success rate of 20-307 for long term cultures. Autologous typing of 75 patients showed IgG on IgM
antibodies in 56. Of these patients with antibody, 4 had
antibody detecting Class 1 antigens, 5 had antibody detecting
Class 2 antigens, and 21 had antibody detecting Class 3 antigens. Analysis of 26 patients is not yet complete.

The antigen detected on the melanoma of the patient AU is an
example of a Class 1 antigen. The patient was a 51-year-old
man with recurrent melanoma who had an unusually long clinical
course. The antibody that detected the Class 1 antigen on the
patient's own melanoma cells was of the IgG class. Antibody
titers were found to rise when the tumor recurred, and to fall
when the tumor was removed (6). The AU antigen could be solubilized by limited papain digestion. It turned out to be a
glycoprotein with a molecular weight in the range of 25,000-
40,000 daltons and has no serological relation to HLA, Ia or
β2 microglobulin (5). Somatic cell hybrids formed by fusing
AU melanoma cells with chinese hamster cells express AU

antigen, independently of HLA and β2 microglobulin. In a
series of hybrids the AU antigen was found to be coded for by
a locus on chromosome 19 (L. Resnick and D. Pravtcheva, unpublished observation). Structural studies and somatic cell hybrid analysis of Class 1 antigens should tell us whether they
represent a family of structurally related molecules with
polymorphic epitopes coded for by a single locus, or totally
unrelated molecules coded for by many loci.

The AH melanoma antigen is an example of a Class 2 antigen.
The patient is a 56-year-old man with recurrent melanoma who
has now been free of disease for 6 years. The antigen is defined by IgM antibody in the patient's serum. Extensive analysis has shown the AH antigen to be present on melanomas and
astrocytomas but not on any other cell (18). Physical characterization indicates that the antigen resides on a glycolipid
moiety and structural studies are underway. One question that
can be asked about antibody to Class 2 antigens is whether
antibody is a consequence of cancer or whether apparently normal individuals can have natural antibodies to this antigen.
An initial survey of over 100 normal non-transfused males has
just been completed. Five of these normal individuals were
found to have IgM antibody to an antigen related to the AH
melanoma antigen, indicating that overt melanoma is not necessary for the development of AH antibody (16).

The serological dissection of human sera tells us which
melanoma cell surface antigens can be recognized as immunogenic by humans. As I mentioned earlier, antisera raised in
animals have not been useful reagents for the serological
analysis of human cancer cells in the past, but this has
changed now that the hybridoma technique has been developed
which permits the production of antibodies of single specificities by single clones of plasma cells (23). The method has
been applied by several groups to the study of human cancer.
Table 2 summarizes information from our ongoing analysis of
mouse monoclonal antibodies to human melanoma cells (10).
Nine systems of melanoma cell surface antigens have been defined by monoclonal antibodies, 6 being glycoproteins and 3
glycolipids. Each shows a characteristic cellular distribution. The antigen defined by R24 antibody has the most restricted distribution of all. Highest reactivity is found
with melanoma and astrocytomas, whereas epithelial cell types,
fibroblasts and hematopoietic cells lack the antigen. As a
consequence of this intense serological scrutiny by our group
and by others (24,45,46), a comprehensive picture of the surface structure of melanoma cells can be expected in the near
future.

There are many ways to put this information from autologous
typing, natural antibodies and monoclonal antibodies to use.

TABLE 2

Cell Surface Antigens of Human
Malignant Melanoma Defined by
Murine Monoclonal Antibodies

Cell Panel	Glycoproteins						Glycolipids		
	GP45 (HLA)	GP28/34 (Ia)	GP95	GP150	M_{19}	R_8	O_5	$K_{9,}$ I_{24}	R_{24}
Melanoma	+	+	+	+	+	+	+	+	+
Epithelial cancer	+	−	+	−	+	+	+	−	−
T-cells	+	−	+	+	−	−	+	+	−
B-cells	+	+	+	+	−	−	+	−	−
Fibroblasts	+	−	+	−	+	−	+	+	−
Fetal brain	+	−	−	+	−	−	+	+	−
Melanocytes	+	−	−	+	+	+	+	+	+

Perhaps the most critical challenge is to determine the range
of melanoma cell surface molecules that are or can be made to
be immunogenic in man. As some of them have been shown to
elicit an immune response in the autologous host, and as serological methods with the resolving power needed to monitor the
specificity of the immune response are now available, it seems
both justified and timely to re-explore the effects of active
specific immunization in melanoma patients. The idea of tumor
cell vaccines is of course not new, and many attempts have
been made over the years to alter the course of cancer by immunization with tumor cells or extracts of tumor cells. But
little if anything can be learned from most of these past
studies because meaningful measurements were not made of the
immune response of vaccinated patients to the vaccine. Therefore, there is no way to know whether these patients received
immunogenic vaccines or not. The first goal of our current
vaccine program is to develop maximally immunogenic forms of
melanoma antigens that can be recognized by human patients,
using serological typing of vaccinated patients as the way to
monitor immunogenicity. In our initial studies, we have used
autologous whole cell vaccines. Only in rare cases did they
elicit formation of antibodies recognizing Class 1 or Class 2
antigens, as shown in the following examples.

Patient BD had initially an IgM antibody against a Class 1
antigen. Antibody titers declined after resection of most but
not all extensive lymph node metastases in both groins and one
axilla. After vaccination with autologous melanoma cells, IgG
antibodies directed against a Class 2 shared melanoma antigen

appeared in the patient's serum (Figure 2). Against all expectations, the patient is still free of recurrence, 4-1/2
years after the vaccine treatment was started.

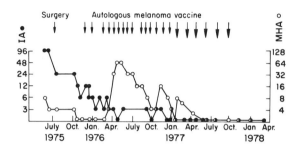

<u>Figure 2.</u>   Autologous melanoma cell vaccine augments sero-
            logical reactivity with autologous melanoma cells
            (BD).

   Patient DM was initially seronegative. He was vaccinated
with allogeneic melanoma cells expressing the AH Class 2 antigen. As expected, the patient as well as many other patients
developed a brisk serological response to the allogeneic cells
in the vaccine, directed against HLA-related antigens. Antibodies were also detected, however, when the patient's serum
was tested on his own melanoma cells (Figure 3). Extensive
absorption analysis showed that these antibodies were directed
against the melanoma-restricted Class 2 antigen of the melanoma cells in the vaccine, an antigen that was shared by the
patient's own melanoma (P. Livingston, T. Watanabe, H.
Takeyama, unpublished observations).

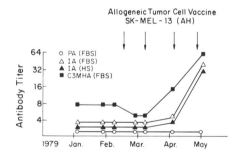

<u>Figure 3.</u>   Allogeneic melanoma cell vaccine (AH) augments sero-
            logical reactivity with autologous melanoma cells
            (DM).

Two points emerge from these observations. First, a melanoma-specific serological response can in fact be induced to
Class 1 or Class 2 melanoma antigens by vaccination. Second,
this has only rarely been accomplished by vaccination with un-
modified whole cells. This fact would not have been established had the patients not been monitored by extensive serological testing, and it throws more doubt on conclusions regarding the lack of therapeutic effects of vaccines derived
from earlier studies. The question then arises how can we
modify the vaccines to increase their immunogenicity. Procedures that have adequate precedent in defined immunological
systems include introduction of foreign helper determinants by
virus infection, chemical modification or hybridization of
melanoma cells with allogeneic melanoma cells, allogeneic B
lymphocytes or cells from animal sources. They also include
the use of isolated Class 1 or Class 2 antigens which is feasible now that serological reagents are available with which we
can monitor purification. We are currently testing modified
vaccines in a sequential fashion for their immunogenicity in
melanoma patients. If an immunogenic vaccine can be found, it
will then be tested for therapeutic effects.

We monitor our patients by serological tests because they
are more precise than currently available tests for cellular
immunity. Although there is a general impression that increased cellular rather than humoral immunity is the desired
endpoint of immunological manipulation in patients with cancer,
we know too little at present to form a judgment about this
matter. In addition, there has been considerable discussion
about the possibility of immunological enhancement of tumor
growth as a consequence of immunotherapy. Once again, our
knowledge about this possibility in man is non-existent.
Antibody-indicated immunological enhancement has never been
convincingly demonstrated with strictly syngeneic or autologous tumors in animals, nor has it been observed in any patient receiving a tumor cell vaccine. Nevertheless, we will
remain alert to this possibility.

While modified cancer cell vaccines no doubt should be explored in attempts to induce or augment an immune response to
cancer antigens, research in basic immunology has unraveled
factors other than the ways in which antigen is presented
that determine the magnitude of the immune response. Until
recently, most immunologists subscribed to the clonal selection theory of one shade or another. According to this concept, the duration and strength of a response depended only on
the number of lymphocyte clones that carried receptor molecules for a particular antigen. Over the past decade, much
evidence has been developed that this view is not correct, and
that regulatory cells play an important part in determining

the magnitude of the immune response, effector cell activity depending on the balance of inducer cell and suppressor cell activity (Figure 4). While B lymphocytes and macrophages no doubt participate in this regulatory network, subsets of T lymphocytes appear to play the major role in the mouse (4,12). With the advent of monoclonal antibodies, a comparable dissection of human T cell subsets has begun (38,40).

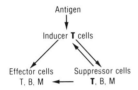

Figure 4. Regulatory network.

Present indications are that subsets of regulator T lymphocytes can be distinguished on the basis of characteristic cell surface phenotypes in both mouse and man, and that immunization may be made more effective by changing the balance of this regulatory system in favor of inducer cells over suppressor cells. Ways by which this has been attempted include the administration of antibodies directed against cell surface antigens considered specific for suppressor cells, chemical modification of antigens that favor stimulation of inducer cells, and utilization of the differential susceptibility of inducer T cells and suppressor T cells to chemotherapeutic agents or radiation. It is far too early to tell how effective these manipulations will be, but there is no doubt that attempts at effective active immunization with cancer antigens must take into consideration the new knowledge of immunoregulation that has been developed by research in basic immunology.

Let us now turn to other approaches to immunotherapy. Transfer of specific immunity, successful in the mouse, has not really been explored in the treatment of human cancer because antisera or sensitized lymphocytes of acceptable specificity have not been available. As progress is made in the dissection of human cancer antigens, and as monoclonal antibodies or cloned sensitized T cells may become available as vehicles of cancer-specific immunity, it may become possible to explore this approach also in the treatment of human cancer.

In the past decade, the field of immunotherapy has been dominated by what has been termed non-specific immunotherapy with immunopotentiators, BCG being the agent that has been most widely investigated. The premise underlying this approach was that agents such as BCG and C. parvum potentiate immunological reactivity on a global basis, and that this results in a more effective specific immune reaction against cancer. While this concept is appealing, its general validity remains to be proven. The overall results of clinical trials with BCG, C. parvum and other such agents have led to current disenchantment with this approach to cancer therapy. Nevertheless, there remains a body of solid observations that requires continued exploration, ranging from the indisputable regressions of cancers associated with bacterial infections or injection of bacterial vaccines (30), to the tumor cell destruction induced by local delayed hypersensitivity reactions (21), to the therapeutic benefit of intratumoral injection of BCG in melanoma patients (29,37).

A more recent example of a potentially useful therapeutic application of BCG is the treatment of patients with bladder cancer. Results of a pilot study by Morales in Canada suggested that intravesical application of BCG delayed recurrence of this disease (28). A prospective randomized trial conducted by our group confirms this suggestion. The patients in this trial had multicentric bladder cancer, Jewett's Stage 0, A or low grade B1, or recurrent papillomas. These patients are known to develop recurrence after local therapy at a very high rate. The patients were randomized to standard local therapy by fulguration, or fulguration followed by BCG. BCG was administered into the bladder through a catheter once weekly for 6 weeks, and also inoculated intradermally at the same time. A significant delay of recurrence was seen in the BCG-treated group (Figure 5), and the number of recurrent tumors was markedly reduced in patients who developed recurrence. There was also a marked decrease in the number of patients with positive cytology in the BCG group (36). Similar results have been obtained by another group (26), and as the side effects are mild, there is every reason to pursue this approach to determine if it leads to long-term clinical benefit.

An understanding of how these agents bring about their effects and what role, if any, specific immune reactions have in the process, has turned out to be far more difficult than originally expected. There is evidence that some of the antitumor effects of these agents are due to mediator molecules released by host cells, and so the question arises whether these mediators are more effective in therapy. Their use would circumvent some of the toxicity of the inducing agents as well as the limitation imposed by the fact that the induction mechanisms become temporarily refractory to continued stimulation.

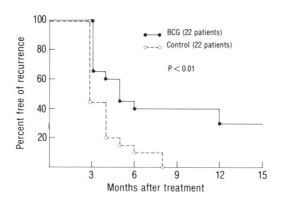

<u>Figure 5</u>.   Delayed recurrence of superficial bladder cancer
              after intravesical application of BCG.

By far the best known members of the group of endogenous
mediators are the interferons. Leukocyte interferon, lymphoblast interferon and fibroblast interferon have been investigated in various clinical trials, and responses have been reported in patients with osteogenic sarcoma, malignant lymphoma,
multiple myeloma, acute leukemia, breast cancer, malignant
melanoma, nasopharyngeal cancer and fibrosarcoma (25). As a
consequence of the difficulty to produce adequate amounts of
interferons, their clinical evaluation is at the earliest
stage and only preliminary results are available. The prospects of treating cancer with interferon are discussed elsewhere in this volume.

Another endogenous mediator of considerable interest is the
tumor necrosis factor found in the serum of mice treated with
endotoxin. One of the most striking phenomena of tumor biology is the hemorrhagic necrosis induced in experimental tumors
by endotoxin. Within a few hours of an intravenous endotoxin
injection, the tumor mass begins to undergo a progressive
darkening in color indicative of tumor cell death and hemor-
rhage, leading in many instances to complete regression. Although extensively investigated over the past 40 years, the
way endotoxin causes tumor destruction is not known. A direct
action is ruled out by the fact that endotoxin lacks toxicity
for tumor cells <u>in vitro</u>.

The suggestion that a mediator molecule was involved came
from the finding that hemorrhagic tumor necrosis could also be
induced by intravenous injection of serum from endotoxin-

treated mice that had been presensitized with BCG or C.parvum
(7). In addition to its tumor necrotizing activity, tumor
necrosis serum was found to have striking effects on the maturation and immunological functions of lymphocytes (15).
With further purification of the tumor-necrotizing activity
and of the activity that enhanced antibody production, they
turned out to be two different entities. The tumor necrosis
factor (TNF), now purified to apparent homogeneity, is a glycoprotein with a molecular weight of 40,000 that has both
tumor-necrotizing activity in vivo and tumor cell killing
activity in vitro (34). The immune response-enhancing activity resides in a protein with a molecular weight of 13,000 (27);
this molecule has a helper function in B cell antibody production and in T cell cytotoxicity. While it was first known as
B cell differentiating factor or lymphocyte activating factor,
it has now been designated Interleukin 1 or IL-1.

The current view of its central role in the regulation of
the immune system is shown in Figure 6. IL-1 is released by
macrophages in response to a T cell signal. This signal can
be replaced by endotoxin (LPS). IL-1 induces maturation of T
and B cell precursors, and stimulates T cells to produce IL-2,
also known as T cell growth factor. IL-2 induces expansion of
antigen-stimulated T and B cell clones, and induces T cells to
produce the so-called T cell replacing factor or TRF which has
been speculated by some to be interferon. It induces effector
cell functions, T cell cytotoxicity and B cell antibody production, in the expanded clones.

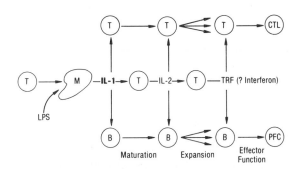

Figure 6. Central role of IL-1 in the regulation of the
immune system.

If we return now to the phenomenon in the mouse, TNF and IL-1, both induced by endotoxin, can be viewed as mediators of two characteristic phases. TNF causes acute necrosis, a phenomenon known to be independent of an immune response; it can be elicited in severely immunosuppressed hosts. IL-1, on the other hand, may play an essential helper role in the second step, complete regression of residual tumor cells, which is known to depend on an intact immune system. Now that these molecules have been characterized, some key questions can be answered such as their relation to other lymphokines and serum factors, the basis for the tumor cell selectivity of TNF, and its possible involvement in the cytotoxic effect of activated macrophages and other classes of killer cells.

Finally, mention should be made of another potent antitumor factor, in this case one that exists in normal plasma. It was first recognized in experiments concerned with the antitumor effects of interferon in AKR mice (18). For control purposes, normal mouse serum was used. The surprising finding was that it had the same antitumor effect as the interferon preparations. The antitumor factor was widespread in other mammalian sera and plasma, but in the mouse it was restricted to strains having the complete set of complement components. Striking and rapid regression of cat lymphoma and dog lymphoma could also be induced by infusions of normal plasma (19).

Although there is no doubt about the involvement of complement in the antileukemic effect of plasma in AKR mice, purification of the factor from normal mouse plasma has shown that it has several characteristics in common with cold insoluble globulin (CIg), also known as fibronectin. Because of this association, it has been suggested (M. Mosessohn, personal communication) that the cryoprecipitated fraction of normal plasma might be active since this plasma fraction, in addition to concentrating the antihemophilic factor, is also rich in CIg. Cat cryoprecipitates have now been tested and found to be as active as whole plasma (G. MacEwen, unpublished observation), and early tests in the clinic with human cryoprecipitate have shown activity in some patients with advanced lymphomas (H. Teitelbaum, unpublished observation).

In closing, it clearly remains for the future to determine what the ultimate contribution of immunological research to the understanding and control of cancer will be. The discipline of cancer immunology is a young one, and to expect major practical applications of its principles and findings at this point would be unrealistic. What we can expect over the next few years is a growing understanding of the nature of tumor-specific antigens and a detailed knowledge of the immune response they elicit. The study of immunology has been profoundly influenced by the realization that genes exert a tight control over immunological reactions, and the genetic control of immune responses to cancer and cancer viruses now needs definition. Learning how to modify or overcome genetic restrictions on immune responses and how to manipulate the intricate regulatory network of the immune system may provide powerful means of preventing tumors from escaping immunological destruction. In research on human cancer the task is to apply the findings derived from the study of animal tumors to human cancer. Among other things this means carefully controlled assessment of the value of immunopotentiators in the treatment of human cancer and rigorous laboratory study to define human cancer antigens as precisely as they have been defined in experimental animals. As we look to the future, neither uncritical optimism nor new waves of doubt and pessimism appear to be justified. Substantial advances have been made. We can expect that immunological investigations will continue to make notable contributions to our understanding of cancer, and that they will guide us to making the host defense against cancer more effective.

REFERENCES

1. Boyse EA, Miyazawa M, Aoki T, Old LJ: Ly-A and Ly-B: Two systems of lymphocyte isoantigens in the mouse. Proc Roy Soc London Ser B 170:175-193, 1968.
2. Boyse EA, Old LJ, Luell S: Antigenic properties of experimental leukemias. II. Immunological studies in vivo with C57BL/6 radiation-induced leukemias. J Natl Cancer Inst 31:987-995, 1963.
3. Boyse EA, Old LJ, Luell S: Genetic determination of the TL (thymus-leukemia) antigen in the mouse. Nature 201:779, 1964.
4. Cantor H: Control of the immune system by inhibitor and inducer T lymphocytes. Ann Rev Med 30:269-277, 1979.
5. Carey TE, Lloyd KO, Takahashi T, et al.: Solubilization and partial characterization of the AU cell surface antigen of human malignant melanoma. Proc Natl Acad Sci USA 76: 2898-2902, 1979.
6. Carey TE, Takahashi T, Resnick LA, et al.: Cell surface antigens of human malignant melanoma. I. Mixed hemadsorption assays for humoral immunity to cultured autologous melanoma cells. Proc Natl Acad Sci USA 73:3278-3282, 1976.
7. Carswell EA, Old LJ, Kassel RL, et al.: An endotoxin-induced serum factor that causes necrosis of tumors. Proc Natl Acad Sci USA 72:3666-3670, 1975.
8. DeLeo AB, Shiku H, Takahashi T, et al.: Cell surface antigens of chemically induced sarcomas of the mouse. I.Murine

leukemia virus-related antigens and alloantigens on cultured fibroblasts and sarcoma cells: Description of a unique antigen on BALB/c Meth A sarcoma. J Exp Med 146: 720-734, 1977.

9. DeLeo AB, Shiku H, Takahashi T, Old LJ: Serological definition of cell surface antigens of chemically induced sarcomas of inbred mice, in Ruddon (ed): Biological Markers of Neoplasia: Basic and Applied Aspects. Elsevier North Holland, Inc., 1978, pp 25-34

10. Dippold W, Lloyd KO, Li LTC, et al.: Cell surface antigens of human malignant melanoma: Definition of six antigenic systems with mouse monoclonal antibodies. Proc Natl Acad Sci USA: in press.

11. Foley EJ: Antigenic properties of methylcholanthrene-induced tumors in mice of the strain of origin. Cancer Res 13:835, 1953.

12. Gershon RK: T cell suppression. Contemp Top Immunobiol 3:1, 1974.

13. Gross L: Intradermal immunization of C3H mice against a sarcoma that originated in an animal of the same line. Cancer Res 3:326, 1943.

14. Hewitt HB, Blake ER, Walder AS: A critique of the evidence for active host defense against cancer based on personal studies of 27 murine tumors of spontaneous origin. Br J Cancer 33:241-259, 1976.

15. Hoffmann MK, Oettgen HF, Old LJ, et al.: Induction and immunological properties of tumor necrosis factor. J Reticuloendocr Soc 23:307-319, 1978.

16. Houghton AN, Taormina MC, Ikeda H, et al.: Serological survey of normal humans for natural antibody to cell surface antigens of melanoma. Proc Natl Acad Sci USA 77: 4260-4264, 1980.

17. Itakura K, Hutton JJ, Boyse EA, Old LJ: Genetic linkage relationships of loci specifying differentiation alloantigens in the mouse. Transplantation 13:239-243, 1972.

18. Kassel RL, Old LJ, Carswell EA, et al.: Serum-mediated leukemia cell destruction in AKR mice. J Exp Med 138:925-938, 1973.

19. Kassel RL, Old LJ, Day NK, et al.: Plasma-mediated leukemic cell destruction: Current status. Blood Cells 3: 605-621, 1977.

20. Kisielow P, Hirst JA, Shiku H, et al.: Ly antigens as markers for functionally distinct subpopulations of thymus-derived lymphocytes of the mouse. Nature (London) 253:219-220, 1975.

21. Klein E: Tumors of the skin. X. Immunotherapy of cutaneous and mucosal neoplasms. N Y State J Med 68:900, 1968.

22. Klein G, Sjögren HO, Klein E, Hellström KE: Demonstration of resistance against methylcholanthrene-induced sarcomas in the primary autochthonous host. Cancer Res 20:1561-1572, 1960.

23. Köhler G, Milstein C: Continuous cultures of fused cells secreting antibody of predefined specificity. Nature (London) 256:495-497, 1975.

24. Koprowski H, Steplewski Z, Herlyn D, Herlyn M: Study of antibodies against human melanoma produced by somatic cell hybrids. Proc Natl Acad Sci USA 75:3405-3409, 1978.

25. Krim M: Towards tumor therapy with interferons, Part I. Interferons: Production and properties. Blood 55:711-721, 1980.

26. Lamm DL, Stogdill VD, Thor DE: Bacillus Calmette-Guerin immunotherapy in superficial transitional cell carcinoma of the urinary bladder. Proc. Am Soc Clin Oncol 21:372, 1980.

27. Männel DN, Farrar JJ, Mergenhagen SE: Separation of a serum-derived tumoricidal factor from a helper factor for plaque-forming cells. J Immunol 124:1106-1110, 1980.

28. Morales A, Ersil A: Prophylaxis of recurrent bladder cancer with Bacillus Calmette-Guerin, in Johnson DE, Samuels ML (eds): Cancer of the Genitourinary Tract. New York, Raven Press, 1979, pp 121-132

29. Morton DL, Eilber FR, Malmgren RA, et al.: Immunological factors which influence response to immunotherapy in malignant melanoma. Surgery 68:158-164, 1970.

30. Nauts HC, Swift WZ, Coley BL: The treatment of tumors by bacterial toxins, as developed by the late William B. Coley, M.D., reviewed in the light of modern research. Cancer Res 6:2505, 1946.

31. Old LJ, Boyse EA, Stockert E: Antigenic properties of experimental leukemias. I. Serological studies in vitro with spontaneous and radiation-induced leukemias. J Natl Cancer Inst 31:977-986, 1963.

32. Old LJ, Stockert E: Immunogenetics of cell surface antigens of mouse leukemia. Ann Rev Genet 11:27-60, 1977.

33. Old LJ, Stockert E: Serological definition of cell surface antigens of mouse leukemia, in Morse HC III (ed): Origins of Inbred Mice. Proceedings of a Workshop. New York, Academic Press, 1978, pp 391-407

34. Oettgen HF, Carswell EA, Kassel RL, et al.: Endotoxin-induced tumor necrosis factor. Recent Results in Cancer Research 75: in press.

35. Pfreundschuh M, Shiku H, Takahashi T, et al.: Serological analysis of cell surface antigens of malignant human brain tumors. Proc Natl Acad Sci USA 75:5122-5126, 1978.

36. Pinsky CM, Camacho FJ, Kerr D, et al.: Treatment of

superficial bladder cancer with intravesical Bacillus Calmette-Guerin (BCG), in Terry WD (ed): Proceedings of the Second International Meeting on Immunotherapy of Cancer, in press.

37. Pinsky CM, Hirshaut Y, Oettgen HF: Treatment of malignant melanoma by intratumoral injection of BCG. Natl Cancer Inst Monogr 39:225-228, 1973.

38. Reinherz EL, Schlossman SF: Characterization of regulatory T cells in man, in Pernis B, Vogel HJ (eds): Regulatory T Cells. P & S Biomedical Sciences Symposia, New York, Arden House: in press.

39. Rowe WP: Leukemia virus genomes in the chromosomal DNA of the mouse. Harvey Lect. 71:173-192, 1978.

40. Schlossman SF, Evans RL, Strelkauskas AJ: Human T-cell subsets with regulatory functions, in Serrou B, Rosenfeld C (eds): Human Lymphocyte Differentiation: Its Application to Cancer. Amsterdam, Elsevier/North-Holland Biomedical Press, 1978, pp 83-92

41. Shiku H, Kisielow P, Bean MA, et al.: Expression of T-cell differentiation antigens on effector cells in cell-mediated cytotoxicity in vitro. Evidence for functional heterogeneity related to the surface phenotype of T cells. J Exp Med 141:227-241, 1975.

42. Shiku H, Takahashi T, Oettgen HF, Old LJ: Cell surface antigens of human malignant melanoma. II. Serological typing with immune adherence assays and definition of two new surface antigens. J Exp Med 144:873-881, 1976.

43. Shiku H, Takahashi T, Resnick LA, et al.: Cell surface antigens of human malignant melanoma. III. Recognition of autoantibodies with unusual characteristics. J Exp Med 145:784-789, 1977.

44. Ueda R, Shiku H, Pfreundschuh M, et al.: Cell surface antigens of human renal cancer defined by autologous typing. J Exp Med 150:564-579, 1979.

45. Woodbury RC, Brown JP, Yeh MY, et al.: Identification of a cell surface protein, p97, in human melanoma and certain other neoplasms. Proc Natl Acad Sci USA 77:2183-2817, 1980.

46. Yeh MY, Hellström I, Brown JP, et al.: Cell surface antigens of human melanoma identified by monoclonal antibody. Proc Natl Acad Sci USA 76:2927-2931, 1979.

Immunogenetics of Cancer in Man and Animals

Frank Lilly

Genetics Department
Albert Einstein College of Medicine
Bronx, N.Y. 10461

ABSTRACT. Both humoral and cellular immune responses are involved in immunologic defenses against cancer, and variations from one individual to another at many genetic loci can influence and alter these immune responses. The highly polymorphic major histocompatibility complex (MHC)—*H-2* in the mouse and *HLA* in man—appears to be the most important of these genetic factors, a finding extensively documented in the mouse but considerably less firmly established in studies of humans. Studies in several laboratories of mouse lymphoma, both spontaneous and virus-induced, have provided the best evidence on this point and have also clearly indicated that more than one gene, closely linked within the MHC, can influence the occurrence of an anti-tumor immune response. It is clear that certain T lymphocytes with anti-tumor cell activity must recognize two different tumor cell-surface molecules (either separately or as a unit) in order to be activated and to exert their effect: (a) a tumor-specific (e.g., viral) molecule and (b) a molecule encoded in the MHC. Evidence suggests that these two molecules must form an appropriate complex on the cell surface in order to elicit a T lymphocyte response, and a given tumor-specific molecule can form such a complex with some but not all allelic products of the relevant MHC genes. Individuals lacking appropriate MHC haplotypes would thus be deprived of the types of immune defenses against their tumor cells which depend on molecular complex formation.

Cell-Mediated Immune Reactions
to Human Cancer Antigens
and Their Regulation

MICHAEL A. BEAN, M.D.

Member and Associate Director
Virginia Mason Research Center
Seattle, Washington 98101

The topic of cell-mediated immune reactions to human tumor antigens has been one that has generated a considerable amount of interest and some controversy. The development in the early and mid 1960's of techniques for the measurement in vitro of cellular immune responses made it possible for investigators to begin asking the question as to whether or not humans developed cellular immune responses to their tumors. In the late 1960's the Hellstrom's (1) were the first to report on the demonstration in vitro of cell-mediated cytotoxicity of blood lymphocytes against human tumors. In their early studies they found that lymphocytes from patients with cancer were cytotoxic for their own tumors or tumors of the same histologic type. And, these cytotoxic blood lymphocytes would not react against tumor cells of different histogenic type. These results were especially exciting as virally induced tumors in mice had cross-reacting tumor associated antigens while chemically induced tumors had unique non cross-reacting antigens. Thus, these data were interpreted at that time as consistent with these human tumors being caused by viruses. The Hellstrom's findings stimulated a massive amount of work in this area and produced a number of different findings that did not seem to reconcile with the early results from their group.

Since studies in murine models had demonstrated that T-cell mediated immunity protected against tumor growth (2), most investigators expected that cytotoxic responses of blood lymphocytes of humans against tumor cells would be T-cell mediated reactions (1). However, it soon became apparent that there were more than just T-cells reacting in the in vitro microcytotoxicity assays. Herberman, Takasugi and their colleagues (3-5) found that normal individuals as well as cancer patients had blood lymphocytes that were capable of cytotoxic reactions against tumor cells in vitro. These cytotoxic lymphocytes did not exhibit the T-cell characteristic of forming stable rosettes with sheep red blood cells and they had Fc receptors (3). Since they were reactive against some tumor cells but not normal cells and were not classic B, macrophage or T-cells, they were named natural killer cells (NK).

These NK cells soon became a primary focus of interest in the cancer immunology field because the accumulating evidence suggested they might comprise a first-line defense system against neoplastic cells (5). It may well be that the "natural cytotoxicity" mediated by NK cells does not fall in the category of a cell-mediated immune reaction if strict immunological definitions are used. To date, there is no definition of antigen specificity for their receptors although future studies may shed some light on this question (6). Much of the current interest in and excitement over NK cells revolves around the fact that interferon and interferon inducers as well as some other immunopotentiators stimulate NK activity in vivo and in vitro (5). This ability to augment NK activity is especially important as NK cells have been shown in murine models to be capable of inhibiting the outgrowth of inoculum of NK sensitive tumor cells.

Antibody-dependent cell-mediated cytotoxicity (ADCMC) has also been found to be the explanation for some of the cytotoxic responses seen with lymphocytes from cancer patients (7). K-cells which mediate ADCMC are non B, non T lymphocytes with high affinity Fc receptors through which they can bind IgG bound to target cells and effect their lysis (3,7). Some of the cytotoxicity of human bladder cancer patients lymphocytes appears to be due to K cells being armed in vivo with antibody or antibody-antigen complexes which are reactive with bladder cancer tumor cell lines (7). The biological significance of ADCMC reactions against tumor cells in vivo is not yet known.

In addition to the above cell types that can be active in the in vitro cytotoxicity assays in humans, it also has become apparent that activated monocytes or macrophages can exert cytostatic and/or cytotoxic effects. Given the complexity of the cell types manifesting cytotoxicity in these assays and the complexity of the assays themselves in terms of whether they measure direct cell killing or a combination of cell killing and cytostatic effects, it is little wonder that there was some confusion over the results coming out of different laboratories (8). And, it is little wonder that the initial question as to whether patients with cancer have cytotoxic T-cells capable of reacting to their own tumor cells has not been fully resolved. The question of cytotoxic T-cells in cancer, which has been greatly overshadowed recently by the study of NK cells would seem likely to soon re-emerge as an area for fruitful investigation.

The more innovative of the recent studies on cytotoxic T-cells directed against human tumors have used experimental protocols designed from results emerging from studies clarifying the cell signal requirements for in vitro generation of cytotoxic T-cells against H-2 and HLA alloantigens. Some investigators have attempted to educate or sensitize the patient's lymphocytes by incubation with the autologous tumor cells in order to detect cytotoxic tumor-reactive T-cells. Zarling, Bach, and co-workers (9,10) have made a number of interesting observations in this regard. They have found that they can induce lymphocytes from some acute myelogenous leukemia patients to become cytotoxic for their own tumor cells by co-incubation of the patient's lymphoid cells with irradiated myeloblasts (as a source of putative tumor antigen) and third party irradiated lymphocytes as a lymphocyte defined signal needed to induce proliferation in order to generate cytotoxic cells reactive to the tumor antigen (9). The resultant cytotoxic lymphocytes lyse autologous tumor but do not lyse autologous normal blasts. And, inhibition studies show the cytotoxicity directed against the tumor cells can only be inhibited by "cold" tumor cells. A confirmation of this phenomenon has been reported by Lee and Oliver (11). In more recent studies, Zarling and associates (10) have found that by priming the patient's lymphocytes to tumor cells with third party stimuli present and then growing the cells for a period of time in T-cell growth factor (TCGF), they could generate T-cell cytotoxicity directed against autologous myeloblasts using lymphocytes from the patients who wouldn't develop detectable cytotoxicity in the culture model without TCGF. These T-cell preparations were also not reactive against autologous normal lymphoblasts indicating the sensitization schema had produced cytotoxic T-cells which possibly could be directed against tumor antigen although it is possible that they could be reactive with a differentiation antigen present on the tumor cell blast and not the lymphoblasts used as control target

cells. The implication of this work is that the in vitro
sensitization procedure did effect sensitization or expanded
pre-existing cytotoxic cells for tumor but that they were
present at too low a frequency to be detected without
further expansion of the reactive clone(s) in TCGF. Using a
related technique with a virus model, Sethi et al. (12) were
successful in expanding clones of HLA restricted cytotoxic
T-cells for HSV and CMV infected target cells. They took
blood from donors recently infected with these viruses,
incubated their lymphocytes with the viral antigen, and then
grew out the cytotoxic T-cells in TCGF. Although exposure
to the viral antigens alone did induce some cytotoxicity, it
was not as strong or as clearly HLA restricted without
further culture in TCGF.

Using a related but different approach using patients with
solid tumors, Vose and his colleagues (13) tried in vitro
stimulation of the patients' blood lymphocytes by exposure
to their autologous tumor cells in co-culture prior to testing for cytotoxic reactions. Some 9 out of 22 blood lymphocyte preparations from patients developed detectable or
augmented cytotoxicity for their tumor cells. Seven of
those nine had no reactivity prior to co-culture. The data
from this study are not sufficient to clarify whether these
cytotoxic cells were tumor specific or NK like.

Approaches using in vitro sensitization or boosting of reactivity of patients' lymphocytes against their own tumor
cells followed then by expansion of the reactive T-cell
clones in TCGF would seem quite likely to produce continuous
lines of human cytotoxic lymphocytes. These cytotoxic cells
then could be used to dissect out whether or not patients
have or can make cytotoxic T-cells to tumor associated antigens, and whether the reactivity to tumor antigens is HLA
restricted. Such cell lines would also be essential for the
determination of whether or not the antigens are unique
(Class I type tumor antigens) or cross-reacting for different types of human tumors. The possibility of using such
"cell lines" for adoptive immunotherapy is a matter of great
interest to us all.

CANCER INDUCED IMMUNOREGULATION

A most important achievement in the area of immunobiology
has been the recognition that the cellular immune system can
regulate itself. It has been clearly demonstrated in animal
models that synthetic antigens, naturally occurring antigens, and tumor antigens can induce immunoregulatory or

"suppressor cells" (2,14). From these studies it seems to be a general rule that when antigen is presented to animals in unusual form, over prolonged periods, or in excessively high doses, the development of suppressor T-cells is a likely outcome. Especially exciting has been the work that has demonstrated that suppressor cells can be transferred to naive animals in which they then abrogate the immune response of these animals to normally immunogenic doses of antigen or tumors. The reports that treatments designed to delete or abolish suppressor cells slow the growth rates and sometimes cause regression of tumors confirm this may be a new approach for immunotherapy (2,14).

Given the above information, it is therefore of considerable interest to ask the question as to whether or not cancer patients have tumor-induced immunoregulatory cells capable of inhibiting their immune responses. There have been a number of recent reports of non-specific suppressor cells in the blood and tumor of cancer patients (15-17). These "suppressor" cells were detected by co-culture of the blood lymphocytes from the patients with lymphocytes from normal donors and determining the effect on the responsiveness of the normal cells. A diminution in the respone of the normal lymphocytes to mitogens was observed in many cases when cells from cancer patients but not control donors were added to the cultures. Although of some interest, these studies do not clearly delineate whether or not humans have the type of antigen specific suppressor cells seen in murine models (2). Those suppressor T-cells are exquisitely antigen specific and in some cases, genetically restricted in contrast to the cells described above in the co-culture experiments.

There have been several reports using human non-tumor models of in vitro detection of antigen specific suppressor T-cells (18-21). Bloom's group (19) has fairly convincingly demonstrated that in the blood of lepromatous leprosy patients, there is a lymphocyte subpopulation of TH2 positive-T-suppressor cells. These cells, when exposed in vitro to lepromanin antigen, suppress the responsiveness of the patient's blood lymphocytes to the mitogen PHA. The same lymphocyte subpopulation from patients with tuberculoid leprosy or normal donors, does not exhibit this suppressor effect.

Engleman et al. (18) have described apparent false typing responses in one-way mixed lymphocyte culture (MLC) as being due to antigen-specific suppressor cells. In the report by Engleman, a homozygous HLA-Dw2 multiparous woman would not respond in MLC typing tests to her husband's homozygous HLA-Dw1 stimulator cells. Yet, her lymphocytes would respond adequately to many other HLA-Dw1 homozygous typing cells. In their analysis of this paradoxical lack of responsiveness, they discovered that anytime HLA-Bw35 or related antigens appeared on the typing cell (stimulator cell) it was sufficient to induce a nonresponsiveness in the woman's lymphocyte population such that her cells would not react in MLC to the HLA-D region stimulating antigens on the stimulator cells. They showed that the cell responsible for this suppression was a T-cell and it would elaborate an antigen specific suppressive factor which was genetically restricted. That is, once the factor was produced by stimulation with the specific antigen it would suppress other normal lymphocytes only if they shared HLA-Dw2 with the suppressor cell. The reason that this woman developed a suppressor T-cell response to the HLA-Bw35 antigen is unknown but may be related to her multiple pregnancies and miscarriages. Nevertheless, this case clearly establishes that antigen specific and genetically restricted suppressor T-cell responses to cell surface antigens can occur in human beings.

During the course of our studies (21,22) on cellular immune responsiveness of cancer patients, we found a patient who had a markedly depressed response to mitogens and in mixed leukocyte culture. When his blood lymphocytes were added to lymphocytes from normal donors, the blastogenic responses of the lymphocytes of a few of those normals (5 of 43) were markedly suppressed or completely abolished. As this pattern of suppression was suggestive of that "genetically restricted" pattern seen in the murine models, we were led to further study of this patient. Our studies (20,21) demonstrated that: 1) a T-cell was responsible for suppressing responsiveness of lymphocytes from the normal donors; 2) those normal donors whose lymphocyte responsiveness was suppressed by the addition of the patient's cells to their culture all bore HLA-B-14 on their cell surface; 3) there was no HLA-D restriction to this phenomenon; 4) this suppressor cell was relatively radio resistant, being abolished by 6,000R but not by 3,000R; and 4) was not due to the patient's blood cells being cytotoxic for the responding lymphocytes bearing HLA-B-14. While it is still not clear why this patient had HLA-B-14 specific suppressor cells, this case was yet another demonstration of the specific type of suppressor response in man.

The above studies prompted us to look in more detail into the question of whether or not cancer patients might have tumor triggered or tumor antigen induced suppressor T-cells regulating their immune responsiveness. Based on our studies (20,21) and those by Engleman and co-workers (18), we were led to hypothesize that if cancer patients had suppressor T-lymphocytes in their blood, we could best demonstrate them by co-incubation of the cancer patient's lymphocytes with the patient's autologous irradiated tumor cells and then ask whether this co-incubation depressed the in vitro cellular immune responsiveness of his lymphocytes (22). As a model of cellular immune response in vitro, we used the one-way mixed leukocyte culture (MLC) reaction. We then tested the MLC responsiveness of the patient's and control lymphocytes in the presence and absence of fresh irradiated tumor cells. Put very simply then, the question was whether the MLC responsiveness of the lymphocytes from the patient would be diminished by exposure of his lymphocytes to his own tumor cells bearing putative tumor antigen.

In a study (cf 22 for preliminary results) of 40 autologous combinations of tumor cells and cancer patients' lymphocytes, we found three patterns of responses elicited by the addition of tumor cells to the MLC cultures. The addition of irradiated autologous tumor cells to the one-way MLC of eight patients augmented or did not otherwise effect their responsiveness. Adding tumor cell preparations depressed the responsiveness of the autologous lymphocytes from eight cancer patients and the lymphocytes from control donors in the same experiments including patients with other cancer and normals. The third and most interesting pattern of results that we observed in 24 cases was that of selective suppression of the lymphocyte blastogenesis of the patient in MLC when his own tumor cells were added whereas addition of the very same tumor cells to cultures from control donors had no effect or increased their blastogenic response. This selective suppression is a pattern analogous to that seen in the murine models of tumor-triggered or tumor antigen specific induction or recall of suppressor cells in in vitro assays (2,14).

Our preliminary studies using cell fractionation techniques have demonstrated that this suppressor response co-purifies with the T-cell fraction. Additional work is necessary to directly prove that this is a tumor antigen triggered suppressor T-cell in this reaction, but the data to date would all be consistent with that interpretation.

Additional control studies, which are difficult at best in man, would best be performed with control subjects matched at the entire HLA complex with the patients in order to demonstrate that people of identical or similar HLA types are suppressed by tumor cells of the same HLA type only if they have been exposed to the tumor.

The importance of development of assays for tumor specific suppressor cells in humans cannot be overemphasized. The ramifications of this concept for immunotherapy are numerous. If exposure of the patient to his tumor (antigen) has induced immunoregulatory cells which are tumor specific, then it would not be logical to vaccinate the patient with tumor antigen without some attempt at eliminating or modulating those suppressor cells. Treatment with immune stimulants and immunopharmacologic agents might produce paradoxical results as they might actually increase suppressor cell activity by either inducing them or by increasing the differentiation of functional T-cell subsets. There are reports in the literature (23) of BCG inducing thymic suppressor T-cells which could prevent the rejection of normally spontaneously regressing MSV tumors.

Therapies of cancer in the mouse with such agents as cytoxan which can be used to eliminate suppressor cells (2) and with antisera to suppressor cell surface antigens such as anti-IJ (2) are very promising approaches. Thus, there might be considerable merit in the possibility of treating cancer patients in such a way as to eliminate the tumor specific suppressor cells and therefore allow the emergence of a heightened cellular immune responsiveness to the tumor. Given the considerable recent developments in making and producing different monoclonal antibodies to human lymphocyte differentiation antigens, such therapeutic strategies may not be in the too distant future.

ACKNOWLEDGMENTS

This work was supported by Grant CA-19165 from the National Bladder Cancer Task Force, Biomedical Research Support Grant from the National Institutes of Health, ROP 5588-15, and Research Faculty Award -169 from the American Cancer Society.

I wish to thank my colleagues Drs. Mitoshi Akiyama, Richard P. Anderson, Vera Brankovan, Bo Dupont, John Hansen, Yoshihisa Kodera, Yuzo Takahashi, and the physicians at Mason Clinic without whose cooperation these studies would not have been possible. In addition I wish to acknowledge the technical assistance of Jean Ewalt, Heather Huppe, Vicki McDonald, and Lyle Sorensen. Finally, the excellent assistance of Harriet Langsford in preparation of this manuscript is gratefully acknowledged.

REFERENCES

1. Hellstrom KE, Hellstrom I: Lymphocyte-mediated cytotoxicity and blocking serum activity to tumor antigens. Adv Immunol 18:209,1974.
2. Greene M: The genetic and cellular basis of regulation of the immune response to tumor antigens, in Contemporary Topics in Immunobiology, Vol. 11, New York, Plenum Press, 1980. (ed. N. Warner).
3. Kay HD, Bonnard GD, West WH, Herberman RB: A functional comparison of human Fc-receptor-bearing lymphocytes active in natural cytotoxicity and antibody-dependent cellular cytotoxicity. J Immunol 118:2058-2066,1977.
4. Takasugi M, Mickey MR, Terasaki PI: Reactivity of lymphocytes from normal persons on cultured tumor cells. Cancer Res 33:3898,1973.
5. Bloom BR: Interferons and the immune system. Nature 284:593-595,1980.
6. Durdik JM, Beck BN, Henney CS: The use of lymphoma cell variants differing in their susceptibility to NK cell mediated lysis to analyze NK cell-target cell interactions, in Herberman RB (ed): Natural Cell-Mediated Immunity Against Tumors. New York, Academic Press, 1980.
7. Troye M, Hansson Y, Paulie S, et al: lymphocyte-mediated lysis of tumor cells in vitro (ADCC), induced by serum antibodies from patients with urinary bladder carcinoma or from controls. Int J Cancer 25:45-51,1980.
8. Bean MA, Kodera Y, Akiyama M: Microcytotoxicity test results with human cells: why the controversy? Israel J Med Sci 14:162-176,1978.
9. Zarling J, Bach FH: Sensitization of lymphocytes against pooled allogeneic cells. I.Generation of cytotoxicity against autologous human lymphoblastoid cell lines. J Exp Med 147:1334-1340,1978.
10. Zarling J, Bach FH: Continuous culture of T cells cytotoxic for autologous human leukaemia cells. Nature 280:685-688,1979.

11. Lee SK, Oliver RTD: Autologous leukemia-specific T-cell-mediated lymphocytotoxicity in patients with acute myelogenous leukemia. J Exp Med 147:912-922,1978.

12. Sethi KK, Stroehmann I, Brandis H: Human T-cell cultures from virus-sensitized donors can mediate virus-specific and HLA-restricted cell lysis. Nature 286:718-720,1980.

13. Vose BM, Vanky F, Fopp M, Klein E: In vitro generation of cytotoxicity against autologous human tumour biopsy cells. Int J Cancer 21:588-593,1978.

14. Broder S, Muul MS, Waldmann MD: Suppressor cells in neoplastic disease. J Natl Cancer Inst 61:5-11,1978.

15. Hersh EM, Patt YZ, Murphy SG, et al: Radiosensitive, thymic hormone-sensitive peripheral blood suppressor cell activity in cancer patients. Cancer Res 40:3134-3140,1980.

16. Jerrells TR, Dean JH, Richardson GL, et al: Role of suppressor cells in depression of in vitro lymphoproliferative responses of lung cancer and breast cancer patients. J Natl Cancer Inst 61:1001-1009.

17. Vose BM, Moore M: Suppressor cell activity of lymphocytes infiltrating human lung and breast tumours. Int J Cancer 24:579-585,1979.

18. Engleman EG, Andrew JM, McDevitt HO: Suppression of the mixed lymphocyte reaction in man by a soluble T-cell factor. J Exp Med 147:1037-1043, 1978.

19. Mehra V, Mason LH, Rothman W, et al: Delineation of a human T cell subset responsible for lepromin-induced suppression in leprosy patients. J Immunol 125:1183-1188.

20. Bean MA, Kodera Y, Cummings KB, Bloom BR: Occurrence of restricted suppressor T-cell activity in man. J Exp Med 146:1455-1460,1977.

21. Bean MA, Akiyama M, Kodera Y, et al: Human blood T lymphocytes that suppress the mixed leukocyte culture reactivity of lymphocytes from HLA-B-14 bearing individuals. J Immunol 123:1610-1614,1979.

22. Akiyama M, Bean MA, Brankovan V, Anderson RP: Suppression of the mixed leukocyte culture (MLC) response of cancer patients triggered by contact with autologous tumor cells. In press, Proc Amer Assoc of Cancer Res, Vol. 21, 1980.

23. Reinisch CL, Andrew SL, Schlossman SF: Suppressor cell regulation of immune response to tumors: Abrogation by adult thymectomy. Proc Natl Acad Sci USA 74:2989-2992,1977.

BIOCHEMISTRY OF HUMAN TUMOR ANTIGENS

Kenneth O. Lloyd, Ph.D.

Associate Member
Memorial Sloan-Kettering Cancer Center
New York, N.Y. 10021

Numerous approaches and techniques have been used to search for components characteristic of human tumors (1,2). However, the basic question as to whether human tumor cells exhibit components expressed only on these cells and not on any other cell or tissue of the body, in any stage of differentiation or development, remains essentially unanswered. Such components would be recognized as being foreign by the tumor-bearing host and could serve as tumor antigens to which the patient could respond with humoral and/or cellular immunity. Studies with experimental tumors in animals have convincingly demonstrated that such tumor-specific antigens, recognized by transplantation techniques, exist in these systems. It has been much more difficult to demonstrate analogous tumor-specific antigens in human tumors. The serologic analysis of human tumor antigens must rely on the immunization of foreign species or on the use of preexisting antibodies in the normal or patient population to provide suitable reagents. The problem of relating antigens detected using these approaches to their role in the biologic behavior of the tumor is hard to resolve. Nevertheless, in recent years considerable progress has been made in the analysis of the cell surface antigens of human tumors and in their biochemical characterization. Three different approaches are discussed in this presentation: (i) the detection of cell surface antigens by antibodies in human sera, (ii) the use of xenogeneic sera including monoclonal antibodies to detect tumor antigens and (iii) a purely biochemical approach to the detection of tumor-restricted components.

I. Antigens detected by human sera

Many sera from both normal individuals and cancer patients

contain antibodies reacting with tumor cells. On further
analysis most of these antibodies can be shown to be directed
towards very common cell surface antigens (Class III). A
number, however, contain antibodies which detect antigens
restricted to tumor cells and/or a few related normal cell
types (Class II) and even to individually-specific antigens
confined to the autologous tumor (Class I). The serological
analysis of these systems is discussed in this volume by
Dr. Herbert F. Oettgen and are described in more detail in
references 3-9. For malignant melanoma, which has received
considerable emphasis, these results are summarized in Table I.

TABLE I: Antigenic systems of malignant melanoma detected by
           human sera.

ANTIGEN CLASS	DESIGNATION	DISTRIBUTION	REFERENCE
Class I (individual)	AU	Only autologous melanoma	3
Class II (shared)	BD-2	Autologous and some allogeneic melanomas	4
	AH	Autologous and some allogeneic melanoma; also normal brain and some astrocytomas	9
Class III (common)	AT	All cultured cells	5
Differentiation antigen	MEL-1	Some melanomas and fetal fibroblasts; some epithelial cancers	8

     The biochemical identification of some of these antigens
is underway in our laboratories. Radioimmunoprecipitation, a
valuable technique for studying many cell surface antigens,
has not, thus far, been effective in characterizing the

antigens detected by these human sera. The reason for this
is not clear but is probably related to the relatively low
titers of the sera or to the low content of the antigens in
the tumor cells. Progress has depended on the fractionation
of tumor cell extracts by standard biochemical techniques and
assay of the antigenic activity by inhibition of the appropriate serological assay. Three of the antigenic systems
have been partially characterized (Table II).

TABLE II: Biochemical characteristics of melanoma antigens
           detected by human sera.

ANTIGEN	BIOCHEMICAL CHARACTERISTICS	REFERENCE
AU	Glycoprotein; Con A$^+$, WGA$^-$	10 and Lloyd - unpub-lished data
BD-2	Glycoprotein; Con A$^+$, WGA$^-$	Lloyd - unpublished data
AH	Acidic glycolipid	9

Both AU and BD-2 antigens can be solubilized from the appropriate cell line by detergent (DOC) extraction. AU specificity was also solubilized by partial proteolytic digestion
with papain and the activity was present in the 25,000-45,000
molecular weight range (10). Both AU and BD-2 activities in
their respective DOC extracts were absorbed by concanavalin A-
Sepharose but not by wheat germ agglutination (WGA)-Sepharose.
It was concluded that both antigens are glycoproteins (but not
highly sialylated glycoproteins, which would bend to WGA-
Sepharose) but further characterization has not thus far been
possible. Progress in this area is hampered by the low antigenic activity of solubilized preparations (in comparison to
the original cell pellet) and further loss of antigenic
activity on subsequent fractionation. A similar comment was
made, by Law *et al.* (11) concerning the purification of mouse
tumor-specific antigens.

In contrast, to these glycoprotein antigens, AH antigen
has recently been shown to be a glycolipid. AH antigenic
specificity is found on a proportion of melanoma cell lines
and on normal and fetal brain; it therefore has the characteristics of a differentiation antigen of neural crest-derived
cells which is, nevertheless, antigenic in humans (9). The
heat and protease-resistance of the antigen gave early indications of its lipid nature. Subsequently, by fractionation of
chloroform-methanol extracts of AH[+] melanoma cells into neutral

and acidic glycolipid fractions, it was shown that antigenic
activity resides in the acidic (ganglioside) fraction (C.
Pukel et al., unpublished data). Inhibition studies using
acidic glycolipids from AH⁺ and AH⁻ cells and tissues showed
complete concordance between the presence or absence of activity in the glycolipid fraction and the original AH typing of
the cell or tissue. AH antigen, therefore, does not exist in
a cryptic situation in AH⁻ cells and tissues. Further studies
on this glycolipid and its relationship to a melanoma glycolipid antigen detected by monoclonal antibodies (see below)
are underway.

II. Antigens detected by xenogeneic immune sera

        Antisera designed to detect tumor antigens have tradi-
tionally been prepared by immunizing an animal with tumor
cells or extracts and subsequently absorbing the resulting
sera with normal cells and tissues. Carcinoembryonic antigen
(CEA) and alphafetoprotein (AFP) are among the tumor-associated antigens to be discovered using this approach. Numerous
other tumor-associated antigens have also been described but
so far none of them have been completely characterized.
        The recent introduction by Köhler and Milstein (12) of
the hybridoma technique for producing xenogeneic monoclonal
antibodies promises to revolutionize this area. Rather than
relying on absorption, this procedure uses selection procedures to identify a hybridoma clone producing antibody of the
required specificity. This is a relatively new procedure and
it is not yet clear whether it will be capable of defining
tumor-specific antigens in human tumors. Early indications
are that the demonstration of specific antigens is as elusive
by this procedure as by classical heteroimmunization but that
the production of antibodies to cell markers which character-
ize different cell types or differentiation states is greatly
facilitated.
        Our own experience with this technique has been mainly in
the analysis of antigens of human malignant melanoma (13).
Other laboratories have also developed monoclonal antibodies
to this tumor (14,15,16). In our study, mice were immunized
with human melanoma cell line (SK-MEL-28) and subsequently 18
hybrid antibody-producing clones were selected. Further analysis using serological and biochemical techniques demonstrated that six of them recognized the same glycoprotein (gp 95),
five identified another glycoprotein (gp 150), two were less
well characterized and the remaining five recognized glycolipid antigens. Despite an initial selection procedure
designed to identify hybrids producing antibodies which

reacted selectively with melanoma as opposed to other cells,
both normal and malignant,   neither of the two glycoproteins
recognized are melanoma-specific antigens.   Gp 95 is a glycoprotein of 95,000 dalton with a pI of 5.0 (Figure 1).   It was
detected by radioimmunoprecipitation on ^{125}I-, $[^{35}S]$-methion-
ine- and $[^{3}H]$glucosamine-labeled melanoma extracts thus
demonstrating that it is a cell surface glycoprotein.   Gp 95
was detected in some but not all melanomas and a similarly
variable number of astrocytomas.   Its distribution on other
cell types is more restricted but it was detected in small
amounts on normal fibroblasts and kidney epithelia.   Although
gp 95 is only a minor component of melanoma membranes it was
the most common specificity detected.   Other workers (15)
have also described a melanoma antigen in the same molecular
weight region which may be same species.   It would appear
that gp 95 is a human melanoma protein which is particularly
antigenic in the mouse and whose tissue distribution is sufficiently restricted for it to be selected in initial screenings for melanoma specificity.   Gp 150 is a somewhat more
widespread antigen than gp 95.   This antigen was detected on
a variable member of melanoma cell lines, on many astrocytomas, on a few epithelial cancers, on normal kidney cells and
melanocytes.   It labels very well with $[^{3}H]$glucosamine which,
together with its low pI (4.2), indicates that it may be a
sialic acid-rich glycoprotein (Figure 1).

   In terms of melanoma specificity, the four monoclonal
antibodies (R_{24} group) recognizing glycolipid antigens are
the most interesting. R_{24} antibody itself is strongly reactive only with melanomas and some astrocytomas and unlike anti-
gp 95 and -gp 150 antibodies, it recognizes all the melanoma
lines tested.   This antigen is absent from a large variety of
other cell lines and tissues tested but may be detected on
normal brain and melanocytes when sensitive techniques are
used.   The first indication of the glycolipid nature of the
antigens detected by the R_{24} group of antibodies came from
heat stability experiments.   More rigorous proof was obtained
by isolating glycolipid fractions from melanomas and other
cells and tissues by standard lipid chemistry techniques.
Fractionation of chloroform:methanol extracts of melanoma cells
into neutral and acidic glycolipid fractions showed that the
R_{24} antigen was an acidic glycolipid (Pukel et al., unpublished
data). Further confirmation of this conclusion came from
showing that R_{24} antigenic activity was destroyed by treating
the melanoma target cells with *Vibrio cholerae* neuraminidase.
Extractions of acidic glycolipids from other cells and tissues
confirmed the results on the distribution of this antigen
obtained by serological studies on intact target cells.   These
experiments also confirmed that although R_{24} antigen is

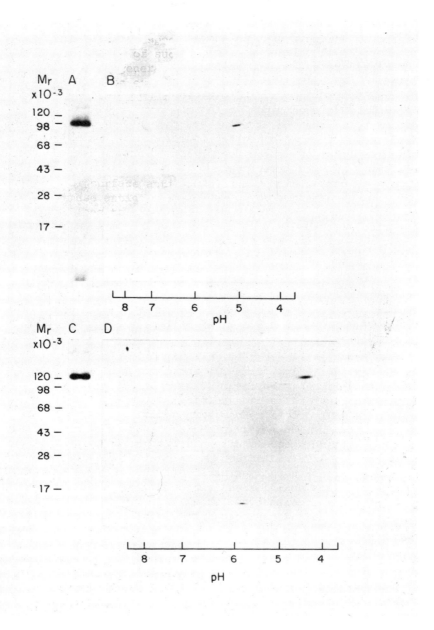

FIGURE I: Autoradiograms of [^{35}S]methionine-labeled glycoproteins from lysates of SK-MEL-28 immunoprecipitated by monoclonal antibody I$_{12}$ (A and B) and by monoclonal antibody Ng (C and D). A and C were analyzed by SDS-PAGE and B and D by 2-D electophoresis. Reproduced by permission of the National Academy of Sciences (ref. 13).

found in substantial amounts only in melanomas (including fresh melanoma tumor), it is present in small amounts in some related normal cell types such as brain and melanocytes.

Since there is some similarity in the distribution of the glycolipid antigen detected by human serum AH (discussed above) and the R_{24} antigen, it is interesting to compare the expression of the two specificities on different cell lines and tissues. Table III summarizes these data obtained from both serological studies and glycolipid isolation.

TABLE III. Distribution of AH and R_{24} antigens among various cell lines and tumors.

AH-POSITIVE	R_{24}-POSITIVE
SK-MEL-13	SK-MEL-13
	SK-MEL-21
	SK-MEL-28
SK-MEL-29	SK-MEL-29
SK-MEL-37	SK-MEL-37
Adult brain	Adult brain (weak)
Astrocytoma AS	
Fetal brain (weak)	Fetal brain (weak)
Bovine brain (weak)	Bovine brain (weak)
	Bovine choroid (weak)
MOLT-4 (weak)	MOLT-4 (weak)

Both reagents are detecting antigens expressed on neural crest-derived but whereas R_{24} is strongly expressed on all melanoma cell lines, AH antigen is found on only a portion of melanomas, on astrocytomas and normal or brain cells. The expression of both AH and R_{24} specificities on MOLT-4 (a T-lymphoid cell line) as well as brain cells is reminiscent of Thy antigen of the mouse (which is also glycolipid antigen, ref. 17).

III. Biochemical comparison of malignant and normal cell glycoproteins

Antibodies, either human or animal, provide reagents for detecting specific components in tumor cells which may be absent in other cell types. Recent advances in biochemical techniques have provided methods to search for differences between normal and malignant cells without relying on immunological reagents. Although a number of studies have been carried out in animal model systems (particularly on normal and virally-transformed mouse fibroblasts), corresponding studies on human cells have been more difficult to carry out because of the unavailability of the normal counterpart to most tumor cell types.

Recently our laboratories have carried out immunological studies on human renal cancer and have developed kidney cancer cell lines and short term cultures of normal kidney epithelial cells, often from the same patient (7). Using the 2-dimensional polyacrylamide gel electrophoresis procedure of O'Farrell (18) we have now compared the [^{3}H]glucosamine-labeled glycoproteins of a number of renal cancer cell lines with those of normal kidney epithelial cells (19). Approximately 70 glycoproteins could be detected, most of which would be expected to be cell surface components. Although the autoradiographic patterns from normal and malignant cells were surprisingly similar (Figure 2A and B), numerous differences could be observed when any two pairs of autoradiograms were compared. Some of these differences involved the absence of a component in the tumor cell pattern which was present in the normal cell profile (e.g. 7 and 11). In the converse direction, most of the tumor cell patterns had a series of basic components, 17, which were missing in the normal pattern. Another possible tumor-specific difference was component 13 - a 100,000 dalton glycoprotein present in six of the eight renal cancer lines examined but absent or very faint in the normal cell patterns. Other minor and less regular divergencies were also observed.

Not all these variations were found in all the cell lines examined and only one difference was consistently observed in comparisons between all the malignant and normal cell patterns. All the tumor cell pattern had three prominent glycoproteins in the 27,500 dalton region with pI's of 5.7, 5.3 and 4.9 respectively (Figure 2A). Normal cells, on the other hand, had a much fainter constellation of six to eight spots in this region (Figure 2B). The two more basic spots (c and e) were present in both tumor and normal cell patterns but the third spot (j) was clearly discernable only in malignant cell patterns. Since this and some of the other differences outlined above were also detected in two pairs of autologous combinations in which both the tumor cells and the normal epithelial cells were derived from the same individual, it is evident that they are not due to allogeneic polymorphisms in the various glycoproteins.

The significance of this characteristic alteration in the 27.5K region glycoproteins is not yet clear but since it is consistently found in all kidney cancer cell lines thus far examined it may be related to the initiation or maintenance of the malignant state in this tumor. As tissue culture techniques improve we are hopeful that similar studies can be carried

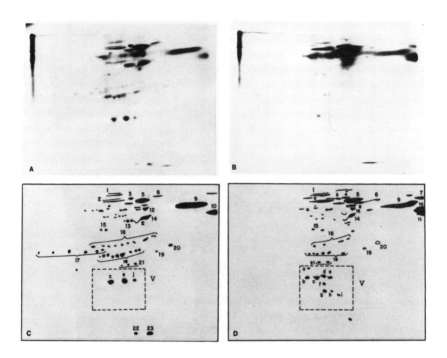

FIGURE 2: Autoradiograms of [³H]glucosamine-labeled glycoproteins from renal cancer and normal kidney epithelial cell
cultures analyzed by 2-D electrophoresis. A: renal cancer
cell line SK-RC-25. B: normal kidney cell culture from the
same individual. C: schematic representation of SK-RC-25
patternd. D: schematic representation of normal pattern.
Reproduced by permission of the National Academy of Science
(ref. 19).

out on other malignant-normal combinations to determine
whether similar alterations are found in other tumor types.

IV. Conclusions

Malignant melanoma has become the best antigenically defined human cell type outside of the lymphoid system.
Numerous antigenic specificities have been identified both by
our laboratories (3-5, 8-10) and by other groups (reviewed in
ref. 20). These include both common antigens such as HLA-A,
-B and -DR (21,22) and fibronectin (23) and more restricted
antigens of the differentiation class (AH, Mel-1). Among
problems which still need to be resolved are the complete
chemical characterization of these antigens, the determination
of their biological significance and function and the better
biochemical definition of the Class I antigens defined by
autologous typing. Studies on the antigenic makeup of other
tumor types, such as renal cancer are rapidly approaching the
level of those on melanoma. Moreover, the application of
recently developed techniques promises a better understanding
of this difficult area in the near future.

Acknowledgments

For the biochemical aspects of this study, I am grateful
to my collaborators: Jennifer Ng, Shun-ichiro Ogata,
Clifford Pukel, Tadashi Tai and Luiz R. Travassos. Serological studies were carried out jointly with Lloyd J. Old,
Herbert F. Oettgen and co-workers. This work was supported
by grants and contracts: CA-08748, CB-74124, CA-19765 and
CA-21445.

References

1. Hellstrőm, K.E. and Brown, J.P. in The Antigens. Ed. M.
    Sela, Vol. V, p. 2-82. Academic Press, New York, 1979.
2. Rosenberg, E.A., Ed. Serologic Analysis of Human Cancer
    Antigens. Academic Press, New York, 1980.
3. Carey, T.E., Takahashi, T., Resnick, L.A., Oettgen, H.F.
    and Old, L.J. Proc. Natl. Acad. Sci. 73:3278-3282 (1976).
4. Shiku, H., Takahashi, T., Oettgen, H.F. and Old, L.J.
    J. Exp. Med. 144:873-888 (1976).
5. Shiku, H., Takahashi, T., Resnick, L.A., Oettgen, H.F.
    and Old, L.J. J. Exp. Med. 145:784-789 (1977).
6. Pfreundschuh, M., Shiku, H., Takahashi, T., Ueda, R.,
    Ransohoff, J., Oettgen, H.F. and Old, L.J. Proc. Natl.
    Acad. Sci. 75:5122-5126 (1978).
7. Ueda, R., Shiku, H., Pfreundschuh, M., Takahashi, T.,

Li, L.T.C., Whitmore, W.F., Oettgen, H.F. and Old, L.J. *J. Exp. Med. 150*:564-579 (1979).

8. Houghton, A.N., Taormina, M.C., Ikeda, H., Watanabe, T., Oettgen, H.F. and Old, L.J. *Proc. Natl. Acad. 77*:4260-4264 (1980).

9. Watanabe, T., Shiku, H., Lloyd, K.O., Pukel, C., Li, L.T.C., Oettgen, H.F. and Old, L.J. *Proc. Natl. Acad. Sci. 78:*

10. Carey, T.E., Lloyd, K.O., Takahashi, T., Travassos, L.R. and Old, L.J. *Proc. Natl. Acad. Sci. 76*:2898-2902 (1979).

11. Law, L.W., Rogers, M.J. and Apella, E. *Adv. Cancer Res. 32*:201-235 (1980).

12. Köhler, G. and Milstein, C. *Nature 236*:495-497 (1975).

13. Dippold, W.G., Lloyd, K.O., Li, L.T.C., Ikeda, H., Oettgen, H.F. and Old, L.J. *Proc. Natl. Acad. Sci. 77:*

14. Koprowski, H., Steplewski, Z., Herlyn, D. and Herlyn, H. *Proc. Natl. Acad. Sci. 75*:3405-3409 (1978).

15. Woodbury, R.G., Brown, J.P., Yeh, M-Y., Hellström, I. and Hellström, K.E. *Proc. Natl. Acad. Sci. 77*:2183-2184 (1980).

16. Brown, J.P., Wright, P.W., Hart, C.E., Woodson, R.G., Hellström, K.E and Hellström, I. *J. Biol. Chem. 255*:4980-4983 (1980).

17. Wang, T.J., Freimuth, W.W., Miller, H.C. and Esselman, W.J. *J. Immunol. 121*:1361-1365 (1978).

18. O'Farrell, P.H. *J. Biol. Chem. 250*:4007-4021 (1975).

19. Ogata, S., Ueda, R. and Lloyd, K.O. *Proc. Natl. Acad. Sci. 77:*

20. Ferrone, S. and Pellegrino, M.A. in *The Handbook of Cancer Immunology.* Ed. H. Waters, Vol. 3, p. 291-327. Garland, STPM Press, New York, 1978.

21. Winchester, R.J., Wang, C-Y., Gibofsky, A., Kunkel, H.F., Lloyd, K.O. and Old, L.J. *Proc. Natl. Acad. Sci. 75:* 6235-6239 (1978).

22. Wilson, B.S., Indiveri, F., Pellegrino, M.A. and Ferrone, S. *J. Exp. Med. 149*:658-668 (1979).

23. Lloyd, K.O., Travassos, L.R., Takahashi, T. and Old, L.J. *J. Natl. Cancer Inst. 63*:623-634 (1979).

The Immunovirology of Dog and Cat
Tumors

WILLIAM D. HARDY, JR.

Laboratory of Veterinary Oncology
Memorial Sloan-Kettering Cancer Center
New York, N.Y. 10021

INTRODUCTION

Tumors similar to those that occur in humans occur in
pet dogs and cats.[1] For example, skin tumors are very common
in both species and mammary tumors and lymphoid tumors also
occur frequently. Like human tumors, most tumors that occur
in pet dogs and cats are thought to be caused primarily by
environmental factors such as chemical and physical agents.
For example, squamous cell carcinomas occur frequently in
white cats exposed to excessive sunlight in the southern[2]
or southwestern areas of the United States. However, there
are some notable differences in the occurrence of certain
types of tumors in pet animals as compared to humans. Lung
and colon cancers are very rare in pet cats and dogs and
their low occurrence is probably attributable to a lack of
smoking and to the diet of pet animals. However, DNA and
RNA viruses cause tumors in cats and dogs.

Acknowledgements
    The author thanks Dr. A.J. McClelland for assistance in
the preparation of this manuscript and E.E. Zuckerman, R.
Markovich, T. Paino and H. Perry for excellent technical
assistance. This work was supported by grants from the
National Cancer Institute CA-16599, CA-19072, and CA-18488,
from the Cancer Research Institute Inc. and from the Special
Projects Committee of the Society of Memorial Sloan-Kettering
Cancer Center. During these studies the author was a Scholar
of the Leukemia Society of America, Inc. I thank the Henry
Bergh Memorial Hospital of the ASPCA and the Animal Medical
Center for use of their clinical facilities and the
National Veterinary Laboratory, Inc. for assistance in
obtaining many cats with lymphosarcoma.

CANINE VIRALLY INDUCED TUMORS

The only known canine virally induced tumor is the benign[2] oral papillomatosis (warts) which occurs in young dogs. Papillomaviruses are DNA viruses and induce only warts in their natural hosts. However, papillomas (warts) can occasionally undergo[3] malignant transformation to squamous cell carcinomas. Warts are hypercornified, papillary tumors of the stratified squamous epithelium. The virus is produced and shed from the superficial cornified cell layers of the tumor and is spread by contact. Canine viral papillomas occur in the oral cavity, cornea, lips and eyelids. The incubation period is about 4 to 6 weeks and, in most cases, they regress after 6 weeks[4] and the animal is then resistant to further papillomas.

There are no known oncogenic RNA viruses in the dog.

FELINE VIRALLY INDUCED TUMORS

There are no known oncogenic DNA viruses in the cat. The cat is one of the few species which appears to be resistant to papillomaviruses or which does not have papillomaviruses,[2] since there have been no reports of feline warts.

Feline Leukemia and Sarcoma Viruses

In the cat the oncogenic RNA virus (oncovirus), the feline leukemia virus (FeLV), and its related virus, the feline sarcoma virus (FeSV), are known to cause both neoplastic and non-neoplastic diseases.[5] The FeLV induced neoplastic diseases are lymphosarcoma, erythroleukemia, erythremic myelosis and granulocytic leukemia, while the degenerative diseases are FeLV anemias, myeloblastopenia, and thymic atrophy. FeLV also causes immunosuppression which leads to chronic secondary diseases. The FeSV induces multicentric fibrosarcomas of the skin in young cats.

Virology

Many animal species have endogenous oncoviruses which are present as nucleic acid sequences in the DNA of normal uninfected cells. At times, these endogenous oncoviruses can escape host control and begin to replicate. Rarely they can escape from their host and infect other species.[6] The FeLV originated as an endogenous oncovirus in the ancestor of rats and, by transpecies transmission, infected the ancestor of present day pet cats about 1 to 10 million years ago.[7] The virus is exogenous in cats, that is, it is not present as complete viral nucleic acid copies in the genome of normal uninfected cat cells, and is spread contagiously among cats. The FeLV envelope has complimentary receptors to the cell surface receptors of the cells of many species. Thus, FeLV can replicate in cat, dog, bovine, guinea pig, mink, primate and human cells.[8] After cell attachment and penetration, FeLV "uncoats" releasing its single strand of RNA and an enzyme, the RNA dependent DNA polymerase (reverse transcriptase), which synthesizes a DNA copy of the FeLV RNA genome.[9,10] The DNA copy (provirus) becomes integrated into the cellular DNA and may then synthesize new viral RNA.[11] After the RNA has been made, new viral proteins are synthesized and new virus particles are assembled. The final stages of FeLV replication occur at the cell membrane from which the virus particles bud and acquire their surface envelope.

The FeSV is a recombinant virus between the FeLV genome and cat cellular sequences.[12] The recombinant FeSV is replication defective because the FeLV genes coding for the reverse transcriptase and the envelope proteins are replaced by cellular transforming sequences. FeSV is an acute transforming virus which transforms cells rapidly. FeLV is present as a helper virus in all FeSV isolates in 10 to 1000 fold excess and it is not known whether FeSV is contagious or whether it is generated de novo in FeLV infected cats.

FeLV Antigens

The FeLV antigens consist of envelope and internal antigens.[13] The major antigen of the FeLV envelope is a 70,000 dalton glycoprotein (gp70). Antibody to the gp70 will neutralize FeLV. A minor component of the FeLV envelope is a protein of 15,000 daltons (p15E). Some host cell material is also incorporated into the FeLV envelope.[14] The envelope antigens distinguish FeLV into 3 subgroups, A, B and C.[15] FeLV A is found in all naturally infected pet cats either alone (50%) or in combination with FeLV B (49%) or with FeLV B and C (1%).[16]

The internal FeLV antigens consist of the viral RNA, viral reverse transcriptase enzyme and the 4 structural proteins p27, p15, p12, and p10. The major internal antigen is the p27. Cats can produce antibody to the internal proteins, but these antibodies are probably not beneficial as they may produce immune complexes and thus induce immunosuppression.[17] The internal FeLV antigens are used as immunological markers in the indirect immunofluorescent antibody (IFA) test for FeLV.[18] This test enables all 3 serotypes of the virus to be readily detected in the peripheral blood or tissues of infected cats. Using this test it has been found that the occurrence of FeLV differs markedly in cats from different exposure environments.[19] For example, FeLV is rare in cats from households containing only 1 cat and in cats living in multiple cat households with no previous history of FeLV diseases. However, approximately one third of cats in multiple cat households with a history of FeLV diseases are infected with the virus. Other seroepidemiologic studies done using the IFA test have shown that about 30% of FeLV exposed cats become persistently infected with the virus, 42% become immune to infection and 28% remain neither infected nor immune.[16] Using the IFA test for FeLV in a test and removal program we have been able to prevent the contagious spread of FeLV among pet cats.[20]

The Feline Oncornavirus Associated Cell Membrane Antigen (FOCMA)

FOCMA is an FeLV and FeSV induced tumor-specific antigen which is present on the cell membrane of FeLV induced lymphosarcoma (LSA), erythroleukemia and myelogenous leukemia cells and FeSV induced fibrosarcoma cells.[21,22] It is present on both FeLV positive and FeLV negative (non-producer) feline LSA cells.[23] FOCMA is not present on FeLV infected nontransformed cells and FeLV antigens do not absorb FOCMA antibody.[22] Thus FOCMA is not an FeLV or FeSV structural antigen. FOCMA isolated from feline LSA cells is present on a 70,000 dalton non-glycosylated protein which is not bound to any FeLV antigens, whereas FOCMA isolated from FeSV transformed cells resides on a polyprotein ranging in size from 85 to 180,000 daltons which also possess FeLV p15, p12, and some p27 determinants.[24,25] Cats can produce antibody against FOCMA which protects them from FeLV and FeSV induced tumors but does not protect them from FeLV non-neoplastic diseases.[5,26]

Immune Response to FeLV and FOCMA

The ability of a cat to respond immunologically to the FeLV antigens and to FOCMA will determine its fate. Pet cats can produce antibody to the FeLV envelope (neutralizing antibody), internal viral proteins (p27, p15, p12), the viral reverse transcriptase and to the tumor-specific antigen FOCMA.[16,17,26,27] Healthy cats can be classified into 6 immune classes based on their FeLV status and their FeLV neutralizing and FOCMA antibody titers (Table 1).[13,16]

TABLE I
Classes of Healthy Pet Cats

FeLV Status	Protective FeLV Neutralizing Antibody ($\geq$1:10)	Protective FOCMA Antibody ($\geq$ 1:32)	Susceptible or Resistant to:	
			FeLV Infection	LSA Development
1 -	-	-	Susceptible	Susceptible
2 -	-	+	Susceptible	Resistant
3 -	+	-	Resistant	Susceptible
4 -	+	+	Resistant	Resistant
5 +	-	-	Infected	Very Suscep.
6 +	-	+	Infected	Resistant

The occurrence of protective FOCMA and FeLV neutralizing
antibody titers is dependent on the FeLV exposure history
of the cat. In a study done by my laboratory, approximately
38% of FeLV uninfected exposed and 25% of FeLV infected,
cats were found to have protective titers of FOCMA antibody,
whereas only 8% of the stray cats, whose FeLV exposure history was unknown, and none of the unexposed cats had protective titers of antibody to FOCMA.[28] Similarly, although 42%
of FeLV uninfected exposed cats had protective titers of
FeLV neutralizing antibody,and thus were immune to FeLV,only
5% of stray cats and none of the unexposed cats tested had
protective FeLV neutralizing antibody titers. We have not
found any FeLV infected cats to have FeLV neutralizing antibody to the serotype(s) with which they are infected. The
results of our study showed that the reaction of the immune
system of cats to FeLV exposure differs from cat to cat.

In some cats the immune system does not, for some unknown reason, respond to FeLV but instead is overwhelmed by
the virus. Such cats are susceptible to LSA, other FeLV
diseases and to secondary diseases related to the immunosuppression caused by FeLV. For example, kittens may develop
thymic atrophy in which FeLV causes a degeneration of the
thymus resulting in a defective T cell mediated immune
response. Kittens with thymic atrophy usually die of secondary bacterial infections within a few weeks of birth.[5]
FeLV can also be immunosuppressive in adult cats.[5,29,30]

For example, about one half of cats with feline infectious
peritonitis, chronic stomatitis, gingivitis, and oral ulcers
are infected with FeLV, as are about 40% of cats with chronic
abscesses and non-healing skin wounds. Also, over half of
the cats with upper respiratory infections, non-responsive
infections, and septicemia are infected with FeLV.[5] More
cats actually die of secondary infections resulting from FeLV
immunosuppression than die of LSA. However, in some cats,[13,16]
exposure to FeLV results in a strong immune response.
Those cats may become immune to FeLV infection, but not to the
development of LSA or may become immune to LSA but not to
FeLV infection. A few cats may even become resistant to both
FeLV infection and LSA (see Table 1).

FeLV Induced FeLV Negative Lymphosarcomas

It should be noted that an effective immune response to
FeLV does not always guarantee that a cat will be protected
from the development of LSA simply as a result of its immunity
to FeLV infection. During local lymphoid infection, the
FeLV genome may become integrated into the chromosomes of a
small number of lymphoblasts before the immune system responds
effectively. Even though the cat may produce FeLV neutralizing antibody and reject the virus (but not produce LSA
protective FOCMA antibody) the integrated FeLV genome may
still be able to transform the "infected" lymphoblast into a
lymphosarcoma cell even without the production of any FeLV
antigens or infectious FeLV. Thus, some transiently infected
pet cats develop LSA but do not replicate or shed any
FeLV.[21,22,23,31] Of the 507 pet cats with LSA that we have
tested for the presence of FeLV, 360 (71%) were FeLV positive
and 147 (29%) were FeLV negative. Most of the FeLV negative[32]
cats with LSA were over 7 years of age. As discussed
earlier, both FeLV positive and negative LSA cells express
the tumor-specific antigen (FOCMA) on their cell
membranes.[21,22,23] We have also found an epidemiologic
association between exposure to FeLV and the development of
FeLV negative LSA similar to that which exists between FeLV
exposure and FeLV positive LSA.[23,32] We observed 1612 pet
cats for the occurrence of LSA. Of these cats, 1074 cats
were controls who had never been exposed to FeLV while 528
cats were exposed to FeLV infected cats under natural conditions in their households. The exposed group of cats consisted of 389 uninfected cats and 149 persistently viremic cats
(Table 2).

TABLE 2
Development of Lymphosarcoma in Pet Cats

FeLV Exposure History	FeLV Status	# of Cats	Obsv. Years	Cases of LSA Obsv.	Significance
Never Exposed	–	1074	3235	0	
Exposed	–	389		11	Less than
	+	149	2334	30	p 0.001
		1612		41	

None of the 1074 unexposed uninfected control cats developed LSA while 11 of the 389 exposed uninfected cats developed FeLV negative LSAs. In addition, 30 of the 149 FeLV infected cats developed FeLV positive LSAs. The difference in LSA occurrence between the uninfected unexposed and uninfected exposed cats is statistically significant at less than p=0.001 by the Chi Square Test. Our findings indicate that FeLV causes both the FeLV positive and negative LSAs of pet cats.

The mechanism by which FeLV induces FeLV negative feline LSA is unknown but three possibilities exist. 1) FeLV DNA recombines with cat cellular gene(s) to form a replication defective acute leukemia virus; 2) only the part of the FeLV genome that is responsible for cell transformation is integrated into the cellular genome or; 3) that FeLV alters the lymphocyte's chromosomes but does not integrate into the cellular genes. The existence of both FeLV positive and negative LSA together with the existence of FOCMA, an immunological marker of viral transformation, provides us with a unique opportunity to study the mechanism(s) by which oncoviruses transform cells. Such studies might enable us to understand how an oncovirus might be able to transform human cells without viral production.

Detrimental Immune Reactivity to FeLV

An effective immune response against FeLV may not, paradoxically, always be beneficial for cats. The persistent viremia of FeLV infected cats is ideal for the development of immune complexes and these immune complexes may lead to glomerulonephritis and immunosuppression. FeLV replication produces an excessive, continuous supply of FeLV antigens

and, if the cat responds to these antigens small nephrotoxic
immune complexes may be formed. [34] We have, in fact, found circulating FeLV-IgG immune complexes in 6 out of the 12 persistently FeLV infected cats that we studied. [5] The continual
formation and circulation of infectious FeLV-FeLV antibody
complexes may result in the deposition of some of these
immune complexes on the glomerular capillary basement membrane
causing inflamatory degeneration of the renal glomeruli
(glomerulonephritis). We have found immune complexes consisting of the internal FeLV proteins with IgG and complement
deposited in the glomeruli of 3 of 12 persistently viremic
cats. [34]   In addition, preliminary clinicopathological studies
suggest that there is a relationship between FeLV infection
and cats that develop clinical glomerulonephritis. [35]

Vaccination Against FeLV

Our understanding of the immunology of FeLV may ultimately lead to the prevention of FeLV diseases by enabling us to
develop an FeLV vaccine. We, and others, have already
successfully immunized some cats with a low dose live FeLV
vaccine. [28,36]   Like some pet cats exposed to low doses of
FeLV in the natural environment, the vaccinated cats developed
high titers of FeLV neutralizing antibody and became resistant
to natural infection with FeLV. Although this live FeLV
vaccine is effective, our recent understanding of the occurrence of FeLV negative LSA indicates that the use of   live
FeLV may be dangerous. That is because :(a) live FeLV may be
a public health risk and (b) because a live FeLV vaccine may
result in the integration of FeLV genes into the cat's chromosomes and thus increase the risk of vaccinated cats developing FeLV negative LSAs. In an attempt to overcome these
problems we are currently investigating the possibility of
a vaccine in which only the outer envelope of FeLV is used
as the immunogen. Since no FeLV RNA would be present in such
a 'subunit' vaccine the public health risks and possibility
that the vaccine would induce FeLV negative LSA are eliminated.

Conclusion

Because of our knowledge of the immunology of FeLV,
feline LSA is a potentially valuable model for studying how
oncoviruses cause cancer and how the spread of the virus can
be controlled. The knowledge obtained by studying feline LSA
may therefore eventually lead to a greater understanding of
the causes and prevention of human leukemia.

REFERENCES

1.   Hardy, W.D., Jr. General concepts of canine and feline tumors. J. Amer. An. Hosp. Assoc. 12: 295-306, 1976.
2.   Hardy, W.D., Jr. The etiology of canine and feline tumors. J. Amer. An. Hosp. Assoc. 12 313-334, 1976.
3.   Watrach, A.M., Small, E., and Case, M.T. Canine papilloma: progression of oral papilloma to carcinoma. J. Natl. Cancer Inst. 49: 915-920, 1970.
4.   Chambers, V.C. and Evans, C.A. Canine oral papillomatosis. I. Virus assay and observations on the various stages of the experimental infection. Cancer Res. 19: 1188-1196, 1959.
5.   Hardy, W.D., Jr. Feline leukemia virus diseases in: Feline Leukemia and Sarcoma Viruses. (Hardy, W.D., Jr., Essex, M. and McClelland, A.J.,Eds.) Elsevier/North Holland, New York, in press.
6.   Todaro, G.J. Interspecies transmission of mammalian retroviruses in: Viral Oncology (G. Klein, Ed.) pp.291-310, Raven Press, New York 1980.
7.   Benveniste, R.E., Sherr, C.J. and Todaro, G.J. Evolution of type C viral genes: origin of feline leukemia virus. Science, 190: 886-888, 1975.
8.   Sarma, P.S., Log, T., Jain, D., Hill, P.R., and Huebner, R.J. Differential host range of viruses of feline leukemia-sarcoma complex. Virology, 64: 438-446, 1975.
9.   Baltimore, D. Viral RNA-dependent DNA polymerase. Nature 226: 1209-1211, 1970.
10. Temin, H.M. and Mizutani, S. RNA-dependent DNA polymerase in virions of Rous sarcoma virus. Nature 226:1211-1213, 1970.
11. Temin, H.M. Nature of the provirus of Rous sarcoma in: Avian Tumor Viruses: National Cancer Institute Monograph 17 (Beard, J.W., Ed.) pp.557-570, NCI, Bethesda, MD 1964.
12. Frankel, A.E., Gilbert, J.H., Porzig, K.J., Scolnick, E.M. and Aaronson, S.A. Nature and distribution of feline sarcoma virus nucleotide sequences. J. Virol. 30: 821-827, 1979.
13. Hardy, W.D., Jr. Immunology of oncornaviruses. Vet. Clinics N. Amer. 4: 133-146, 1974.
14. Azocar, J. and Essex, M. Incorporation of HLA antigens in the envelope of RNA tumor viruses grown in human cells. Cancer Res. 39: 3388-3391, 1979.
15. Sarma, P.S. and Log, T. Subgroup classification of feline leukemia and sarcoma viruses by viral interference and neutralization tests. Virology 54: 160-170, 1973.

16. Hardy, W.D., Jr., Hess, P.W., MacEwen, E.G., McClelland, A.J., Zuckerman, E.E., Essex, M., and Cotter, S.M. The biology of feline leukemia virus in the natural environment. Cancer Res. 36: 582-588, 1976.

17. Noronha, F., de, Post, J.E., Norcross, N.L. and Rickard, C.G. Induction of group-specific interspecies antibody in a cat by immunization with disrupted feline leukemia virus. Nature 235: 14-15, 1972.

18. Hardy, W.D., Jr.,Hirshaut, Y. and Hess, P. Detection of feline leukemia virus and other mammalian oncornaviruses by immunofluorescence in: Unifying Concepts of Leukemia(Dutcher R.M. and Chieco-Bianchi, G., Eds.) pp.778-799, Karger, Basel, 1973.

19. Hardy, W.D., Jr., Old, L.J., Hess, P.W., Essex, M. and Cotter, S.M. Horizontal transmission of feline leukemia virus in cats. Nature 244: 266-269, 1973.

20. Hardy, W.D., Jr., McClelland, A.J., Zuckerman, E.E., Hess, P.W., Essex, M., Cotter, S.M., MacEwen, E.G. and Hayes, A.A. Prevention of the contagious spread of feline leukemia virus and the development of leukemia in pet cats. Nature 263: 326-328, 1976.

21. Hardy, W.D., Jr., Zuckerman, E.E., MacEwen, E.G., Hayes, A.A., and Essex, M. A feline leukemia and sarcoma virus induced tumor virus specific antigen. Nature 270: 249-251, 1977.

22. Essex, M., Cotter, S.M., Stephenson, J.R., Aaronson, S.A. and Hardy, W.D., Jr. Leukemia, lymphoma and fibrosarcoma of cats as models for similar diseases of man in: Origins of Human Cancer (Hiatt, H.H., Watson, J.D., and Winsten, J.A., Eds.) pp.1197-1214, Cold Spring Harbor Laboratory, Cold Spring Harbor, N.Y. 1977.

23. Hardy, W.D., Jr., McClelland, A.J., Zuckerman, E.E., Snyder, H.W., Jr., MacEwen, E.G., Francis, D. and Essex, M. Development of virus non-producer lymphosarcomas in pet cats exposed to FeLV. Nature, in press.

24. Snyder, H.W., Jr., Hardy, W.D., Jr., Zuckerman, E.E. and Fleissner, E. Characterization of a tumor-specific antigen on the surface of feline lymphosarcoma cells. Nature 275: 656-658, 1978.

25. Sherr, C.J., Sen, A., Todaro, G.J., Sliski, A., and Essex, M. Feline sarcoma virus particles contain a phosphorylated polyprotein (pp85) with p15, p12 and FOCMA antigens. Proc. Natl. Acad. Sci. 75: 1505-1509, 1978.

26. Essex, M., Sliski, A., Cotter, S.M., Jakowski, R.M. and Hardy, W.D., Jr. Immunosurveillance of naturally occurring feline leukemia. Science 190: 790-792, 1975.

27. Jacquemin, P.C., Saxinger, C., Gallo, R.C., Hardy, W.

D., Jr., and Essex, M.   Antibody response in cats to feline leukemia virus reverse transcriptase under natural conditions of exposure to the virus.   Virology 91: 472-476, 1978.
28. Hardy, W.D., Jr.   The immunology and epidemiology of the feline leukemia virus in: Feline Leukemia and Sarcoma Viruses (Hardy, W.D., Jr., Essex, M., and McClelland, A.J. Eds.) Elsevier/North Holland, New York, in press.
29. Perryman, L.E., Hoover, E.A. and Yohn, D.S.   Immunological reactivity of the cat: immunosuppression in experimental feline leukemia.   J. Natl. Cancer Inst. 49: 1357-1365, 1972.
30. Mathes, L.E., Olsen, R.G., Hebebrand, L.C., Hoover, E.A. and Schaller, J.P.   Abrogation of lymphocyte blastogenesis by a feline leukemia virus protein.   Nature 274: 687-689, 1978.
31. Hardy, W.D., Jr., Geering, G., Old, L.J., de Harven, E. Brodey, R.S. and McDonough, S.   Feline leukemia virus: occurrence of viral antigen in the tissues of cats with lymphosarcoma and other diseases.   Science 166: 1019-1021, 1969.
32. Hardy, W.D., Jr., McClelland, A.J., Zuckerman, E.E., Snyder, H.W., Jr., MacEwen, E.G., Francis, D.P. and Essex, M.   The immunology and epidemiology of feline leukemia virus non-producer lymphosarcomas in: Viruses in naturally occurring cancers (Essex, M., Todaro, G. and ZurHausen, H. Eds.) Cold Spring Harbor Laboratory, Cold Spring Harbor, N.Y., in press.
33. Gallo, R.C., Saxinger, W.C., Gallagher, R.E., Gillespie, D.H., Aulakh, G.S. and Wong-Staal, F.   Some ideas on the origin of leukemia in man and recent evidence for the presence of type-C viral related information in: Origins of Human Cancer (Hiatt, H.H., Watson, J.D., and Winsten, J.A., Eds.) pp.1253-1285, Cold Spring Harbor Laboratory, Cold Spring Harbor, N.Y, 1977.
34. Wexsler, M.E., Ryning, F.W. and Hardy, W.D., Jr.   Immune complex disease in cancer.   Clinical Bull. 5: 109-113, 1975.
35. Cotter, S.M., Hardy, W.D., Jr. and Essex, M.   Association of feline leukemia virus with lymphosarcoma and other disorders in the cat.   J. Amer. Vet.Med. Assoc. 166:449-454, 1975.
36. Jarrett, W., Mackey, L., Jarrett, O., Laird, H.M., and Hood, C.   Antibody response and virus survival in cats vaccinated against feline leukemia.   Nature 248: 230-232, 1974.

Prospects for the Treatment of Cancer with Interferon

SUSAN E. KROWN, M.D.

Assistant Attending Physician
Clinical Immunology Service
Memorial Sloan-Kettering Cancer Center
New York, New York

INTRODUCTION

Interferons are a family of inducible glycoproteins produced by a wide range of vertebrate cells in response to viral infections and a variety of other stimuli. They are intercellular messages with a restricted host range which bind to specific cell surface receptors and direct the expression of an interferon-induced phenotype characterized by viral resistance and a variety of non-antiviral activities. Interferons have shown inhibitory effects on a wide variety of animal tumors, and recent clinical trials have demonstrated antitumor effects in man as well. The precise mechanism of interferon's antitumor effect is not known, although several possibilities have been suggested, some acting directly on tumor cells and others mediated by the tumor-bearing host.

This review will briefly describe the current evidence for antitumor activity of interferons in animals and in man, and will consider some of the possible mechanisms by which interferons, acting as modifiers of a variety of biological responses, may mediate tumor regression. The ways in which clinical trials of interferons have deviated from the traditional scheme for new drug development, and some of the unique problems faced in evaluating interferons in clinical trials will be considered. This approach will identify some of the unresolved issues that remain to be dealt with before the ultimate role of interferons in cancer therapy can be defined.

Supported in part by NIH grants CA-19267 and CA-08748 and an American Cancer Society Junior Faculty Clinical Fellowship. Reprint requests: Susan E. Krown, M.D., 1275 York Avenue, New York, N.Y. 10021.

ANTITUMOR EFFECTS IN ANIMALS

The antitumor effects of interferons in experimental animals have been described in detail in several recent reviews (1-3) and will simply be summarized here. Because of the antiviral effects of interferon, the initial animal tumors chosen for investigation were those where a viral etiology was known or suspected. In the case of tumors induced by nonproductive transforming viruses (e.g. Polyoma, Shope), interferon appears to inhibit an early virus-dependent event leading to cell transformation, and has been effective when given just prior to, together with, or immediately after virus challenge. In the case of tumors releasing transforming virus particles (e.g. Friend and Rauscher leukemias), where repeated cycles of virus multiplication and shedding occur throughout the animal's life, interferon shows antitumor effects only when given at high doses, daily, and over long periods of time, suggesting that its main effect may be in reducing viremia. Host-mediated defense mechanisms or direct inhibition of the rate of tumor cell multiplication may also contribute in part to interferon's antitumor effects in virally induced tumors.

Although interferon's effects on viral oncogenesis are not likely to be particularly relevant to human neoplasia, its effects on transplantable tumors and those induced by carcinogens may be of greater relevance. Interferon preparations have inhibited tumor growth in a wide variety of transplantable mouse tumors (including Ehrlich ascites, EL-4, L1210, RC19, Lewis lung and sarcoma 180), as well as transplantable tumors in the rabbit and rat. In such tumors, high doses of interferon, small tumor burden and close contact between interferon and tumor cells are factors which promote interferon's effectiveness, while pretreatment with interferon is ineffective. Interferon has also been reported to delay or inhibit development of methylcholanthrene induced tumors, and to decrease the incidence of lymphomas in irradiated mice. Although the effects of interferon in combination with other antineoplastic therapies has not been extensively studied, synergistic antitumor effects have been described when interferon was combined with cytoreductive chemotherapy or surgery, or with an immunopotentiator, isoprinosine (4). Malignant cells of human origin, transplanted into nude mice, have been found susceptible to human interferon but not mouse interferon, suggesting a direct antitumor effect rather than a host-mediated one.

One feature which is common to most of these examples in experimental animals is the fact that, with rare exceptions, interferon has succeeded only in delaying tumor progression or prolonging survival, but has not caused regression of established tumors. Another point worth emphasizing before considering clinical trials is the type of interferon preparation used. In most of the studies mentioned so far, mouse L-cell interferon has been used, whereas clinical trials have, for the most part, employed human leukocyte interferon. The mouse seems to lack an equivalent of human leukocyte interferon (5), and mouse type I interferon, like human fibroblast interferon, has a more rapid clearance from the circulation and is inactivated by muscle extracts (6). Thus, as will be discussed below, the results of preclinical studies with mouse interferon preparations may not permit extrapolation to the design of trials with leukocyte or lymphoblastoid interferons in man.

ANTITUMOR EFFECTS IN MAN

To date, most clinical studies of systemic antitumor activity have been with human leukocyte interferon. With rare exceptions, these studies have used interferon preparations with a specific activity of no more than 10^6 units of interferon per mg of protein (equivalent to approximately one part in one thousand of interferon). These preparations have, in most cases, been administered by intramuscular injection, daily, at doses of from 3 X 10^6 to 10 X 10^6 U per day for periods of from several weeks to several months.

In solid tumors, the first trial was reported by Strander and his colleagues at the Karolinska Institute who used leukocyte interferon as an adjuvant to surgery in primary osteosarcoma. Compared to both historical and concurrent non-randomized controls, the interferon-treated group showed a significant reduction in lung metastases and improvement in long-term survival (7). Although Strander has not observed regression in metastatic osteosarcoma, Kishida has reported short-lived regression of lung metastases in 2 of 3 patients treated with doses $\geq 10^7$ U/day (8). Responses have been observed in breast cancer by Gutterman et al. (9), who reported that 7 of 17 patients showed partial or minor responses, and by Borden et al. (10) reporting on the American Cancer Society sponsored cooperative trial where 5 of 23 patients showed major objective tumor regression. In neither of these studies was there evidence suggesting that higher doses of interferon (9 X 10^6 U/day) were more effective than lower ones (3 X 10^6 U/day). In the former study (9), response to interferon was positively correlated with response to prior chemotherapy or hormonal therapy, and was seen only in patients who developed at least moderate leukopenia, suggesting that interferon's antiproliferative activity played an important role. In our

own trial in previously treated patients with non-small cell
lung cancer, none of 19 evaluable patients showed an objective response after daily treatment for 30 days (11). Over
half of these patients had responded previously to combination chemotherapy regimens, and three showed objective responses in subsequent chemotherapy trials. Strander has reported excellent therapeutic responses in 7 of 7 children
with benign recurrent laryngeal papillomas (7), where it is
likely that interferon's antiviral activity plays a role.
At a recent conference, Hersh, speaking for the M.D. Anderson group, reported 2 of 9 partial responses in patients with
colon cancer, none of 9 responses in previously treated ovarian cancer patients, and one of 8 responses in prostatic cancer (12).

Patients with a variety of hematologic malignancies have
also been treated with human leukocyte interferon. Several
clinical trials have been undertaken in multiple myeloma,
following the encouraging initial report by Mellstedt et al.
(13) of complete or partial responses in all 4 patients
treated. In a subsequent study from the Karolinska Institute (cited in 3), partial or complete responses were observed in 7 of 8 previously untreated patients with intermediate tumor mass, no responses in 4 previously untreated
patients with high estimated tumor mass, and one partial response in 4 patients previously treated with chemotherapy.
Gutterman et al. (9) have reported complete or partial response in 3 of 10 myeloma patients, plus significant improvement (less than partial response) in another 3. Osserman,
reporting on a cooperative trial sponsored by the American
Cancer Society, showed only 4 objective responses in 14 patients (14). It has been suggested that differences in response rates in these trials may have been due to loss of activity in some lots of lyophilized interferon, and this possibility is being investigated further.

Excellent therapeutic responses have been reported in nodular poorly differentiated lymphomas (9,15), and in some cases the response has persisted for over one year without
maintenance therapy. The results in diffuse histiocytic lymphoma have been poor in the few patients treated to date (9,
15), and too few patients with other types of lymphoma have
been treated to reach any conclusions, although case reports
have appeared of responses in Hodgkin's disease (16) and
chronic lymphocytic leukemia (9). After brief courses of intravenously administered leukocyte interferon, Hill et al.
(17) have also described a decrease in circulating and bone
marrow blasts in several patients with acute leukemias. Direct intratumoral injection of human leukocyte interferon
has reportedly induced regression of cutaneous breast cancer
metastases (18), while human fibroblast interferon injected

into cutaneous metastases of breast cancer, malignant melanoma and prostatic cancer has also caused regression of injected, but not uninjected lesions (19).

Although most studies reported so far have used leukocyte
interferon, reports are beginning to appear of clinical trials with lymphoblastoid and fibroblast interferon preparations. Niethammer (20) has recently presented preliminary
results of ongoing studies in Germany using intravenously administered fibroblast interferon. Of 4 patients with nasopharyngeal carcinoma with high antibody titers to Epstein-
Barr virus, one showed a major objective response, 2 showed
stabilization of growing tumors and one progressed. These
investigators have also begun a cross-over study to test whether fibroblast and leukocyte interferon preparations have
different spectra of therapeutic activity. Patients with
multiple myeloma or laryngeal papilloma are first treated
with human fibroblast interferon. Those who fail to respond
are then treated with human leukocyte interferon. So far,
2 patients with laryngeal papillomas showed no response to
fibroblast interferon, but responded to a subsequent course
of leukocyte interferon. One patient with multiple myeloma
responded to fibroblast interferon, while another responded
to neither preparation. This type of study design may eventually prove important in determining whether different interferon preparations have different tissue specificities, a
possibility that has been suggested in at least one in vitro
study (21).

Finally, Priestman (22) has recently reported on the first
clinical trial using human lymphoblastoid interferon in man.
The interferon preparations used had specific activities some
20 to 50 times higher than the leukocyte interferon preparations used in clinical trials to date. This study represents
the first systematic Phase I study with any interferon preparation designed to establish the maximum tolerated dose of
the preparation and to define its side effects using both
single doses and long-term daily administration. A dose of
3×10^6 U/M^2 body surface area (BSA) was the maximum tolerated single dose, limiting toxicity consisting of fever and
mild transient hypotension. When given in repeated daily doses, fever decreased over the first 5 days, permitting escal-
ation of the dose to as high as 7.5×10^6 U/M^2 BSA. Dose reduction was eventually required in the majority of patients
because of either leukopenia, nausea and malaise or abnormal
liver function tests. Other side effects included hypertension (associated with rapid temperature elevation), anemia,
thrombocytopenia, confusion and muscle weakness. These side
effects are similar to those seen in trials of less purified
leukocyte interferon, and are similar to those seen in acute
viral illness, suggesting that interferon itself, rather than

impurities in the preparations, may account for the toxicity observed. Intravenous hydrocortixone was shown capable, in this study, of abolishing rigors, without affecting subsequent fever, while pretreatment with salicylates reduced the degree of fever. Two patients, one with malignant melanoma who received 2.5 X 10^6 U/M^2 BSA for 30 days, and the other with gastric carcinoma who had the interferon dose escalated to 7.5 X 10^6 U/M^2 BSA, showed partial but short-lived tumor regression.

POTENTIAL MECHANISMS OF ANTITUMOR ACTIVITY

Both direct effects on tumor cells, and indirect, host-mediated effects, may account for interferon's antitumor activity (reviewed in 23-25). One of the well characterized properties of interferons is their ability to inhibit cell multiplication, and this applies to both tumor cells and normal cells. For example, mouse interferon inhibits, in a dose-dependent manner, the in vitro multiplication of mouse Ll210 leukemia cells, while Ll210R cells, selected for resistance to the antiviral action of interferon (and which are unable to bind interferon) are also resistant to the cell multiplication inhibitory actions of interferon (24). Human interferon preparations have been shown capable of inhibiting the differentiation of granulocyte precursors in vitro (26), and it is likely that this accounts for the leukopenia observed in clinical trials. The mechanism by which interferons inhibit cell multiplication and differentiation is far from clear, and it is likely that a variety of effects on cellular metabolism are involved. While interferon preparations do not appear to have direct cytotoxic effects, interferon-treated cells often plateau at lower saturation density than do normal cells and the intermitotic time appears to be progressively increased rather than arrested. In any case, while a direct effect on the rate of cell multiplication is probably a significant factor in mediating in vivo tumor regression, in the case of Ll210R cells, despite their lack of sensitivity to interferon in vitro, their growth is inhibited by interferon in vivo, implying indirect effects of interferon which are mediated by the tumor-bearing host (24).

Interferons have also been shown to have a variety of effects on cell surfaces. Of particular interest are its effects on the expression of cell surface antigens (25). An increase in the expression of cell surface antigens on tumor cells might render them more susceptible to recognition and elimination by the host. For example, pretreatment of Ll210 leukemia cells with interferon in vitro elicited an increased cell mediated response in vivo (27). Changes in the expression of histocompatibility antigens have also been observed

in effector cell populations after interferon treatment, including an increase in H-2K and H-2D antigens on mouse thymocytes and splenic lymphocytes, and an increase in HLA-A, B
and DR antigens on human peripheral blood lymphocytes (28).
Although increases in expression of histocompatibility antigens may relate to changes in subpopulations of immune reactive cells or to the role that such antigens play in the presentation of tumor associated antigens, thus far these changes have not correlated with therapeutic activity in clinical
trials (11,29).

Finally, interferons have been shown to affect the specialized functions of cells involved in immune reactions.
Thus, under appropriate circumstances, interferons have been
shown to increase (30) or decrease (31) antibody responses,
to decrease the proliferative response of lymphocytes to mitogens and alloantigens (32), to decrease (33), or in some
cases, increase (34) delayed hypersensitivity reactions, to
delay (35) or accelerate (36) graft rejection, to enhance
macrophage phagocytic activity (37) and macrophage mediated
tumor cell cytotoxicity (38), and to increase both specific
(39) and spontaneous (40) cell mediated cytotoxicity. These
activities have been demonstrated in in vitro and murine systems, and some are now being confirmed in clinical trials in
man. For example, in our study of human leukocyte interferon
in non-small cell lung cancer (11), 12 of 13 patients who
were tested serially showed a significant increase in peripheral blood natural killer cell activity against K-562 target
cells within one week of starting treatment. Increases occurred in patients with both low and normal pretreatment natural killer cell activity, but in this study occurred in the
absence of tumor regression.

PROBLEMS AND PROSPECTS

With this background we can begin to consider interferon's
future prospects in cancer therapy and the direction that
clinical trials with these preparations ought to take in the
next few years. Traditionally, before undergoing preliminary
clinical trials, a potential new anticancer agent is screened
in a variety of experimental tumor systems and then undergoes
further preclinical development including toxicology studies
and pharmacologic studies to determine optimal dose schedules (41). In the case of interferon preparations, unique
problems are encountered even at this early stage of drug development, because of the restricted host range of interferon
preparations, and pharmacokinetic differences among different
types of interferons. Thus, it is difficult to predict,
based on animal studies, either the toxicity or optimal
schedules when human interferon preparations are used in man.

Another factor which hampers interpretation of preclinical
and clinical pharmacology studies is the purity of interferon
preparations. Thus, the same stimuli that result in interferon induction also induce the release of a wide variety of
factors (e.g. lymphokines, monokines, prostaglandins) (42)
which are present in varying amounts in interferon preparations and which exert a variety of effects on cells. These
factors may contribute both to the toxicity of interferon
preparations and to their therapeutic activity (or lack of
it). One should not infer that these impurities are necessarily undesirable nor that they, rather than interferon itself, are responsible for all of the biological response modifications that may be involved in mediating therapeutic responses. Rather, the presence of these factors in currently
available interferon preparations must be acknowledged, and
one must question whether all the information gained in trials with relatively impure preparations will be applicable to
later trials where more highly purified preparations are
used.

The development of potential new anticancer drugs usually
proceeds in an orderly sequence of phases (41). In the first
phase, clinical pharmacology studies are performed to determine dosage regimens that are not too toxic. Generally, with
chemotherapeutic agents, one wishes to define a maximum tolerated dose, and to identify the type of toxicity, whether it
is predictable and whether it can be modified or reversed.
Usually one also tries to explore more than one schedule of
administration. Phase II is usually a screen for antitumor
activity in patients where a therapeutic response can be
clearly defined. The dose and schedule of drug administration is selected based on the preceding clinical pharmacology
studies, and the drug is screened in groups of patients with
various types of tumors. In evaluating whether a drug goes
on to Phase III trials, factors in addition to the percent
response rate must also be considered. Thus, drugs without
significant bone marrow toxicity or those capable of killing
non-proliferating cells might be candidates for further study
even in the absence of high objective response rates. Finally, a drug may go on to Phase III trials, where it may be
compared with other agents in randomized trials, or where it
may be combined with other drugs of proven efficacy to determine whether additive or synergistic therapeutic effects occur.

In evaluating interferon preparations, particularly leukocyte interferon, clinical studies have taken a somewhat
different course. Generally speaking, with little data concerning the clinical pharmacology of interferons, disease-
oriented Phase II studies using fixed doses and schedules of
interferon administration have been performed in a variety of

tumors. Most studies to date, with the possible exception of those in breast cancer, myeloma and lung cancer, have included too few patients to make any realistic estimate of true response rates. The fact that therapeutic responses have been observed under these circumstances with interferon preparations of low specific activity is extraordinary, and certainly has and should encourage further investigation.

This brings us back to the need for Phase I studies to define the optimal dose and schedule of interferon administration. In the long run, the optimal dose and schedule will be defined as the one which most often gives us the desired endpoint, tumor regression. In approaching this endpoint we could, on the one hand, concentrate on defining the maximum tolerated dose, assuming that this dose, given repeatedly, would result in maximum antiproliferative effects. On the other hand, we could assume that interferon's effects on cells involved in immune reactions were most important, and we might wish to explore the effects of different interferon doses and schedules on a variety of immune responses. In the latter case, it would be important to know which immune responses were involved in mediating tumor regression in man, and to what degree they ought to be modified, and these facts are as yet unknown. Finally, in trying to establish tolerable treatment regimens, we might wish to modify some of the toxic effects of interferon preparations through pharmacologic manipulations. The use of drugs such as corticosteroids, salicylates and indomethacin seems logical, based on the acute and chronic toxic effects observed in clinical trials to date. However, it is possible that the addition of such drugs may decrease the therapeutic activity of interferon. For example, one of the ways in which interferon is thought to regulate cell growth is by stimulating the release of prostaglandin E (43), and this may account as well for some of the toxic reactions observed in patients. Yaron et al. (43) have reported that the addition of cortisol and indomethacin, inhibitors of prostaglandin E production, also prevented the inhibitory effect of interferon on the growth of cultured human fibroblasts. In another study by Schultz et al. (38), the addition of hydrocortisone suppressed the ability of interferon-treated mouse macrophages to kill tumor cells in vitro.

What can we conclude about interferon's prospects in cancer treatment? It is already clear that interferon is a potent modifier of biological responses. The fact that tumor regression has been documented in patients with macroscopic tumor using impure preparations under circumstances where neither the optimal dose and schedule of treatment nor the primary mechanism of action has been defined is clearly promising, particularly when one considers that in experimental

animals interferon is most successful when the tumor burden
is minimal. It is likely that interferon's potential in man
will also be best realized not as a single agent, but rather
in combination with chemotherapy or as an adjuvant to surgery
when tumor burden is low. Attaining this end, and realizing
interferon's full potential, will require continued investigation of the mechanisms by which interferons mediate tumor
regression, possible variations in therapeutic activity of
different types of interferon, and clinical trials with interferon preparations of increasing purity.

REFERENCES

1. Gresser I: Antitumor effects of interferon, in: Cancer - A
   Comprehensive Treatise (Chemotherapy, Vol. 5). New York,
   Plenum, 1977, pp 525-571.
2. Stewart WE II: Antitumor activities of interferons in animals, in: The Interferon System. New York, Springer-Verlag, 1979, pp 292-304.
3. Krim M: Towards tumor therapy with interferons. Part II:
   Interferons: In vivo effects. Blood 55:875-884, 1980.
4. Cerutti I, Chany C, Schlumberger JF: Isoprinosine increases the antitumor action of interferon. Int J Immuno-
   pharmacol 1:59-63, 1979.
5. Paucker, K: Comparison of lymphoid and non-lymphoid Type I
   mouse interferon, in: Krim M, Edy VG, Oettgen H, Stewart
   WE II (eds): IInd International Workshop on Interferons.
   New York, Rockefeller Univ. Press, (in press).
6. Hanley DF, Wiranowska-Stewart M, Stewart WE II: Pharmacology of interferons. I. Pharmacologic distinctions between
   human leukocyte and fibroblast interferons. Int J Im-
   munopharmacol 1:219-226,1979.
7. Strander H: in: Krim M, Edy VG, Oettgen H, Stewart WE II
   (eds): IInd International Workshop on Interferons. New
   York, Rockefeller Univ Press, (in press).
8. Kishida T: in: Krim M, Edy VG, Oettgen H, Stewart WE II
   (eds): IInd International Workshop on Interferons. New
   York, Rockefeller Univ Press, (in press).
9. Gutterman JU, Blumenschein GR, Alexanian R, et al.: Leukocyte interferon-induced tumor regression in human metastatic breast cancer, multiple myeloma, and malignant lymphoma. Ann Int Med 93:399-406,1980.
10. Borden E, Dao T, Holland J, et al.: Interferon in recur-
    rent breast carcinoma: Preliminary report of the American
    Cancer Society clinical trials program. Proc Amer Assoc
    Cancer Res 21:187, 1980.
11. Krown SE, Stoopler MB, Gralla RJ, et al.: Phase II trial
    of human leukocyte interferon in non-small cell lung can-
    cer - preliminary results, in: Terry WD, Rosenberg SA

(eds): Immunotherapy of Cancer - Current Status of Trials in Man. Proceedings of the Second International Conference on Immunotherapy of Cancer. New York, Elsevier North-Holland, (in press).

12. Hersh EM: Clinical trials with leukocyte interferon at the M.D. Anderson Hospital. Presented at the First International Conference on Immunopharmacology, Brighton, U.K., July 30, 1980.

13. Mellstedt H, Bjorkholm M, Johansson B, et al.: Interferon therapy in myelomatosis. Lancet 1:245-247,1979.

14. Osserman EF, Sherman WH, Alexanian R, et al.: Preliminary results of the American Cancer Society (ACS)-sponsored trial of human leukocyte interferon (IF) in multiple myeloma (MM). Proc Amer Assoc Cancer Res 21:161, 1980.

15. Merigan TC, Sikora K, Breeden JH, et al.: Preliminary observations on the effect of human leukocyte interferon in non-Hodgkin's lymphoma. N Engl J Med 299:1449-1453, 1978.

16. Blomgren H, Cantell K, Johansson B, et al.: Interferon therapy in Hodgkin's disease. Acta Med Scand 199: 527-532, 1976.

17. Hill NO, Loeb E, Pardue AS, et al.: Human leukocyte interferon responsiveness of acute leukemia. J Clin Hematol Oncol 9: 137-149, 1979.

18. Habif D: in: Krim M, Edy VG, Oettgen H, Stewart WE II (eds): IInd International Workshop on Interferons. New York, Rockefeller Univ Press, (in press).

19. Horoszewicz JS, Leong SS, Ito M, et al.: Human fibroblast interferon in human neoplasia: Clinical and laboratory study. Cancer Treat Rep 11: 1899-1906, 1978.

20. Niethammer D: Clinical trials; antitumor studies; phase II with fibroblast interferon. Presented at the First International Conference on Immunopharmacology, Brighton, U.K., July 30, 1980.

21. Einhorn S, Strander H: Is interferon tissue-specific? Effect of human leukocyte and fibroblast interferons on the growth of lymphoblastoid and osteosarcoma cell lines. J Gen Virol 35:573-577, 1977.

22. Priestman T: Initial evaluation of human lymphoblastoid interferon in patients with advanced malignant disease. Lancet 2:113-118, 1980.

23. Stewart WE II: Non-antiviral actions of interferons, in: The Interferon System. New York, Springer-Verlag, 1979, pp 223-256.

24. Gresser I, Tovey MG: Antitumor effects of interferon. Biochim Biophys Acta 516:231-247, 1978.

25. Krim M: Towards tumor therapy with interferons. Part I: Interferons: Production and properties. Blood 55:711-722, 1980.

26. Verma DS, Spitzer G, Gutterman JU, et al.: Human leuko-
    cyte interferon preparation blocks granulopoietic differ-
    entiation. Blood 54:1423-1427, 1979.
27. Skurkovich SB, Kalinina IA, Eremkina EI, et al.: Enhance-
    ment of the immune response following immunization with
    L1210 cells preliminarily incubated with interferon.
    Biull Eksp Biol Med 81:706-707, 1976.
28. Pollack MS, Krown S, Oettgen H, Dupont B: Interferon in-
    duced quantitative and qualitative changes in expression
    of HLA-A,B,C and DR alloantigens on lymphocyte subpopula-
    tions. Proc Amer Soc Microbiol, abstract E85, 1980.
29. Krown SE, Kerr D, Stewart WE II, et al.: Phase I trial of
    poly ICLC in patients with advanced cancer, in: Hersh EM,
    Chirigos MA, Mastrangelo MJ (eds), Augmenting Agents in
    Cancer Therapy, New York, Raven, (in press).
30. Braun W., Levy MB: Interferon preparations as modifiers
    of immune responses. Proc Soc Exp Biol Med 141: 769-773,
    1972.
31. Brodeur BR, Merigan TC: Suppressive effect of interferon
    on the humoral immune response to sheep red blood cells
    in mice. J Immunol 113:1319-1325, 1974.
32. Lindahl-Magnusson P, Leary P, Gresser I: Interferon in-
    hibits DNA synthesis induced in mouse lymphocyte suspen-
    sions by phytohemagglutinin or by allogeneic cells. Na-
    ture New Biol 237:120-121, 1972.
33. DeMaeyer E, DeMaeyer-Guignard J, Vandeputte M: Inhibition
    by interferon of delayed-type hypersensitivity in the
    mouse. Proc Nat Acad Sci USA 72:1753-1758, 1975.
34. Holden H: Immunomodulation by interferons. Presented at
    the First International Conference on Immunopharmacology,
    Brighton, U.K., July 30, 1980.
35. Hirsch MS, Ellis DA, Black PH, et al.: Immunosuppressive
    effect of an interferon preparation in vivo. Transplan-
    tation 17:234-236, 1974.
36. Chernyakhovskaya I, Slavina E: Lymphocyte activation by
    interferon. Vopr Virusol 4: 329-333, 1972.
37. Huang KY, Donahoe RM, Gordon FB, Dressler HR: Enhancement
    of phagocytosis by interferon-containing preparations.
    Infect Immun 4: 581-588, 1971.
38. Schultz RM, Pavlidis NA, Stylos WA, Chirigos MA: Cytotox-
    ic activity of interferon-treated macrophages studied by
    various inhibitors. Cancer Treat Rep 62:1889-1892, 1978.
39. Zarling JM, Sosma J, Eskra L, et al.: Enhancement of T
    cell cytotoxic responses by purified human fibroblast in-
    terferon. J Immunol 121:2002-2004, 1979.
40. Herberman RB, Djeu JY, Ortaldo JR, et al.: Role of inter-
    feron in augmentation of natural and antibody-dependent
    cell-mediated cytotoxicity. Cancer Treat Rep 62:1893-1896,
    1978.

41. Carter SK, Goldsmith M: The development and clinical
    testing of new anticancer drugs at the National Cancer
    Institute - Example cis platinum (II) diamminedichloride
    (NSC 119875), in, Connors TA, Roberts JJ (eds), Platinum
    Coordination Complexes in Cancer Chemotherapy. Recent
    Results in Cancer Res, Vol 48, New York, Springer-Verlag,
    1973, pp 137-144.
42. Stewart WE II: Interferon inducers, in The Interferon
    System, New York, Springer-Verlag, 1979, pp 27-57.
43. Yaron M, Yaron I, Gurari-Rotman D, et al.: Stimulation of
    prostaglandin E production in cultured human fibroblasts
    by poly I·C and human interferon. Nature 267:457, 1977.

Genetics

Genetics and Cancer

ALFRED G. KNUDSON, JR., M.D., Ph.D.

Director
The Institute for Cancer Research
The Fox Chase Cancer Center
Philadelphia, PA

During the decade of the National Cancer Program there has
been astonishing progress in our understanding of genetics.
Some of this new knowledge has already been utilized in the
investigation of cancer, but it seems to many of us that we
are just now on the threshold of achieving the most important
applications of this knowledge and that these applications
will in turn advance our understanding of genetics itself. So
far we have learned a great deal about the role of heredity in
the etiology of human cancer, but it is likely that the new
genetics can now be employed in the explication of the fundamental defects of cancer cells. With this accomplished there
may be new opportunities for prevention, for treatment, and
for the science of developmental biology. Here I wish to
discuss the current status of the somatic mutation hypothesis
of carcinogenesis, genetic states that predispose to cancer,
and the existence and nature of cancer genes.

SOMATIC MUTATION AND CANCER

The idea that somatic mutations may be important in carcinogenesis was first clearly stated by Boveri, but it has only
been in the past decade that significant evidence has been

This work was supported by Public Health Service Grants No.
CA-06927 and No. RR-05539 from the National Cancer Institute
and by an appropriation from the Commonwealth of Pennsylvania.
Reprints may be obtained by writing to Dr. Alfred G. Knudson,
Jr. at The Institute for Cancer Research, The Fox Chase Cancer
Center, 7701 Burholme Avenue, Philadelphia, PA 19111.

accumulated in its favor. Capitalizing upon the discovery
that some carcinogens require activation, Ames was able to
show that, although unactivated carcinogens are not mutagenic
in bacterial systems, many activated carcinogens are mutagenic.[1] Since then the circles of mutagens and carcinogens
have increasingly overlapped. Another line of evidence in
support of somatic mutation has been the discovery of the
induction by carcinogens of alterations in DNA that can
explain this mutagenic activity.

New findings in radiobiology also support the somatic mutation hypothesis. Much of this work has borrowed from previous
work on photorepair in microbial systems. One of the most
heuristic discoveries came from the laboratory of Cleaver
shortly before the beginning of the National Cancer Program.[8]
This was the finding that repair of damage to DNA by ultraviolet light occurs in human cells and is defective in
patients with the genetic disease, xeroderma pigmentosum.
Because these patients are at greatly increased risk of basal
and squamous cell carcinoma and melanoma, this discovery
provided direct evidence in support of the idea that somatic
mutation can lead to cancer. Since then it has been demonstrated that specific locus mutation rates are increased, in
vitro, as anticipated.[36]

For ionizing radiation there is also a genetic susceptibility in man. Following reports that patients with ataxia
telangiectasia, and cells from such patients, are unusually
sensitive to X-rays, Paterson demonstrated a defect in the
repair of DNA lesions caused by ionizing radiation, a defect
quite separable from that of xeroderma pigmentosum.[42] It is
still not clear how this defect is related to the specific
immunologic abnormalities seen in this disease or to the susceptibility to tumors, notably lymphomas.

For radiation we have seen how heredity and environment can
interact in carcinogenesis. A similar circumstance applies to
chemical carcinogenesis. Thus, the activation of carcinogens
itself is a genetically controlled process. In mice there are
mutations that interfere with activation and so impart resistance to the carcinogenic activity of some agents. One enzyme
that has been particularly well studied is aryl hydrocarbon
hydroxylase.[40] A claim that susceptibility to lung cancer
induced by cigarette smoking results from genetically determined inducibility of this enzyme has not been substantiated,
although recent studies do suggest that there may be some
basis for the conclusion after all.[25] The findings for both
chemicals and radiation greatly complicate any attempt to
assign a cause to cancer; are cancers caused in this way
hereditary or environmental?

The study of mutations induced by chemicals and by irradiation has been associated with an improved understanding of mutations that occur "spontaneously" and account for "background" mutation rates. These mutations show a different array of DNA lesions from those induced by carcinogens, just as the arrays for different carcinogens vary. The "causes" of spontaneous mutation are incompletely known, although cosmic radiation and thermal effects are among them. According to a somatic mutation hypothesis there will always be a "background" incidence of cancer, attributable to spontaneous mutations.[30] Since the agents of cause of spontaneous mutations do not vary greatly geographically, the incidence of any cancer should be relatively constant world-wide if spontaneous mutations are the sole cause of cancer. The fact that epidemiologists have found that very few cancers display such a distribution indicates that environmental mutations are operating and/or other mechanisms can affect cancer incidence.[4] Nevertheless, it is important to realize that cancer cannot be eliminated as a problem as long as there are spontaneous mutations.

An important implication of the somatic mutation hypothesis is that there are specific genes in the genome that are targets of spontaneous and induced mutations. Certainly mutation at just any genetic locus would not impart a susceptibility to cancer. What then are the genetic sites that are critical? How many are there and where are they located? Does each cancer have its own genetic locus? Are there in fact "cancer genes"?

The answers to these questions are still unknown, but the cytogeneticists have made some observations in the past decade that seem to be germane.[16,48] The existence of cancer genes was suggested by the discovery of the Philadelphia chromosome of chronic myeloid leukemia by Nowell and Hungerford in 1960.[41] The introduction a decade ago of new techniques for discerning bands in chromosomes has made possible an analysis of the fine structure of such aberrations. Rowley has thus shown that the Philadelphia chromosome results from a translocation of part of chromosome 22 to another chromosome, usually number 9.[46] The fact that the recipient chromosome can vary strongly suggests that there is a critical site in chromosome 22 whose normal function is disrupted by this translocation. Is this site the locus of a "cancer gene"?

The development of a new methodology spurred a renewal of the search for other chromosomal aberrations that might be related to specific cancers. The result is that several examples have been uncovered in the past few years. Tumor cells from patients with Burkitt's lymphoma very often show a translocation between chromosomes 8 and 14. This aberration is found in both the African and the American forms of this disease, whether EB virus is present or not.[28] Recently a few cases have been found in which the translocation involves chromosome 8 and some other chromosome than 14. As with chronic myeloid leukemia a specific chromosomal site, in this case on the long arm of chromosome 8, seems to be critical to the development of a specific cancer. Is this the site of another "cancer gene"?

Other forms of lymphoreticular cancer also seem to show specific change. Thus the leukemic cells of many cases of acute promyelocytic leukemia show a specific translocation between chromosomes 15 and 17, of acute myeloblastic leukemia, between 8 and 21, and of various lymphoid tumors, between 14 and some other chromosome.[18,47,48] These findings may also mark the location of specific "cancer genes".

Similar progress has not been made with other kinds of cancer, with just a few exceptions. This is undoubtedly related to the fact that nearly all cancers show so many chromosomal aberrations, obviously associated with tumor growth and progression, that detailed analyses of this kind are difficult to perform. In the leukemias and lymphomas these other abnormalities are reduced in number and sometimes no other aberration is present, as is usual for chronic myeloid leukemia at the time of diagnosis. Other aberrations are often also few in benign tumors and in the embryonal tumors of children. Unfortunately, the mitotic index of benign tumors is so low that the results of cytogenetic analysis are scanty. In the case of meningioma Mark has found a specific abnormality, absence of one chromosome 22, in many of the tumors. Few studies have been performed on the embryonal tumors, but it has been found that in some cases of retinoblastoma there is a deletion in the long arm of chromosome 13.[20] The significance of this finding is great in view of the occurrence of retinoblastoma in genetically predisposed individuals in whom every cell in the body shows the same deleted segment.

Even though these karyotypic changes are specifically related to individual cancers, can we conclude that they precede the development of cancer and are in fact causative? Although the answer is probably no at this time, the finding of such aberrations preceding the development of neoplasm would strengthen the presumption of causation, and in fact there are some reports of this kind for the Philadelphia chromosome. In any case the specificities of changes noted so far are striking and strongly indicative of some functional significance.

In some cases of these same cancers there is no specific aberration.[18,48] This fraction is small for chronic myeloid leukemia but is approximately 50 per cent for acute

promyelocytic leukemia. There are two possible explanations;
one is that these cases arise in some other fashion; the
other, that the same genetic loci are affected by an abnormality that is not visible microscopically. This latter possibility would hardly be surprising in view of the many examples
from genetics of phenotypic effects associated with a spectrum
of changes from intragenic aberrations as small as point mutations to visible deletions that eliminate the entire gene and
adjacent genes as well.

There is, then, much to support the somatic mutation hypothesis. On the one hand carcinogenic chemicals and radiation
can cause mutations, and, on the other hand, some cancers
demonstrate specific genetic abnormalities that seem to point
to the changes that these mutations can bring about. If the
latter idea is correct, then the same aberration should be
observed whether a specific cancer results from spontaneous or
induced mutation. This is indeed the case for chronic myeloid
leukemia. Both the cases with no identifiable causation and
those almost certainly caused by radiation or chemicals show
the Philadelphia chromosome. We strongly suspect that there
are sensitive sites at which mutation must occur in order for
cancer to ensue.

GERMINAL MUTATIONS AND CANCER

Awareness of heritable states that predispose to human
cancer has increased sharply during the past
decade.[19,23,30,35,39] Some of these conditions, including
xeroderma pigmentosum and ataxia telangiectasia, are recessive, while others, including polyposis coli and neurofibromatosis, are dominantly transmitted. We are especially
interested in dominantly inherited cancer, because the cells
of the gene carriers may be altered by germ cell mutations
that occur in the same genes altered by somatic mutations. It
now appears that for every cancer site there is a dominant
hereditary and a nonhereditary form.[33] Thus two genes that
predispose to colon cancer are well known: one for polyposis
coli and one for the heritable colon cancer first described by
Warthin, in which there are no polyps; Anderson believes that
there are five well defined dominantly heritable states that
predispose to colon cancer. Together they may account for
about 10 per cent of colon cancer in the United States. At
least three forms of hereditary breast cancer can be discerned
from the patterns of associated tumors; ovarian cancer or no
other cancer with one, endometrial cancer with a second, and
brain tumors and/or sarcomas with a third. Again, these may
total 10 per cent or so of all breast cancer in the U.S.A.

For some tumors, particularly childhood cancers, the
hereditary fraction may be higher; for example, the heritable
form of retinoblastoma constitutes approximately 40 per cent
of all cases.[29] The information on heritable forms of cancer
is increasing rapidly and it will not be surprising if the
distinctly dominant forms exceed 100 in number.

Any estimate of the contribution of heredity to the burden
of human cancer is impossible of course until we have a better
understanding of genetic and environmental interactions. As
mentioned earlier, if there were a polymorphism for aryl
hydrocarbon hydroxylase that imparts a strong predisposition
to lung cancer in smokers, most cases could result from such
an interaction. But it is clear that there are four categories of cancer that are defined by the contributions of
heredity and environment, if we understand by environment
those influences that are not universally distributed, such as
cosmic radiation and body temperature, which seem to play an
important role in spontaneous or background cancer.[30] Suppose, then, that we assume that environmental variables can
account for as much as 80 per cent of cancer in the United
States,[28] purely genetic cancer about 5 per cent, and spontaneous cancer about 15 per cent. Environmental cancer should be
partitioned then into a fraction that is purely environmental
and one that is interactive with heredity (Fig. 1). We have
no idea how this should be done
at present. It may even
develop that most cancer is of
the interaction type.[19,35,39]
For example, Swift has reported
that heterozygous carriers for
ataxia telangiectasia, who may
comprise one per cent of the
population, have an increased
susceptibility to cancer.[50] If
this predisposition is mediated
via a defect in repair of
damage to DNA that is inflicted
by an environmental agent, then
just that one gene would contribute a significant fraction
of all cancer.

DISTRIBUTION OF CANCER BY CAUSE

SPONTANEOUS (~15%)

GENETIC (~5%)

INTERACTIVE (X%)

ENVIRONMENTAL (80-X%)

Figure 1

There is a great problem
even in those instances of what
may be called the purely genetic forms of cancer, in that
phenotypically identifying features are absent in most
instances. How, for example, can we tell whether a particular
offspring of a person with familial colon cancer (without
polyposis) carries the gene or not? That offspring will

usually even reproduce before colon cancer develops. What is
needed is a laboratory means for identifying such persons.
For example, retinoblastoma occurs in a heritable form and in
a nonhereditary form. The risk of tumor in a carrier of the
retinoblastoma mutation is 100,000 times greater than it is
for the child who does not carry the gene.[30] All bilateral
cases are genetic, but some unilateral cases are genetic and
some are not. Can we identify those at risk of passing the
mutation on to their offspring?

Some recent investigations may prove to be useful in this
regard. Two groups of investigators have reported that skin
fibroblasts from patients with the hereditary form of retinoblastoma are sensitive to the lethal effects of ionizing
radiation, although not to the extent that cells from persons
with ataxia telangiectasia are.[52] Unfortunately, this indicator cannot discriminate between normal and abnormal in all
cases. For polypsis coli Kopelovich has reported that skin
fibroblasts grow to greater than normal density in vitro,
tolerate low serum concentrations in the medium, and can be
transformed by phorbol esters into colonies able to grow in
agar or in the anterior chamber of the eye of the nude
mouse.[34] These findings offer for another genetic cancer the
possibility that laboratory identification may be possible.

In a few instances the genetic abnormality that predisposes
to cancer can be visualized cytogenetically. A unique family
with renal carcinoma in 10 of its members was recently
reported in which the affected individuals available for study
all showed in their lymphocytes a translocation between chromosomes 3 and 8.[9] In two cases the tumor was found as a
result of knowing that the translocation was present. In this
family then the finding of normal karyotype can be very reas-
suring, whereas the finding of the abnormality is associated
with an approximately 90 per cent risk of a specific cancer.
No other pedigrees with renal carcinoma show such a karyotypic
abnormality, so most hereditary cases probably result from
sub-microscopic alterations in some gene, perhaps the same
gene that is critical in the translocation pedigree.

Some small fraction of patients with retinoblastoma also
shows a karyotypic abnormality, a deletion in the long arm of
chromosome 13 (13 q$^-$). The deletions vary in size but all
include band 14 (13 q 14). With a new technique for extending
chromosomes and thereby greatly increasing the number of
visible bands, Yunis has identified one case in which there is
a subband deletion within band 14.[53] It may be that cases
thought previously not to show such a deletion will now do so.
The best interpretation of the data available is that in some
instances of the genetic form of retinoblastoma band 14 is
deleted, in others, mutated in a way that is not visible

microscopically. A spectrum of changes from point mutation to
deletion could be expected.

As noted earlier, this same deletion, 13 q 14, has also
been observed in the tumor cells of some patients with the
nonhereditary form of retinoblastoma; in these instances the
lymphocytes and fibroblasts are normal. It seems then that
some initial change can occur in the same specific chromosomal
site in both hereditary and nonhereditary cases; germinal and
somatic mutation affect the same target locus. Is this locus
a "retinoblastoma gene"? Does the presence of the normal
allele at this site ensure that retinoblastoma will not occur,
its absence, greatly increase the chance that it will. We
note in passing that in the genetic cases, including the constitutional deletion cases, all of the somatic cells carry the
mutation, yet only a few of those in the primary target tissue
become tumor cells. The mutation is not sufficient; it only
increases greatly the probability that tumor will occur.

Similar information has recently become available for
Wilms' tumor. This tumor is also known in a hereditary and
nonhereditary form. In a few cases, the patient also has
congenital aniridia. Strong and I proposed that such cases
might be due to a deletion, in all cells, that includes both
an "aniridia" gene and a Wilms' tumor gene.[32] In fact a
deletion in the short arm of chromosome 11 was discovered by
Riccardi in several cases, and, again, a precise karyotypic
localization, 11 p 13, has been established.[15,44] We now
predict that deletions of this locus will also be found in
only the tumor cells of some nonhereditary cases.

We cannot reasonably expect that any substantial fraction
of genetic cases of cancer will show cytogenetic abnormality,
even with highly refined techniques. Perhaps in the future we
shall be able to identify carriers of cancer genes by
alterations in DNA, but for now we must rely on other means.
In addition to the phenotypic and karyotypic methods already
mentioned, there is another genetic technique that may be
useful in a given pedigree. This is the method of genetic
linkage, which has recently been applied to the analysis of
breast cancer. This method depends upon the close proximity
on the same chromosome of the gene of interest and a gene
whose product is known, and which demonstrates significant
genetic variation (polymorphism) in a population. This method
can be applied to a cancer family when the cancer gene carriers show two forms of the adjacent gene, because this means
that the member of this particular chromosome pair that
carries the cancer gene will be associated (linked) with one
form of the adjacent gene and the member that does not carry
the cancer gene will be linked with the other form of the
adjacent gene. The products of the adjacent gene can

therefore serve as markers for the presence or absence of the cancer gene in a given pedigree. By this method King and colleagues have demonstrated that one genetic form of breast cancer is linked to the gene for serum glutamate-pyruvate transaminase (GPT).[26] Therefore, in some families GPT may be used as a marker for the presence of the breast cancer gene. Since the GPT gene is thought to be located on the short arm of chromosome 10, it may be that the tumor in some cases of breast cancer will actually show a deletion there and that in some few families there may even be an aberration at that site in all somatic cells. Linkage analysis is a promising method for revealing the location of cancer genes. Unfortunately it is useful only in families with cancer, and then only if polymorphic neighboring genes are available. This latter difficulty may be ameliorated by the application of restriction enzyme mapping, as recently described by Botstein and colleagues.[6]

HUMAN CANCER GENES

The picture that has emerged from the study of environmental and hereditary cancers is that mutation, somatic or germinal, occurs at specific genetic sites and is followed later by the development of a cancer from one or more mutant cells. In the classical parlance of environmental carcinogenesis the cell has been "initiated". So initiation can be somatic or germinal, spontaneous or induced. However, we cannot say that all cancers follow upon initiating mutations. The reversible teratocarcinomas of mice seem to originate in some other way, perhaps through some functional activation or inactivation of the same gene sites at which mutation can initiate carcinogenesis.[37] It may also be that the oncogenic viruses act through quite other pathways. If activation of oncogenes, either viral or host, can lead to cancer, then viral oncogenesis entails the <u>presence</u> of some function, whereas an initiating chromosomal deletion obviously involves loss of a function, albeit perhaps regulatory.[5] It seems unlikely that the two can be identical. It is possible, however, that the class of dominantly heritable cancer genes regulate the class of oncogenes as suggested by Comings.[10]

The problem of the generation of neoplasms from initiated cells is a central one in carcinogenesis. Early experiments in animals demonstrated that large doses of initiating carinogens could generate cutaneous carcinomas. On the other hand, benign papillomas are produced when low doses of carcinogens are combined with repeated applications of chemical promoters that themselves are not carcinogenic or mutagenic.

Only occasional carcinomas develop and the papillomas themselves regress when promoter is discontinued. These experiments stimulated the notion of a two-stage sequence for
carcinogenesis.[3]

So whether a cell is initiated by a germinal mutation or by
a somatic mutation, that event is insufficient to produce a
malignant tumor. The same conclusion has been reached by
epidemiologists who have studied the age-dependent increase in
age-specific incidence of various human cancers.[11] The chief
controversy concerns the number of "events" that lie between
initiation and detectable tumor and whether these events are
genetic or not genetic. Finding conclusive evidence that
bears on the controversy is very difficult, however. It could
be extremely helpful to be able to transform initiated cells
into malignant cells in vitro, under conditions where the
kinetics and cell biology of the transformation can be
analyzed.

The most intriguing possibility regarding further steps is
that only one rare event is involved in transforming an initiated cell into a malignant one.[21] If the kinetics of tissue
formation from stem cells and multiplication of the latter are
taken into account, a model based on two events can be shown
to be consistent with the results of experimental carcinogenesis and, in its mathematical form, able to be fitted to
all of the epidemiological features of three tested tumors:
retinoblastoma, breast cancer and lung cancer.[38] According to
this model the intermediate, initiated cells may multiply at
different rates from the target cells from which they arise
(Fig. 2) thus causing benign tumors such as papillomas,
adenomatous polyps, or neuro-
fibromas, or hyperplastic
lesions such as the C-cell
hyperplasia found in Sipple's
disease.[2,13,24] A second event
is responsible for the emergence of the corresponding
malignant tumors, carcinoma of
the skin or colon, neurofibro-
sarcoma, or medullary carcinoma
of the thyroid.

The matter of the kinetics
of multiplication, differentiation, and death of normal and
intermediate cells underscores
the importance of not concentrating only upon the transformation events themselves.
Agents that do not effect the

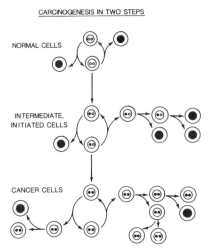

CARCINOGENESIS IN TWO STEPS

NORMAL CELLS

INTERMEDIATE,
INITIATED CELLS

CANCER CELLS

Figure 2

transformation steps directly may bear more on human carcinogenesis even than initiators do. For example, infection with
EB virus may operate upon the kinetics of cells rather than
the transformation process. The study of a sex-linked recessive disorder, Duncan's disease, and a related condition has
shed light on the origin of Burkitt's lymphoma.[43] Children
with these hereditary diseases often develop a fatal, progressive hyperplasia of lymph nodes in response to EB virus infection. In some instances recovery is followed by the
development of Burkitt's lymphoma, which is then associated
with the usual translocation between chromosomes 8 and 14.
Recent investigations suggest that EB virus normally stimulates B lymphocytes to undergo more than the usual number of
cell divisions, but the process is then modified by killer and
suppressor T cells.[45,49] It is this T cell response that
seems to fail in the hereditary diseases, thus leading to
progressive hyperplasia or to the emergence of a clone of
Burkitt's lymphoma cells. Perhaps this discovery will lead to
elucidation of the mechanism by which several hereditary
immunodeficiency diseases predispose to cancer, especially of
the lymphoreticular system.[14]

A second event – an event that converts an initiated intermediate cell into a cancer cell – does seem to be essential in
carcinogenesis. A specific suggestion regarding the nature of
a second event is that it involves the replacement or loss of
the corresponding normal gene that is in the homologous chromosome; i.e., a cancer cell is recessively defective for a
single gene. Such an outcome could arise in one of three
ways: mutation, loss by nondisjunction, or somatic recombination. This last possibility has been offered as an explanation for the high incidence of cancers of various kinds in
Bloom's syndrome, where homologous chromosome exchange is
known to occur, and for the production of carcinomas by chemical promoters.[12,27]

Regardless of the number or nature of subsequent events, it
is apparent that the initiating mutation is extremely important. If the recessive gene hypothesis is correct, there is
only one genetic defect, present in the homozygous state.
Even if that idea is not correct, we could still learn much
about the pathophysiology of cancer by discovering the normal
function of the genes in which mutation initiates cancer.
From the heritable cancers we learn that these genes show
great tissue specificity and are almost certainly important
differentiation genes. Clearly the isolation and characterization of such a gene could illuminate the basic defect in a
cancer and at the same time the genetic control of
development.[31]

Isolation of a gene whose product is unknown provides a great challenge. Yet there are some rays of hope.' Thus the procedure of chromosome sorting by flow cytometry may permit the isolation and concentration of chromosomes that carry cancer genes. In fact chromosome 13, carrier of the retinoblastoma gene, has been reported to be the chromosome obtainable in purest form by this method.[7] Another procedure entails isolation of hybrids between human and rodent cells that have eliminated all except one human chromosome. In this way chromosome 11, the carrier of a Wilms' tumor gene, has been isolated from other human chromosomes.[51] Once obtained, can particular genes be isolated? Perhaps the best opportunity is provided by chromosome 11, whose short arm carries not only the Wilms' tumor gene, but also, in an adjacent band, the β-globin gene complex, and for which there are already some DNA probes.[17] Application of the technology of "gene walking" may yet be possible, although the distance between the Wilms' tumor gene and any known gene may still be too great. Still it is conceivable that by proper use of deleted, mutant, and normal chromosomes isolation will be accomplished. From there it might be possible to transcribe the DNA and discover for the first time the product of a human cancer gene. Such a product might in turn provide a new approach to the treatment of cancer.

CONCLUDING REMARKS

During the past decade the genetic analysis of human cancer has provided new support for the concept that somatic mutation, both spontaneous and induced by environmental mutagens, play a major role in its origin. The existence of genetic states that predispose to environmental mutagenesis reminds us that the interaction of heredity and environment is important in carcinogenesis. The specificity of chromosomal aberrations in some cancers strongly suggests that certain genetic loci are the target for cancer-inducing mutations, whether these are somatic or germinal in origin and that they can be considered as "cancer genes". The pathway from initiated cell to cancer is not well understood, but it offers other sites for the interactions of heredity and environment. Two major tasks in the genetic study of cancer are the explication of events on this pathway and the isolation and characterization of cancer genes. Both have major implications not only for cancer biology but also for the prevention, diagnosis, and treatment of cancer.

REFERENCES

1. Ames BN, Durston WE, Yamasaki E, Lee FD: Carcinogens are mutagens: a simple test system combining liver homogenates for activation and bacteria for detection. Proc Natl Acad Sci USA 70:2281-2285, 1973.

2. Baylin SB, Hsu SH, Gann DS, Smallridge RC, Wells SA: Inherited medullary thyroid carcinoma: a final monoclonal mutation in one of multiple clones of susceptible cells. Science 199:429-431, 1978.

3. Berenblum I: The two-stage mechanism of carcinogenesis in biochemical terms, in Shubik P (ed): The Physiopathology of Cancer, Vol. 1: Biology and Biochemistry. Basel:Kanger, 1974, pp 393-402.

4. Berg JW: World-wide variations in cancer incidence as clues to cancer origins, in Hiatt HH, Watson JD, Winsten JA (eds): Origins of Human Cancer. Cold Spring Harbor, Cold Spring Harbor Laboratory, 1977, pp 15-19.

5. Bishop JM, Gonda T, Hughes SH, et al: The genesis of avian retrovirus oncogenes, in Genes, Chromosomes, and Neoplasia. Thirty-third Annual Symposium on Fundamental Cancer Research. M.D. Anderson Hospital and Tumor Institute, 1980, (in press).

6. Botstein D, White RL, Skolnick M, Davis RW: Construction of a genetic linkage map in man using restriction fragment length polymorphisms. Am J Hum Genet 32:314-331, 1980.

7. Carrano AV, Gray JW, Langlois RG, et al: Measurement and purification of human chromosomes by flow cytometry and sorting. Proc Natl Acad Sci USA 76:1382-1384, 1979.

8. Cleaver JE: Defective repair replication of DNA in xeroderma pigmentosum. Nature 218:652-656, 1968.

9. Cohen AJ, Li FP, Berg S, et al: Hereditary renal-cell carcinoma associated with a chromosomal translocation. N Engl J Med 301:592-595, 1979.

10. Comings DE: A general theory of carcinogenesis. Proc Natl Acad Sci USA 70:3324-3328, 1973.

11. Doll R: The age distribution of cancer: implications for models of carcinogenesis. J Royal Stat Soc Ser A 134:133- 166, 1971.

12. Festa RS, Meadows AT, Boshes RA: Leukemia in a black child with Bloom's syndrome: somatic recombination as a possible mechanism for neoplasia. Cancer 44:1507-1510, 1979.

13. Fialkow PJ: Clonal origin and stem cell evolution of human tumors, in Mulvihill JJ, Miller RW, Fraumeni JF Jr. (eds): Genetics of Human Cancer. New York, Raven Press, 1977, pp 439-453.

14. Filipovich AH, Spector BD, Kersey J: Immunodeficiency in humans as a risk factor in the development of malignancy. Preventive Med 9:252-259, 1980.

15. Francke U, Holmes LB, Atkins L, Riccardi VM: Aniridia-Wilms' tumor association: evidence for specific deletion of 11p13. Cytogenet Cell Genet 24:185-192, 1979.

16. German J. (Editor): Chromosomes and Cancer. New York, John Wiley and Sons, 1974, pp 601.

17. Gusella JF, Keys C, Varsanyi-Breiner A, et al: Isolation and localization of DNA segments from specific human chromosomes. Proc Natl Acad Sci USA 77:2829-2833, 1980.

18. Harnden DG, Taylor AMR: Chromosomes and neoplasia, in Harris H, Hirschhorn K (eds): Advances in Human Genetics, Vol. 9. New York, Plenum Press, 1979, pp 1-70.

19. Harris CC, Mulvihill JJ, Thorgeirsson SS, Minna JD: Individual differences in cancer susceptibility. Ann Intern Med 92: 809-825, 1980.

20. Hashem N, Khalifa SH: Retinoblastoma: a model of hereditary fragile chromosomal regions. Hum Hered 25:35-49, 1975.

21. Hethcote HW, Knudson AG: A model for the incidence of embryonal cancers: application to retinoblastoma. Proc Natl Acad Sci USA 75:2453-2457, 1978.

22. Higginson J, Muir CS: The role of epidemiology in elucidating the importance of environmental factors in human cancer. Cancer Detect Prev 1:79-105, 1976.

23. International Cancer Research Data Bank, National Cancer Institute: Genetic Predisposition to Cancer in Man (Oncollogy Overview), Knudson AG (ed). Springfield, VA, National Technical Information Service, 1980, pp 143.

24. Jackson CE, Block MA, Greenawald KA, Tashjian AH: The two-mutational-event theory in medullary thyroid cancer. Am J Hum Genet 31:704-710, 1979.

25. Kellermann G, Shaw CR, Luyten-Kellermann M: Aryl hydrocarbon hydroxylase inducibility and bronchogenic carcinoma. New Engl J Med 289:934-937, 1973.

26. King MC, Go RCP, Elston RC, Lynch HT, Petrakis NL: Allele increasing susceptibility to human breast cancer may be linked to the glutamate-pyruvate transaminase locus. Science 208:406-408, 1980.

27. Kinsella A, Radman M: Tumor promoter induces sister chromatid exchanges: relevance to mechanisms of carcinogenesis. Proc Natl Acad Sci USA 75:6149–6153, 1978.

28. Klein G: Lymphoma development in mice and humans: diversity of initiation is followed by convergent cytogenetic evolution. Proc Natl Acad Sci USA 76:2442–2446, 1979.

29. Knudson AG: Mutation and cancer: statistical study of retinoblastoma. Proc Natl Acad Sci USA 68:820–823, 1971.

30. Knudson AG: Genetics and etiology of human cancer. Adv Hum Genet 8:1–66, 1977.

31. Knudson AG: Human cancer genes, in Genes, Chromosomes, and Neoplasia. Thirty-third Annual Symposium on Fundamental Cancer Research. M.D. Anderson Hospital and Tumor Institute, 1980, (in press).

32. Knudson AG, Strong LC: Mutation and cancer: a model for Wilms' tumor of the kidney. J Natl Cancer Inst 48:313–324, 1972.

33. Knudson AG, Strong LC, Anderson DE: Heredity and cancer in man. Prog Med Genet 9:113–158, 1973.

34. Kopelovich L, Bias NE, Helson L: Tumour promoter alone induces neoplastic transformation of fibroblasts from humans genetically predisposed to cancer. Nature 282:619–621, 1979.

35. Lynch HT: Genetics, etiology and human cancer. Preventive Med 9:231–243, 1980.

36. Maher VM, Ouellette LM, Curren RD, McCormick JJ: Frequency of ultraviolet light-induced mutation is higher in xeroderma pigmentosum variant cells than in normal human cells. Nature 261:593–595, 1976.

37. Mintz B: Genetic mosaicism and in vivo analyses of neoplasia and differentiation, in Saunders GF (ed): Cell Differentiation and Neoplasia. New York, Raven Press, 1978, pp 27–53.

38. Moolgavkar SH, Venzon DJ: Two-event model for carcinogenesis: incidence curves for childhood and adult tumors. Math Biosci 47:55–77, 1979.

39. Mulvihill JJ, Miller RW, Fraumeni JF: Genetics of Human Cancer. New York, Raven Press, 1977, pp 519.

40. Nebert DW, Robinson JR, Niwa A, et al: Genetic expression of aryl hydrocarbon hydroxylase activity in the mouse. J Cell Physiol 85:393–414, 1975.

41. Nowell PC, Hungerford DA: A minute chromosome in human chronic granulocytic leukemia. Science 132:1497, 1960.

42. Paterson MC, Smith BP, Lohman PHM, et al: Defective excision repair of X-ray damaged DNA in human (ataxia telangiectasia) fibroblasts. Nature 260:444-447, 1976.
43. Purtilo DT, Cassel CK, Yang JPS, et al: X-linked recessive progressive combined variable immunodeficiency (Duncan's disease). Lancet i:935-940, 1975.
44. Riccardi VM, Sujansky E, Smith AC, Francke U: Chromosomal imbalance in the aniridia-Wilms' tumor association: 11p interstitial deletion. Pediatrics 61:604-610, 1978.
45. Robinson JE, Brown N, Andimann W, et al: Diffuse polyclonal B-cell lymphoma during primary infection with Epstein-Barr virus. N Engl J Med 302:1293-1297, 1980.
46. Rowley JD: A new consistent chromosomal abnormality in chronic myelogenous leukemia identified by quinacrine fluorescence and Giemsa staining. Nature (London) 243:290- 293, 1973.
47. Rowley JD, Golomb HM, Dougherty C: 15/17 translocation, a consistent chromosomal change in acute promyelocytic leukemia. Lancet 1:549-550, 1977.
48. Sandberg AA: The Chromosomes in Human Cancer and Leukemia, New York, Elsevier North Holland Inc, 1980, pp 748.
49. Schwartz RS: Epstein-Barr virus - oncogen or mitogen? New Engl J Med 302:1307-1308, 1980.
50. Swift M, Sholman L, Perry M, Chase C: Malignant neoplasms in the families of patients with ataxia-telangiectasia. Cancer Res 36:209-215, 1976.
51. Waldren C, Jones C, Puck TT: Measurement of mutagenesis in mammalian cells. Proc Natl Acad Sci USA 76:1358-1362, 1979.
52. Weichselbaum RR, Nove J, Little JB: X-ray sensitivity of diploid fibroblasts from patients with hereditary or sporadic retinoblastoma. Proc Natl Acad Sci USA 75:3962-3964, 1978.
53. Yunis JJ, Ramsay N: Retinoblastoma and subband deletion of chromosome 13. Am J Dis Child 132:161-163, 1978.

Genetic Epidemiology of Human Cancer

Mary-Claire King, Ph.D.

Assistant Professor of Epidemiology
School of Public Health
University of California
Berkeley, California

A DEFINITION OF GENETIC EPIDEMIOLOGY

Virtually since cancer has been recognized, physicians have observed, treated, and tried to counsel families in which the disease appears much more frequently than one would expect by chance. But why does cancer sometimes appear to cluster in families? Are there genetic factors inherited in such families that increase susceptibility to certain cancers? Or do many relatives in these families share cultural practices, dietary habits, or poor health behaviors that might increase their risk of cancer at specific sites? Or have many members of the same family been exposed to the same environmental carcinogen? Certainly, the answers to these questions will differ for various high-risk families and for different neoplastic diseases.

The goal of genetic epidemiology is to unravel the genetic, cultural, and environmental contributions to cancer susceptibility in families with significantly high incidence of the disease. The tools of genetic epidemiology are statistical genetics and epidemiology. For the past several years, we have been using this approach to study breast cancer and cancers associated with breast in extended families at extraordinarily high risk of the disease.

THE FAMILIAL NATURE OF BREAST CANCER

Until very recently, breast cancer was considered too "difficult" a disease to be susceptible to analysis by the methods of genetic epidemiology. Breast cancer is, after all, clearly complex epidemiologically, probably heterogeneous etiologically, and highly variable in age of onset. However, timely developments in three rather different fields lead us

to believe that the problem of disentangling the genetic and
environmental causes of breast cancer in families could be
effectively approached. These contributions were (1) the epidemiologic demonstration of the familial nature of breast cancer, (2) the creation of statistical tools for testing genetic
and environmental models of disease susceptibility in large
pedigrees, and (3) the development of a large repertoire
of clinically innocuous, polymorphic genetic markers which
allow us to test whether a hypothesized allele for increased
susceptibility to breast cancer is chromosomally linked to a
known locus.

Breast cancer has historically been a prominent lesion for
epidemiologic studies, both because it is so common and because
it is relatively easily recognized and accurately diagnosed
compared to other cancers. Pedigrees of families with many
cases of breast cancer have been reported since the 19th century. However, it has not always been certain that breast
cancer actually clusters in families. This uncertainty was
due primarily to the high prevalence of breast cancer in the
general population, so that it was not clear that occasional
examples of familial concentration were not merely due to
chance. Investigators therefore began recording information
from series of breast cancer patients, noting the incidence
(or mortality) of this disease among the patients' relatives
in comparison to its incidence (or mortality) among the relatives of cancer-free women[11]. Convincing epidemiologic evidence
now indicates that probably the single factor most dramatically
increasing a woman's risk of breast cancer is the presence of
the disease in her immediate family, especially if more than
one relative has had breast cancer, or if the relative was
affected bilaterally or at a young age[1,2].

STATISTICAL MODELS OF DISEASE SUSCEPTIBILITY

Parallel advances in mathematical tools from the field of
human genetics have allowed us to apply the techniques of
segregation and linkage analysis to family studies[5]. Specifically, we can determine whether breast cancer in high-risk
families occurs in a pattern consistent with a disease largely
determined by a putative "breast cancer susceptibility gene."
Such a hypothetical susceptibility gene must segregate according to Mendelian Laws; could be dominant or recessive on the
X chromosome or an autosome; and would be strongly influenced
in its expression by the sex and age of family members of the
susceptible genotypes. In 14 of the high-risk families we
have studied so far, the pattern of occurrence of breast cancer is consistent with the inheritance of an autosomal dominant allele greatly increasing susceptibility to breast cancer

in women. Under this model, susceptibility to breast cancer could be inherited from either the father or mother, though in general only women would be susceptible. Furthermore, women in these families who do not carry a susceptibility allele are at no increased risk of breast cancer[6].

The consistency of a genetic model with the pattern of breast cancer occurrence in a family needs to be interpreted cautiously, however. Cultural inheritance can, and frequently does, mimic genetic inheritance[4]. For example, families with many cases of lung cancer may appear, not because of genetic susceptibility, but because the smoking habit is passed from parents to children. In other words, smoking--and therefore susceptibility to lung cancer--is culturally inherited in such families. Though no comparable cultural influence is known for breast cancer, it is nevertheless necessary to verify the genetic model in these families.

LINKAGE ANALYSIS

An effective means of verifying a model of genetic transmission is through linkage analysis[12]. The principle of linkage analysis is that if a hypothetical allele influencing disease susceptibility exists, then it must be a length of DNA on one of the 23 pairs of human chromosomes. If the chromosomal location of the susceptibility allele can be determined, then the susceptibility allele exists, even if its protein product remains unknown.

In order to map the chromosomal location of a hypothetical susceptibility gene, we use marker genes whose chromosomal locations are known, to tract the inheritance of each of the 23 autosomes and the X and Y chromosomes through a family. If one allele of one of these marker genes is consistently inherited with breast cancer susceptibility within a family, then a susceptibility allele for breast cancer may be chromosomally linked to that marker gene in that family. The hypothetical family in Figure 1 illustrates this approach. Suppose the results of segregation analysis indicate that an autosomal model for breast cancer transmission is consistent with the observed pattern of breast cancer occurrence in this extended family. Some family members will, of course, no longer be living, but suppose that for every person in the pedigree, we know the current age or age at death, whether the individual had cancer, and if so, at what site. Suppose also that we obtain blood samples for genetic marker analysis from each living member of the family. Possible results for a genetic marker with three common alleles A, B and C might be as illustrated in Figure 1. The putative autosomal dominant allele

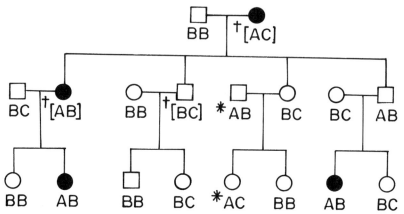

Figure 1. *A hypothetical family with breast cancer, analyzed at a genetic marker with alleles A, B, and C. Dark circles represent women with breast cancer, whose disease suscepti- bility is consistent with autosomal dominant inheritance. Crosses indicate deceased individuals, whose genotypes at marker loci can be assigned probabilistically, based on the marker genotypes of their relatives (such "reconstructed" geno- types are in brackets).*

increasing susceptibility to breast cancer among women in this family may be linked to the $\underline{A}$ allele at the marker locus on one of the grandmother's chromosomes. A much larger family than this one, or several families each demonstrating the same trend, would be required to confirm the linkage. Other fami- lies in which linkage of breast cancer susceptibility and this marker locus appears likely will not necessarily show linkage to the $\underline{A}$ allele. Furthermore, possession of an $\underline{A}$ allele at the marker locus does not necessarily indicate the presence of the breast cancer susceptibility allele in this family (see * in the figure)--only if the A allele represents the grandmother's chromosome (and recombination between the susceptibility allele and the marker locus has not occurred). In other words, link- age between a susceptibility allele and a marker locus does not imply that any particular genotype at the marker locus will be associated with disease susceptibility in the general popu- lation or even among a group of high-risk families. The marker locus cannot be used to screen for breast cancer risk in the general population--only within certain extended, high- risk families.

The usefulness of linkage analysis depends not only on the power and efficiency of the statistical techniques employed, but also on the number of polymorphic markers available for analysis. That is, even if a breast cancer susceptibility allele is segregating in a family, it is only possible to demonstrate linkage to a marker locus if such a polymorphic marker locus happens to be on the same chromosome as the susceptibility gene, and to be reasonably close to it. Furthermore, since not all genetic markers are segregating in informative patterns in all families, a great many marker systems would be required to "cover" the 23 chromosomes. While the human genome is by no means completely "covered" by markers at present, a great deal of progress has been made in the last decade, so that many markers are now available, and blood storage techniques are sufficiently advanced that samples can be saved for long periods and new markers tested as they are developed. Figure 2 indicates the chromosomal location of each of the polymorphic marker loci currently analyzed by electrophoretic and immunologic techniques[10]. Some chromosomes

POLYMORPHIC GENETIC MARKERS OF THE HUMAN GENOME

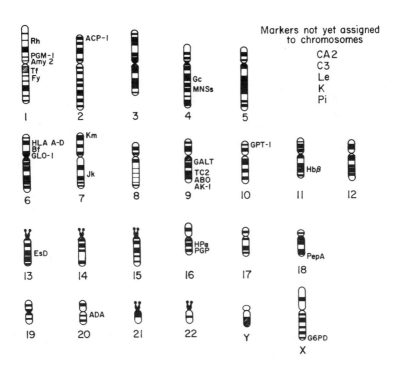

Figure 2.

include several marker genes, so that if a susceptibility
allele happens to lie on such a chromosome, we are very likely
to detect linkage to a marker locus. Other chromosomes include no currently detectable polymorphic genetic markers, or
include markers polymorphic only in certain populations. For-
tunately, the development of DNA mapping techniques should
offer us the possibility of detecting many more polymorphisms
within the next few years[3]. Linkage analysis of the families
at high risk of breast cancer indicates that the marker gene
glutamate-pyruvate transaminase may be close to a dominant
allele increasing susceptibility to breast cancer in some
families [8-7] (Figure 3). The results are highly significant

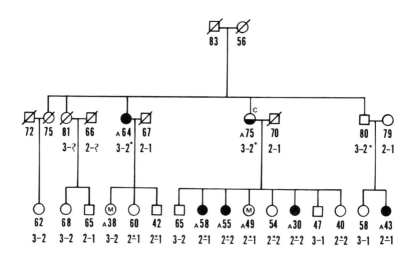

Figure 3. Linkage of GPT to a dominant allele increasing susceptibility to breast cancer in a Mormon family. Filled circles indicate breast cancer cases; half filled circle is a colon cancer patient; M indicates women who had prophylactic bilateral mastectomies. The age presented for each relative is
that person's age at diagnosis, if the person has had cancer;
their age at surgery if they had surgery, their present age,
if they are still alive and cancer free; and their age at
death if they died without having been a cancer patient. In
other words, each person's number of breast cancer-free years
is indicated. The genotype at the GPT locus is also indicated
for each person for whom it could be determined. An * indicates the GPT 2 allele that appears to be linked to the dominant allele for breast cancer susceptibility.

statistically: the odds in favor of linkage between GPT and a susceptibility gene are greater than 400 to one. The GPT locus has been provisionally mapped on chromosome 10, but no other markers polymorphic in Caucasian populations have been located on that chromosome. As polymorphic markers linked to GPT are discovered, they can be tested for linkage to the hypothesized susceptibility allele in the present families.

BIOLOGICAL IMPLICATIONS OF THE LINKAGE RESULT

In biological terms, it is now quite likely that an autosomal dominant allele strongly influencing breast cancer susceptibility exists and is responsible for the high incidence of breast cancer in some families. We believe this to be the first demonstration of the existence of a gene increasing susceptibility to breast cancer. In families in which this susceptibility gene is present, our results predict that women carrying the susceptibility allele have a 12 percent risk of breast cancer by age 35, a 50 percent risk of breast cancer by age 50 and an 87 percent risk of breast cancer by age 80, while their female relatives who do not carry the susceptibility allele have no increased risk of breast cancer[5]. Furthermore, fathers can carry the susceptibility allele and pass the increased risk to their daughters.

However, GPT cannot be used as a screening test for breast cancer. Glutamate-pyruvate transaminase has no physiological relationship to breast cancer. The GPT gene simply marks the chromosomal region where a susceptibility gene of still-unknown function may be located in some families. In the general population, there is no association between a woman's GPT genotype and her risk of breast cancer. Furthermore, there are clearly some families at high risk of breast cancer in which increased susceptibility is not inherited as a gene linked to GPT. The GPT-linked susceptibility appears in families with relatively, though not extremely, young ages of breast cancer diagnosis, and an increased frequency of ovarian cancer. However, at least two other types of breast cancer families have appeared in our studies so far: families with elderly breast cancer patients and increased risk of endometrial cancer, and families with very young breast cancer patients and increased risk of many other cancers affecting young people, including sarcomas, leukemias, brain tumors, and adenocarcinomas[6-9]. It is very likely that the cancer susceptibility in these families is also genetically influenced, but that the genes increasing susceptibility in those families are not linked to GPT. Susceptibility genes in these families may be found on other chromosomes.

We are also investigating why not all genetically-susceptible women develop breast cancer. The influence of cultural
and environmental factors on breast cancer risk in the general
population is well established. Do these same factors modify
the increased risk of genetically-susceptible women, or do
other factors, perhaps of less importance in the general population, protect some genetically-susceptible women from development of breast cancer? We are now investigating these questions using epidemiological methods.

Finally, what are the biochemical and physiological mechanisms by which a gene increases breast cancer susceptibility?
The linkage of GPT and breast cancer susceptibility in some
families may offer an excellent opportunity to elucidate
breast cancer etiology. Using linkage analysis, it is possible
to identify genetically-susceptible young women who have not
yet developed breast cancer, and other young women in the same
family who are at low risk. By comparing appropriate immunological, biochemical, and endocrinological profiles of these
high-and low-risk young women, it may be possible to determine
the mechanism of expression of the breast cancer susceptibility
allele linked to GPT. If we can determine how susceptibility
genes for breast cancer are expressed, we can begin then to
investigate how to alter this expression to prevent the development of breast cancer in these families.

REFERENCES

[1] Anderson DE: A genetic study of human breast cancer. J Nat
Cancer Inst 48:1029-1034, 1972.

[2] Anderson DE: Genetic study of breast cancer: Identification
of a high-risk group. Cancer 34:1090-1097, 1974.

[3] Botstein D,White RL,Skolnick M,Davis RW: Construction of a
genetic linkage map in man using restriction fragment length
polymorphisms. Amer J Hum Genet 32:314-331, 1980.

[4] Cavalli-Sforza LL,Feldman MW: Cultural versus biological inheritance: phenotypic transmission from parents to children.
Amer J Hum Genet 25:618, 1973.

[5] Elston RC,Go RCP,King MC,Lynch HT: A statistical model for
the study of familial breast cancer, in Lynch HT (ed): Genetics and Breast Cancer, 1980.

[6] Go RCP,King MC,Elston RC,Lynch HT: Genetic epidemiology of
breast and associated cancers in high risk families.
I.Segregation analysis. J Nat Cancer Inst-submitted.

[7] King MC,Bishop DT: Preliminary analysis for linkage of glu-
tamate pyruvate transaminase and breast cancer susceptibility
in a Mormon kindred. in Banbury Report 4: Cancer Incidence in
Defined Populations. Cold Spring Harbor, New York, 1980.

[8] King MC,Go RCP,Elston RC,Lynch HT,Petrakis NL: Allele increasing susceptibility to human breast cancer may be linked to glutamate-pyruvate transaminase locus. Science 208:406-408 1980.

[9] Lynch HT,Mulcahy GM,Harris RE,Guirguis HA,Lynch JF: Genetic and pathologic findings in a kindred with hereditary sarcoma, breast cancer, brain tumors, leukemia, lung, laryngeal, and adrenalcortical carcinoma. Cancer 41:2055-2064, 1978.

[10] McKusick VA: Anatomy of the human genome. Amer J Med 69:267-276, 1980.

[11] Petrakis NL,Ernster VL,King MC: The epidemiology of breast cancer, in Schottenfeld DS,Fraumeni JF (eds):Cancer Epidemiology and Prevention. Philadelphia, Saunders, 1980.

[12] Vogel F,Motulsky AG: Chapter 3 in Human Genetics: Problems and Approaches, New York, Springer, 1979.

This work has been supported by the Breast Cancer Task Force of the National Cancer Institute (grants CA-13556 and CA-27632 and contracts CB-44003 and CB-84274).

Specific fine structural chromosome defects in human neoplasia

JORGE J. YUNIS, M.D.

Professor
Laboratory Medicine and Pathology
University of Minnesota
Minneapolis, Minnesota

Cancer cells have been found to exhibit a wide range of chromosome defects that vary in both degree and number among different cells in the same tissue. These abnormalities include aneuploidy, polyploidy, and numerous types of structural chromosome defects. Until recently, it was believed that chromosomal abnormalities in human cancer represented a non-specific and secondary phenomenon of neoplasia. This was due, in part, to the fact that, except for the association of the Philadelphia chromosome with chronic myelogenous leukemia, no chromosome defect was consistently observed (German, 1974).

Since the advent of banded chromosome techniques in 1971, approximately 20 specific types of tumors (Rowley, 1978; Yunis and Ramsay, 1978, 1980; Mark et al., 1979, 1980; Sandberg, 1980; Wake et al., 1980; Sokal et al, 1980; Yunis, 1981) have been found to exhibit a consistent chromosome defect, most often represented by a reciprocal translocation between two chromosomes in which one remains constant and breaks at a specific site (donor chromosome), while the other varies in type and breakpoint (receptor chromosome). The recent application of high resolution chromosome analysis of synchronized cells (Yunis, 1976) to the study of neoplasia has made it possible to obtain a large number of finely banded mitoses with which we can visualize previously undetectable chromosome defects and determine, at a refined level, the specific site where some cancer genes appear to be localized

This work was supported in part by NIH grant GM26800 and grant No. 1-568 from the National Foundation. Dr. Clara Bloomfield's kind referral of bone marrow samples is gratefully acknowledged. Reprint address: Box 198, University of Minnesota Hospitals, Minneapolis, MN 55455.

(Yunis and Ramsay, 1978, 1980). The increased resolution of
the new techniques dispells the earlier finding that, for
example, approximately 50% of acute non-lymphocytic leukemias
have a normal karyotype (Rowley, 1978; Mitelman, 1980;
Sandberg, 1980).

Based on available evidence from somatic and germinal
mutations in cancer, it has been postulated that cancer results from a mutation of one of some 100 to 200 cancer genes
present in the human genome (Knudson, 1980). With the un-
covering of a minute chromosomal loss in some embryonic carcinomas and specific reciprocal translocations in various
neoplasias, it may become possible to determine the precise
location of many cancer genes in man. In addition, the finding of several specific types of balanced translocations
among groups of patients with acute non-lymphocytic leukemia,
acute lymphocytic leukemia and non-Hodgkin's non-Burkitt's
lymphoma now makes it possible to subdivide these malignancies
into several entities, each with a different clinical course
and response to treatment.

CHRONIC MYELOGENOUS LEUKEMIA

Approximately 90 percent of adult patients suffering with
CML can easily be identified by chromosome analysis; they
exhibit a small chromosome 22 (Philadelphia or Ph^1) (Nowell
and Hungerford, 1960) in which the "missing" distal segment of
the long arm is often translocated to the end of the long arm
of chromosome 9 t(9;22)(q23;11) (Rowley, 1973a; Yunis, 1981).
In approximately five percent of the cases, the distal end of
the long arm of chromosome 22 is translocated to a chromosome
other than No. 9, and almost every chromosome of the human
complement has been involved (Rowley, 1980). Since the small
chromosome 22 and not the abnormal No. 9 is the consistent
defect found in CML, it is evident that chromosome 22 represents the donor chromosome, and possibly an affected gene at
the breakpoint site (band 22q11) may be responsible for the
development of CML. Indeed, finding the Philadelphia chromosome in CML is of prognostic importance: Ph^1-positive
patients respond better to chemotherapy than Ph^1-negative ones
and survive significantly longer periods of time (42 months
for Ph^1-positive compared with 15 months for Ph^1-negative
patients).

ACUTE NON-LYMPHOCYTIC LEUKEMIA (ANLL)

Recent evidence suggests that there are four or five
clinical subgroups of ANLL that can be identified by the type

of chromosome defect found. One group is represented by approximately 10-15 percent of all ANLL patients (Kamada et al., 1976; Golomb et al., 1978) and has a translocation involving the long arm of chromosomes 8 and 21 with breakpoints at band q22 in both chromosomes (Rowley, 1973b). These patients have a hematological picture of acute myelogenous leukemia (AML). They are clinically recognized because the leukemic process has a younger onset age (average age 37 years) and approximately two-thirds of the myeloblasts have Auer rods and low alkaline phosphatase activity. Patients with this disorder respond well to treatment and have a relatively good prognosis (32 weeks average life) (Kamada et al., 1976).

A second group is represented by patients with acute promyelocytic leukemia (APL) in which a translocation involving the long arm of chromosomes 15 and 17 was found (Rowley et al., 1977; Okada et al., 1977; Kaneko and Sakurai, 1977; van den Berghe et al., 1979b) with breakpoints in band q21 of chromosome 17 and band q26 of chromosome 15 (Yunis, 1981). Patients with APL have hypergranular promyelocytes and a tendency to develop intravascular coagulation unless prompt diagnosis is made and heparin therapy initiated (Golomb et al., 1979). Although there is no definitive information, chromosome 17 appears to be the donor chromosome since in one of the patients reported by van den Berghe et al. (1979b) there was a "deletion" in the long arm of chromosome 17 and the two chromosomes 15 were normal, suggesting a "hidden" translocation of chromosome 17 to a different chromosome.

A third group of patients with ANLL shows a Ph[1] chromosome, has a poor response to therapy and a significantly short survival period (two months survival) (Bloomfield et al., 1977, 1978). Because these patients show the same 9;22 translocation found in CML, it has been postulated that Ph[1]-positive AML represents a defect of a more primitive stem cell line than the one involved in CML (Janossy et al., 1976; Bloomfield et al., 1978).

In addition to the three main groups of ANLL patients with a clearly defined translocation, we have recently found three patients with acute myelomonocytic leukemia (AMMoL) and a reciprocal translocation involving chromosome 11 with breakpoints occurring at band q23 (Yunis, 1981). In these patients, contracted mid-metaphases gave equivocal results and the abnormality could only be delineated with elongated chromosomes. In two of the patients the translocation involved a receptor chromosome 6 with breakpoint in band q27 and the translocation of the third patient involved a receptor chromosome 9 with breakpoint at band p22. These cases suggest that among patients with AMMoL a new group with a specific translocation involving chromosome 11 with breakpoint in band q23 may be found.

At present, the largest subgroup of ANLL reported to have a chromosomal abnormality does not appear to contain specific reciprocal translocations. Instead, they exhibit a variety of non-random structural or numerical chromosome defects, including in 85% of the cases, one or more of four particular changes: monosomy or partial deletion of chromosome 5, monosomy or partial deletion of chromosome 7, trisomy 8, and trisomy 21 (Sakurai and Sandberg, 1973; Rowley, 1978; Mitelman and Levan, 1978). Mitelman and Levan (1978) proposed that these chromosomes, whether in a monosomic or trisomic state, confer proliferative advantage to the leukemic cells and may explain the short survival of affected patients (average survival = 2 months). Mitelman has also suggested that patients in this group generally have a history of exposure to chemical solvents and insecticides (Mitelman et al., 1978, 1979b).

In the literature, it is widely accepted that approximately 50% of all cases of ANLL have a normal karyotype (Mitelman and Levan, 1978; Sandberg, 1980; Rowley, 1980). Using high resolution chromosome analysis, we studied 25 untreated adults with ANLL and found chromosomal abnormalities in all cases. In six of the cases, however, between 65 and 73% of the analyzed mitoses were normal, while a small population of poor quality mitotic spreads showed a chromosome defect. In 5 additional cases an abnormality was found in most cells, but the defect was not clear in contracted metaphases and could only be delineated through careful analysis of finely banded chromosomes (Yunis, 1981). This study suggests that with the use of new techniques, the majority of ANLL patients will probably be found to have structural and/or numerical chromosome abnormalities.

ACUTE LYMPHOCYTIC LEUKEMIA (ALL)

A reciprocal translocation (4;11) recently revealed in ALL can now be added to the list of specific chromosome defects in malignancies presently known. This translocation has been observed in 9 out of 117 patients with ALL (Oshimura et al., 1977; van den Berghe et al., 1979a; Prigogina et al., 1979). In four of the nine reported cases, the patients were babies with inborn leukemia and high white blood cell count (> 100,000 mm^3) (Prigogina et al., 1979). The t(4;11) form of ALL seems to carry a poor prognosis (< 12 months survival). Commonly, the breakpoints in chromosomes 4 and 11 involve bands q21 and q23, respectively. In two cases of this disorder, however, the translocation involved a chromosome other than No. 11 (van den Berghe, H., personal communication), suggesting chromosome 4 as donor.

Ph[1]-positive ALL is a common occurence representing 25% of adults with ALL (Bloomfield et al., 1977, 1978; Catovsky et al., 1979) and 2 to 10% of children with ALL (Secker Walker et al., 1976; Priest et al., 1980). Finding of the Ph[1] chromosome in ALL is important, since it is a sign of poor prognosis (median survival = 11 months). Since the Ph[1] chromosome is found in most cases of CML and in a large group of patients with ANLL and ALL, it has been postulated that a common carcinogen affects chromosome 22. ALL results when the agent attacks a lymphoid (presumably multi-potent) stem cell, AML when a primitive myeloid stem cell is affected, and CML when the carcinogen acts on a more differentiated myeloid stem cell (Janossy et al., 1976; Bloomfield et al., 1978).

Recently, Berger et al. (1979) and Mitelman et al. (1979a) emphasized the occurrence of B-cell ALL. The leukemic cells resemble those of Burkitt's lymphoma and have a reciprocal translocation 8;14. In these chromosomes, the breakpoints are the same as those found in Burkitt's lymphoma (8q24.1 and 14q32.3; Mitelman et al., 1979a). This variety of ALL is estimated to represent 1-2% of all ALL and occurs more frequently in children than adults (Berger et al., 1979). The presence of an identical t(8;14) translocation and of typical Burkitt's cells in both ALL and Burkitt's lymphoma, suggests a common etiologic factor similar to that responsible for the Ph[1]-positive CML, ANLL and ALL.

NON-HODGKIN'S LYMPHOMA

As in the case of AML, it is becoming evident that non-Hodgkin's lymphomas can be subdivided into several subgroups depending on the type of chromosome translocation involved. In Burkitt's lymphoma, for example, tumor cells of most cases of this disease have a marker chromosome 14 with an extra long long arm (14q+) (Manolov and Manolova, 1972), which is now known to be the product of a translocation between chromosomes 8 and 14 (8;14)(q24;q32) (Zech et al., 1976; Manolova et al., 1979). The 8;14 abnormality has been found in both the African and non-African forms of Burkitt's lymphoma (Zech et al., 1976; McCaw et al., 1977; Douglass et al., 1980) and in a group of patients with B-cell acute lymphocytic leukemia, representing the leukemic counterpart of the lymphomatous process (Berger et al., 1979). As in the case of the Ph[1] chromosome in CML, in a few patients of Burkitt's lymphoma the distal end of the long arm of the donor chromosome 8 translocates to a chromosome other than the common receptor chromosome 14 (van den Berghe et al., 1979c; Miyoshi et al., 1979). This strongly suggests that the breakpoint in band 8q24 (subband 24.1; Manolova et al., 1979) is critical in the development of this neoplasia.

As in Burkitt's lymphoma, there is increasing evidence that patients with non-Hodgkin's non-Burkitt's lymphoma may be found to be associated with relatively consistent types of reciprocal chromosome translocations. For example, several patients with non-Burkitt's non-Hodgkin's lymphoma have been reported to have a translocation involving the long arm of chromosomes 18 and 14; t(14;18)(q32;q21) and a histologic pattern of poorly differentiated lymphocytic malignant lymphoma with typical small cleaved cells (Reeves, 1973; Fukuhara et al., 1979).

Until the present time, emphasis has been placed on the frequent finding of a marker chromosome 14 (14q+) in non-Hodgkin's non-Burkitt's lymphoma (McKaw et al., 1977; Mark et al., 1977; Mitelman and Levan, 1978; Sandberg, 1980). This relates to the frequent occurrence of this defect and ease of detection. Indeed, the marker chromosome 14 has been found in 31 out of 77 of all reported cases of non-Hodgkin's non-Burkitt's lymphoma. In better chromosome preparations and when attention is paid to the donor chromosome, however, it is found to involve with approximately similar frequency chromosomes 1, 8, 11, 14 and 18 with specific breakpoints in bands q23, q22, q13, q24 and q21, respectively (Reeves, 1973; Fleischman and Prigogina, 1977; Fukuhara et al., 1979; Mark et al., 1977, 1978, 1979). If confirmed, these findings may make it possible to classify non-Hodgkin's non-Burkitt's lymphomas into several clinically significant subtypes as is now the case with acute leukemia.

EMBRYONIC CARCINOMAS

The solid tumor that has been most thoroughly studied cytogenetically is retinoblastoma. As an isolated finding, this tumor occurs sporadically (unilateral) (Fuhrmann and Vogel, 1976) or is transmitted in an autosomal dominant fashion (usually bilateral) (Knudson et al., 1975). In a few cases (about 1% of all cases of retinoblastoma, usually associated with congenital defects and/or mental retardation) all the somatic cells of the patient show a deletion in the long arm of chromosome 13 (13q-). A comparative study of these cases shows that one band, 13q14, is always affected and with more refined banding methods it has been shown that the middle third of band 13q14 is the critical site at which a retinoblastoma gene appears to be located (Yunis and Ramsay, 1978). There is now evidence that a related abnormality occurs just in the tumor cells of patients with either unilateral or bilateral retinoblastoma present as an isolated finding and in

whom other cells of the body have a normal chromosome constitution. Using non-banded chromosomes Hashem and Khalifa
(1974) reported a deletion in a D(13-15) group chromosome in
four of five tumors. We have very recently studied the tumor
cells from a patient with bilateral retinoblastoma whose
karyotypes were normal in cultured lymphocytes. In five
chromosome spreads analyzed in detail we found them to show a
subtle reciprocal translocation between chromosomes 13 and 22,
involving breakpoints in bands q14 and q12, respectively
(Yunis, 1981). Also, in an established retinoblastoma cell
line kindly provided by Dr. F. Gilbert, Philadelphia, a reciprocal translocation involving chromosomes 13 and 8 was found.
Unfortunately, however, it is not clear yet if the breakpoint
on chromosome 13 involves band p11 or q14. Balaban-Malenbaum
et al. (1980) has also reported in brief that in tumor
cells from four retinoblastomas, both unilateral and bilateral,
each tumor had one normal and one abnormal chromosome 13 and
that the abnormality on chromosome 13 consistently involved
band p14. These preliminary observations are significant
since they suggest the possibility that the same gene site is
affected in retinoblastoma as part of the 13q deletion syndrome and in retinoblastoma patients in which the tumor appears as an isolated finding (Knudson, 1980).

Similar to the cases of retinoblastoma with the 13q deletion syndrome, Wilms' tumor associated with bilateral
aniridia has been found associated with an interstitial deletion of the short arm of chromosome 11, including band p13
(Riccardi et al., 1978; Francke et al., 1979). In most of
these cases, a deletion involving either bands p11-13 or
p13-15 of the short arm of chromosome 11 was found. With the
use of finely banded chromosomes we have studied four additional cases which only show a loss of the distal half of
band p13 and the small subband p14.1, suggesting that the
critical segment in the aniridia-Wilms' tumor syndrome represents the distal half of band p13 (Yunis and Ramsay, 1980;
Yunis, 1981). These findings provide support to the concept
that there are genes for aniridia and Wilms' tumor which are
located close to each other (Knudson and Strong, 1972) and a
deletion eliminates both. Unlike retinoblastoma, where the
same chromosome site may be affected in most cases, the
possibility exists that there may be different genes that
predispose to Wilms' tumor since the neoplastic process can
be observed as an isolated finding or sometimes associated
with hemihypertrophy, pseudohermaphroditism, glomerulonephritis, aniridia or macroorgans (Beckwith-Wideman syndrome).

Thus far, one short term and one long term cell lines
from patients with Wilms' tumor without associated defects
have been examined in our laboratory. These cell lines,

Wiltu-2 in its 10th passage and SK-NEP-1 in the 39th passage,
were both kindly provided by Dr. Jørgen Fogh, New York, and
showed no deletion or translocation involving band 11p13.
This goes along with the concept that, unlike retinoblastoma,
Wilms' tumor, when present as an isolated finding, may not
involve a genetic abnormality at the same site found for
the Aniridia-Wilms' tumor syndrome.

SUMMARY

With the use of newer chromosome banding techniques, the
last few years of cancer research has yielded the impressive
finding of specific chromosome defects in approximately 20
neoplasias.
In patients with retinoblastoma associated with the 13q-
syndrome, a prezygotic deletion of band q14 of a chromosome
13 has been consistently observed. Further, in the more
common sporadic and hereditary types of retinoblastoma there
is preliminary evidence that a similar chromosome defect (e.g.
reciprocal translocation affecting band 13q14) is found just
in tumor cells. These findings point to the presence of a
retinoblastoma gene which is deleted in constitutional retinoblastoma and altered in sporadic and hereditary cases.
The remarkable finding of specific reciprocal chromosome
translocations in several classes of acute leukemias and non-
Hodgkin's lymphomas, each with a specific breakpoint in the
donor chromosome, also suggests that a given cancer gene may
become affected during the process of chromosomal rearrangement. If this proves correct, it would become possible, for
the first time, to learn about the site and general function
of a large number of cancer genes in man.
Whatever the molecular mechanism involved in the translocation process and its role in the etiology of neoplasia,
there is no doubt that the chromosome defects observed have
already proven useful as prognostic indicators in some neoplasias. In CML, for example, the Ph[1] chromosome, often the
only chromosome abnormality observed, has been shown to be
present throughout the entire course of the disease, and is a
sign of good prognosis when compared with Ph[1]-negative CML.
Likewise, the occurrence of 8;21 translocation in ANLL is a
sign of good prognosis when compared to other types.
Until now, it had not been possible to detect a chromosome
defect in approximately half of all cases of ANLL, ALL and
non-Hodgkin's non-Burkitt's lymphomas. However, the recent
use of high resolution chromosomes to the study of ANLL shows
that most patients have a structural or numerical chromosome
defect that could not be detected with standard techniques.

Also, other improvements in cytogenetic techniques for the study of solid tumors now make it possible to link a specific chromosome translocation in papillary cystoadenocarcinoma of the ovary t(6;14)(q21;q24) (Wake et al., 1980) and mixed parotid gland tumors with early cancerous transformation t(3;8)(p25;q21) (Mark et al., 1980). Obviously, the field of cancer cytogenetics is coming of age and will no doubt bring important new information regarding the role of chromosomes in the etiology, subclassification and treatment of malignancy.

REFERENCES

Balaban-Malenbaum G, Gilbert F, Nichols W: Abnormalities in
  chromosome 13 in direct preparations from human retinoblastoma. Am. Soc. Human Genet., 31st annual mtg., p. 62A,
  Sept. 24-27, 1980.
Berger R, Berhneim A, Brouet JC et al.: t(8;14) translocation
  in a Burkitt's Type of Lymphoblastic Leukemia (L3). Br J
  Haematol 43:87-90, 1979.
Bloomfield CD, Peterson LC, Yunis JJ et al.: The Philadelphia
  chromosome (Ph^1) in adults presenting with acute leukemia:
  a comparison of Ph^1+ and Ph^1- patients. Br J Haematol 36:
  347-358, 1977.
Bloomfield CD, Brunning RD, Smith KA et al.: The Philadelphia
  chromosome in acute leukemia. Virchows Arch B Cell Path 29:
  81-91, 1978.
Catovsky D: Ph^1-positive Acute Leukemia and Chronic Granulocytic Leukemia: One or Two Diseases? Br J Haematol 42:
  493-498, 1979.
Douglass EC, Magrath IT, Lee EC, et al.: Cytogenetic studies
  in Non-African Burkitt Lymphoma. Blood 55(1):148-155, 1980.
Fleischman EW, Prigogina EL: Karyotypic peculiarities of
  malignant lymphomas. Humangenetik 35:269-279, 1977.
Francke U, Holmes LB, Atkins L et al.: Aniridia-Wilms' tumor
  association: evidence for specific deletion of 11p13.
  Cytogenet Cell Genet 24:185-192, 1979.
Fuhrmann W, Vogel F: *Genetic Counseling* (ed 2). New York,
  Springer-Verlag, 1976, pp 31-36.
Fukuhara S, Rowley JD, Variakojis D et al.: Chromosome ab-
  normalities in poorly differentiated Lymphocytic Lymphoma.
  Canc Res 39:3119-3128, 1979.
German J (ed): *Chromosomes and Cancer.* New York, Wiley, 1974.
Golomb HM, Vardiman JW, Rowley JD et al.: Correlation of
  clinical findings with quinacrine-banded chromosomes in 90
  adults with acute non-lymphocytic leukemia. New Engl J
  Med 299: 613-619, 1978.
Golomb HM, Testa JR, Vardiman JW et al.: Cytogenetic and
  ultrastructural features of de novo acute promyelocytic
  leukemia; the University of Chicago experience (1973-1978).
  Cancer Genet Cytogenet 1: 69-78, 1979.
Hashem N, Khalifa Sh: Retinoblastoma: a model of hereditary
  fragile chromosomal regions. Hum Hered 25: 35-49, 1975.
Janossy G, Greaves MF, Lister TA et al.: Blast crisis of
  chronic myeloid leukaemia (CML). II. Cell surface marker
  analysis of 'lymphoid' and myeloid cases. Br J Haematol 34:
  179-192, 1976.
Kamada N, Okada K, Oguma N et al.: C-G translocation in acute
  myelocytic leukemia with low neutrophil alkaline phosphatase
  activity. Cancer 37: 2380-2387, 1976.

Kaneko Y, Sakurai M: 15/17 translocation in acute promyelo-
cytic leukaemia. Lancet I: 961, 1977.
Knudson AG, Jr.: Human Cancer Genes. Thirty-Third Annual
Symposium on Fundamental Cancer Research at M.D. Anderson
Hospital and Tumor Institute of the University of Texas
System Cancer Center. March 4-7, 1980.
Knudson AG, Strong LC: Mutation and cancer: a model for
Wilms' tumor of the kidney. J Natl Cancer Inst 48: 313-324,
1972.
Knudson AG, Meadows AT, Nichols WW et al.: Chromosomal de-
letion and retinoblastoma. New Engl J Med 295: 1120-1123,
1976.
Manolov G, Manolova Y: Marker band in one chromosome 14 from
Burkitt lymphomas. Nature (Lond.) 237: 33-34, 1972.
Manolova Y, Manolov G, Kieler J et al.: Genesis of the 14q+
marker in Burkitt's lymphoma. Hereditas 90: 5, 1979.
Mark J, Ekedahl C, Hagman A: Origin of the translocated seg-
ment of the 14q+ marker in non-Burkitt lymphomas.
Hum Genet 36: 277-282, 1977.
Mark J, Ekedahl C, Dahlenfors R: Characteristics of the
banding patterns in non-Hodgkin and non-Burkitt lymphomas.
Hereditas 88: 229-242, 1978.
Mark J, Dahlenfors R, Ekedahl C: Recurrent chromosomal aber-
rations in non-Hodgkin and non-Burkitt lymphomas. Cancer
Genet Cytogenet 1: 39-56, 1979.
Mark J, Dahlenfors R, Ekedahl C et al.: The mixed salivary
gland tumor - a usually benign human neoplasm frequently
showing specific chromosomal abnormalities. Cancer Genet
Cytogenet (in press), 1980.
McCaw BK, Epstein AL, Kaplan HS et al.: Chromosome 14 trans-
location in African and North American Burkitt's lymphoma.
Int J Cancer 19: 482-486, 1977.
Mitelman F, Brandt L, Nillson PG: Relation among occupational
exposure to potential mutagenic/carcinogenic Agents, Clinical findings, and Bone Marrow Chromosomes in Acute non-
lymphocytic Leukemia. Blood 52(6): 1229-1237, 1978
Mitelman F, Levan G: Clustering of aberrations to specific
chromosomes in human neoplasms. III. Incidence and geographic distribution of aberrations in 856 cases.
Hereditas 89: 207-232, 1978.
Mitelman G, Andersson-Anverg M, Brandt L et al.: Reciprocal
8;14 translocation in EBV-negative B-cell acute lymphocytic
leukemia with Burkitt-type cells. Int J Cancer 24: 27-33,
1979a.
Mitelman F, Nilsson PG, Brandt L et al.: Chromosomes,
Leukaemia, and Occupational Exposure to Leukaemogenic
Agents. Lancet: 1195-1196, 1979b.

Mitelman F: Cytogenetics of experimental neoplasms and non-random chromosome correlations in man. Clin Haematol 9(1): 195-219, 1980.

Nowell PC, Hungerford DA: A minute chromosome in human chronic granulocytic leukemia. Science 132: 1497, 1960.

Okada M, Miyazaki T, Kumota K: 15/17 translocation in acute promyelocytic leukaemia. Lancet i: 961, 1977.

Oshimura M, Freeman AJ, Sandberg AA: Chromosomes and causation of human cancer and leukemia. XXVI. Banding studies in acute lymphoblastic leukemia (ALL). Cancer 40: 1161-1172, 1977.

Prigogina EL, Fleischman EW, Puchkova GP et al.: Chromosomes in Acute Leukemia. Hum Genet 53: 5-16, 1979.

Priest JR, Robison LL, McKenna RW et al.: Philadelphia chromosome positive childhood Acute Lymphoblastic Leukemia. Blood 56(1): 15-22, 1980.

Reeves BR: Cytogenetics of malignant lymphomas: studies utilizing a Giemsa-banding technique. Humangenetik 20: 231-250, 1973.

Riccardi VM, Sujansky E, Smith AC et al.: Chromosomal imbalance in the aniridia-Wilms tumor association: 11p interstitial deletion. Pediatrics 61: 604, 1978.

Rowley JD: A new consistent chromosomal abnormality in chronic myelogenous leukemia identified by quinacrine fluorescence and Giemsa staining. Nature 243: 290-293, 1973a.

Rowley JD: Identification of a translocation with quinacrine fluorescence in a patient with acute leukemia. Annales Genet (Paris) 16: 109-112, 1973b.

Rowley JD, Golomb HM, Vardiman J et al.: Further evidence for a non-random chromosomal abnormality in acute promyelocytic leukemia. Int J Cancer 20: 869-872, 1977.

Rowley JD: Chromosomes in leukemia and lymphoma. Seminars Hematol 15: 301-319, 1978.

Rowley JD: Ph[1]-positive leukaemia, including chronic myelogenous leukaemia. Clin Haematol 9(1): 54-86, 1980.

Rowley JD: Chromosome abnormalities in acute lymphoblastic leukemia. Cancer Genet Cytogenet 1: 263-271, 1980.

Sakurai M, Sandberg AA: Prognosis of acute myeloblastic leukemia: chromosomal correlation. Blood 41: 93-104, 1973.

Sandberg AA: *The Chromosomes in Human Cancer and Leukemia.* Elsevier North Holland, Inc., 1980.

Secker-Walker LM, Hardy JD: Philadelphia chromosome in acute leukemia. Cancer 38: 1619, 1976.

Sokal G, Michaux JL, van den Berghe H: The Karyotype in Refractory Anemia and Pre-leukaemia. Clin Haematol 9(1): 129-139, 1980.

van den Berghe H, David G, Broeckaert-Van Orshoven A et al.: A new Chromosome Anomaly in Acute Lymphoblastic Leukemia (ALL). Hum Genet 46: 173–180, 1979a.

van den Berghe H, Louwagie A, Boreckaert-Van Orshoven A et al.: Chromosome abnormalities in aucte promyelocytic leukaemia (APL). Cancer 43: 558–562, 1979b.

van den Berghe H, Parloir C, Gosseye S et al.: Variant translocation in Burkitt lymphoma. Cancer Genet Cytogenet: (in press), 1979c.

Wake N, Hreshchyshyu MW, Piver SU et al.: Specific cytogenic changes in ovarian cancer. Canc Res: (in press), 1980.

Yunis JJ: High Resolution of Human Chromosomes. Science 191: 1268, 1976.

Yunis JJ, Ramsay N: Retinoblastoma and subband deletion of chromosome 13. Am J Dis Child 132: 161–163, 1978.

Yunis JJ, Ramsay N: Familial occurrence of the aniridia-Wilms' tumor syndrome with deletion 11p13–14.1. J Ped 96(6): 1027–1030, 1980.

Yunis JJ: Fine structural chromosome defects, cancer genes and human malignancy. J Natl Canc Inst: (In press), 1981.

Zech L, Haglund U, Nilsson K et al.: Characteristic chromosomal abnormalities in biopsies and lymphoid cell lines from patients with Burkitt and non-Burkitt lymphomas. Int J Cancer 17: 47–56, 1976.

Clinical Features and Management
of Genetic Cancers

FREDERICK P. LI

Clinical Epidemiology Branch
National Cancer Institute

Department of Biostatistics and Epidemiology
Sidney Farber Cancer Institute
Boston, MA

In our technological era, the medical history and
physical examination remain the principal approaches to
discovery of cancer genes in humans (1). Every clinician
possesses these skills and can contribute to knowledge of
the genetic etiology of human cancers. This chapter describes the use of clinical observation to identify cancer
genes that can be further examined in epidemiologic and
laboratory studies. In addition, potentials for cancer
control through prevention and early detection of genetic
cancers are outlined.

One gene can confer nearly 100 percent risk of a specific
cancer (2). Cancer genes are more potent than strong
environmental carcinogens, which usually induce cancer in
only a small fraction of exposed persons after latent
periods of years to decades. Cancer is the sole or
principal manifestation of some of these genes, such as
that for hereditary retinoblastoma of the eye (3). This
cancer is a model of autosomal dominant cancers in humans
because a high proportion of retinoblastoma is hereditary
and penetrance of the gene is high. In addition, retinoblastoma is usually curable with treatments that do not
reduce fertility, and is diagnosed early in life. Studies
have shown that approximately 1 retinoblastoma in 3 is
inherited as an autosomal dominant trait with penetrance
of 90 percent (3). The remaining two-thirds of cases are
non-hereditary. Clinically, retinoblastoma may be unifocal
or multifocal in one or both eyes. Non-hereditary retinoblastomas are nearly always unifocal and, therefore,

cytoma develops on average 15 years earlier in non-familial cases. The familial forms of these neoplasms also tend to develop as multiple primary cancers in individual patients. In multiple endocrine neoplasia (MEN) type I, tumors develop most often in the pituitary, parathyroids, and pancreatic islet cells, but thyroid, adrenal cortex and other endocrine organs may also be involved (7). In MEN type II, medullary thyroid carcinoma, often bilateral, develops in association with pheochromocytoma and para-thyroid lesions. Patients with MEN type III have medullary thyroid carcinoma, pheochromocytoma and multiple mucosal neuromas. One hypothesis suggests that these constellations of hereditary tumors result from embryonic origin in common of the affected tissues (7). In 2 forms of cancer of the kidney, Wilms' tumor and clear cell adenocarcinoma, bilater-ality and earlier ages at diagnosis are clues of the heredi-tary forms of these neoplasms (2, 8). Future search for hereditary cancers should focus on young patients with multifocal, bilateral or multiple primary cancers who should be evaluated for other evidence of genetic susceptibility.

The clinical features of hereditary cancers have been explained by a 2-mutation model, as proposed by Knudson and modified by others (2, 3, 9). According to the model, patients with hereditary cancer inherited a first (germinal) mutation from one parent. Cancerous clues develop from cells that undergo a second somatic mutation. Somatic mutations in several cells in one organ produce multifocal or bilateral neoplasms, whereas mutations in cells of several organs produce multiple primary cancers. Non-herediatry cancers develop in the rare single cell that undergoes 2 somatic mutations. One somatic mutation in a susceptible person requires less times on average than 2 somatic mutations, and result in earlier age at diagnosis of hereditary cancers.

Neoplasia is the principal manifestation of the genes for retinoblastoma and other hereditary cancers. Other predisposing genetic diseases have a broader range of manifestations, and cancer is only one component or a com-plication of a genetic syndrome. These predisposing genetic disorders can be recognized in the history and physical examination by associated disorders that are pre-neoplastic or other manifestations of the gene. The skin, which is accessible to examination, is an important source of clues to genetic predisposition to cancer (10). More than 50 inherited or inborn disorders affect the skin and predispose to neoplasia, but nosologic classifications of these conditions lack uniformity. Von Recklinghausen's

unilateral. In contrast, hereditary retinoblastoma can be
unilateral or bilateral; bilaterality is a marker of
hereditary retinoblastoma and up to 50 percent of offspring
of these patients are likely to be affected (2). The gene
for retinoblastoma per se is insufficient for development
of the disease because only one or several retinal cells
undergo neoplastic transformation. The additional steps
appear to be time-dependent, and hereditary retinoblastoma
develops nearly 1 year earlier on average than non-hereditary
retinoblastoma. In patients with hereditary retinoblastoma,
organs other than the eyes may be susceptible to cancer and
studies have shown increased risk of osteogenic sarcoma (4).
The bone cancer occurs excessively both within and outside
the field of radiotherapy for the eye tumor. By comparison,
few patients with unilateral disease have developed second
primary neoplasms (4). The finding suggests that the
retinoblastoma gene has pleiotropic effects and can
produce multiple primary cancers.

The location of the gene for retinoblastoma is not known
with certainty. However, reports of the cancer in patients
with deletion of band 14 on the long arm of chromosome 13
(13q 14) suggest that genes in this region have an etiologic role (5). Patients with the deletion usually have
mental retardation, growth retardation, and microcephaly,
presumably because of loss of adjacent genes.

Studies of retinoblastoma and other cancers have revealed
several clinical characteristics of autosomal dominantly
inherited neoplasms. In general, hereditary cancers tend
to develop at earlier ages than usual for the neoplasm,
arise in several foci in one organ or bilaterally in paired
organs, and predispose to development of multiple primary
cancers such as retinoblastoma and osteogenic sarcoma. In
adenomatosis of the colon and rectum, multiple polyps appear
in early adulthood, usually in the second or third decade
of life (6). Median age at diagnosis of colon cancer in
these patients is approximately 40 years, or 15-20 years
earlier than colon cancer in general. Within the lower
intestines, multiple synchronous or metachronous cancers
may develop. In a related polyposis disorder, Gardner's
syndrome, cancer risk extends outside the colon and patients
can also develop adenocarcinoma of the ampulla of Vater
and benign and malignant tumors of bone and soft-tissues (6).
Within the endocrine system, hereditary forms of medullary
thyroid carcinoma, carotid body tumors, pheochromocytoma,
parathyroid tumors, and neuroblastoma may be bilateral and
multifocal; corresponding non-hereditary forms of these
neoplasms are usually unifocal (2). Familial pheochromo-

neurofibromatosis, tuberous sclerosis, von Hippel-Lindau
disease, and Sturge-Weber syndrome are phacomatoses, autosomal dominant diseases that predispose to tumors of the
nervous and vascular systems. These syndromes are recognized by the presence of characteristic hamartomas of the
skin and other dermatologic manifestations. Other dominant
diseases that predispose to cancer also feature skin abnormalities: epidermal cysts, pits in nevoid basal cell carcinoma syndrome; BK moles in hereditary melanoma; angiomas,
lipomas and cysts in Cowden's disease associated with cancers
of the breast, thyroid and other sites; and tylosis of the
palms and soles associated with esophageal cancer (10).
Autosomal recessive diseases with skin abnormalities and
elevated cancer risk include xeroderma pigmentosum, Werner's
syndrome, albinism, and dyskeratosis congenita.

Birth defects may indicate the presence of a genetic
disease that predisposes to cancer. These associated
defects may be anatomical or functional. Laboratory studies
have identified defects in common among genetic diseases
that predispose to specific cancers and suggest biologic
mechanisms of carcinogenesis in these organs. Inborn defects
in immunologic function are associated with high risk of
lymphomas in several recessive diseases: ataxia-telangiectasia, Wiskott-Aldrich syndrome, and X-linked immunodeficiency diseases (11, 12). Chronic hereditary tyrosinemia,
alpha-1-antitrypsin deficiency and hemochromatosis are
associated with the development of cirrhosis and hepatic
cancer (11). Genetic disease that predispose to acute
leukemia can be diagnosed clinically and features associated
chromosome abnormalities: trisomy 21 in Down's syndrome,
and chromosome fragility in autosomal recessive Fanconi's
anemia and Bloom's syndrome (12). Evidence has been shown
that other associations between birth defects and cancer
may have a genetic basis. In Wilms' tumor associated with
aniridia, a deletion of chromosome 11 p13 has been identified (13). Retinoblastoma develops in patients with
deletion of chromosome 13 q14 (5).

Family history is an important source of clues to cancer
etiology. Relatives of patients with diverse forms of
cancer have been found to have a 2-3 fold increase in risk
of the specific cancer in the index patient (12). Familial
aggregation of cancer may result from genetic factors or
carcinogenic exposures in common among relatives, such as
the tendency for concordance of cigarette smoking habits
within families. Furthermore, aggregation of prevalent
forms of cancer in a few families may be due to chance or
biased selection. In the U.S. 1 person in 4 develops cancer

during a lifetime, and among the tens of millions of families in this nation virtually any aggregation of cancers might be due to chance. Other areas of the world are endemic for cancers of the liver and esophagus, and some families can be expected to have large numbers of these cancers. Difficulties in interpreting familial data are exemplified by a recent report from the People's Republic of China (14). In a high rate area for esophageal cancer, the neoplasm developed in 46 members of one family of 613 persons, whereas familial esophageal cancer is rare elsewhere. No evidence was found for predisposing tylosis (11). However, 1 person in 6 in this area of China dies from esophageal cancer, and mortality rate of the cancer exceeds 1 per 100 persons per year in the elderly age groups. In large Chinese families with several hundred members, 46 cancers may not exceed chance frequency. In addition, genetic factors are difficult to distinguish from environmental factors in this endemic area for esophageal cancer. Geographic clustering of the cancer in China suggests the role of carcinogens in the environment, but the family aggregates may also have underlying genetic predisposition to esophageal cancer. In these families, spouses of family members were seemingly affected with high frequency, a finding more consistent with environmental factors. Demonstration of excess risk in prospective studies of high risk and low risk family members and their spouses may distinguish between alternative explanations for the familial aggregates.

Comparable analytic issues in familial neoplasia are encountered in studies of breast cancer and other common cancers in the U.S. The lifetime risk of breast cancer among women is approximately 1 in 15 (15). Studies indicate that a family history of breast cancer elevates the risk by several fold, but much of the data come from speciality centers (15). Patients at these centers are selected, perhaps partly because of knowledge about breast cancer that had affected a close relative. In some families, breast cancers have clustered with other adenocarcinomas, particularly of the endometrium, ovary and colon (16). These cancers comprise a high proportion of all cancers in U.S. women, and chance aggregation has to be excluded by other consideration. Relevant findings include the early age at diagnosis of cancer within affected families, tendency to develop multiple primary cancers, segregation into affected and unaffected family lineages, and detection of excess cancers through screening and prospective observation of asymptomatic family

members (16, 17). These features have been examined in a
second, less common familial cancer syndrome that comprises
carcinomas of the breast associated with sarcomas, leukemia
and brain tumor in childhood (19). In the initial study of
4 families with these neoplasms, chance aggregation was
considered unlikely because of the rarity in the general
population of most component lesions, including breast
cancer before 35 years of age. Follow-up data have been
available in 3 of the families and revealed the development
of 8 additional cancers over 7 years among approximately
50 persons at risk. In one of the families, 3 cancers
were identified initially in 2 generations in 1969
(Figure 1). By 1975, 3 additional primary breast cancers
had developed in 2 women under 40 years of age. In 1980,
2 additional sarcomatous malignancies and 1 additional
breast cancer developed in the 2 generations, and a child
in the third generation died with acute nonlymphocytic
leukemia. The high frequency of additional cancers
including multiple primary cancers in children and
young adults cannot be explained in a chance basis, and
selection bias is excluded by the prospective nature of
the observations.

The contribution of genetic and environmental influences
in breast cancer families is difficult to discern
clinically. The role of diet in cancers of the breast,
female reproductive organs and colon has been suggested by
migrant studies (19). Among ethnic Chinese and Japanese,
breast cancer rates are low in Asia but rise with migration
to the U.S., a nation with high rate of breast cancer.
Genetic factors in breast cancer may have been clarified
recently by segregation and linkage analysis of 11 breast
cancer families (20). Six of the families provided
evidence of close linkage to the glutamine-pyruvate transaminase locus, which has tentatively been assigned to
chromosome 10. Thus laboratory studies of cancer families
can confirm genetic etiology that is suspected on clinical
grounds.

In a recently studied family with renal cell carcinoma,
genetic etiology was established through another laboratory
study, i.e., chromosome analysis (8). As usual, the clinical
findings provide the initial evidence of a cancer gene.
The proband in the family developed bilateral renal cell
carcinoma at age 37 years. Only 1 to 2 percent of renal
cell carcinomas in general are bilateral and median age at
diagnosis is 60 years. These differences suggested possible
genetic etiology and family history revealed renal cell
carcinoma in several relatives. Eventually 6 other family

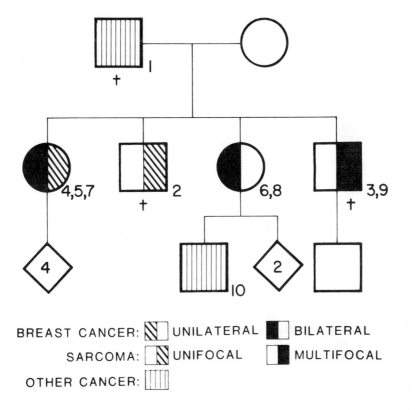

BREAST CANCER: ⊠ UNILATERAL ◨ BILATERAL

SARCOMA: ⊡ UNIFOCAL ◨ MULTIFOCAL

OTHER CANCER: ▥

Figure 1. Prospective observations of a family with breast cancer-sarcoma syndrome. By 1969, 3 cancers had developed: fatal skin cancer at age 47 years (cancer 1), sarcoma at age 2 (cancer 2), and sarcoma at age 11 (cancer 3). Cancers 4, 5, and 6 were breast carcinomas that developed at ages 30, 36, and 32 between 1970 and 1975. By 1979, 4 additional cancers had been diagnosed. Cancer 7 was a sarcoma at age 40, cancer 8 a breast carcinoma at age 35, cancer 9 a sarcoma at age 26, and cancer 10 was acute leukemia at age 14.

members affected at ages 44 to 59 years were identified.
Karyotype studies revealed a familial translocation between
chromosomes 3 and 8, t(3;8) (p21;q24), which was present
in noncancerous somatic cells of all evaluable family
members with renal carcinoma. The finding provided
additional evidence of the genetic origin of the familial
cancer. The translocation also served as a marker for
identification of clinically unaffected family members who
are likely to develop cancer. Through screening of these
individuals asymptomatic bilateral renal carcinomas were
found in 3 women, ages 39-44 years, with the translocation.
Each has been rendered free of tumor by surgery, although
future induction of cancer in the kidney remnant remains
a possibility. Additional renal cell carcinomas can be
expected in younger family members with the translocation
as they reach the age of high cancer risk.

Early detection through screening for renal cell carcinoma in the affected family represents one approach to
the control of genetic cancers. High risk families
eligible for periodic screening comprise those with
hereditary cancers of other sites that can be treated more
readily at early stages of disease. Suspected carriers
of genes for cancers of breast, colon, stomach, genito-
urinary tract, musculoskeletal tissues and several endocrine
and other organs may benefit from early cancer detection (21).
Selective screening of these high risk persons appears more
cost-effective than general population screening in which
many need to be screened to find one early cancer. For
other cancers such as acute leukemia and perhaps lung
cancer, earlier diagnosis has not been shown to substantially
alter longevity.

Cancers that develop from an interaction of genetic and
environmental influences can be prevented through avoidance
of the environmental carcinogen. Children with xeroderma
pigmentosum, an autosomal recessive disorder with defective
excision repair of ultraviolet light-induced DNA damage,
have successfully avoided skin cancer through protection
from sunlight exposure (22). Patients with ataxia-telangiectasia have analogous sensitivity to ionizing radiation
and should avoid unnecessary exposure, even at low doses.
Studies of host interaction with chemical carcinogens are
in early stages, but humans clearly differ in metabolism
of pharmacologic agents and endogenous products (23). It
is likely that enzyme activation of carcinogens differs
within humans, as illustrated by studies of aryl hydrocarbon hydroxylase (AHH) inducibility in relation to lung
cancer among cigarette smokers. Despite the paucity of

data on biologic mechanisms host factors have been implicated
in the development of lung cancer, and cessation of cigarette smoking is particularly important for persons with a
family history of the neoplasm. Persons who had cancer in
childhood and were treated with radiotherapy or chemotherapy also appear to have high risk of the carcinogenic
effect of cigarette smoking. However, rates of cigarette
smoking in one series of these patients were comparable
to those for the general population (24).

In a few instances, prophylactic removal of the organ
at extraordinary risk of a genetic cancer appears to be
indicated despite the damage from the surgery. In polyposis
coli, the risk of colon cancer approaches 100% by 60 years
of age (6). At present, prophylactic colectomy is recommended for persons found to have familial polyposis coli.
Whether total proctocolectomy with permanent ileostomy
should be performed is unclear. Some have recommended
sparing the lower rectum in those patients with few rectal
polyps at initial evaluation. These patients require
regular proctoscopic examinations for the remainder of
their lives, and some will eventually require ileostomy.
In MEN, type III, the finding of multiple mucosal neuromas
indicates extraordinarily high risk of medullary thyroid
carcinoma and prophylactic thyroidectomy has been recommended. Hyperparathyroidism in patients with family
history of MEN type II may serve as a comparable marker of
cancer susceptibility. An alternative approach to management in these MEN syndromes is periodic calcitonin studies,
which provide a sensitive assay for the cancer or precancerous hyperplasia of thyroid C-cells (25). In familial
aggregates of breast cancer the lifetime risk in affected
lineages can vary between 25 and 50 percent, and prophylactic
mastectomy may be recommended to some patients. Prophylactic
oophorectomy has been performed in familial ovarian cancer
and in predisposing gonadal dysgenesis with a Y chromosome (26). Cryptorchism is associated with testis cancer
and surgical correction in the first years of life appears
to reduce but not eliminate the cancer risk (27).

Carriers of cancer genes may benefit from genetic
counseling, although the reduction in cancer frequency is
not realized for many years. However, the delay may not
be longer than that associated with removal of environmental carcinogens, which tend to produce oncogenic effects
decades after the exposure. Recent advances in prenatal
diagnosis of genetic diseases can be applied to the
identification of carriers of cancer genes. The marker
in fetal cells may be a chromosome defect in individual

families with hereditary retinoblastoma or renal cell carcinoma, or defective repair processes in xeroderma pigmentosum (8, 13, 28). Opportunities for in-utero diagnosis will increase with clarification of biologic mechanisms of action of cancer genes.

REFERENCES

1. Li FP: Clinical studies of cancer etiology. Cancer 40: 445-447, 1977.
2. Knudson AG Jr, Strong LC, Anderson DE: Heredity and cancer in man. Prog Med Genet 9:13-158, 1973.
3. Knudson AG Jr: Retinoblastoma: A prototypic hereditary neoplasm. Semin Oncology 5:57-60, 1978.
4. Kitchin FD, Ellsworth RM: Pleiotropic effects of the gene for retinoblastoma. J Med Genet 11:244-246, 1974.
5. Wilson MG, Ebbin AJ, Towner, JW, Spencer WH: Chromosomal anomalies in patients with retinoblastoma. Clin Genet 12:1-8, 1977.
6. Erbe RW: Inherited gastrointestinal-polyposis syndromes. N Engl J Med 294:1101-1104, 1976.
7. Bolande RP: The neurocristopathies: A unifying concept of disease arising in neural crest maldevelopment. Hum Pathol 5:409-429, 1974.
8. Cohen AJ, Li FP, Berg S et al: Hereditary renal-cell carcinoma associated with a chromosomal translocation. N Engl J Med 301:592-595, 1979.
9. Matsunaga E: Hereditary retinoblastoma: Delayed mutation or host resistance? Am J Hum Genet 30: 406-424, 1978.
10. Lutzner MA: Nosology among the neoplastic genodermatoses, in Mulvihill JJ, Miller RW, Fraumeni JF Jr (eds): Genetics of Human Cancer. New York, Raven Press, 1977, pp 145-167.
11. Mulvihill JJ: Genetic repertory of human neoplasia, in Mulvihill JJ, Miller RW, Fraumeni JF Jr (eds): Genetics of Human Cancer. New York, Raven Press, pp 137-143.
12. Li FP: Host factors in the development of childhood cancers. Semin Oncology 5:17-23, 1978.
13. Yunis JJ, Ramsay NK: Familial occurrence of the aniridia-Wilms tumor syndrome with deletion 11p13-14.1. J Pediatr 96:1027-1030, 1980.
14. Li FP, Shiang EL: Cancer mortality in China. J Natl Cancer Inst 65:217-221, 1980.
15. Anderson DE: Breast cancer in families. Cancer 40:1855-1860, 1977.

16. Fraumeni JF Jr: Family cancer syndromes, in Severi L
    (ed): Tumours of Early Life in Man and Animals. Perugia,
    Italy, Perugia Quadrennial International Conferences on
    Cancer, 1978.
17. Lynch HT, Krush AJ: Cancer family "G" revisited: 1895-
    1970. Cancer 27:1505-1511, 1971.
18. Li FP, Fraumeni JF Jr: Familial breast cancer, soft-
    tissue sarcomas, and other neoplasms. Ann Intern Med
    83:833-834, 1975.
19. MacMahon B, Cole P, Brown J: Etiology of human breast
    cancer: A review. J Natl Cancer Inst 50:21-42, 1973.
20. King MC, Go RCP, Elston RC et al: Allele increasing
    susceptibility to human breast cancer may be linked to
    the glutamate-pyruvate transaminase locus. Science 208:
    406-408, 1980.
21. Williams C: Management of malignancy in "cancer
    families." Lancet 1:198-199, 1978.
22. Lynch HT, Frichot BC III, Lynch JF: Cancer control in
    xeroderma pigmentosum. Arch Dermatol 113:193-195, 1977.
23. Harris CC, Mulvihill JJ, Thorgeirsson SS, Minna JD:
    Individual differences in cancer susceptibility. Ann
    Intern Med 92:809-825, 1980.
24. Corkery JC, Li FP, McDonald JA et al: Kids who really
    shouldn't smoke. N Engl J Med 300:1279, 1979.
25. Graze K, Spiler IJ, Tashjian AH Jr et al: Natural history
    of familial medullary thyroid carcinoma: Effect of a
    program for early diagnosis. N Engl J Med 299:980-
    985, 1978.
26. Fraumeni JF Jr, Grundy GW, Creagan ET, Everson RB:
    Six families prone to ovarian cancer. Cancer 36:364-
    369, 1975.
27. Gehring GG, Rodriguez FR, Woodhead DM: Malignant
    degeneration of cryptorchid testes following orchiopexy.
    J Urol 112:354-356, 1974.
28. Halley DJJ, Keijzer W, Jaspers NGJ et al: Prenatal
    diagnosis of xeroderma pigmentosum (group C) using
    assays of unscheduled DNA synthesis and postreplication
    repair. Clin Genet 16:137-146, 1979.

Chromosome 14: A Step In The Development of Lymphoid Malignancies

FREDERICK HECHT, M.D.

Director
The Cancer Research and Genetics Centers of
Southwest Biomedical Research Institute
Tempe, Arizona

BARBARA KAISER-MCCAW, Ph.D.

Associate Director
The Cancer Research and Genetics Centers of
Southwest Biomedical Research Institute
Tempe, Arizona

INTRODUCTION

In 1975 we first proposed that rearrangement of the long arm (q) of chromosme 14 might be a step in the development of lymphoid malignancies (McCaw et al., 1975). As with a number of ideas, this hypothesis was set forth intuitively on the basis of rather sparse data. In the intervening 5 years, evidence has steadily accumulated in support of this idea.

ATAXIA-TELANGIECTASIA: HISTORY OF AN IDEA

Our interest in chromosome 14 dates back to a curious set of coincidences. At a local pediatric meeting in 1966 one of us (F.H.) accidently sat down next to a visitor. The visitor was, it turned out, Robert W. Miller from the National Cancer Institute. Learning of our interest in medical genetics, Dr. Miller suggested that we look up an unusual family. The family had lost two children with acute lymphocytic leukemia and had a surviving child with "cerebral palsy". Dr. Miller wondered if the child might not have ataxia-telangiectasia (A-T), a genetic disease associated with an increased risk of cancer. In 1966 we looked up the family just to oblige

433

Dr. Miller. The surviving child with "cerebral palsy" did indeed have classical A-T and the deceased leukemic sibs clearly had A-T also by history.

Next we found that children with A-T have markedly increased chromosome breakage (Hecht et al., 1966). The chromosome breaks present in their lymphocytes are randomly distributed throughout the genome. Neither chromosome 14 nor any other chromosome appear to have a "hot spot". As of the end of the sixties we thus knew that A-T, an autosomal recessive disease with an impaired immune system, was accompanied by chromosome breaks and oftimes cancer, especially lymphomas and lymphocytic leukemias. Early in the seventies a new graduate student (B.K.-McC.) became intrigued with A-T and initiated a series of new chromosome studies. She observed in an A-T patient more than one cell with the same translocation. If two or more cells have the same translocation (or any other chromosome marker), this suggests a "clone". The clone had a translocation involving chromosome 14. The patient was Bob Miller's "cerebral palsy" boy with A-T.

In 1973 we reported longitudinal chromosome studies of this A-T boy, showing the proliferation of a clone of lymphocytes with a chromosome 14 translocation (Hecht et al., 1973). The translocation was due to exchange of material between chromosome 14 and the homologous chromosome 14. The abnormal lymphoid clones in A-T always involve chromosome 14 (McCaw et al., 1975). Usually the translocation is between two no. 14 chromosomes, although in rare cases the translocation may entangle chromosome 14 and another chromosome, such as no. 7 or the X. But at least one no. 14 chromosome is always in the act.

The proportion of the no. 14 translocation rises with time, occasionally to almost 100% (of phytohemagglutinin-responsive lymphocytes). Nonetheless, the A-T child may not have leukemia. Apparently these chromosomally marked clones may proliferate benignly, at times.

Now there is increasing evidence that lymphocytic leukemia may arise from the benignly proliferating clone with a rearrangement of chromosome 14 in A-T (McCaw et al., 1975). In other words, a benign chromosome 14 rearrangement precedes the conversion to malignancy. (We will return later to A-T as a model.)

BURKITT'S LYMPHOMA

At the time we first proposed that changes in chromosome 14 might be involved with the development of lymphoid malignancies, we knew the work of Manolov and Manolova (1972) that biopsies and cells cultured from Burkitt's lymphoma have extra material on the long arm of chromosome 14. This was then the other major clue. Subsequently the extra material on 14q in Burkitt's lymphoma was found to come from a translocation with 8q (Zech et al., 1976; McCaw et al., 1977a). The chromosomal event in Burkitt's is a balanced, reciprocal 8q-;14q+ translocation. Work has now been done on enough Burkitt's lymphomas to state that virtually all cases show this translocation. The breakpoint is near the end of the long arm (q) of chromosome 14: in band 14q32.

The Epstein-Barr virus (EBV) is, of course, closely associated with Burkitt's lymphoma. Some have said that EBV causes Burkitt's lymphoma. But how about the 8;14 translocation? It, too, is intimately associated with Burkitt's lymphoma. One piece of evidence may be important: that even without detectable EBV, the translocation is present in Burkitt's lymphoma (McCaw et al., 1977a). In any event, the no. 14 translocation in Burkitt's lymphoma marks a proliferating clone of lymphocytes with B-cell surface characteristics.

NON-BURKITT'S LYMPHOMAS AS A GROUP

The single most common chromosome abnormality in non-Burkitt's lymphoma is the 14q+ marker chromosome. It is noted in about 50% of patients. The other chromosomes in the translocation with no. 14 in non-Burkitt's lymphomas vary. Chromosome 8 may be the translocation partner; as may be chromosome 1, 11, 18 (Fukuhara et al., 1978) and others (Mark et al., 1978).

DIFFUSE HISTIOCYTIC LYMPHOMAS (DHL)

Twelve cell lines from DHL patients were studied cytogenetically in collaboration with Henry Kaplan and Alan Epstein. From each cell line 100-200 metaphases were analyzed. The results are presented in Table 1.

The 14q+ translocation was found in 8 of the 12 cell lines. The breakpoint in chromosome 14 in each of these cell lines was in band 14q32. The cell surface markers of the 12 DHL lines were characterized: 8 lines were B-cell, 2 were histiocytic and 2 were null-cell.

Most interesting is the correlation of the 14q+ translocation with cell surface markers (Table 2). All 8 of

TABLE 1
Chromosome abnormalities in DHL cell lines

SU-DHL Cell Line	1	2	3	6	7	8	11	12	13	14	18	Y	Markers
1				q−							t		+
2				q−									+
3			p+							q+			+
4			p+			+				q+	q−		+
7				q−						q+			+
8						q+	+						+
9		+		q−		+	+	+					+
10					q+	t				q+		t	
11	q+					q−				q+			+
12	p+	−				q+	p+			q+			+
13										q+			+
14										q+			+

*Abbreviations − p: short arm; q: long arm; + or − after p or q: addition or deletion of material; + or − alone: extra or missing chromosome; t: translocation. Markers are unidentified extra chromosomes.

TABLE 2
14q+ Chromosome translocation and cell type in DHL cell lines*

SU-DHL Cell Line	14q+ chromosome translocation	Cell type
3	+	B
4	+	B
7	+	B
10	+	B
11	+	B
12	+	B
13	+	B
14	+	B
1	−	H
2	−	H
8	−	N
9	−	N

*Abbreviations − + or −: 14q+ translocation present or absent; ?: chromosome 14 missing; B, H and N: B-cell, histiocytic and null-cell.

the lines with a 14q+ translocation were of B-cell origin.
The 4 lines without the 14q+ translocation were null or
histiocytic. We do not know whether T-cell DHL's have the
14q+ translocation, since none were studied. However, it
appears clear that null and histiocytic DHL's probably do not
possess this chromosome marker, while B-cell DHL's do.

HODGKIN'S DISEASE

More than 75% of cases with Hodgkin's disease show
chromosome abnormalities, usually in the triploid or
tetraploid range (Sandberg, 1980), attesting to the malignant
nature of Hodgkin's disease.
In collaboration with Henry Kaplan at Stanford we have
studied cells established in long-term culture from a patient
with Hodgkin's disease. The patient is an adult male with
Stage IIIA disease. A cell line cultured from his pleural
effusion disclosed a near triploid mode with a number of
marker chromosomes, none of them involving no. 14. Three
clones were obtained from the pleural effusion line (SU-HD-1).
All 3 clones also have a near triploid mode with the same
marker chromosomes, none involving 14. The clones were
studied up to passage 25 and appear chromosomally very
similar to the original culture, speaking for its chromosome
stability. Although there is a suggestive increase in the
number of whole copies of chromosome 14 (up to 5-6 per cell)
there is no rearrangement of chromosome 14, consistent with a
non-lymphoid origin for Hodgkin's disease.

MYCOSIS FUNGOIDES

Hyperdiploid cells from a lymph node from a patient with
mycosis fungoides and from peripheral blood cultured with
PHA had a structural anomaly of the long arm of chromosome 14
(14q+) (Fukuhara et al., 1978). This finding suggests that
mycosis fungoides is a type of malignant lymphoma and that
rearrangement of 14q may prove to be characteristic.

MONOCLONAL GAMMOPATHIES: MULTIPLE MYELOMAS
AND PLASMA CELL LEUKEMIAS

Multiple myeloma is a B-cell disease. Direct preparation
of the bone marrow and PHA-stimulated blood cultures have
been analyzed. A 14q+ chromosome marker has been reported in
6 cases (Liang and Rowley, 1978; Wurster-Hill et al., 1978).

It is impossible to determine the exact incidence yet of this abnormality in the monoclonal gammopathies.

ACUTE LYMPHOCYTIC LEUKEMIA (ALL)

There are three classes of ALL: T-cell, B-cell and null-cell. About 4% of ALL cases are of B-cell origin. As in the non-Burkitt's lymphomas, many cases of ALL have unstable karyotypes, making chromosome analysis difficult.

A 14q+ translocation has only been reported in those cases of ALL classified as B-cell. Again, band 14q32 is involved in the translocation. The other chromosome involved is usually chromosome 11, as in the non-Burkitt's lymphomas (Cimino et al., 1979).

CHRONIC LYMPHOCYTIC LEUKEMIA (CLL)

Cytogenetic studies of patients with CLL have been numerous, but often uninformative. This may have been due, in part, to the fact that about 95% of CLL cases are B-cell. Most cytogenetic studies were done with PHA (primarily a T-cell mitogen) stimulated cells. EBV can be used to stimulate CLL cells and to establish transformed lymphoblast lines with B-cell characteristics and, in several cases recently the 14q+ marker was observed (Najfeld et al., 1980). The 14 was also reported in two rare cases of CLL characterized as T-cell. In one case, material from chromosome 18 was translocated to 14q and in the second case, part of no. 11 was translocated onto 14q (Nowell et al., 1980).

We predict that additional work will demonstrate the 14q+ marker in both T- and B-cell CLL in the nineteen eighties.

ATAXIA-TELANGIECTASIA (A-T) AS A MODEL

In benign lymphocyte clones in A-T the rearrangement of chromosome 14 always involves a proximal break: in band 14q12. The remainder of 14q is translocated to the other no. 14, where it attached at 14q32, or to another chromosome. When the translocation is to 14q32, the clone may have malignant potential. When the translocation is to another site, the clone remains benign.

The first case of A-T with leukemia had CLL of the T-cell type. The translocation was between the two number 14 chromosomes: 14q12 and 14q32 were the breakpoints (McCaw et al., 1975). The second case of A-T with leukemia had subacute atypical LL with T-cell markers. The identical chromosome rearrangement was present (Levitt et al., 1978). The third case of A-T with leukemia also had T-cell LL. The rearrangement between the two 14's was identical (Saxon et al., 1979). A case of A-T with Burkitt's lymphoma (B-cell) had the classic 8;14 translocation associated with Burkitt's lymphoma (McCaw et al., 1977b). Again the breakpoint in 14 was distal: in band 14q32.

CHROMOSOME 14 TRANSLOCATIONS IN NORMAL CULTURED LYMPHOCYTES

Translocations with non-random involvement of chromosome 14 have been observed in peripheral blood lymphocyte cultures (Hecht et al., 1975; Welch and Lee, 1975; Beatty-DeSana et al., 1975). We have now collected data from clinical cytogenetic laboratories in different parts of North America and Europe, indicating that these no. 14 translocations are found routinely in about 1 in every 100-150 individuals. The breakpoint in chromosome 14 is always proximal, located in band 14q12, and the translocated material is usually on chromosome 7, never on the homologous no. 14 (Hecht et al., 1979; Kaiser-McCaw et al., 1979). None of these translocations to our knowledge is in any way associated with malignancy.

BENIGN AND MALIGNANT BREAKPOINTS IN CHROMOSOME 14

It appears therefore that there are two key breakpoints in chromosome 14 in lymphoid cells. One breakpoint is proximal: in band 14q12. The other breakpoint is distal in band 14q32. No case with a break solely in band 14q12 has yet been reported with cancer. All cases with cancer and a chromosome 14 translocation have had a break in the distal band: 14q32.

We therefore designate: (1) the proximal breakpoint at 14q12 as benign; and (2) the distal breakpoint at 14q32 as malignant in keeping with earlier suggestions we (McCaw et al., 1977b) and Tischler (1979) made (Fig. 1).

MECHANISM OF ACTION OF CHROMOSOME 14: POSITION EFFECT

How does a translocation involving band 14q32 cause a change in the cell? Let us take the 8;14 translocation marking Burkitt's lymphoma as a model. Several laboratories, including ours, demonstrated that the breakpoints in Burkitt's were at bands 8q24 and 14q32 (Kaiser-McCaw et al., 1977b; Zech et al., 1976). The mechanisms of action must therefore pertain to the region around 8q24 and/or region around 14q32. Three general mechanisms of action can be envisaged: (1) loss (or gain) or chromosome material; (2) misreading near the breakpoint(s); or (3) position effect. However, we noted that the 8;14 translocation was reciprocal with no evidence visually or by semi-automated photodensitometry for loss or gain of chromosome material (Kaiser-McCaw et al., 1977a). Misreading near the breakpoint is a possibility, one which has not yet been tested.

Position effect (Kaiser-McCaw et al., 1977b; Hecht et al., 1978) is the leading possibility. Position effect is a change in the location of genetic material. The effect of a gene(s) may depend on its neighboring gene(s). Active genes may thus become inactive or inactive genes may be activated. The neighborhood counts.

Evidence for the concept of position effect was first presented when we noticed that the segment of no. 8 translocated onto 14 appeared to have altered fluorochromatic staining properties with acridine orange (Kaiser-McCaw et al., 1977b; Hecht et al., 1978). Acridine orange in this respect is an intriguing stain, since it presumably reflects the state of the DNA: whether it is normal double-stranded DNA or whether it is denatured into a single-stranded state. The same phenomenon of altered staining of the 14q+ region was noted with quinacrine (Hecht et al., 1978). We suggested that if this were confirmed it would constitute the first cytologic evidence for position effect in malignant human cells. Confirmation has come from an interesting perspective. Manalova et al. (1979) examined late prophase and prometaphase chromosomes in Burkitt's lymphoma and state that with G-banding "it was noticed that the segment of no. 8, translocated onto no. 14, exhibited somewhat different morphologic features in translocated than in normal position". Thus, with acridine orange, quinacrine and G-banding the same phenomenon has been observed. There is a change in the banding pattern of the material translocated onto chromosome 14.

We have proposed (Hecht et al., 1978) and we repeat the proposal that the change in banding pattern reflects a change in gene action, as has been proven with experiments in Drosophila. We predict that in this decade the final proof for position effect in malignant 8;14 and other no. 14 translocations will be produced. The final proof, of course, is inappropriate production of a gene product (or the converse).

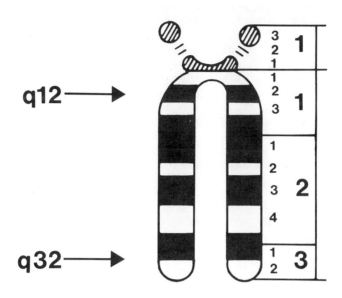

q12——▶

q32——▶

Figure 1. Breakpoints leading to translocations of
chromosome 14 are indicated by the two arrows. The upper
arrow points to the "benign" breakpoint at 14q12 and the
lower arrow indicates the "malignant" breakpoint at 14q32.

     Further, we predict that position effect will be found to
hold for the other transloctions characteristic of cancer
cells. These translocations include the 8;21 translocation,
the 15;17 translocation and the best known of them all: the
9;22 Philadelphia translocation.

SUMMARY AND THE FUTURE

     It is clear in 1980 that rearrangement of the long arm (q)
of chromosome 14 is, indeed, a step in the development of many
lymphoid malignancies. Supporting evidence stems from
cytogenetic studies of Burkitt's lymphoma, diffuse histiocytic
lymphomas (B-cell types), other non-Burkitt's lymphomas, acute
and chronic lymphocytic leukemias, mono-clonal gammopathies,
mycosis fungoides and other lymphoid cancers. The 14q+
chromosome is the key cytogenetic marker in many of these
malignancies of the lymphoid system. Current data indicate
that the 14q+ chromosome is found in B-cell and T-cell

lymphoid cancers. Data presented here on DHL that the 14q+
marker is not found in null-cell or histiocytic tumors. The
14q+ is not closely associated with Hodgkin's disease, as
illustrated by cytogenetic studies we report here on a
permanent cell line established by Dr. Henry Kaplan. The
genetic disease, ataxia-telangiectasia (A-T), has yielded
much information about chromosome 14. A-T is characterized
by benignly proliferating lymphocyte clones marked by a 14q-
chromosome with a break at band 14q12. A-T patients with
lymphocytic leukemia have been studied and have a 14q+
chromosome with a break at band 14q32. Burkitt's lymphoma
studies have shown that most (or all) cases have an 8;14
translocation with the breakpoint at 14q32, irrespective of
whether they show evidence of EBV. From the composite data,
it can now be seen that there is (1) a "benign" breakpoint
in no. 14 at band 14q12; and (2) a "malignant" breakpoint in
no. 14 at band 14q32. The mechanism of action of the
"malignant" breakpoint in chromosome 14 is probably, we
suggest, via position effect. Genetic material translocated
onto 14q32 shows altered fluorochromatic staining properties
and altered banding patterns. This is consistent with the
idea that genes translocated onto 14q32 are altered in
activity. They become inappropriately active or inactive.

One area of future work will pertain to learning what
genes are located, for example, on the segment of chromosome
8 translocated to 14q32 in Burkitt's lymphoma. Likewise, we
need to know the genetic information contained in 14q32 and
in the neighboring region. Work in this direction will in
turn yield information concerning the genodemographic
hypothesis (Hecht and Kaiser-McCaw, 1977), which states that
the chromosome changes we observe in cancer cells are
permissible ones that do not kill the cell. These
chromosome changes specifically involve facultative genes,
genes where loss or gain of gene activity is permitted.

Cytogenetic studies on lymphoid cancers are running 5-10
years behind analogous research on myeloproliferative
disorders. The reason is clear: the work in many ways is
more difficult. Still it is to be hoped that the eighties
will see new light shed on chromosome 14 and its role in the
development of lymphoid cancers.

REFERENCES

Beatty-DeSana, J., Hoggard, M.J. and Cooledge, J.W.: Non-random occurrence of 7;14 translocation in human lymphocyte cultures. Nature 255:242 (1975).

Cimino, M.C., Roth, D.G., Golomb, H.M., Rowley, J.D.: A chromosome marker for B-cell cancers. N. Engl. J. Med. 298:1422 (1978).

Cimino, M.C., Rowley, J.D., Kinnealey, A., Variakojis, D., Golomb, H.M.: Banding studies of chromosomal abnormalities in patients with acute lymphocytic leukemia. Cancer Res. 39:227-238 (1979).

Fukuhara, S., Rowley, J.D.: Chromosome 14 translocations in non-Burkitt lymphomas. Int. J. Cancer 22:14-21 (1978).

Fukuhara, S., Rowley, J.D., Variakojis, D.: Banding studies of chromosomes in a patient with mycosis fungoides. Cancer 42:2262-2268 (1978).

Hecht, F., Koler, R.D., Rigas, D.A., Dahnke, G.S., Case, M.P., Tisdale, V., Miller, R.W.: Leukemia and lymphocytes in ataxia-telangiectasia. Lancet ii, 1193 (1966).

Hecht, F., McCaw, B.K., Koler, R.D.: Ataxia-telangiectasia. Clonal growth of translocation lymphocytes. N. Engl. J. Med. 289:286-291 (1973).

Hecht, F., McCaw, B.K., Peakman, D., Robinson, A.: Non-random occurrence of 7;14 translocations in human lymphocyte cultures. Nature 255:243-244 (1975).

Hecht, F., Kaiser-McCaw, B., Patil, S., Wyandt, H.: Are balanced translocations really balanced? Preliminary evidence for position effect in man. Birth Defects: Original Article Series. Vol. XIV 6C:281-286 (1978).

Hecht, F., Kaiser-McCaw, B.: Chromosomes and genes in human cancer cells: Multidisciplinary approaches to a unitary genodemographic hypothesis. Chromosomes Today 6, 357-361 (1977).

Hecht, F., Kaiser-McCaw, B., Peakman, D., Robinson, A.: New translocations in human lymphocytes: A mutagen monitoring system. Environ. Health Perspectives 31:19-22 (1979).

Kaiser-McCaw, B., Epstein A.L., Overton, K.M., Kaplan, H.S., Hecht, F.: The cytogenetics of human lymphomas: Chromosome 14 in Burkitt's diffuse histiocytic and related neoplasms. Chromosomes Today 6. A. de la Chapelle and M. Sorsa, eds. 1977b Elsevier/North Holland pp. 282-390.

Kaiser-McCaw, B., Peakman, D., Hecht, F., and Robinson, A.: Recurrent somatic 7;14 translocations in lymphocytes. Amer. J. Human Genet. 31(6):99A (1979).

Levitt, R., Pierre, R.V., White, W.L., and Kiekert, R.G.: Atypical lymphoid leukemia in ataxia-telangiectasia. Blood 52:1003-1011 (1978).

Liang, W., Rowley, J.D.:   14q+ marker chromosomes in multiple myeloma and plasma-cell leukemia. Lancet i, 96 (1978).

McCaw, B.K., Hecht, F., Harnden, D.G., and Teplitz, R.L.: Somatic rearrangement of chromosome 14 in human lymphocytes. Proc. Natl. Acad. Sci. 72, 2071-2075 (1975).

Kaiser-McCaw, B., Epstein, A.L., Kaplan, H.S., and Hecht, F.: Chromosome 14 translocation in African and North American Burkitt's lymphoma. Int. J. Cancer 19, 482-486 (1977a).

Manlov, G., Manlova, Y.: Marker band in one chromosome 14 from Burkitt lymphomas. Nature 237, 33-34 (1972).

Manlova, Y., Manlov, G., Kieler, J., Levan, A. and Klein, G.: Genesis of the 14q+ marker in Burkitt's lymphoma. Heriditas 90, 5-10 (1979).

Mark, J., Ekedahl, C., Dahlenfors, R.: Characteristics of the banding patterns in non-Hodgkin and non-Burkitt lymphomas. Hereditas 88, 229-242 (1978).

Najfield, V., Fialkow, P.J., Karande, A., Klein, G., Nilsson, K.:   Cytogenetics of lymphoid cell lines derived from patients with chronic lymphocytic leukemia (CLL). Abst. 31st Annual Meeting Amer. Soc. Hum. Gen. Sept. 24-27, 1980, p. 82A.

Nowell, P., Daniele, R., Rowlands, D., Finan, J.: Cytogenetics of chronic B-cell and T-cell leukemia. Cancer Genetics and Cytogenetics I, 273-280 (1980).

Sandberg, Avery A.:   The chromosomes in human cancer and leukemia. Elsevier North Holland, Inc. p. 387-393 (1980).

Saxon, A., Stevens, R.H., Golde, W.: Helper and suppressor T-lymphocytic leukemia in ataxia telangiectasia. N. Engl. J. Med. 300, 700-704 (1979).

Sparkes, R.S., Komo, R., Golde, D.W.: Cytogenetic abnormalities in ataxia telangiectasia with T-cell chronic lymphocytic leukemia. Cancer Genetics and Cytogenetics I, 329-336 (1980).

Tishler, Peter: Chromosomal abnormality in lymphoreticular tumors: N. Engl. J. Med. 301 (7) p. 383 (1979).

Welch, J.P., and Lee, C.L.Y.: Non-random occurrence of 7;14 translocations in human lymphocyte cultures. Nature 255:241 (1975).

Wurster-Hill, D.M., McIntyre, O.R., Cornwell, G.G.III: Chromosome studies in myelomatosis. Virchows Arch. B. Cell Pathol. 29, 93-97 (1978).

Zech, L., Haglund, U., Nilsson, K., Klein, G.: Characteristic chromosomal abnormalities in biopsies and lymphoid cell lines from patients with Burkitt and non-Burkitt lymphomas. Int. J. Cancer, 17, 47-56 (1976).

Cell Biology and Cancer

The contribution that the study of
cell biology may make to the
treatment and prevention of cancer.

JOHN CAIRNS

Imperial Cancer Research Fund
Burtonhole Lane, London NW7 1AD

Cancer research is supported by organizations whose
stated objective is the conquest of the disease – either by
prevention or treatment or some combination of the two. But
it encompasses some very advanced biology that is being
pursued by people whose prime interest, quite properly, is
in the niceties of science rather than the practicalities of
the cancer problem. As one might expect, communication
between the separate wings of this advancing army is often
a rather tenuous affair, especially as each group is inclined
to underestimate the difficulties being encountered by the
others. The epidemiologists and clinicians keep hearing
about the great advances in molecular biology, and yet
nothing ever seems to come of this knowledge. Conversely,
the laboratory worker is astonished to hear that, although
we already know how we might prevent about a third of all
cancer deaths (by attacking the cult of the cigarette), few
nations are willing to put this information into practice.

I believe that much of the confusion arises because we
are thinking of the war against cancer in quite the wrong
way. It has been presented as a matter of a few years'
effort, but it is surely going to last much longer than that.
So far, after 50 years of cold war and 10 years of highly
publicized warfare, no major inroads have been made into the
overall death rate from cancer. To be specific, each year
each of us still has about the same overall probability of
dying from some non-respiratory cancer as our parents had
when they were our age; and thanks to the efforts of the
tobacco companies, our chance of dying of lung cancer has
unfortunately become far greater than it was in our parents'
day, so that overall we are, at least in respect of
mortality, worse off than our parents were.

Once we accept the idea that the war against cancer is
going to be a very long haul, certain changes in strategy

445

become inevitable. While we are waiting for the advances in
biology that will lead to the invention of really effective
treatments for cancer (analogous, if you like, to the
antibiotics that completed the conquest of the bacterial
diseases), we should wage the war on the only major front
available to us, namely prevention. So we support basic
biology because that is the long route to the cure of cancer
and we seek out the causes of cancer because that is the
short route to prevention. I think it is useful therefore
to step back occasionally from considering the details of
each branch of cancer research and instead ask how it fits
in to these two overall strategies. I will therefore try
now to show how work on the biology of the cancer cell may
eventually bear upon treatment and prevention.

When we consider the biology of the cancer cell we are, I
think, asking two separate questions. What is wrong with the
cells and how did they get to be that way ? If we knew the
answer to the first question and really understood all about
the phenotype of the cancer cell, we might be in a good
position to rectify its defects or intervene in some other
way. If we knew the answer to the second question and had
discovered what classes of event had occurred in the history
of the typical cancer cell, it should be much easier to
identify the agents in our environment that cause cancer and
therefore much easier to devise a lifestyle that would free
us from most cancers. In this article, I shall discuss in
very general terms our progress towards these two objectives.

The Phenotype of the Cancer Cell

It has, I suppose, been the dream of many people that
cancer cells will be found to have one particular thing wrong
with them that lies at the root of their undisciplined
behavior, because one could then imagine devising a broad-
spectrum treatment that would attack this common feature. As
might be expected, the tendency has always been to hope that
the defect lies in whatever branch of cell activity has most
recently become understood. As long as biochemistry was
largely confined to the study of intermediary metabolism,
we had to be content with theories couched in those terms.
Looking back, it is hard to imagine how anyone could ever
have believed that a cell became cancerous once it went over
to anaerobic glycolysis; yet for a time that was an accepted
theory. For the last 30 years, however, the balance of
power has swung over to the molecular geneticists. As a
result, we now know a lot about the ways a cell can control
and regulate its behavior. But the research has been almost

exclusively concerned with the biology of bacteria. So it is therefore unlikely to lead directly to a full understanding of a disease that represents an error in the organization of a multicellular system. Before we can hope to work out the molecular genetics of cancer we are going to have to learn more about multicellular biology. The defect of a cancer cell lies in the way it interprets its environment. Like its normal counterpart, it multiplies and may undergo terminal differentiation, but it does not respect the rules that determine the clone size and territory of normal cells. If we knew something about those rules, we might be able to guess what gene products are abnormal in cancer cells.

Perhaps the most useful overview of the biology of the cancer cell is therefore not to discuss any work actually done with cancer cells, but to approach the subject from the other direction by reviewing briefly what is known about the way cells interpret their environment. The creation and maintenance of every tissue and organ of the body must depend upon the relaying of some form of "positional information", and by considering that subject we may get some idea of how much research in basic biology will have to be done before we can expect to understand what is wrong with a cancer cell.

The most easily investigated example of a cell's response to positional information is that of a motile bacterium swimming up a concentration gradient of a substrate such as galactose. It sounds simple enough. Yet who would have thought that the process involves a battery of special receptors coupled to a memory system (based, if you please, on the reversible methylation of certain proteins) plus a program for changing the direction of swimming, the whole being coupled to a set of reversible induction motors, each placed at the base of a flagellum. A few years ago, no one would have believed such a preposterous story; yet that is roughly how bacterial chemotaxis works.

The kind of positional information that determines the form and behavior of multicellular systems is probably even more complicated because it usually involves separate measurements in several dimensions and depends on communication between different sets of cells rather than simply the detection of some fortuitous concentration gradient. The best understood example, at least in terms of the method of signalling, is the agglutinative reaction of certain slime molds that is the first step in the sequence of events which convert a scattered collection of single amebae into an organized multicellular animal. The process requires each cell to carry out repeatedly a quite elaborate program in which it somehow senses and memorizes the direction of the

signal's concentration gradient, sends out a similar signal
in all directions, and then moves for a predetermined period
along the memorized axis of the gradient. With hindsight, it
is easy to see that some signal-relaying program like this
would be needed if single cells are to be drawn together
from a very large area. But all the same it has been a
surprise to find such ingenuity at work.

The example of the slime molds is especially illuminating
because it represents the transition from chaos to order and
therefore may be a good analog (in reverse) of the process
that makes a cancer cell. It is worth considering, for
example, what particular defects in cell function would
interrupt this transition. Apart from certain obvious
defects, such as a fault in the surface receptor that detects
the signalling substance or some fault affecting motility,
we would have to list all changes that affect the listen-
memorize-signal-move program. The list would probably be
rather long because the similar but simpler program used for
bacterial chemotaxis is known to involve some 50 gene
products. And this is the message that comes from the
analogy. If we were presented with some variant of the
slime molds that did not aggregate properly but went
wandering off on its own in a completely unorganized way, we
would have little chance of finding out what was wrong with
it if we knew nothing about the program which brings about
aggregation. For this reason, I believe that we cannot hope
to understand what is wrong with most cancer cells until we
have learnt something about the programs that determine the
structure of the organs and tissues of the body.

So far the study of positional information in higher
animals has proved to be extremely difficult. Some tissues
in certain animals, such as the nematodes, appear to be set
up in a determinstic way; i.e., the fate of each cell is
determined at the time of its birth by information contained
within the cell rather than derived from outside. But most
tissues are probably under the control of gradients of some
form of signalling substance. Unfortunately, the nature of
these substances has proved very elusive. In most tissues
the signals that determine cell behavior and multiplication
must be very localized, present in low concentration and
therefore hard to isolate.

We can, however, hope for some success with those tissues
(such as the various endocrine glands, the liver and the bone
marrow) that serve a general function and so have to be
under the control of some system that monitors the total mass
of the tissue rather than its local concentration. The
signals that pass to-and-fro between such cells have to

circulate in the bloodstream and therefore are easily accessible to investigation. It is already clear, for example, that one of the first requirements in making a successful clone of leukemic cells is that they should be either insensitive to some negative repressing signal or supersensitive to a positive stimulatory signal that normally governs the total mass of such cells. Similarly, there seems to be selection within most solid cancers for cells that can send out signals which summon an adequate blood supply. But the most important signals are presumably those that determine each cell's interaction with its more immediate neighbors, because it is presumably these signals that normally restrain the multiplying cells in epithelia from competing with each other for territory, and it must be some insensitivity to these signals that starts off the initial growth of a cancerous or precancerous clone. About such signals we really know nothing.

The next step in the determination of cell behavior is the transduction of the signal into some course of action. It is easy to see how this might be done. There are several rather well investigated instances in bacteria where a simple substance triggers a major alteration in the program of macromolecular synthesis; perhaps the best known is the response of stringent bacteria when an aminoacid becomes in short supply. But it does not follow that the regulation of gene function will occur in the same way in eukaryotes.

As yet, rather little is known about the molecular biological basis for major acts of differentiation, except in a few special cases such as the change between mating types in yeast and the genesis of antibody diversity in B lymphocytes. Much has been made of certain nuclear transplantation experiments which have been taken to indicate that the differentiated cells of vertebrates still retain a fully functional set of genes. However, the fact remains that although it is easy to produce a normal animal using the nucleus taken from a fertilized egg or an early blastula cell, no one has ever succeeded in producing a normal animal using the nucleus taken from a somatic cell of an adult. So when we are drawing up a list of mechanisms for differentiation and the control of gene expression, we should therefore not leave out genetic rearrangement as one of the possible devices.

This overview of what we know about the control of cell phenotype in multicellular systems may seem unduly pessimistic, but it is meant to have a practical outcome. If, as I suspect, we are really very far away from understanding (or even investigating in a sensible fashion) the defects

responsible for the uncontrolled behavior of most cancer
cells, then we should be supporting more research into the
underlying biology of cell communication - that is to say,
the field usually called developmental biology. For, until
this subject is much better understood and we are starting to
learn what is wrong with most cancer cells we cannot hope to
devise specific ways of treating cancer. While we wait for
the developmental biologist to provide the underpinings for
this branch of cancer research, we can concentrate on trying
to find out at least what kinds of event change a normal cell
into a cancer cell. For if we knew this it should be easier
to identify what factors in our environment and lifestyle
are likely to be important in determining the national
incidence of cancer.

The Molecular Biology of Carcinogenesis

Unlike the biology of the cancer cell phenotype, the
molecular biology of carcinogenesis appears to be a
reasonably accessible subject. The study of carcinogenesis
in experimental animals has shown that cancers can be
produced in many different ways. Some of the protocols
simply involve prolonged exposure to conventional mutagens;
certain cancers can apparently arise as the result of
reversible changes in gene regulation, and are therefore
thought of as being "epigenetic"; and others arise from a
sequence of steps, some of which are probably mutations and
some are not. Lastly, certain cancers can arise in
experimental animals as the result of changes in the quantity
of the food that the animals eat, rather than its quality;
here the mechanism of carcinogenesis is completely obscure.
When we come to consider the causes of human cancer, we
therefore have several scenarios to choose from.
    In the western world the two commonest cancers are cancer
of the skin and the lung, and each of them happens to be so
strongly dependent on a single factor (namely, sunlight and
tobacco) that their cause could be identified without the
need for any understanding of the underlying mechanism of
carcinogenesis (i.e., without any help coming from
experimental cancer research). But the preventable causes of
the other common cancers are less clearcut, and most people
feel that some understanding of mechanism may be needed if
we are to single out the causes from among the multitude of
variables in our environment and lifestyles.
    The classical stratagem for disclosing the mechanism
underlying any obscure biological reaction is to ask what
kinds of mutation affect the process, and this would seem to

be the best way of finding out what classes of biochemical event tend to be rate-limiting in human carcinogenesis. The results of such an approach are, however, rather surprising.

If the conventional dogma were correct and human cancers were usually being initiated by localized somatic mutations produced by the chemical mutagens in our environment, we would expect inherited defects in DNA repair to have a marked effect on the incidence of the common cancers. But this turns out not to be true. The disease xeroderma pigmentosum (XP) is equivalent in its effects to the *uvr* mutations of *Escherichia coli* and *Salmonella typhimurium* which make these bacteria into exquisitely sensitive tester strains for most chemical carcinogens. Thus the cells of an XP patient are defective in the excision-repair pathway that deals with all bulky lesions and distortions of the DNA double helix, and as a result they are very sensitive to the lethal and mutagenic actions of most mutagens. However, although XP patients have a very high incidence of skin cancer due to ultraviolet light (i.e., confined to those areas of their skin that are exposed to sunlight), they do not seem to suffer any excess of the common internal cancers.

TABLE 1.1
Deaths From Internal Cancers. Observed (expected)

Age	XP Patient Years	XP Internal Cancer	Bloom's Syndrome Patient Years	Bloom's Syndrome Leukemias Lymphomas	Carcinomas
0- 4	640	0 (.059)	340	1 (.013)	0 (.017)
5-14	886	0 (.055)	640	3 (.020)	0 (.019)
15-24	450	0 (.036)	327	2 (.011)	0 (.016)
25-34	213	0 (.035)	108	2 (.005)	2 (.013)
35-44	109	0 (.038)	16		1 (.008)
45-54	54	0 (.107)	3		1 (.005)
Total		0 (.330)		12 (.127)	

The figures for Bloom's syndrome come from a series of 89 patients (James German, personal communication). The figures for xeroderma pigmentosum come from various published reports that are summarized elsewhere (Cairns, 1980). The expected values were calculated from the current age-specific death rates from cancer in England and Wales.

In the published collections of cases that I have found in
the literature, about half the patients had had one or more
skin cancers but there was not one recorded death from an
internal cancer. This suggests firstly that the main source
of localized mutagenic lesions in our DNA is ultraviolet
light, and secondly that the common internal cancers are not
caused by the kind of lesions in DNA that XP patients (and
bacterial *uvr* mutants) are unable to repair.

The inherited defects that do raise the incidence of a
wide range of common cancers are the chromosome-instability
diseases - namely, Bloom's syndrome, ataxia telangiectasia
and Fanconi's anemia. As the accompanying table shows,
Bloom's syndrome results in roughly a 100-fold increase in
age-specific death rate both from the leukemias and
lymphomas and from the carcinomas. This suggests that large-
scale changes in the genome, such as rearrangements and
deletions, are much more hazardous than the local changes
produced by conventional mutagens.

Although these conclusions are in conflict with the
current dogma, they are not really so unreasonable. Most of
the cancers, for which an analysis of karyotype is possible,
tend to show characteristic rearrangements of chromosomes,
and sometimes these changes have been observed to arise very
early in the sequence of events that finally leads to overt
cancer; so rearrangement plainly is taking part in the
process. Furthermore, we should not be surprised by this.
To judge from the studies of biochemical evolution, most
local changes in DNA base sequence tend either to be lethal
(when they inactivate some essential gene) or to be
relatively innocuous, and that is why sequence changes
accumulate at a roughly constant rate in each species
irrespective of its rate of evolution; by contrast, when
morphological evolution is occurring rapidly it tends to be
associated with chromosomal changes, because change in
morphology means large changes in program (i.e., when are
various genes expressed, and for how long) rather than small
changes in gene products. So perhaps we should have expected
to find that cancer often arises as the result of
rearrangement and seldom as the result of sequence changes.

At this point, I should introduce a cautionary note,
because I do not want to be misunderstood. Obviously
conventional mutagens are dangerous and can cause cancer,
and so I am not advocating any relaxation in the standards
controlling our exposure to mutagens. Rather, I am
suggesting that such agents are only a minor cause of cancer
and that we are not likely to achieve a major reduction in
cancer death rate by an attack on the factors in our

environment that cause local changes in base sequence.

At the moment, the factors that cause genetic transposition are obscure. And this is where the experimentalist comes in. The molecular biology of transposition is just starting to be understood. This has suddenly become a subject of great interest and intense activity. But so far there has been no systematic study of the external factors that switch on the various enzymes (transposases) responsible for site-specific transpositions.

Summary

In this brief review I have discussed what I think are some of the ways basic studies in cell biology may contribute to the solution of the cancer problem. My first conclusion is that the organizations which support cancer research should make certain that the field of developmental biology is being adequately supported, because it will be as a result of discoveries in that area that the defects of the cancer cell will eventually come to be understood; once the defects are known, it should be possible to devise specific methods of treatment. My second conclusion is that most human cancers are the result of large-scale genetic rearrangements rather than the local base changes that are produced by conventional mutagens, and so I believe that there is a pressing need for more information about the molecular biology of such rearrangements and what it is that provokes them.

REFERENCES

Cairns, J. Cancer: the case for preventive strategies, in *Healthy people. The Surgeon General's Report on Health Promotion and Disease Prevention.* DHEW (PHS) publication No. 79-55071A, 1979, pp157-171

Cairns, J. On the origin of human cancers, to be published 1980

Calos, M.P. & Miller, J.H. Transposable elements. Cell 20: 579-595, 1980

Koshland, D.E. A response regulation model in a simple sensory system. Science, 196: 1055-1063, 1977

Loomis, W.F. *Dictyostelium discoideum. A developmental system.* New York:Academic Press, 1975

Slack, J.M.W. A serial threshold theory of regeneration. J Theoret Biol 82:105-140, 1980

Wilson, A.C., Carlson, S.S. & White, T.J. Biochemical evolution. Ann Rev Biochem 46:573-639, 1977

EVOLUTION OF THE MALIGNANT CELL PHENOTYPE

Daniel Medina

Department of Cell Biology
Baylor College of Medicine
Houston, Texas USA 77030

INTRODUCTION: A neoplastic cell population develops as a consequence of sequential alterations from normal cells through
various degrees of atypia to neoplastic cells. Over the past
decade, it has become increasingly clear that the majority of
epithelial tumors arise through sequential precursor populations.[6] Mouse mammary epithelial tumorigenesis is one of the
best-illustrated cases of sequential changes leading to neoplasia.[1,10] The availability of discrete precursor populations induced by hormones, chemical and viral carcinogens, and
the ability to examine the morphogenetic and growth properties
in an orthotopic site (the mammary fat pad) in syngeneic hosts
has provided a unique opportunity to study the host and cellular factors which modulate the evolution of the neoplastic
cell. An early scheme for the evolution of mammary tumors
emphasized the role of the alveolar hyperplasia (HAN) as the
precursor to mammary tumors induced by the mouse mammary tumor
virus (MMTV).[1]

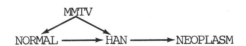

These precursor lesions were defined as preneoplastic
because they possessed a greater tumor-producing capability
that normal mammary epithelial cells. Subsequent studies demonstrated that chemical carcinogens can also induce preneoplastic HAN and that viral and chemical carcinogens can enhance
both the induction of HAN and the evolution of neoplastic cells
from existing HAN. Within the framework of this model, some
of the important questions concerning the evolution of the
neoplastic phenotype have been addressed in the past decade:

1. Are there alternative pathways to mammary neoplasias?

2. What factors modulate the expression of preneoplastic transformed cells from the normal population?

3. What factors modulate the expression of neoplastic transformed cells from the HAN population?

4. Is the primary tumor a homogeneous population with respect to its growth properties?

Alternative pathways to mammary neoplasms? In the mouse, chemical carcinogens induce at least 3 morphological types of precursor lesions:[10] (1) HAN, which have similar properties as viral-induced HAN; (2) Keratinizing nodules, (KN), which are alveolar hyperplasias with a marked degree of epidermoid differentiation; and (3) Ductal hyperplasis (DH), which are alterations of the ductal epithelial. Both HAN and DH have markedly increased tumor-producing capabilities, whereas KN have very low tumor-producing capabilities. However, prolonged hormone stimulation of KN can select out hyperplastic epithelial cells with increased tumor-producing capabilities suggesting that these lesions are alveolar in origin and may be a special variant of HAN.

In the rat, the major mammary lesions are intraductal proliferations which give rise to adenocarcinomas.[18] These lesions are induced by 7,12-dimethylbenzanthracene (DMBA) in great quantity, are produced from the growing distal tip of the mammary gland and develop into mammary adenocarcinomas. In humans, Wellings and Jensen[20] have proposed that a significant number of adenocarcinomas arise from atypical lobules. Progressive lobular distension due to epithelial cell proliferation gives the appearance of ducts in conventional, 2-dimensional histologic slides. During the morphological progression from atypia to adenocarcinomas, these early lesions resemble ductal carcinoma in situ. Wellings and Jensen[20] refer to the site of origin of these lesions as the terminal ductal lobular unit (TDLU). Thus, the model developed in the mouse has both general applicability and specific correlates in other species, including human. Depending on the etiological agent and the species, one or another pathway may predominate.

Factors which modulate expression of the preneoplastic transformed state: The interacting roles of viruses and hormones in the genesis of mammary tumors has been recognized for a long time.[16] A puzzling aspect of mammary tumorigenesis has been the relatively long latent period, particularly since the oncogenic agent (MMTV) is present in the host since birth.

Recent experiments by DeOme and co-workers have shed some light on this puzzle[2] (Figure 1). In virgin BALB/cfC3H female mice (MMTV-positive), precursor populations (HAN) start to appear at about 9 months of age. However, the preneoplastic cells can be shown to be present at 2-3 months of age. In these experiments, normal mammary gland tissue was enzymatically dissociated to yield a single cell suspension. A fixed number of cells was injected into the mammary fat pads of syngeneic hosts. Eight weeks later (the chronological age of the injected cells is 5 months), a significant number of the implants produced hyperplastic outgrowths which were shown to be preneoplastic by morphological and transplantation analysis. Thus, these experiments demonstrated that inapparent preneoplastically transformed cells were present in the poplation of normal mammary gland cells long before they were detectable as small hyperplastic foci; also, the number of inapparent transformed cells increased with the age of the host. Factors which modulate the expression of inapparent preneoplastic cells become important to the overall emergence of a neoplasm. Subsequent experiments demonstrated that one of the effects of hormones was to enhance the expression of inapparent preneoplastic cells into detectable hyperplastic foci.[3] The mechanism of this hormonal effect is unknown and may involve alterations of growth kinetic properties or cell-cell interactions.

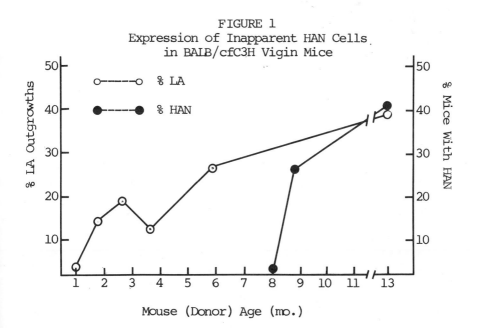

FIGURE 1
Expression of Inapparent HAN Cells
in BALB/cfC3H Vigin Mice

Mouse (Donor) Age (mo.)

TABLE 1
Induction and Neoplastic Transformation
of Preneoplastic HAN

Agent	Induction of HAN		Tumor Incidence in HAN	
	No. Mice Positive / No. Treated	%	No. Tumors / No. Transplants	%
γ-Irrad-iation (225R)	0/80	0	27/36	75
Urethan	0/40	0	30/32	94
DMBA	2/40	5	31/33	94
Melphalan	0/40	0	24/32	75

Modulation of expression of the neoplastic phenotype: The induction and/or expression of the neoplastic phenotype from the
preneoplastic cell population is very sensitive to numerous
factors, both carcinogenic and non-carcinogenic.[10] One of the
ways to study this question is to use preneoplastic outgrowth
lines which have been derived by serially transplanting HAN
originally found in old retired BALB/c breeders. Since BALB/c
mice are free of the exogeneously transmitted MMTV, the effect
of MMTV and other factors on the tumor-producing capabilities
of these outgrowth lines can be evaluated and compared to the
ability of these same agents to transform normal cells.

Agents which under defined experimental conditions, have
a minimal capability to transform normal mammary cells, have a
significant capability to modulate the neoplastic transformation from preneoplastic cell populations (Table 1). Agents
such as urethan, melphalan, DMBA, γ-irradiation and prolactin
enhance significantly the rate of neoplastic transformation
in the absence of exogenous MMTV.[10] So far, there is no indication that these agents activate an endogenous MMTV in this
system.[5,14,15,19] Another approach which examined the expression of neoplastic cells from preneoplastic cell populations
was to enzymatically dissociate the tissue and follow the
morphogenetic and growth properties of the cells injected
back into the mammary fat pads[13] (Table 2). Surprisingly,
the procedure of disrupting these cells was sufficient to increase their tumor potential. The hypothesis was formulated
that enzymatic dissocation disrupted cell-cell interactions
required for normal homeostasis of the preneoplastic cell
population. Neoplastic cells are generated at a constant
rate from preneoplastic cell populations, although their expression (multiplication) can probably be regulated by adjacent

TABLE 2
Inhibition of Mammary Tumor Formation by Normal Mammary Cells[a]

Group	Outgrowth Line [Ratio Normal:Nodule]	No. of Tumors/ No of Transplants	% Tumors
Intact	D1	6/30	20
Cell Suspension	10^5 D1	8/18	44
Mixed Cell Suspension	(3:1)	3/17	18
Intact	D2	25/37	68
Cell Suspension	10^5 D2	14/14	100
Mixed Cell Suspension	(2:1)	12/21	57

[a] Experiment terminated at 10 months

normal or preneoplastic cells. Disruption of the microenviron-
ment followed by injection of a single cell suspension confered
a selective advantage for the growth of neoplastic cells, thus
the rate of tumor formation was enhanced by this procedure.
The number of emerging neoplastic foci per unit time must not
be great since the tumor-producing capabilities of enzymatical-
ly-dissociated preneoplastic cell lines revert to a normal
background rate upon serial transplantation.

If a hypothetical interaction exists between preneoplastic
and normal cells, can this be demonstrated experimentally?
There are at least 2 experiments where such an interaction
has been documented. Experiments by Faulkin and DeOme[7] demonstrated that preneoplastic cells will stop growing in the presence of adjacent normal mammary cells. A second experiment
demonstrated that normal mammary cells mixed with preneoplastic cells in a single cell suspension inhibited the rate of
tumor formation from preneoplastic cells[13] (Table 2). Thus,
the data are consistent with the hypothesis that the emergence
of neoplastic cells and preneoplastic cells can be modulated
by cellular interactions and by chemical agents.

Heterogeneity of primary tumors: The primary tumor as it develops in the host is often assumed to be homogeneous in its
properties and of clonal origin. Although the neoplastic component may be of clonal origin, simple histological analysis
has documented the morphological heterogeneity of the primary
tumor population. It seems likely that the cell population
contains both neoplastic and non-neoplastic components. For

TABLE 3
Growth Properties of Mammary Cells
Grown in Primary Monolayer Cell Cultures

Growth Property	Normal	Preneo- plastic	Primary Tumor	Transplanted Tumor
CB-induced multi- nucleation[a]	4%	3%	34%	68%
In vivo growth of multi- cellular spheroids[b]	25%	63%	25%	100%
In vitro growth in low Ca^{++} medium[c]	No	No	No	Yes

[a] Percent of cells with number of nuclei > 3.
[b] Percent of transplants in the mammary fat
    pads which successfully produced outgrowths
    typical of the starting phenotype.
[c] Cells were grown in standard Dulbecco's modified
    Eagles medium under serum-free conditions and with
    1.4 mM or 0.09 mM Ca^{++} (11).

instance, the growth capabilities of primary tumors in vitro
suggest a heterogeneous population. Several results illustrate
this point (Table 3). Tumor cells generally show a relaxed
control of DNA synthesis and nuclear division compared to normal cells. Cytochalasin B is a drug used to probe cellular
control of DNA synthesis.[12,17] DNA synthesis in normal and
preneoplastic cells is inhibited by cytochalasin B; in primary
tumors, DNA synthesis is inhibited in 66% of the cells; whereas in transplanted tumors, DNA synthesis is inhibited in 30%
or less of the cells. Thus, the primary tumor contains many
cells which are non-cycling or otherwise regulated cells. With
serial transplantation, the cycling neoplastic cells soon predominate. A similar conclusion arises if one examines the
ability of cells to grow as multicellular aggregates in liquid
suspension. Normal, preneoplastic, and neoplastic cells grow
readily as multicellular aggregates in suspension; however,
if the aggregates are transplanted back into the cleared fat
pads, primary tumors grow very poorly. Only 25% of the implants from primary tumors grown in vitro produce tumors in
vivo, whereas 100% of the implants from serially transplanted
tumors grown in vitro produce tumors in vivo. Another marker

for neoplastic transformation is the ability to grow in low
[Ca^{++}] medium. Whereas transplanted tumors will grow in low
[Ca^{++}] medium, primary tumors require high [Ca^{++}] levels.
Thus, analyses of the growth characteristics of primary tumors
suggest a heterogeneous population with the neoplastic component being perhaps a minor component. Analysis of the be-
havorial properties of the neoplastic component suggest that
in early tumors, even this component is markedly heterogeneous
for a diverse set of properties, such as growth rate, immunogenicity, virus expression, sensitivity to chemotherapeutic
drugs, and metastatic potential.[4,9]

CONCLUSION: The evolution of the neoplastic phenotype in mammary
cancer may be summarized in the following scheme:

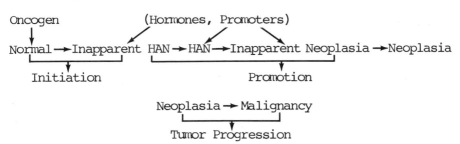

Putting this scheme in concepts of modern tumor biology, one
can visualize the oncogenic agent (MMTV, chemical carcinogens)
as an initiating agent which alters the normal cell to form
unexpressed HAN cells. Subsequent insults, by hormones, chemicals, irradiation, and non-specific stimuli act to promote subsequent steps in the pathways to the ultimate emergence of the
neoplastic phenotype. Finally, the emergence of the malignant
phenotype is the result of changes in the neoplastic phenotype
perhaps driven by karyotpyic instability which is a consequence
of the neoplastic phenotype. This latter step has been termed
"tumor progression" and is characterized by the emergence of
cell variants and selection of those cells optimally suited to
their environment.[8] Several important corallaries emerge from
this view of the evolution of the malignant cell. First, from
the data given earlier, it is clear that each of these populations is heterogeneous and contains elements of the immediate
precursor population. The recognition of cellular interactions
in the emergence of the neoplastic phenotype, whether these be
normal cell-transformed cell interactions or transformed cell-
stromal cell interactions has been belated and will provide
fruitful new information for the control of neoplastic growth.
Secondly, chemopreventive intervention is more likely to be
successful in those phenotypic states where the cell is still
closely regulated, i.e. the preneoplastic or early neoplastic

lesion. A previous review summarized this latter point succinctly: "A new and productive approach to the problem of breast cancer would be to focus more attention on the induction and transformation of preneoplastic lesions rather than the emphasis on the progression to metastasis."[21]

With the emerging methodology on the ability to grow normal and preneoplastic mammary cells in vitro, some fundamental questions about the evolution of the neoplastic phenotype can be approached systematically:

1. How do normal cells regulate the expression of the preneoplastic and neoplastic transformed phenotypes?

2. Is the appearance of the neoplastic cell phenotype a result of the induction of a new phenotype from the preneoplastic phenotype or do neoplastic cells already pre-exist in the preneoplastic population?

3. Can one develop chemopreventive agents which act on the expression of early stages of transformed cells?

4. What is the molecular nature of the alteration in the neoplastic cell phenotype which confers upon the cell the ability to divide independently from local growth regulatory factors?

5. What is the mechanism of action of promoting agents (i.e. hormones, phorbol estes) on the emergence of preneoplastic and neoplastic cell variants?

These questions are currently under investigation not only in the mammary tumor system, but in other epithelial cell tumor systems (skin, respiratory, liver, bladder) where sequential alterations have been documented in the evolution of the neoplastic phenotype.

REFERENCES

1. DeOme, K.B.: The mouse mammary tumor system, in Neyman, J. (ed.): Proc. 5th Berkeley Symp. on Mathematical Statistics and Probability. Univ. of Calif. Press, Berkeley, 1967, pp. 649-655.

2. DeOme, K.B., Miyamoto, M.J., Osborn, R.C. et al.: Detection of inapparent nodule-transformed cells in the mammary gland tissues of virgin female BALB/cfC3H mice. Cancer Res. 38: 2103-2111, 1978.

3. DeOme, K.B., Miyamoto, J.J., Osborn, R.C. et al.: Effect of parity on recovery of inapparent nodule-transformed mammary gland cells in vivo. Cancer Res. 38:4050-4053, 1978.
4. Dexter, D.L., Kowalski, J.M., Blazar, B.A. et al.: Heterogeneity of tumor cells from a single mouse mammary tumor. Cancer Res. 38:3174-3181, 1978.
5. Dusing-Swartz, S., Medina, D., Butel, J.S. et al.: Mouse mammary tumor virus genome expression in chemical carcinogen-induced mammary tumors in a low and high tumor incidence mouse strain. Proc. Natl. Acad. Sci. USA 76:5360-5364, 1979.
6. Farber, E., Sporn, M., eds.: Symposium on "Early Lesions and the Development of Epithelial Cancer". Cancer Res. 36:2475-2706, 1976.
7. Faulkin, L.J., Jr., DeOme, K.B.: Regulation of growth and spacing of gland elements in the mammary fat pad of the C3H mouse. J. Natl. Cancer Inst. 24:953-969, 1960.
8. Foulds, L.: The histologic analysis of mammary tumors in mice. J. Natl. Cancer Inst. 17:701-801, 1956.
9. Heppner, G.H., Dexter, D.L., DeNucci, T., et al.: Heterogeneity in drug sensitivity among tumor cell subpopulations of a single mammary tumor. Cancer Res. 38:3758-3763, 1978.
10. Medina, D.: Preneoplasia in breast cancer, in McGuire, W.L. (ed.): Breast Cancer. New York, Plenum Publishing Company, 1978, pp. 47-102.
11. Medina, D., Oborn, C.J.: Growth of preneoplastic mammary epithelial cells in serum-free medium. Cancer Res. (in press).
12. Medina, D., Oborn, C.J., Asch, B.B.: Distinction between preneoplastic and neoplastic mammary cell populations in vitro by cytochalasin B-induced multinucleation. Cancer Res. 40:329-333, 1980.
13. Medina, D., Shepherd, F., Gropp, T.: Enhancement of the tumorigenicity of preneoplastic mammary nodule lines by enzymatic dissociation. J. Natl. Cancer Inst. 60:1121-1126, 1978.
14. Michalides, R., VanDeemter, L., Nusse, R., et al.: Involvement of mouse mammary tumor virus in spontaneous and hormone-induced mammary tumors in low-mammary-tumor mouse strains. J. Virology 27: 551-559, 1978.
15. Michalides, R., VanDeemter, L., Nusse, R., et al.: Induction of mouse mammary tumor virus RNA in mammary tumors of BALB/c mice treated with urethane, X-irradiation, and hormones. J. Virology 31:63-72, 1979.
16. Nandi, S., McGrath, C.M.: Mammary neoplasia in mice. Adv. Cancer Res. 17:353-414, 1973.
17. O'Neill, F.J.: Control of nuclear division and chromosomal abnormalities in cytochalaisn B-treated normal and transformed cells, in Tanenbaum, S.W. (ed.): Cytochalasins, New

York, North-Holland Publishing Co., 1978, pp. 217-255.

18. Russo, J., Saby, J., Isenberg, W.M., et al.: Pathogenesis of mammary carcinomas induced in rats by 7,12-dimethylbenz-(a)anthracene. J. Natl. Cancer Inst. 59:435-445, 1977.

19. Smith, G.H., Pauley, R.J., Socher, S.H., et al.: Chemical carcinogenesis in C3H/StWi mice, a worthwhile experimental model for breast cancer. Cancer Res. 38:4504-4509, 1978.

20. Wellings, S.R., Jensen, J.M.: On the origin and progression of ductal carcinoma in the human breast. J. Natl. Cancer Inst. 50:1111-1118, 1978.

21. Welling, S.R., Jensen, H.M., Marcum, R.G.: An atlas of subgross pathology of the human breast with special reference to precancerous lesions. J. Natl. Cancer Inst. 55:231-273, 1975.

ACKNOWLEDGEMENTS

Figure 1 was used with permission of the author, Kenneth B. DeOme and the publisher, Cancer Research.

Suppression of Myeloid Leukemic Cells by Biological Regulators

DONALD METCALF

Head, Cancer Research Unit,
Walter and Eliza Hall Institute of Medical Research,
Melbourne, Australia.

While encouraging progress has been achieved in the past 20
years in the treatment of lymphoid and myeloid leukemias by
chemotherapy, it is recognized that such therapy is limited
by the profound toxicity for normal hemopoietic tissues of
the drugs used.   It is becoming apparent that further advances in the therapy of leukemia will depend on the development
of ancillary therapeutic approaches, the most logical of which
is to suppress leukemic cell proliferation by manipulation of
the regulatory factors controlling the production and differentiation of normal and leukemic cells.

CONTROL OF NORMAL GRANULOCYTE-MACROPHAGE CELLS

Studies in the last decade using semisolid culture systems
have shown that the production of neutrophilic granulocytes
and monocyte-macrophages is under the control of a glycoprotein humoral regulator - granulocyte-macrophage colony stimulating factor (GM-CSF) (see reviews[1,2]). GM-CSF is necessary
for the survival in vitro of granulocyte-macrophage (GM) progenitor cells, activates them into cycle if non-cycling, and
must be present continuously for all cell divisions from the
GM progenitor cells to the post-mitotic end cells: metamye-
locytes, polymorphs and monocyte-macrophages.

High GM-CSF concentrations shorten cell cycle times,stimu-
late the formation of progeny clones of large size and, where
progenitor cells are bipotential, force cells to enter or to
remain in the differentiation pathway of granulocyte formation.[3]   Conversely, low GM-CSF concentrations stimulate progenitors to divide more slowly and to form relatively small
numbers of progeny, most of which differentiate to macrophages.
These effects of GM-CSF can be demonstrated using GM-CSF purified to homogeneity and in cultures of single cells in serum-free medium. From this it can be concluded that the regulator acts directly on target GM cells.

No other proliferative stimulus has been identified for GM cells and all agents modifying GM proliferation appear to do so either by modifying GM-CSF concentrations or by modifying the responsiveness of GM cells to GM-CSF.

While the essential role of GM-CSF in GM proliferation is firmly established, it is less well appreciated that this regulator has profound effects on the differentiation of GM cells. Two types of effects have been documented: (a) stimulation of end cell functional activity, e.g. of RNA and protein synthesis by polymorphs,[4,5] of synthesis of PGE-1 and plasminogen-activator by macrophages,[6,7] of phagocytosis and killing of microorganisms by macrophages,[8] and (b) the concentration-dependent influence determining G or M differentiation referred to above.[3] It has also been shown that GM-CSF has a curious ability to stimulate the initial proliferation of multipotential hemopoietic cells and early cells of the erythroid, eosinophil and megakaryocytic series without altering their commitment to non-GM pathways of differentiation,[9,10] a functional activity of potential relevance to human myeloid leukemia where the leukemic clone arises in the multipotential, stem cell, compartment.

Analysis of the regulatory effects of GM-CSF on GM cells has been complicated by the facts that there is more than one molecular form of GM-CSF and that GM progenitor cells exhibit marked heterogeneity in their proliferative capacity and responsiveness to stimulation. Certain subsets of GM progenitor cells appear to respond preferentially to distinct subsets of GM-CSF molecules.

Normal GM progenitor (colony-forming) cells appear to have essentially no capacity for self-replication as opposed to their ability to generate differentiating clones of up to 10^4 progeny cells. Because of this, it has not been possible so far to determine whether GM-CSF can influence self-replication of normal GM-progenitor cells as distinct from the formation of daughter cells of a more highly differentiated nature.

THE BIOLOGICAL NATURE OF MYELOID LEUKEMIA

The myeloid leukemias in man are accepted with some reservations as being neoplasms of GM populations. They exhibit the capacity for progressive proliferation characteristic of neoplasms and, like many neoplasms, are clonal in origin, the leukemic population clearly representing progeny of a single initiating cell. Two unique features set the myeloid leukemias apart from all other cancers: (a) in acute myeloid leukemia, the leukemic population can, for a time, be suppressed almost completely (usually following chemotherapy) with the re-emergence and dominance of previously suppressed normal hemopoietic populations - the phenomenon of remission in-

duction, and (b) the cell initiating the myeloid leukemic
clone is multipotential and the phenotypically normal erythroid, megakaryocytic and B-lymphoid cells in the patient
are members of the same clone. The phenotypic behavior of
neoplasia exhibited by the GM members of the clone appears to
be dependent on cells entering the GM pathway of differentiation.

Both these aspects of the biology of myeloid leukemia suggest strongly that the myeloid leukemias are unusually dependent on biological regulators for both their initiation and
progressive proliferation and that useful therapeutic intervention might be feasible by manipulating these regulators.

It has been known for many years that myeloid leukemic
cells often possess an impressive capacity for generating differentiating progeny. However from the critical viewpoint of
controlling the population size of a tumor, it is of little
importance whether tumor cells can or cannot form differentiating progeny. Control of a tumor population can only be
achieved if the capacity of the tumor stem cells for extensive self-replication can be restricted. The semilogarith-
mic (Gompertzian) size increase in a neoplastic population is
influenced very little by mean cell cycle times or whether
some cells can differentiate to end cells. If more than 50%
of the progeny of the stem cells within the population retain
the proliferative characteristics of the parent stem cells,
such a population will expand exponentially regardless of
other parameters. Control of any neoplastic population, including the myeloid leukemias, therefore hinges in the last
analysis on control of the pattern of proliferation of the
stem cells within the population.

WEHI-3B MYELOMONOCYTIC LEUKEMIA

Cells of this transplantable leukemia of BALB/c mice[11] are
able to form colonies in semisolid culture and, when initially tested, colony formation was largely dependent on stimulation by GM-CSF.[12] The cells forming colonies in culture
were shown to be stem cells of the leukemic population and to
have a variable capacity for self-replication in vivo according to their location in the body.[13] The true dependency of
WEHI-3B leukemic cells on GM-CSF is difficult to assess because these leukemic cells are unusual in themselves being
able to synthesize GM-CSF.[12,14]

After 10 years of continuous culture in vitro including
cloning, a variant population has emerged, the cells of which
form large colonies of undifferentiated blast and promyelocytes without the addition of exogenous GM-CSF. Individual
colony-forming cells exhibit an extensive capacity for self-
replication within developing colonies. Addition of purified GM-CSF forced cells in a significant proportion of col-

onies to differentiate to identifiable granulocytes and macrophages.   Such differentiated colonies contained sharply reduced numbers of colony-forming (stem) cells.[15]   However in
the presence of purified GM-CSF, some colonies remained undifferentiated and this form of GM-CSF was unable to completely suppress the exponential expansion of the leukemic population.

Serum from mice injected with endotoxin is known to contain
high concentrations of GM-CSF[16,17] and, even at high dilutions,
was found to enforce a marked degree of differentiation in
WEHI-3B colonies.   Serial reculture of WEHI-3B colony cells
in the presence of endotoxin serum led to complete clonal suppression of the leukemia within 2 - 6 passages.[18]   When 10^4
pooled colony cells grown in the presence of endotoxin serum
were injected into syngeneic BALB/c mice, a consistent suppression of their leukemogenicity was observed, particularly
if the mice had received an injection of endotoxin at the time
of transplantation of the leukemic cells (Metcalf, D., unpublished data).   Analysis of the nature of the factor with this
exceptional differentiation-enforcing activity revealed that
it was not the major type of GM-CSF in the serum but activity
cofractionated with a minor subset of GM-CSF molecules selectively stimulating G colony formation by normal cells (Burgess,
A.W. and Metcalf, D., unpublished data).

Ml AND R453 MYELOID LEUKEMIAS

Cells of the continuous mouse myeloid leukemia cell line Ml
were demonstrated to form colonies of undifferentiated cells
in semisolid culture in the absence of added GM-CSF.   Such
colony cells could be forced to exhibit extensive differentiation to granulocytes and macrophages by addition of materials
now known to contain GM-CSF.[19,20]   Endotoxin serum, mouse
lung conditioned medium and GM-CSF purified from the latter
source were all shown to enforce differentiation of Ml cells
both by morphological criteria and by the use of a wide variety of surface markers, functional and biochemical criteria
(see review Sachs[21]).

Differentiation after exposure to GM-CSF-containing materials was associated with a marked suppression of the capacity
to form colonies in vitro and to produce progressively growing leukemic populations after transplantation to syngeneic
recipients.[19,22,23]

Essentially similar results have been obtained with the
more recently developed R453 myeloid leukemic cell line.[24]
Studies using Ml cells demonstrated that relatively stable
subclones could be derived that either exhibited a capacity to
differentiate in the presence of GM-CSF (D+ cells) or an in-

ability to differentiate (D⁻ cells).[21]   Extended proliferation of the D⁻ cells could not be suppressed by GM-CSF.

These latter observations raised the likelihood that attempts to enforce differentiation in myeloid leukemic populations would encounter the familiar problems of genetic resistance with the emergence of subclones unresponsive to further regulatory control.   It is of considerable interest therefore that exposure of the D⁻ M1 cells to a number of cytotoxic drugs used clinically in the treatment of myeloid leukemia appears to convert such cells to D⁺ cells that are then responsive to the differentiation-enforcing effects of GM-CSF-containing materials.[25,26]

HUMAN CHRONIC MYELOID LEUKEMIA

Chronic myeloid leukemic populations in man are characterized by their exceptionally high content of cells able to form GM colonies in semisolid culture.   CML colony-forming cells have been identified as myeloblasts in the leukemic population and can be distinguished from normal GM progenitor (colony-forming) cells by differences in cell cycle status, sedimentation rate and particularly buoyant density (see review Metcalf[27]).   However the colonies they generate in vitro are essentially indistinguishable from normal GM colonies in growth rate, size and the differentiation of colony cells.   In distinction from the situation with the mouse myeloid leukemic cell lines, the colony-forming cells in CML have no detectable capacity for self-replication, again closely resembling the behavior of normal colony-forming cells.

Of the many hundreds of CML patients analyzed, in no instance have CML cells been detected that are able to proliferate in vitro in the absence of GM-CSF.   This complete dependency of CML cells does not alter during the course of the disease.   The dose-response curves for CML cells indicate that they are essentially normal in their responsiveness to GM-CSF.[28,29]   The situation following acute transformation is not entirely clear, since often the cells fail to grow or grow poorly in vitro.   Acute transformation often appears to be associated with loss of ability of the cells proliferating in vitro to exhibit normal differentiation but apparently the cells remain responsive to, and dependent on, GM-CSF.[30]

The GM population in CML has therefore been characterized as exhibiting   extreme hyperplasia of the precursor population but with individual progenitor cells closely resembling normal cells.   Since GM-CSF levels are normal or above normal in CML[1,27] and CML cells respond normally to regulatory control in vitro, why does the GM population show a progressive size increase in an untreated patient?   The answer presumably lies in the fact that the GM precursors originate

from the true stem cells of the leukemic population that are
located in the multipotential stem cell compartment.   The
implication is that the generation of GM precursors by such
stem cells is not subject to adequate regulatory control.
Although techniques have now been developed for cloning hemopoietic stem cells in vitro,[31,32,33] these methods have not
yet been applied to analyze the situation in CML and to determine the level at which regulatory control is inadequate.

HUMAN ACUTE MYELOID LEUKEMIA

   Cells from patients with acute myeloid or myelomonocytic
leukemia can be cloned in semisolid medium but the plating
efficiency varies over very wide limits and growth is frequently very restricted.   As is the case with CML cells, the
AML cells proliferating in culture can be distinguished from
normal GM progenitor cells on the basis of cell cycle status,
sedimentation velocity, and density abnormalities.[27,30] AML
cells are as dependent on GM-CSF for proliferation as normal
cells, although in some instances the dose-response curves to
CSF vary slightly from normal.[29,30,34]
   The situation with AML is essentially similar to that just
discussed for CML cells.   The more differentiated cells in
the leukemic clone should be responsive to control by GM-CSF
and the basis for the progressive size increase in the AML
population that actually occurs needs to be investigated in
the stem cell compartment of the leukemic population. Some
progress has been made in developing a cloning system for undifferentiated blast cells in the AML population[35] and, as
there is evidence that these cells are capable of extended
self-generation,[36] this system may allow an investigation of
the responsiveness of these cells to regulatory control.
Since blast colony formation requires stimulation by leukocyte conditioned medium,[35,36] the provisional conclusion is
that such blast cells are not autonomous and may well be controllable by molecules analogous with GM-CSF.
   It is unclear whether GM-CSF levels are normal or subnormal in AML.   There is evidence that patients at special risk
of AML development have a subnormal capacity to produce GM-
CSF as do certain patients with AML, particularly those not
responding well to chemotherapy.[37,38]
   The mechanisms underlying the suppression by AML cells of
normal hemopoietic populations are obviously complex and are
not well understood.[39]   Some evidence has been presented for
inhibition of normal GM cells by AML cells in cocultures and
a factor has been described as being produced by leukemic
cells that can inhibit the proliferation of normal GM precursors.[40]   Whatever the mechanisms involved in suppression,
the subsequent regeneration of normal hemopoietic populations

following destruction or suppression of leukemic cells may not require the operation of any novel regulatory systems, simply the removal of leukemic cells.

STRATEGIES FOR REGULATORY CONTROL OF MYELOID LEUKEMIC POPULATIONS

Since both AML and CML populations are dependent on GM-CSF for proliferation, a possible method for controlling leukemic cell proliferation is by suppression of GM-CSF. The only reported method for suppressing serum GM-CSF levels is the injection of cortisone[41] and it is of some interest that this agent is included in most chemotherapeutic regimes for the induction of remission in AML.   However, suppression of GM-CSF is unlikely to be a realistic approach since the formation of normal GM cells is equally dependent on GM-CSF and patients require GM cells to combat infections.

At the present, the opposite procedure of deliberately elevating GM-CSF levels seems a more logical approach since this might be expected to suppress or minimize stem cell replication with the added advantage at least temporarily of forcing the production of more differentiated, and thus more functionally active, cells.

Although short-term elevations of serum GM-CSF levels can be achieved using injections of bacterial cell-wall products, repeated injection of such agents rapidly leads to an unresponsive state.[16,42,43]   There is an urgent need to develop methods capable of elevating GM-CSF levels for several weeks so that these could be used during the initial induction of a remission by chemotherapy.

From the observed half-life of GM-CSF in mice (2 - 7 hours) [44,45] it is unlikely that significantly elevated levels could be sustained in man by injected GM-CSF unless an enormous logistics problem of GM-CSF mass-production can be solved, perhaps by cloning the message for human-active CSF-production, since present methods for GM-CSF production would be quite inadequate.

A final possibility is that agents will be discovered that are able to render leukemic GM cells hyperresponsive to existing GM-CSF levels, thereby effectively elevating GM-CSF levels.

It should be added for completeness that GM populations are clearly controlled by the interaction of a matrix of regulatory factors.   While GM-CSF is the dominant component in this matrix, manipulation of other components e.g. various inhibitory factors, may also prove useful in the control of leukemic populations.

REFERENCES

1. Metcalf, D. Hemopoietic colony stimulating factors.
    In "Tissue Growth Factors" Ed. R. Baserga. Springer
    New York (in press) 1980.
2. Moore, M.A.S. Humoral regulation of granulopoiesis. In
    "Clinics in Haematology" Ed. L.J. Lajtha Vol.8,p.287-
    309, 1979.
3. Metcalf, D. Clonal analysis of the proliferation and
    differentiation of paired daughter cells: Action of
    GM-CSF on granulocyte-macrophage precursors. Proc.Natl.
    Acad.Sci.(USA) (in press) 1980.
4. Burgess, A.W. and Metcalf, D. The effect of colony
    stimulating factor on the synthesis of ribonucleic acid
    by mouse bone marrow cells in vitro. J.Cell.Physiol. 90,
    471-484, 1977.
5. Burgess, A.W. and Metcalf, D. Colony-stimulating factor
    and the differentiation of granulocytes and macrophages.
    In "Experimental Hematology Today" Eds. S. J. Baum and
    G. D. Ledney. Springer-Verlag. New York. pp 135-146,
    1977.
6. Kurland, J., Broxmeyer, H.E., Pelus, L.M., Bockman, R.S.
    and Moore, M.A.S. Role for monocyte-macrophage derived
    colony stimulating factor and prostaglandin E in the
    positive and negative feedback control of myeloid stem
    cell proliferation. Blood 52, 388-407, 1978.
7. Lin, H-S, Gordon, S. Secretion of plasminogen activator
    by bone marrow-derived mononuclear phagocytes and its
    enhancement by colony-stimulating factor. J.Exp.Med.
    150, 231-245, 1979.
8. Handman, E., and Burgess, A.W. Stimulation by granulo-
    cyte-macrophage colony stimulating factor of Leishmania
    tropica killing by macrophages.   J.Immunol. 122,1134-
    1137, 1979.
9. Metcalf, D., Johnson, G. R. and Burgess, A.W. Direct
    stimulation by purified GM-CSF of the proliferation of
    multipotential and erythroid precursor cells. Blood 55,
    138-147, 1980.
10. Metcalf, D., Burgess, A.W. and Johnson, G. R. Stimula-
    tion of multipotential and erythroid precursor cells by
    GM-CSF. In "Experimental Hematology 1979" Ed. S. J.
    Baum. Springer Verlag, New York (in press) 1980.
11. Warner, N.L., Moore, M.A.S. and Metcalf, D. A trans-
    plantable myelomonocytic leukemia in BALB/c mice: cytol-
    ogy, karyotypic and muramidase content. J.Natl.Cancer
    Inst.43,963-982, 1969.

12. Metcalf, D., Moore, M.A.S. and Warner, N.L. Colony formation in vitro by myelomonocytic leukemic cells. J.Natl.Cancer Instit. 43,983-1001, 1969.

13. Metcalf, D. and Moore, M.A.S. Factors modifying stem cell proliferation of myelomonocytic leukemic cells in vitro and in vivo. J.Natl.Cancer Instit.44,801-808, 1970.

14. Williams, N., Eger, R.R., Moore, M.A.S. and Mendelsohn, N. Differentiation of mouse bone marrow progenitor cells to neutrophil granulocytes by an activity separated from WEHI-3 cell conditioned medium. Differentiation 11, 59-63, 1978.

15. Metcalf, D. Clonal analysis of the action of GM-CSF on the proliferation and differentiation of myelomonocytic leukemic cells. Int.J.Cancer 24,616-623, 1979.

16. Metcalf, D. Acute antigen-induced elevation of serum colony stimulating factor (CSF) levels. Immunology 21, 427-436, 1971.

17. Staber, F.G. and Burgess, A.W. Serum of lipopolysaccharide treated mice contains two types of colony-stimulating factor, separable by affinity chromatography. J.Cell.Physiol. 102,1-10, 1980.

18. Metcalf, D. Clonal extinction of myelomonocytic leukemic cells by serum from mice injected with endotoxin. Int. J.Cancer 25,225-233, 1980.

19. Ichikawa, Y. Differentiation of a cell line of myeloid leukemia. J.Cell.Physiol. 74,223-234, 1969.

20. Ichikawa, Y. Further studies on the differentiation of a cell line of myeloid leukemia. J.Cell.Physiol.76,175-184, 1970.

21. Sachs, L. Control of normal cell differentiation and the phenotypic reversion of malignancy in myeloid leukaemia. Nature 274,535-539, 1978.

22. Fibach, E. and Sachs, L. Control of normal differentiation of myeloid leukemic cells. VII Induction of differentiation to mature granulocytes in mass culture. J.Cell.Physiol. 86,221-230, 1975.

23. Honma, Y., Kasukabe, T., Okabe, J. and Hozumi, M. Prolongation of survival time of mice inoculated with myeloid leukemia cells by inducers of normal differentiation. Cancer Res. 39,3167-3171, 1979.

24. Ichikawa, Y., Maeda, M. and Horiuchi, M. In vitro differentiation of Rauscher virus-induced myeloid leukemia cells. Int.J.Cancer 17,789-797, 1976.

25. Okabe, J., Honma, Y. and Hozumi, M. Inhibition of RNA and protein syntheses make non-differentiating mouse myeloid leukemia cells sensitive to a factor stimulating differentiation. Int.J.Cancer 20,933-940, 1977.

26. Hayashi, M., Okabe, J. and Hozumi, M. Sensitization of
    resistant myeloid leukemia clone cells by anticancer
    drugs to factor stimulating differentiation. Gann 70,
    235-238, 1979.
27. Metcalf, D. Hemopoietic Colonies. In Vitro Cloning of
    Normal and Leukemic Cells. Springer Verlag Berlin/
    New York, 1977.
28. Metcalf, D., Moore, M.A.S., Sheridan, J.W. and Spitzer,G.
    Responsiveness of human granulocytic leukemic cells to
    colony stimulating factor. Blood 43,847-859, 1974.
29. Francis, G.E., Berney, J.J., Chipping, P.M. and Hoffbrand,
    A.V. Stimulation of human haemopoietic cells by colony
    stimulating factors - sensitivity of leukaemic cells.
    Brit.J.Haemat.41,545-562, 1979.
30. Moore, M.A.S. In vitro studies in the myeloid leukemias.
    In Advances in Acute Leukemia, Eds. Cleton, F.J., Crow-
    ther, D., Malpas, J.B. North-Holland. Amsterdam. p 161,
    1975.
31. Johnson, G.R. and Metcalf, D. Pure and mixed erythroid
    colony formation in vitro stimulated by spleen condit-
    ioned medium with no detectable erythropoietin. Pro-
    ceedings National Academy of Sciences USA 74,3879-3882,
    1977.
32. Metcalf, D., Johnson, G.R. and Mandel T.E. Colony for-
    mation in agar by multipotential hemopoietic cells.
    J.Cell.Physiol. 98,401-420, 1979.
33. Fauser, A.A. and Messner, H.A. Identification of mega-
    karyocytes, macrophages and eosinophils in colonies of
    human bone marrow containing neutrophilic granulocytes
    and erythroblasts. Blood 53,1023-1027, 1979.
34. Brennan, J.K., Di Persio, J.F., Abboud, C.N. and Licht-
    man, M.A. The exceptional responsiveness of certain
    human myeloid leukemia cells to colony-stimulating acti-
    vity. Blood 54, 1230-1239, 1979.
35. Minden, M.D., Till, J.E. and McCulloch, E.A. Prolifera-
    tive state of blast cell progenitors in acute myelo-
    blastic leukemia (AML). Blood 52,592-600, 1978.
36. Buick, R.N., Minden, M.D. and McCulloch, E.A. Self-
    renewal in culture of proliferative blast progenitor
    cells in acute myeloblastic leukemia. Blood 54,95-104,
    1979.
37. Greenberg, P.and Mara, B. Microenvironmental influences
    on granulopoiesis in acute myeloid leukemia. In Dif-
    ferentiation of Normal and Neoplastic Hematopoietic Cells.
    Eds. Clarkson, B., Marks, P.A., Till, J.E. Cold Spring
    Harbor Laboratory New York, p.405, 1978.

38. Hornsten, P., Granstrom, M., Wahren, B. and Gharton, G.
     Prognostic value of colony-stimulating and colony-form-
     ing cells in peripheral blood in acute non-lymphoblastic
     leukemia.   Acta Med.Scand. 201, 405-410, 1977.
39. Broxmeyer, H.E. and Moore, M.A.S. Communication between
     white cells and the abnormalities of this in leukemia.
     Biochim.Biophys.Acta 516,129-166, 1978.
40. Broxmeyer, H.E., Jacobsen, N., Kurland, J., Mendelsohn,
     N. and Moore, M.A.S. In vitro suppression of normal
     granulocytic stem cells by inhibitory activity derived
     from human leukemia cells. J.Natl.Cancer Instit.60,497-
     511, 1978.
41. Metcalf, D. Cortisone action on serum colony-stimulating
     factor and bone marrow in vitro colony-forming cells.
     Proc.Soc.Exp.Biol.132,391-394, 1969.
42. Metcalf, D. Depressed responses of the granulocyte-
     macrophage system to bacterial antigens following pre-
     immunization. Immunology 26,1115-1125, 1974.
43, Quesenberry, P., Halperin, J., Ryan, M. and Stohlman,F.
     Tolerance to the granulocyte releasing and colony stimu-
     lating factor elevating effects of endotoxin. Blood 45,
     789-800, 1975.
44. Burgess, A.W. and Metcalf, D. Serum half-life and organ
     distribution of radiolabeled colony stimulating factor
     in mice. Exp.Hemat.5,456-464, 1977.
45. Shadduck, R.K., Waheed, A., Porcellini, A., Rizzoli, V.
     and Pigoli, G. Physiologic distribution of colony stim-
     ulating factor in vivo.   Blood 54,894-905, 1979.

Properties of Metastatic Tumor Cells

GARTH L. NICOLSON

Professor and Chairman
Department of Tumor Biology
University of Texas System Cancer Center
M.D. Anderson Hospital and Tumor Institute
Houston, Texas 77030

INTRODUCTION

The spread of tumors or metastasis contributes in a major way to clinical fatalities due to cancer (Salsbury, 1975; Sugarbaker, 1979). Although cancer metastasis is one of the most important events in the pathogenesis of cancer, there have been proportionately few comprehensive studies of this important phenomenon in man or experimental animal models. However, with the development of tumor transplantation, cell tissue culture and sophisticated biochemical, immunological, genetic and ultrastructural techniques we know far more about the pathogenesis of tumor metastasis. It is now well established that metastasis involves a complex series of sequential steps whereby malignant tumor cells invade adjacent tissues and penetrate into lymphatic and circulatory systems, detach from the primary tumor mass, spread to near and distant sites, arrest and invade at these secondary sites and finally proliferate to form new tumor foci (reviews: Fidler and Nicolson, 1980; Fidler et al., 1978; Poste and Fidler, 1980; Sugarbaker, 1979; Weiss, 1977; Zeidman, 1957). That this phenomenon is the end result of several highly selective sequential steps where fewer and fewer tumor cells survive to finally form secondary growth is an important concept in the pathogenesis of metastasis (Fidler and Nicolson, 1980; Poste and Fidler, 1980). This concept suggests that the actual cells that are capable of forming metastases such as distant secondary tumor colonies may actually represent a very minor

Supported by National Cancer Institute grants 7RO1-CA-28867, 7RO1-CA-29571 and 1RO1-CA-28844.

subpopulation of the cells that comprise the primary tumor
mass. Evidence in support of cell subpopulations will be
discussed below.

Metastasis usually begins when a tumor mass extends or
invades surrounding tissues; this loss of proper cell positioning and cell-cell interactions characterizes the malignant state (Nicolson and Poste, 1976). Invasion is thought
to occur by mechanical extension (Eaves, 1973) or enzymatic
destruction of extracellular tissue matrix (Dresden et al.,
1972; Hashimoto et al., 1973) or both.

During the course of invasion neoplastic cells can detach and be transported away from the original tumor mass.
The far more important routes in this process are the blood
vessels and lymphatics where penetrating tumors can release
multiple cell emboli. The release of such emboli into the
blood is known to be affected by venous pressure, blood flow
and trauma due to surgery or other manipulations (Fisher et
al., 1967). However, the presence of malignant cells or cell
emboli in the blood is not an indication that subsequent distant metastases will form (Salsbury, 1975), probably because
most tumor cells die rapidly in the circulation, and only a
small fraction survive to form secondary tumors (reviewed in
Fidler et al., 1978).

During transport in the blood malignant cells undergo
cellular interactions with themselves, other circulating host
cells, soluble blood components and the vascular endothelium.
Cellular interactions that affect tumor cell arrest and subsequent survival include homotypic adhesion of tumor cells to
form multicell emboli (Fidler, 1973a; Liotta et al., 1976;
Winkelhake and Nicolson, 1976), heterotypic adhesion such as
that of tumor cells to platelets (Gasic et al., 1973; Warren,
1973), lymphocytes (Fidler, 1975; Fidler and Bucana, 1977) or
endothelial cells (Kramer and Nicolson, 1979; Kramer et al.,
1980) and interactions of tumor cells with blood components
such as fibrinogen (or fibrin) (Chew et al., 1976; Warren,
1973). Although mechanical factors such as tumor emboli size
and capillary deformability modify lodgement properties in
the first capillary bed encountered (Sato and Suzuki, 1976;
Zeidman and Buss, 1952), malignant cells often pass through
capillaries after initial arrest (Fidler and Nicolson, 1976,
1977; Fisher and Fisher, 1967a; Zeidman and Buss, 1952).

Mechanical considerations alone are insufficient to explain the non-random blood-borne arrest and survival patterns
of various malignant cells. In man there are numerous examples where tumors tend to metastasize to particular secondary locations (Regato, 1977; Salsbury, 1975; Sugarbaker,
1979). In addition, many experimental animal tumor systems

show organ preference of secondary tumor colonization (Dunn,
1954; Fidler and Nicolson, 1976; Hart and Fidler, 1980;
Kinsey, 1960; Potter et al., 1957; Sugarbaker, 1952) suggesting that metastasis is influenced by unique tumor cell
and/or host properties. Recognition of unique capillary
vascular endothelial cell surface determinants by circulating malignant cells could result in implantation at specific
sites (Nicolson and Winkelhake, 1975), or the subsequent
growth of arrested tumor cells may be site-dependent (Hart
and Fidler, 1980).

After implantation of blood-borne tumor cells in the
microcirculation the most common step is extravasation or
secondary invasion of the endothelium and its underlying
basement membrane. This process may (Chew et al., 1976;
Wood, 1964) or may not (Fisher and Fisher, 1967b; Ludatscher
et al., 1967) involve deposition and dissolution of a fibrin
matrix around the arrested tumor cell(s). Penetration of
the vascular endothelium may in some cases occur by diapede-
sis or intracellular penetration (Dingemans, 1973), but the
usual route appears to be penetration at points of endothelial cell retraction (Kramer and Nicolson, 1979; Ludatscher
et al., 1967). The retraction of vascular endothelial cells
caused by tumor cell-endothelial cell interactions and exposure of underlying basement membrane results in net movement
of malignant cells to the basement membrane surface of higher
adhesive potential (Kramer et al., 1980). Cell surface secreted tumor enzymes may be responsible for subsequent invasion (Dresden et al., 1972; Hashimoto et al., 1973; Koono
et al., 1974; Strauch, 1972; Sylven, 1973), and tissue damage
or tumor cell secretion of angiogenesis factor(s) (Folkman,
1974) may be responsible for vascularization of the secondary
colony resulting in rapid growth.

TUMOR CELL AND HOST PROPERTIES AND METASTASIS

Animal tumor mocels have been successfully used to study the
role of tumor cell properties in metastasis. Since tumor
cell lines exist with common genetic heritage but differing
in metastatic phenotype, certain aspects of metastasis may
be traceable to distinct cellular characteristics. Koch
(1939) was the first to select tumor cell variants for malignant properties, but potentially the most useful techniques
for obtaining malignant cells with differing metastatic properties were developed by Fidler (1973b). By sequential
selection of variant tumor cell lines for enhanced abilities
to form blood-borne experimental pulmonary metastases in syngeneic hosts Fidler (1973b) developed a series of variant
B16 melanoma cell lines with increasing lung colonization

TABLE 1

In Vivo Selection for Altered Metastatic Behavior

Tumor Type	Selection for Site of Metastasis	References
Carcinoma	Lung	Koch, 1939
Carcinoma	Lung	Klein, 1955
Carcinoma	Lung	Kerbel et al., 1978
Melanoma	Lung	Fidler, 1973b
Melanoma	Brain	Brunson et al., 1978
Melanoma	Brain	Raz & Hart, 1980
Melanoma	Brain	Nicolson et al., 1981
Melanoma	Ovary	Brunson & Nicolson, 1979
Melanoma	Liver	Tao & Burger, 1977
Lymphoma	Liver	Schirrmacher et al., 1979
Sarcoma	Lung	Nicolson et al., 1978
Sarcoma	Lung	Salk & Lanza, 1979
Lymphosarcoma	Liver	Brunson & Nicolson, 1978
Lymphosarcoma	Lung	Belloni & Nicolson, 1980
Adenocarcinoma	Lung, RLN	Neri et al., 1979
Adenocarcinoma	Ascites, lung	Takahashi et al., 1978
Adenocarcinoma	Lung	Talmadge et al., 1979

abilities. Several types of B16 melanoma selections have now
been performed, and B16 sublines are available that show enhanced abilities to colonize lung, liver, ovary or brain
(Table 1). Some of these in vivo selections were performed
by implanting tumor cells subcutaneously and allowing the
implanted cells to spontaneously metastasize (Neri et al.,
1979). It is interesting that when these experiments were
repeated without the requirement for blood-borne or lymphatic
tumor cell arrest, variants with enhanced metastatic properties were not obtained. For example, sequential adaptation
of B16 melanoma cells for brain survival and growth by direct
intracerebral implantation did not result in variant cell
lines with enhanced blood-borne brain implantation, survival
and growth properties (Brunson and Nicolson, 1980).

Selection for metastatic variant tumor cell lines has
also been accomplished by selection in vitro (Table 2). For
example, it has been possible to select in vitro for tumor
cell properties such as loss of sensitivity to lymphocyte-
mediated cellular toxicity (Fidler et al., 1976), decreased
binding to immobilized lectins (Reading et al., 1980), increased invasiveness of tissue (Hart, 1979) or veins (Poste
et al., 1980) as well as other cellular properties (Table 2).
Often these selections have resulted in concomitant modifi-

TABLE 2

In Vitro Selection for Altered Metastatic Behavior

Cell Type	Mode of Selection	References
B16 Melanoma	Resistance to lympho-cyte killing	Fidler et al., 1976
B16 Melanoma	Detachment from plastic	Briles & Kornfeld, 1978
B16 Melanoma	Resistance to lectin toxicity	Tao & Burger, 1977
B16 Melanoma	Attachment to collagen	Liotta et al., 1978
B16 Melanoma	Invasion of tissue	Poste et al., 1980
B16 Melanoma	Invasion of bladder	Hart, 1979
RAW117 Lymphosarcoma	Loss of lectin binding	Reading et al., 1980

cations in malignant phenotype (Table 2). In each case variant sublines were eventually obtained with altered in vivo metastatic properties indicating that successful selections do not require organ site selection.

Host properties are also important in tumor metastasis. In many clinical and experimental tumor situations endocrine state appears to play an important role in metastasis. Analogous to the situation in many patients with malignant melanoma (Cochran, 1973), Proctor et al. (1976) found that B16 melanoma grew more slowly and metastasized less often in female compared to male mice. However, these differences were abrogated by oblation of female hormonal systems. Traumatization, inflammation or damage of host tissues can lead to increased arrest and survival of blood-borne tumor cells to form metastases (Fisher et al., 1967). One of the more interesting properteis is immunologic recognition and destruction of metastatic cells. Although some experimental metastases are susceptible to immunodestruction (reviewed in Castro, 1978; Fidler and Nicolson, 1980), the mere fact that metastasis occurs is thought to be a good indication that inherent host anti-tumor immunity is insufficient to prevent this process. Indeed, experimental studies on the role of host immunity have been somewhat antithetical; that is, in some cases host immune status appears to be linked to the incidence of metastasis such that depression of anti-tumor immune state enhanced metastasis (Alexander, 1976), while in others depression of host immune status has no effect (Fidler et al., 1979) or even a negative effect on metastasis (Fidler and Nicolson, 1978; Vaage, 1978). Clearly, there is

TABLE 3

Heterogeneity of Malignant Neoplasms

Tumor Type	Characteristic	Experiment	References
Melanoma	Metastasis	Clones	Fidler & Kripke, 1977
Mammary tumor	Metastasis	Clones	Dexter et al., 1978
Fibrosarcoma	Metastasis	Clones	Suzuki et al., 1978
Sarcoma	Metastasis	Clones	Nicolson et al., 1978
Lymphosarcoma	Metastasis	Clones	Reading et al., 1980b
Carcinoma	Metastasis	Clones	Talmadge et al., 1979
Fibrosarcoma	Metastasis	Clones	Kripke et al., 1978
Melanoma	Drug response	Sublines/clones	Lotan & Nicolson, 1979
Hepatoma	Drug response	Sublines	Barranco et al., 1978
Melanoma	Drug response	Sublines	Barranco et al., 1972
Carcinoma	Metastasis/drug response	Sublines	Dexter et al., 1978
Carcinoma	Metastasis/drug response	Sublines	Heppner et al., 1978
Carcinoma	Antigens	Sublines	Fogel et al., 1979
Sarcoma	Antigens	Sublines	Pimm & Baldwin, 1977
Sarcoma	Antigens	Sublines	Byers & Johnston, 1977
Carcinoma	Radiation sensitivity	Sublines	Revesz & Norman, 1963

no simple relationship between host immunity and metastasis, and much needs to be done in this area in order to eventually understand complex tumor-host relationships.

TUMOR HETEROGENEITY AND METASTASIS

As discussed above, metastasis is a highly selective pheno-menon such that only a small fraction of the total cells in a primary lesion are probably able to complete the entire process. Nowell (1976) has proposed that as tumor progres-sion occurs tumor cell variants arise within the lesion; these variants are subjected to host selection pressures re-sulting in the overall emergence of rare sublines with en-hanced malignant potentials. The abilities of various

investigators to select in vivo or in vitro metastatic variant sublines is consistent with this proposal, but the most
convincing data have come from cloning experiments. Fidler
and Kripke (1977) were the first to clone tumors such as the
B16 melanoma. They compared individual clones for their
metastatic potentials and found that experimental metastases
formed in animals receiving melanoma cells intravenously
varied widely among the different clones and also when compared to the parental B16 melanoma line. Fidler and Kripke
(1977) concluded that cell subpopulations with high metastatic potential existed in the parental B16 tumor and were not
produced by the cloning techniques. That tumors are heterogeneous and are made up of cell subpopulations of widely different metastatic potential and phenotypes has been seen in
a variety of neoplasms (Table 3). If tumors are monoclonal
in origin, this suggests that heterogeneity could result from
random phenotypic drift. In fact, there is evidence for
metastatic drift in cell clones of B16 melanoma (Fidler
and Nicolson, 1980), 13762 adenocarcinoma (A. Neri and
G.L. Nicolson, in preparation) and RAW117 lymphosarcoma
(C.L. Reading and G.L. Nicolson, unpublished observations)
suggesting that an important property of malignant tumor
cells might be their ability to change or drift phenotypically at much higher rates compared to normal cells or benign
tumor cells.

The heterogeneity of tumor cell populations has important implications for the treatment of cancer. The success
of anti-tumor therapy could well depend on the ability of
various treatments to eliminate the possibly rare, highly
metastatic tumor cell subpopulations that exist within a
neoplasm (Fidler, 1978). Differences in radiation sensitivity (Revesz and Norman, 1963), susceptibility to cytotoxic
(Fuji and Mihich, 1975; Heppner et al., 1978; Nicolson et al.,
1980) or cytostatic (Lotan and Nicolson, 1979) drugs, as well
as differences in immunogenicity (Pimm and Baldwin, 1977) may
pose serious problems for cancer management, if highly metastatic variant subpopulations that are refractory to various
treatment strategies persist after the treatments are terminated (Goldin and Johnson, 1977; Olsson and Ebbesen, 1979).
The usefulness of combination therapies has been well established and is considered in detail in other sections of this
monograph. What may be necessary in the future could well
be the development of such therapies for the exclusive treatment of highly metastatic variant cell subpopulations that
ultimately cause the most problems in terms of cancer management. Research on the development of metastatic tumor
models should play an increasingly important role in the

development and testing of new therapeutic concepts that
concentrate on the destruction and prevention of metastases.

REFERENCES

Alexander, P. Dormant metastases which manifest on immunosuppression and the role of macrophages in tumours. In L.
   Weiss (Ed.), Fundamental aspects of metastasis. Amsterdam:
   North-Holland Publishing Co., 1976, 227-239.
Barranco, S.C., Ho, D.H.W., Derwinko, B. et al. Differential
   sensitivities of human melanoma cells grown in vitro to
   arabinosylcytosine. Cancer Res., 1972, 32, 2733-2736.
Barranco, S.C., Haenelt, B.R., & Gee, E.L. Differential sen-
   sitivities of five rat hepatoma cell lines to anticancer
   drugs. Cancer Res., 1978, 38, 656-660.
Belloni, P.N., & Nicolson, G.L. Unpublished observations,
   1980.
Briles, E.G., & Kornfeld, S. Isolation and metastatic prop-
   erties of detachment variants of B16 melanoma cells. J.
   Natl. Cancer Inst., 1978, 60, 1217-1222.
Brunson, K.W., & Nicolson, G.L. Selection and biologic prop-
   erties of malignant variants of a murine lymphosarcoma.
   J. Natl. Cancer Inst., 1978, 61, 1499-1503.
Brunson, K.W., & Nicolson, G.L. Selection of malignant melanoma variant cell lines for ovary colonization J. Supramol. Struct., 1979, 11, 517-528.
Brunson, K.W., & Nicolson, G.L. Experimental brain metastasis
   In L. Weiss, H. Gilbert & J.B. Posner (Eds.), Brain metas-
   tasis. Boston: G.K. Hall & Co., 1980, 50-65.
Brunson, K.W., Beattie, G., & Nicolson, G.L. Selection and
   altered tumour cell properties of brain-colonising meta-
   static melanoma. Nature, 1978, 272, 543-545.
Byers, V.S., & Johnston, J.O. Antigenic differences among
   osteogenic sarcoma tumor cells taken from different loca-
   tions in human tumors. Cancer Res., 1977, 37, 3173-3183.
Castro, J.E. (Ed.) Immunologic aspects of cancer. Baltimore:
   University Pak Press, 1978.
Chew, E.C., Josephson, R.L., & Wallace, A.C. Morphologic
   aspects of the arrest of circulating cancer cells. In L.
   Weiss (Ed.), Fundamental aspects of metastasis. Amsterdam:
   North-Holland Publishing Co., 1976, 121-150.
Cochran, A.J. Malginant melanoma. A review of ten years ex-
   perience in Glasgow, Scotland. Cancer, 1973, 23, 1190-1199.
Dexter, D.L., Kowalski, H.M., Blazar, B.A. et al. Hetero-
   geneity of tumor cells from a single mouse mammary tumor.
   Cancer Res, 1978, 38, 3174-3181.

Dingemans, K.P. Behavior of intravenously injected malignant lymphoma cells: A morphologic study. J. Natl. Cancer Inst., 1973, 51, 1883-1897.

Dresden, M.H., Heilman, S.A., & Schmidt, J.D. Collagenolytic enzymes in human neoplasms. Cancer Res., 1972, 32, 993-996.

Dunn, T.B. Normal and pathologic anatomy of the reticular tissue in laboratory mice, with a classification and discussion of neoplasms. J. Natl. Cancer Inst., 1954, 14, 1281-1433.

Eaves, G. The invasive growth of malignant tumors as a purely mechanical process. J. Pathol., 1973, 109, 233-237.

Fidler, I.J. The relationship of embolic homogeneity, number, size and viability to the incidence of experimental metastasis. Eur. J. Cancer, 1973a, 9, 223-227.

Fidler, I.J. Selection of successive tumor lines for metastasis. Nature New Biol., 1973b, 242, 148-149.

Fidler, I.J. Biological behavior of malignant melanoma cells correalted to their survival in vivo. Cancer Res., 1975, 35, 218-224.

Fidler, I.J. Tumor heterogeneity and the biology of cancer invasion and metastasis. Cancer Res., 1978, 38, 2651-2660.

Fidler, I.J., & Bucana, C. Mechanism of tumor cell resistance to lysis by syngeneic lymphocytes. Cancer Res., 1977, 37, 3945-3956.

Fidler, I.J., & Kripke, M.L. Metastasis results from pre-existing variant cells within a malignant tumor. Science, 1977, 893-895.

Fidler, I.J., & Nicolson, G.L. Organ selectivity for implantation, survival and growth of B16 melanoma variant tumor lines. J. Natl. Cancer Inst., 1976, 57, 1199-1202.

Fidler, I.J., & Nicolson, G.L. Tumor cell and host properties affecting the implantation and survival of blood-borne metastatic variants of B16 melanoma. Israel J. Med. Sci., 1978, 14, 38-50.

Fidler, I.J., & Nicolson, G.L. The immunobiology of experimental metastatic melanoma. Cancer Biol. Rev., 1980, in press.

Fidler, I.J., Gersten, D.M., & Budman, M.B. Characterization in vivo and in vitro of tumor cells selected for resistance to syngeneic lymphocyte-mediated cytotoxicity. Cancer Res., 1976, 36, 3160-3165.

Fidler, I.J., Gersten, D.M., & Hart, I.R. The biology of cancer invasion and metastasis. Adv. Cancer Res., 1978, 28, 149-250.

Fidler, I.J., Gersten, D.M., & Kripke, M.L. The influence of immunity on the metastasis of three murine fibrosarcomas of differing immunogenicity. Cancer Res., 1979, 39, 3816-3821.

Fisher, B., & Fisher, E.R. The organ distribution of dis-
    seminated ^{51}Cr-labeled tumor cells. Cancer Res., 1967a,
    27, 412-420.
Fisher, B., & Fisher, E.R. Anticoagulants and tumor cell
    lodgement. Cancer Res., 1967b, 27, 421-425.
Fisher, B., Fisher, E.R., & Feduska, N. Trauma and the local-
    ization of tumor cells. Cancer, 1967, 20, 23-30.
Fogel, M., Gorelik, E., Segal, S., & Feldman, M. Differences
    in cell surface antigens of tumor metastases and those of
    local tumor. J. Natl. Cancer Inst., 1979, 62, 585-588.
Folkman, J. Tumor angiogenesis. Adv. Cancer Res., 1974, 19,
    331-358.
Fuji, H., & Mihich, E. Selection for high immunogenicity in
    drug-resistant sublines of murine lymphomas demonstrated
    by plaque assay. Cancer Res., 1975, 35, 946-952.
Gasic, G.J., Gasic, T.B., Galanti, N. et al. Platelet-tumor
    cell interaction in mice. The role of platelets in the
    spread of malignant disease. Int. J. Cancer, 1973, 11, 704-
    718.
Goldin, A., & Johnson, R.K. Resistance to antitumor agents.
    In H.J. Tagnon and M.J. Staquet (Eds.), Recent advances in
    cancer treatment. New York: Raven Press, 1977, 155-169.
Hart, I.R. The selection and characterization of an invasive
    variant of B16 melanoma. Am J. Pathol., 1979, 97, 587-600.
Hart, I.R., & Fidler, I.J. The role of organ selectivity in
    the determination of metastatic patterns of B16 melanoma.
    Cancer Res., 1980, in press.
Hashimoto, K., Yamanishi, Y., & Dabbous, Y. Electron micro-
    scopic observations of collagenolytic activity of basal
    cell epithelioma of the skin in vivo and in vitro. Cancer
    Res., 1972, 32, 2561-2567.
Hashimoto, K., Yamanishi, Y., Maeyens, E. et al. Collageno-
    lytic activities of squamous cell carcinoma of the skin.
    Cancer Res., 1973, 33, 2790-2801.
Heppner, G.H., Dexter, D.L., DeNucci, T. et al. Heterogeneity
    in drug sensitivity among tumor cell subpopulations of a
    single mammary tumor. Cancer Res., 1978, 38, 3758-3763.
Kerbel, R.S., Twiddy, R.R., & Robertson, D.M. Induction of
    a tumor with greatly increased metastatic growth potential
    by injection of cells from a low metastatic H-2 heterozy-
    gous tumor cell line into an H-2 incompatible parental
    strain. Int. J. Cancer, 1978, 22, 583-594.
Klein, E. Gradual transformation of solid into ascites tumors.
    Evidence favoring the mutation-selection theory. Exp. Cell
    Res., 1955, 8, 188-212.
Koch, F.E. Zur fragoder metastasenbildung bei impflumorin.
    Krebsforsch, 1939, 48, 495-507.

Koono, M., Ushijima, K., & Hayashi, H. Studies on the mechanisms of invasion in cancer. III. Purification of a neutral protease of rat ascites hepatoma cell associated with production of chemotactic factor for cancer cells. Int. J. Cancer, 1974, 13, 105-115.

Kramer, R.H., & Nicolson, G.L. Interactions of tumor cells with vascular endothelial cell monolayers: A model for metastatic invasion. Proc. Natl. Acad. Sci. U.S.A., 1979, 76, 5704-5708.

Kramer, R.H., Gonzalez, R., & Nicolson, G.L. Metastatic tumor cells adhere preferentially to the extracellular matrix underlying vascular endothelial cells. Int. J. Cancer, 1980, in press.

Kripke, M.L., Gruys, E., & Fidler, I.J. Metastatic heterogeneity of cells from an ultraviolet light-induced murine fibrosarcoma of recent origin. Cancer Res., 1978, 38, 2962-2967.

Liotta, L.A., Kleinerman, J., & Saidel, G.M. The significance of hematogenous tumor cell clumps in the metastatic process. Cancer Res., 1976, 36, 889-894.

Liotta, L.A., Vembu, D., Saini, R.K., & Boone, C. In vivo monitoring of the death rate of artificial murine pulmonary micrometastases. Cancer Res., 1978, 38, 1231-1236.

Lotan, R., & Nicolson, G.L. Heterogeneity in growth inhibition by β-trans-retinoic acid of metastatic B16 melanoma clones and in vivo-selected cell variant lines. Cancer Res., 1979, 39, 4767-4771

Ludatsher, R.M., Luse, S.A., & Suntzeff, V. An electron microscopic study of pulmonary tumor emboli from transplanted Morris hepatoma 5123. Cancer Res., 1967, 27, 1939-1952.

Neri, A., Ruoslahti, E., & Nicolson, G.L. Relationship of fibronectin to the metastatic behavior of rat mammary adenocarcinoma cell lines and clones. J. Supramol. Struct., 1979, (suppl. 3), 444.

Nicolson, G.L., & Poste, G. The cancer cell: Dynamic aspects and modifications in cell-surface organization. New Engl. J. Med., 1976, 259, 197-203 and 253-258.

Nicolson, G.L., & Winkelhake, J.L. Organ specificity of blood-borne tumour metastasis determined by cell adhesion? Nature, 1975, 255, 230-232.

Nicolson, G.L., Brunson, K.W., & Fidler, I.J. Specificity of arrest, survival and growth of selected metastatic variant cell lines. Cancer Res., 1978, 38, 4105-4111.

Nicolson, G.L., Lotan, R., & Rios, A. Tumor cell heterogeneity and the in vitro sensitivities of metastatic B16 melanoma sublines and clones to retinoic acid or BCNU.

Cancer Treatment Reports, 1980, in press.

Nicolson, G.L., Miner, K.M., & Reading, C.L. Tumor cell heterogeneity and blood-borne metastasis. In Fundamental Mechanisms in cancer immunology. New York: Elsevier/North Holland, Inc., 1981, in press.

Nowell, P.C. The clonal evolution of tumor cell populations. Science, 1976, 194, 23-28.

Olsson, L., & Ebbesen, P. Natural polyclonality of spontaneous AKR leukemia and its consequences for so-called specific immunotherapy. J. Natl. Cancer Inst., 1979, 62, 623-627.

Pimm, M.V., & Baldwin, R.W. Antigenic differences between primary methylcholanthrene-induced rat sarcomas and post-surgical recurrences. Int. J. Cancer, 1977, 20, 37-43.

Poste, G., & Fidler, I.J. The pathogenesis of cancer metastasis. Nature, 1980, 283, 139-146.

Poste, G., Doll, J., Hart, I.R., & Fidler, I.J. In vitro selection of murine B16 melanoma variants with enhanced tissue invasive properties. Cancer Res., 1980, 40, 1636-1644.

Potter, M., Rahey, J.L. & Pilgrim, H.I. Abnormal serum protein and bone destruction in transmissible mouse plasma cell neoplasm (multiple myeloma). Proc. Soc. Exp. Biol. Med., 1957, 94, 327-333.

Proctor, J.W., Auclair, B.G., & Stokowski, L. Endocrine factors and the growth and spread of B16 melanoma. J. Natl. Cancer Inst., 1976, 57, 1197-1198.

Raz, A., & Hart, I.R. Murine melanoma. A model for intracranial metastasis. Brit. J. Cancer, 1980, in press.

Reading, C.L., Belloni, P.N., & Nicolson, G.L. Selection and in vivo properties of lectin-attachment variants of malignant murine lymphosarcoma cell lines. J. Natl. Cancer Inst., 1980a, 64, 1241-1249.

Reading, C.L., Brunson, K.W., Torrianni, M., & Nicolson, G.L. Malignancies of metastatic murine lymphosarcoma cell lines and clones correlate with decreased cell surface display of RNA-tumor virus envelope glycoprotein gp70. Proc. Natl. Acad. Sci. U.S.A., 1980, in press.

Regato, J.A., Jr. Pathways of metastatic spread of malignant tumors. Sem. Oncol., 1977, 4, 33-38.

Revesz, L., & Norman, L. Relationship between chromosome ploidy and radiosensitivity in selected tumor sublines of common origin. J. Natl. Cancer Inst., 1963, 25, 1041-1063.

Salk, P., & Lanza, R.P. In vitro growth characteristics, motility and adhesive properties of metastatic variant PW20 cell lines. J. Supramol. Struct., 1979, (suppl 3): 182.

Slasbury, A.J. The significance of the circulating cancer cell. Cancer Treatment Rev., 1975, 2, 55-72.

Sato, H., & Suzuki, M. Deformability and viability of tumor cells by trans-capillary passage, with reference to organ affinity of metastasis in cancer. In L. Weiss (Ed.), Fundamental aspects of metastasis. Amsterdam: North-Holland Publishing Co., 1976, 311-317.

Schirrmacher, R., Shantz, G., Clauer, K. et al. Tumor metastases and cell-mediated immunity in a model system in DBA/2 mice. I. Tumor invasiveness in vitro and metastasis formation in vivo. Int. J. Cancer, 1979, 23, 233-244.

Strauch, L. The role of collagenases in tumor invasion. In D. Tarin (Ed.), Tissue interactions in carcinogenesis. New York: Academic Press, 1972, 399-434.

Sugarbaker, E.V. The organ selectivity of experimentally induced metastasis in rats. Cancer, 1952, 5, 606-612.

Sugarbaker, E.V. Cancer Metastasis: A produce of tumor-host interactions. Curr. Prob. Cancer, 1979, 3, 3-59.

Suzuki, N., Withers, H.R., & Koehler, M.W. Heterogeneity and variability of artificial lung colony-forming ability among clones from a mouse fibrosarcoma. Cancer Res., 1978, 38, 3349-3351.

Sylven, B. Biochemical and enzymatic factors involved in cellular detachment. In S. Garattini & G. Franchi (Eds.), Chemotherapy of cancer dissemination and metastasis. New York: Raven Press, 1973, 129-138.

Takahashi, S., Konishi, Y., Nakatanli, K. et al. Conversion of poorly differentiated human adenocarcinoma to ascites form with invasion and metastasis in nude mice. J. Natl. Cancer Inst., 1978, 60, 925-927.

Tao, T-W., & Burger, M.M. Non-metastasising variants selected from metastasising melanoma cells. Nature, 1977, 270, 437-438.

Vaage, J. A survey of the growth characteristics of and the host reactions to one hundred C3H/He mammary carcinomas. Cancer Res., 1978, 38, 331-338.

Warren, B.A. Environment of the blood-borne tumor embolus adherent to vessel wall. J. Med., 1973, 4, 150-177.

Weiss, L. A pathobiologic overview of metastasis. Sem. Oncol., 1977, 4, 5-19.

Winkelhake, J.L., & Nicolson, G.L. Determination of adhesive properties of variant metastatic melanoma cells to BALB/3T3 cells and their virus-transformed derivatives by a monolayer attachment assay. J. Natl. Cancer Inst., 1976, 56, 285-291.

Wood, S., Jr. Experimental studies of the intravascular dissemination of ascitic V2 carcinoma cells in the rabbit,
with special reference to fibrinogen and fibrinolytic
agents. Bull. Schweiz. Akad. Med. Wiss., 1964, 20, 92-121.

Zeidman, I. Metastasis: A review of recent advances. Cancer
Res., 1957, 17, 157-162.

Zeidman, I., & Buss, J.M. Transpulmonary passage of tumor
cell emboli. Cancer Res., 1952, 12, 731-733.

High Efficiency, Kinetics and Numerology

of Transformation by Radiation in vitro

ANN R. KENNEDY

Assistant Professor of Radiobiology

JOHN B. LITTLE

Professor of Radiobiology

Laboratory of Radiobiology
Harvard University, School of Public Health
Boston, Massachusetts 02115

It is now clear that ionizing radiation is a potent human carcinogen (2). There is growing concern from both the public and regulatory agencies concerning the carcinogenic risks from low-level radiation exposures. Up to the present time, most of the relevant studies on radiation carcinogenesis in animals or in human populations have yielded little information concerning the mechanism involved in radiation carcinogenesis. Understanding of the mechanism involved in the conversion of a cell from the normal state to malignancy is essential if we are to develop a rational approach to cancer prevention. We have been examining the mechanism of radiation carcinogenesis in an in vitro transformation assay system in which cellular exposure and environmental conditions can be precisely controlled. This paper reviews some of our current data on the induction of malignant transformation and its modification by chemical agents in cultured mammalian cells.

MATERIALS AND METHODS

The experiments reported here have used the C3H mouse em-

This research was supported by NIH Grants CA-22704 and ES-00002. Address reprint requests to Dr. Ann R. Kennedy at the above address.

bryo fibroblast cell line designated 10T 1/2, clone 8, developed
for studies of chemical transformation by Reznikoff et al.
(18,19), and adapted for studies of radiation transformation
(12,21). Details of radiation transformation experiments have
been previously described.

RESULTS AND DISCUSSION

    As shown in the top line of Fig. 1 (5), our usual experi-
ment involves the irradiation of dishes seeded 24 hrs before
with sufficient cells to yield about 300 viable cells per dish
(12,21). These cells then undergo about 13 divisions to reach
confluence - a density of about 2 x 10^6 cells per 100 mm Petri
dish. The cells are then allowed to remain in the confluent
stationary phase of growth until visible transformed foci de-

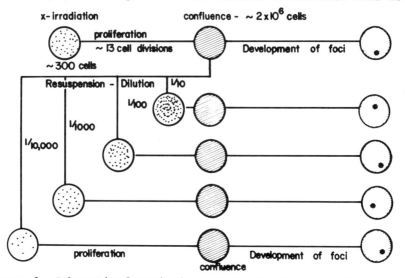

Figure 1. Schematic description of the development of transformation in vitro (as occurs in routine experiments) is
shown in the top line. The number of cells initially seeded
is such that about 300 viable cells per 100 mm Petri dish
(left) result. The cells are irradiated the following day and
allowed to proliferate until confluence is reached and cell
division ceases 10-14 days later (center). Transformed foci
appear 4-5 weeks later (right) overlying the confluent monolayer. The lower lines schematically describe the resuspen-
sion of individual dishes at confluence and reseeding at different dilutions. The cells in each of the reseeded dishes
then proliferate until confluence is reached a second time,
and incubation is continued for 4 additional weeks until foci
develop. (from Ref. 5).

velop. This quiescent phase takes about 4-5 weeks; thus the
whole experiment takes about 6-7 weeks post-irradiation before
visible foci can be scored. In certain experiments we reduced
the initial cell density to as low as about 1 viable cell per
dish. In other experiments, 300 viable cells per dish were
seeded and irradiated, and the cells allowed to proliferate to
confluence. At this point, the confluent dishes were trypsin-
ized and new dishes seeded at various dilutions; after confluence was reached a second time, the cells were maintained in
the quiescent phase until transformed foci developed.

   The remarkable observation in all these experiments is that,
for a given dose of radiation, the number of foci that finally
develop in each confluent plate is approximately constant
(Fig. 1). As shown in Fig. 2 (from Ref. 5), the yield of
transformed foci per dish remained constant even when the number of viable cells seeded per dish was varied over a range
of 5 orders of magnitude;   this yield was equal to the frequency of transformation observed on undisturbed dishes. These
results suggest that the cellular alteration that leads to the
formation of a clone of transformed cells is not an immediate,
direct consequence of exposure to X-rays such as is usually

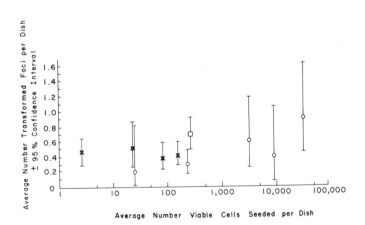

Figure 2. Results of experiments involving subculture (as dia-
grammed in Fig. 1). Transformation induced by 400-600 rads of
X-rays as a function of the number of cells initially seeded or
reseeded following subculture at first confluence. Symbols:
     □ - 400 rads, initial cell density; O - 400 rads,
subcultured groups;   X   - 600 rads, initial cell density;
(Data and fig. from Ref. 5).

associated with a single gene mutation. For example, if the
ultimate transformed focus were the direct result of a mutational change induced by X-rays in an occasional cell, resus-
pension of the irradiated population would give rise to many
transformed foci per dish if the population were reseeded at
high cell densities, and the number of transformed foci per
dish would decline when the population was reseeded at progressively lower cell densities. This is the result seen when
variants are arising by rare mutations (15), but it was not
seen in our experiments on transformation.

Our observations can, however, be accounted for by making
the assumption that a two-stage process is responsible for
radiation induced transformation. Our working hypothesis is
that exposure to x-rays (in the dose range of 400-600 rads)
produces in all or nearly all of the surviving cells a functional or metabolic change which is inherited by all their
progeny (perhaps an inherited epigenetic change like that described in certain bacterial systems (16). We assume that this
functional change increases the probability of a second, perhaps mutational, transforming event when the cells are being
maintained under conditions of confluence (5).

Other explanations are possible for our results shown in
Fig. 2. One explanation for the apparent reduction in the
yield of transformants per surviving cell at high initial
(or reseeded) cell density is the previous observation that
the presence of large numbers of normal cells can inhibit the
phenotypic expression of transformed or potentially transformed cells as foci (8,20). It seems unlikely, however, that this
mechanism could explain the increasing yield of transformants
(as measured on a per surviving cell basis) observed in low
density cultures (1-200 viable cells/dish), because the cells
were so sparsely seeded even at the highest density.

As proliferation has been shown to be essential for the
phenotypic expression of transformation following carcinogen
exposure (12) another possible explanation could be that the
additional cell proliferation possible in the low density
cultures enhanced the expression of transformation[1], leading
to the higher transformation frequencies per surviving cell
from a given dose of radiation as the cell density decreased.
It appears, however, that this effect is not simply related
to the increased capacity for cell division if one considers
the results obtained for different initial and reseeded cell
densities together, or the results of experiments outlined in
Fig. 1. In experiments involving 300 surviving cells initially and reseeding to 300 viable cells (or about a 1/1000 dilu-

[1]The lower the cell density, the more cells must proliferate
until confluence is reached, as shown in Fig. 1.

tion (5), the cells have undergone two proliferative phases or, with about 13 divisions for each proliferative phase, a total of 26 divisions. With 26 divisions, the resultant transformation frequency per surviving cell is about the same as that observed in undisturbed cultures in which the cells underwent only 13 divisions (at 1 focus per plate, about 3.3 x 10^{-3} transformants per surviving cell). In cultures in which the initial cell density was as low as 1 cell per dish (5), the initial treated cell goes through about 23 divisions before confluence is reached, and the transformation frequency per surviving cell approaches 100% (at about 1 focus per dish resulting from the treatment). Thus, the number of divisions this treated single cell goes through is less than the 26 divisions the cells underwent in the reseeding experiments described above, and yet the transformation frequency per surviving cell is considerably higher in the low cell density (i.e. one cell per dish) experiment.[1]

To account for our observations described above, and shown in Figs. 1 and 2, by these other mechanisms would require the remarkable coincidence that the suppressing effect of normal cells on the growth of transformed or potentially transformed cells (or the rate of phenotypic reversion) were precisely compensated for by dilution over at least 4 decades and over a wide range of growth experience from 13 to 29 cellular generations (5).

We have previously shown that X-ray transformation can be enhanced by incubating the irradiated cells with the known phorbol ester promoting agent, 12-0-tetradecanoyl-phorbol-13-acetate (TPA) (6-11,13), which is not carcinogenic in itself. TPA is most effective in enhancing radiation transformation when added to proliferating cells which have been exposed to a low dose of radiation that would ordinarily lead to little or no measurable transformation by itself (10,11). TPA has little or no enhancing effect when added after cells have reached the confluent state of growth (11). We have performed a series of dilution experiments involving a relatively low dose of radiation (100 rads) and TPA treatment, similar to the ones described above for radiation treatment (400-600 rads) alone. One series of successive dilution experiments involved the presence of TPA for the entire time, another involved the presence of TPA only until the first confluence was reached.

We analyzed the 100 rad-TPA dilution results in the same

[1]An additional factor to be considered in analyzing the effect of proliferation in such transformation assays is the known phenomenon of phenotypic reversion of the transformed phenotype when transformed cells are passaged at low cell density (1,17).

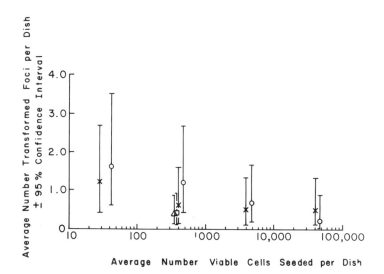

Figure 3. Results of subculture experiments. Transformation
induced by 100 rads of X-rays with subsequent incubation with
TPA as a function of the number of cells reseeded following
subculture at first confluence. Initial cell density of undisturbed cultures shown for comparison. Symbols:
☐ - undisturbed dishes - TPA removed at confluence; △ -
undisturbed dishes - TPA present for whole experiment; X -
subcultured dishes - TPA removed at first confluence; O -
subcultured dishes - TPA present for whole experiment.

manner as the high-dose radiation alone results (shown in Fig.
2) in terms of the average number of transformed foci per dish;
we observed the same lack of a relationship between the number
of foci per dish and the average number of cells seeded per
dish. These results are shown in Fig. 3, and described in detail elsewhere (9). Thus, it seems possible that a low dose
of radiation, coupled with TPA treatment, produces a similar
effect to high doses of radiation alone (400-600 rads) and
that a similar mechanism may be involved (9).
     The question arose, in such dilution experiments involving
the presence of TPA, whether the yield of transformants following subculture to low cell densities might be higher (left -
Fig. 3) than that observed for cultures reseeded at higher densities (right - Fig. 3). We addressed this question in a series of experiments designed to study the transformation yield
as a function of initial cell density for 100 rads followed by
TPA treatment. The transformation yields following x-ray exposure, TPA treatment and varying cell densities at the time
of irradiation of 10T½ cells are shown graphically in Fig. 4;

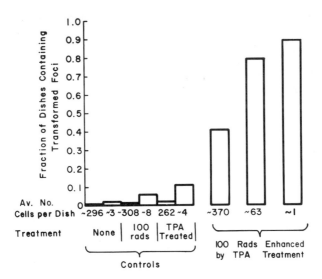

<u>Figure 4</u>. Increased yield of transformants, measured here in terms of the fraction of dishes containing transformed foci, when irradiation of 100 rads of X-rays is followed by TPA treatment compared to no treatment, 100 rads or TPA alone for cultures of varying initial cell densities. (Data from Ref. 9)

the results are described in detail elsewhere (9).

It can be seen in Fig. 4 that the yield of transformants was very low in cultures seeded at different cell densities and exposed to either 100 rads or TPA alone. When cultures exposed to 100 rads were subsequently incubated with TPA, how-ever, a large increase in the yield of transformants occurred. The effect of TPA appears to have been further enhanced (about a two-fold increase) when the initial cell density was de-creased from 370 to <100 cells per dish. This latter result suggests that TPA may have a greater enhancing effect on low cell density cultures. This would be expected if, as sugges-ted by previous experiments, the primary effect of TPA is on actively proliferating cells (11). When cells are seeded at low cell density, they are able to undergo more divisions be-fore confluence is reached; thus, TPA has more time while the cells are proliferating in its presence to exert its effect.

Our finding of very high "transformation frequencies" per surviving cell (approaching 100%) in 10T½ cells seeded at an initial density of about one cell per dish (Fig. 4) and ex-posed to 100 rads and TPA is similar to that previously repor-ted by Mondal and Heidelberger for chemical transformation <u>in vitro</u> of C3H mouse prostate cells (14). It should be noted,

however, that in such experiments involving single cell exposure to carcinogens, we do not in reality find transformation
amongst 100% of the progeny of the initially treated cells.
Rather, occasional transformed foci develop on a monolayer of
normal appearing cells many generations after the carcinogen
treatment of single cells. In other words, the treated cell
gives rise initially to a confluent monolayer of cells; a few
of these progeny eventually undergo transformation such that
the fraction of dishes containing transformed foci approaches
100% .

There is some evidence that normal diploid cells in vivo
behave similarly to the in vitro response of the 10T½ cell
line as described above. Terzaghi and Nettesheim (22) have
shown that a large fraction of rat tracheal mucosa cells exposed to DMBA in vivo have neoplastic potential when cultured
in vitro (80-90% of cultures); however, only a small number of
tumors develop from carcinogen exposed cells left in the host
animals. Similarly, the number of irradiated C3H 10T½ cells
which have neoplastic potential appears to be much greater in
number than those which in fact express the transformed phenotype under the conditions of our usual low-dose radiation
transformation experiment (in which about 300 viable cells are
seeded per dish treated with 100 rads without subsequent exposure to promoting agents).

Thus, it appears from our results that a very large fraction of cells irradiated with a high dose of X-rays alone or
a low radiation dose followed by TPA treatment have been altered in a heritable fashion such that one or more of their
progeny will undergo transformation.

This finding challenges the notion that the initial step
in the malignant conversion of a cell involves a rare event
in a target cell; rather it suggests that the initial cellular
alteration produced by the carcinogen is a common event occurring in most if not all of the cells exposed to the carcinogen. This frequency is several orders of magnitude higher than those associated with the induction of a single gene
mutation by X-rays (4). The probability of the second event
(which usually occurs after confluence and leads to the expression of the transformed phenotype) is, however, small
($<10^{-6}$).

There appear to be many factors secondary to the initial
radiation exposure which operate between the initial cellular
alteration and the emergence of a fully transformed cell in
the multi-stage process of carcinogenesis (3). These secondary factors may be particularly important in determining
the expression of X-ray transformation. They include the relation of the cell to its neighbors, the capacity for adequate

cellular proliferation, and the presence of agents which either promote or inhibit carcinogenesis. Our own studies on the inhibition of radiation transformation in vitro suggest indeed that carcinogenesis is an ongoing process that can be arrested, even at late times after cellular exposure to a carcinogen, by such agents as protease inhibitors (6-8,13). Perhaps a more careful study of the actions of agents that modify the expression of carcinogenesis at its later stages might be more fruitful in our attempts to prevent cancer than the study of compounds one by one for their ability to induce mutations in vitro or tumors in experimental animals.

REFERENCES

1. Brouty-Boyé D, Gresser I and Baldwin C: Reversion of the transformed phenotype to the parental phenotype by subcultivation of x-ray transformed C3H/10T½ cells at low cell density. Int. J. Cancer 24:253-260, 1979.
2. Committee on the Biological Effects of Ionizing Radiations, National Research Council, The Effects on Populations of Exposure to Low Levels of Ionizing Radiation. (BEIR Report). National Academy of Sciences, Washington, D.C. 1980.
3. Foulds, L. Neoplastic Development. Academic Press, New York, 1969.
4. Hsie AW, O'Neill JP, Couch DB, SanSebastian JR, Brimer PA, Machanoff R, Fuscoe JC, Riddle JC, Li AP, Forbes NL, and Hsie MH: Quantitative analyses of radiation- and chemical-induced lethality and mutagenesis in Chinese hamster ovary cells. Radiation Res. 76:471-492, 1978.
5. Kennedy AR, Fox M, Murphy G and Little JB: On the relationship between X-ray exposure and malignant transformation in C3H 10T½ cells. Proc. Natl. Acad. Sci. USA (in press).
6. Kennedy AR and Little JB: Effects of protease inhibitors suppress radiation-induced malignant transformation in vitro. Nature 276:825-826, 1978.
7. Kennedy AR and Little JB: Radiation transformation in vitro: Modification by exposure to tumor promoters and protease inhibitors. In: Radiation Biology in Cancer Research, Raven Press, New York, 1980, pp. 295-307.
8. Kennedy AR and Little JB: Effects of protease inhibitors on radiation transformation in vitro. Cancer Res. (submitted).
9. Kennedy AR and Little JB: An investigation of the mechanism for the enhancement of radiation transformation in vitro by TPA. Carcinogenesis (submitted).
10. Kennedy AR, Mondal S, Heidelberger C and Little JB: En-

hancement of X-ray transformation by 12-0-tetradecanoyl-phorbol-13-acetate in a cloned line of C3H mouse embryo cells. Cancer Res. 38:439-443, 1978.

11. Kennedy AR, Murphy G and Little JB: The effect of time and duration of exposure to 12-0-tetradecanoyl-phorbol-13-acetate (TPA) on x-ray transformation of C3H 10T½ cells. Cancer Res. 40:1915-1920, 1980.

12. Little JB: Radiation carcinogenesis in vitro: Implications for Mechanisms. In: Origins of Human Cancer, Hiatt HH, Watson JD and Winston JA (eds), Cold Spring Harbor Conferences on Cell Proliferation Vol.IV, 1977, pp.923-939.

13. Little JB, Nagasawa H and Kennedy AR: DNA repair and malignant transformation: Effect of X-irradiation, TPA and protease inhibitors on transformation and sister chromatid exchanges in mouse 10T½ cells. Radiat Res 79:241-255, 1979.

14. Mondal S and Heidelberger C: In vitro malignant transformation by methylcholanthrene of the progeny of single cells derived from C3H mouse prostate. Proc Natl Acad Sci USA 65:219-225, 1970.

15. Newcombe, HB: Origin of bacterial variants. Nature 164: 150-151, 1949.

16. Novick A and Weiner M: Enzyme induction as an all-or-none phenomenon. Proc Natl Acad Sci USA 43: 553-566, 1957.

17. Rabinowitz Z and Sachs L: Control of the reversion of properties in transformed cells. Nature 225:136-139, 1970.

18. Reznikoff CA, Bertram JS, Brankow DW and Heidelberger C: Quantitative and qualitative studies of chemical transformation of cloned C3H mouse embryo cells sensitive to postconfluence inhibition of cell division. Cancer Res. 33: 3239-3249, 1973.

19. Reznikoff CA, Brankow DW and Heidelberger C: Establishment and characterization of a cloned line of C3H mouse embryo cells sensitive to postconfluence inhibition of cell division. Cancer Res. 33:3231-3238, 1973.

20. Sivak A and VanDuuren BL: Phenotypic expression of transformation: Induction in cell culture by a phorbol ester. Science 157:1443-1444, 1967.

21. Terzaghi M and Little JB: X-radiation-induced transformation in a C3H mouse embryo-derived cell line. Cancer Res. 36:1367-1374, 1976.

22. Terzaghi M and Nettesheim P: Dynamics of neoplastic development in carcinogen-exposed tracheal mucosa. Cancer Res. 39:4003-4010, 1979.

Hormones, anchorage and oncogenic cell growth

ROBERT POLLACK

Professor
Department of Biological Sciences
Columbia University
New York, NY 10027

When objects on the exterior membrane press,
The alarm runs in most thro' each dark recess,
Impulsive strikes the corresponding springs,
And moves the accord of sympathetic strings...
Henry Brooke
Universal Beauty, iv, 41-44

ABSTRACT

Oncogenic transformation of cultured cells is thought to mimic the heritable loss of growth control that is the earliest step in the development of a neoplasm. While the mechanism of oncogenic transformation remains unknown, current phenomenology provides boundaries sufficient to permit the construction of a hypothesis. According to this hypothesis, the critical event in normal growth control is the restriction by cell anchorage of lateral movement of different hormone receptors in the cell membrane. This hypothesis generates a series of experimentally testable predictions for the roles of oncogenic viral gene products.

INTRODUCTION

The in vivo and in vitro endpoint assays applied to cells after exposure to a potential oncogenic transforming agent are cellular tumorigenicity and transformation. Tumors are a failure of in vivo growth control; transformations are failures of in vitro growth control. Many agents cause tumors in vivo, many agents transform normal cultured cells, and some agents do both. However, even when caused by a single agent, the in vivo and in vitro endpoint assays show only a partial

501

overlap. For example, with papovaviruses only some but not all virus-induced tumors will grow as transformed cells in culture, and only some but not all _in vitro_ transformants will be tumorigenic upon injection into susceptible animals[1,2]. Recently we have described a subset of _in vitro_ phenotypic changes matching _in vivo_ tumorigenicity for one agent capable of acting in both assays, the papovavirus SV40[3,4]. I will detail this subset, and then present a hypothesis to link its parts as perturbations of a single mechanism of growth control operating in normal cultured cells.

SUBSET OF CELLULAR CHANGES YIELDING TUMORIGENIC TRANSFORMATION

1) Serum requirement reduced

Many tumor cells, and some normal cell lines, can be grown in defined media with mixtures of hormones, in lieu of serum[5,6,7]. We will adopt Sato's term and say that all cells have a hormone "address", consisting of the sum of hormones necessary for cell proliferation. This address may be more or less complex, but all fibroblast lines studied to date, whether normal or transformed, need at least two hormones for growth in the absence of serum. Complete deprivation of any one of the hormones in the address is sufficient to prevent the growth of a normal cell.

2) Anchorage requirement reduced

A normal cell must spread out in order to proceed through the cycle[8,9]. The anchorage assay deprives a cell of a substrate on which to spread, and thereby prevents cell division. The normal point of spreading is at the M/G1 boundary[10] close or identical to the point of blockade by hormone deprivation[11]. Anchorage-transformed cells are almost always found to have acquired the ability to grow in low serum, but not _vice versa_[12,13]. This suggests that a change in hormone address may be prerequisite to a loss of the need to spread in order to divide. Tumorigenicity and anchorage-independence are well correlated, both qualitatively[1,2,14] and quantitatively[3,15,16]. Tumorigenic cells by this correlation have the ability to proceed past the M/G1 boundary without spreading.

3) Saturation density increased

A population of normal cells can maintain a stable maximum cell density despite repeated feeding with fresh

nutrients[17-20]. Both the serum and anchorage requirements
contribute to this saturation of cell density[8]. The cells
of any dense culture are actually less well spread than those
in a sparse culture[8]. Since anchorage dependence means that
cell thickness must be reduced to a threshold before normal
cells can divide, saturation is likely to be the cell density
for a given serum concentration at which the spreading that
occurs cannot reduce cell thickness to this degree. Saturation
densities of both normal and transformed cells increase with
serum concentration[17]. This ability of increased serum to
counter the requirement for spreading suggests that spreading
may be a necessary part of a normal cells's mechanism for
making efficient use of limiting amounts of serum growth
hormones.

4) Fibronectin is decreased

In the normal cell, the secreted glycoprotein fibronectin
covers regions of cell anchorage, both to substrate and to
other cells[21,22]. Transformation is sometimes accompanied by
reduction of about 10 to 100-fold in surface associated FN[23].
FN can be crosslinked by transglutaminases (eg clotting factor
XIII) to an extracellular matrix that contains collagen and
glycosaminoglycans[24]. FN can be released from the cell surface by mild denaturation (in urea) or very low concentrations
of certain proteases[25]. The proteases do not cleave FN, but
rather disrupt as yet undefined FN receptor proteins at the
cell surface[21,24].

5) Cytoskeleton is disorganized

The major intracellular protein of both normal and transformed cells is actin[26,27]. The actin of a normal spread cell
is partitioned by cofactors into four major states[26,28,29].
These states are a soluble complex that is unable to participate in the formation of long chains of F-actin,[28,30] and
three different macromolecular states that have double-helical
F-actin as a core. The microfilament gel consists of poly-
actin, an actin-binding protein such as filamin[31] and the Ca
binding protein calmodulin[32]. The gel is located just under
the membrane[29]. Microfilament cables contain poly-actin,
myosin, α-actinin and tropomyosin[33]. In normal cells, cables
are located primarily at the adherent side of the cells just
under the surface[34]. Thus, they share a localization with
that part of the microfilament gel which also lies under the
adherent surface. Finally, an isotropic matrix of single
microfilaments fills the cytoplasm, interacting with

microtubules[35], and intermediate filaments[36-39]. In tumorigenic anchorage-transformed cells, the actin is repartitioned
among these four states. More of the actin is found in microfilament gel, and less of it in the cables[40,41]. This last
event is most dramatic because the cables, mostly in one plane
of focus, are easily visualized by immunofluorescence microscopy[39,42,43].

6) Lateral mobility of trans-membrane proteins is increased

Freeze-fracture studies of normal cells show that trans-
membrane proteins (TMPs) are evenly distributed in the cell
surface[30,44,45]. Binding of a number of agents to the extracellular portion of TMPs eventually leads to directed lateral
migration and finally to clustering of the TMPs in patches on
the cell surface. Lectins, antibodies and hormones are examples of patching agents[46-48]. Clustering and patching are very
slow in normal, spread cells compared to the response in transformed cells[48,49]. This difference underlies the classic observation that transformed cells are agglutinated by lectins
more rapidly and efficiently than normal cells: in the presence of lectins, patches of lectin-receptor are observed at
regions of cell-cell sticking[46].

7) Proteases are secreted

A normal, well spread fibroblast releases little if any
proteolytic activity into the medium. Such cells also have
little capacity to proteolyse a variety of substrates on which
they can spread, including fibrin and FN, so it is also unlikely that most cells have appreciable proteolytic activity
associated with their outer surfaces[50]. However, for a brief
period, as normal cells proceed through G2 to M, they do surround themselves with proteolytic activity[51]. Presumably this
proteolysis is a necessary part of rounding. Most tumorigenic
transformed cells synthesize copious amounts of neutral serine
protease, plasminogen activator (PA)[13,52]. Synthesis occurs
throughout the cell cycle, not just at the G2/M interface[53,54].
While the substrates for plasmin are limited, they include FN
as well as fibrin. In the presence of plasminogen, a transformed cell making PA becomes bathed in plasmin[52]. Thus a
normal cell in mitosis, and a transformed cell at all times,
usually are surrounded by higher than normal amounts of the
two proteases PA and plasmin.

8) Cell cycle transition probability increases

Normal cells, restricted by serum deprivation or by

suspension without anchorage, have an extremely low probability of progressing through mitosis into the S period.   When
this probability is low enough, it becomes experimentally indistinguishable from a synchronizing block at Gl.   Nevertheless under all degrees of restriction the probability of transition from M to S is random and shows first-order kinetics[55].
For normal cells this transition probability can be experimentally raised by increasing anchorage or serum concentration.
Upon transformation, the transition probability remains stochastic, but becomes higher than for normal cells under equivalent amounts of anchorage and serum[56,57].

A UNIFYING HYPOTHESIS

    The relation of TMP motility to growth control begins
with the observation that hormone receptors are TMPs whose
lateral movement seems prerequisite to their function[58,59].
For the insulin receptor, the formation of cluster is sufficient for normal hormone action[59].   Whole IgG directed against
insulin receptor, or the (Fab)2 fragment antibody, will both
suffice to stimulate a full lipogenic response in 3T3-Ll adipocytes. No insulin is necessary[59]. Monovalent Fab prepared
from the same antibody has no stimulatory effect in the absence of insulin.   Though it binds to the receptors, it cannot
cross-link to bring on the formation of a cluster of receptor
molecules[60-62].   Similar results have been reported with antibody to EGF and an inactivated EGF fragment[62].
    When one population of TMP is specifically clustered by
an antibody or lectin, other classes of TMPs are not in general brought along into that cluster[49].   In lymphoid cells,
for example, anti kappa caps H2-K, but not H2D molecules.   In
fibroblasts, three separate TMPs have been each separately
clustered by their respective antibodies, without coclustering
of the other two[47].
    In all cases of cellular functions that require TMP
clustering studied to date, one hormone has been sufficient
for stimulation. Thus, in the adipocyte, insulin or antibody
to insulin receptor both stimulate specific protein phosphorylation with similar kinetics[63].   Therefore a cluster with
only one type of TMP is presumably a minimal signal for cellular response.   Hormone-induced clustering is likely to require
a specific state of actin on the inside of the cell.   In the
lymphocyte, the transplantation antigen H2 molecule is physi-
cally linked to actin and this linkage is enhanced by agents
that patch H2 molecules[26].

A Paradox

The decision to proceed from M to S is regulated in normal cells by an address of more than one polypeptide hormone. Polypeptide hormones bind to specific receptors and receptor movement (clustering) is a prerequisite to hormone response. What then keeps a normal cell from responding to merely a single one of the hormones of its growth address? If any of the hormones of the address formed a receptor cluster, the cellular response would not be division, but differentiation. The problem is real, since some hormones (e.g. insulin) do act alone, through clustering to stimulate differentiated responses. Thus paradoxically, any one-hormone response must be restricted, if the complex multi-hormone signal for growth is to be received.

How can a normal cell ever get the whole address? Let us make the conservative guess that the cellular response to a signal of many hormones, is still one TMP patch or cluster. This one cluster would then be heterogeneous, containing receptors for each of the hormones of the growth address. By this hypothesis, the cell machinery that carries out clustering need not be different for stimuli requiring one, or more than one, hormone.

An immediate consequence of this hypothesis is that lateral movement of any one class of receptors participating in a multi-hormone response must be restricted from clustering until the probability is high that the full address has been received somewhere on the cell surface. By extension then, all such receptors must have restricted mobility. Otherwise, premature clustering of one or more receptor types into homogeneous patches will occur. These patches, by removing a receptor from the pool of molecules available for a heterogeneous patch, would lower formation of the probability of the latter, and hence of the signal. The probability of a passage from M to S would then be the probability of getting receptors of all necessary specificities into one heterogeneous cluster, before any one kind is self-clustered. Such competition would lead to a predictable average probability, but its outcome would be unpredictable for any one cell.

In the normal cell, spreading permits a complex hormone address to be read

Spreading, with the concomittant appearance of FN and actin cables, slows the formation of clusters. This could be sufficient to raise the probability of the critical heterogeneous cluster being formed. Cross-linking of FN (to itself or by factor XIII for example) would have an additive effect, slowing patch formation by non-specific clogging. Once all receptors required by the address have been found by hormones and co-clustered, the cell would be past its indeterminant phase. Events from S to M are stereotyped. Protease synthesis and secretion are part of this stereotyped response; G2 cells synthesize and secrete proteases (including PA) to aid in their retraction from substrate prior to mitosis.

In summary, regulation of the normal cell cycle is hypothesized to be the result of the following mechanism linking serum and anchorage requirements.

1) polypeptide hormone receptors are TMP's
2) TMP linked to cytoskeletal actomyosin mesh
3) mesh needed to translocate TMP's into patch
4) patch is signal that hormone is received
5) normal spreading alters actomyosin mesh: cables form
6) spread configuration necessary to permit receptor patch

Therefore, rounded normal cells cannot divide even in presence of serum.

Transformations

There should be as many different transformants as there are ways to break the normal sequence outlined above. All of the transformants so far discovered fit easily into scheme, at the following different points of disruption.

Serum-transformation

This phenotype would be the consequence of any cellular change which increased the probability of heterologous cluster formation but which did not reduce the complexity of the hormonal signal for growth. Coordinate increases in hormone receptor number or affinity would be examples of such changes. However, the complexity of the address will still demand the restriction of receptor lateral motility, which will be detected as a retained anchorage requirement[12].

Density transformation

Saturation would be the density at which the probability of formation of a heterologous receptor cluster signalling growth drops sharply, due to the inability of crowded cells to become fully spread. Simple density-transformants that retain

an anchorage requirement for growth, would be cells whose
ability to spread on each other permits them to receive hormone signals properly at higher than normal cell density.
Saturation density would always remain proportional to serum
concentration for such cells; that is, the probability of
formation of the receptor cluster signalling growth would go
up with increasing concentrations of required hormones.

Anchorage Transformation

Cells already transformed by the above criteria are not
always able to grow without anchorage [12,13]. Yet only cells
that can grow without anchorage will express the full in vitro
syndrome associated with cellular tumorigenicity[16]. Release
of the anchorage requirement, whatever its mechanism, must
therefore represent a qualitatively different event from
either of the two transformations already discussed.

I have proposed that the function of anchorage is to restrict formation of patches of certain TMPs. The most direct
way to lose the anchorage requirement would be to bypass this
function. Were a cell to acquire the internal submembranous
actin-gel organization characteristic of a heterogeneous receptor patch, it would be "blinded" to both the hormone and
anchorage requirements normally prerequisite to the development of this configuration of its cytoskeleton. There are two
direct but different ways to accomplish this: via proteases
and via the cytoskeleton.

Proteases

The sequence of events in the growth of a normal cell is
proposed to include a proteolytic event which occurs before
mitosis, but after the signal generated by the heterogeneous
cluster of hormone receptors. If a major consequence of the
cluster is to signal the eventual synthesis of a protease,
then a cell constitutively synthesizing the protease might
cycle whether or not a cluster is formed. The stochastic
event could occur even without serum, or any of the hormones
of the normal cell's address. All parts of normal cell behavior given over to maintaining the restriction of receptor
movement would then become gratuitous. In addition to release
from the anchorage requirement for growth, the consequences of
out-of-phase PA production would include the following. Cell
bound FN would be reduced by the activity of plasmin and PA.
Lectin agglutinability would rise as a consequence of increased TMP mobility. Cytoskeletal organization would be disrupted as a consequence of the protease[64], but could in any

event become disrupted for any other reason, such as altered
TMP motility. Indeed they would have to be gratuitous, since
the effect of the premature protease precisely would be to
free the TMP receptors to form independent clusters. This
would provide an explanation for the fact that many tumors
remain differentiated, since rapid independent clustering is
a prerequisite to hormone-stimulated differentiation.

Cytoskeleton

Not all anchorage-transformed, tumorigenic cells show an
increase in production of plasminogen activator, or any other
protease[54,65]. Such an increase would be unnecessary in a
cell that had discovered any other means of signalling to itself that all its hormone-receptors were clustered into a
joint TMP patch. The most direct way to do this would be to
change the mechanism of TMP clustering, so that receptors trap
each other and the cluster forms spontaneously. Then the
first hormone received would make the required heterogeneous
patch and signal the cell.

Since TMP movement is a function of the submembraneous
actin gel, a partitioning of excess actin into the gel at the
expense of the cables might generate a hyper-clustering state.
Under these circumstances the protease would still be necessary for the transition from G2 to M, but its synthesis would
remain consequential, and part of the sterotyped cell cycle.

TMP biochemistry

By either the protease or the cytoskeleton pathway,
anchorage-transformed and normal cells should differ from each
other in TMP clustering responses when presented with a single growth hormone, or with the normal cell's whole address
of hormones. Isolation of the hormone-receptor-actin-complex
should show these differences. With lymphoid cells, myosin
mesh can trap the TMP H2, via actin[26]. If such a mesh can be
used to trap the above complex, then a direct biochemical
test of the hypothesis will be possible.

Contributions of viral genes to transformation

Perhaps the most direct function for a viral gene product would be the capacity to interfere with heterogeneous TMP
patch formation. A close alternative role would be to induce
the synthesis or activate a cell protein made in the normal
course of events only as a result of patch formation. Recent
work on the transforming gene products of SV40 and ASV is

consistent with these proposed functions[66,67]. If a single
hormone can become a sufficient growth signal, then synthesis
and secretion of such a hormone, or of a compound that binds
to such a hormone's receptor, would accomplish anchorage-
transformation. Perhaps the EGF-receptor-binding compound of
Ki(MSV) transformed cells[68], works this way.

Differentiation

Many differentiated states are induced by single hormones. In some cases, such a hormone (e.g., insulin) is also
part of the address signalling cell division. Without ad hoc
assumptions, the hypothesis explains the common observation
that in normal cells such differentiations are accompanied by
a reduced transition probability. A transformation that destroyed the growth-regulatory utility of a heterogeneous
patch of hormone receptors would free those receptors for
homogeneous patch formation. That is the hypothesis predicts
the observation that differentiation combined with
continued growth is a characteristic of abnormal
cell behavior. Indeed, almost all tumors retain the differentiated markers of their cell of origin.

The successful signal of differentiation necessarily
would remove a receptor from the pool of TMP's available for
the heterogeneous, growth-signalling cluster. Agents that
enhance patching of a single class of receptors should then
direct normal cells from growth to differentiation. This can
be tested with antibody to insulin receptor.

REFERENCES

1. Shin S, Freedman VH, Risser R, Pollack R: Tumorigenicity
    of virus-transformed cells in nude mice is correlated
    specifically with anchorage independent growth in vitro.
    Proc. Nat. Acad. Sci. 72:4435-4439, 1975.
2. Kahn P, Shin S: Cellular tumorigenicity in nude mice II.
    Test of associations among loss of cell surface fibronectin
    anchorage independence and tumor forming ability. J. Cell
    Biol. 82:1-16, 1979.
3. Steinberg B, Rifkin D, Shin S et al.:The tumorigenic syn-
    drome in revertants from an SV40-transformed line. J.
    Supramol. Struct.11:539-546, 1979.
4. Pollack R, Kopelovich L: The cytoskeleton in cultured
    cells: coordinate in vitro regulation of cell growth and
    shape. Meth.and Achiev. in Exper. Path. 9:207-230, 1979.
5. Leffert HL, Koch KS: Proliferation of hepatocytes. In

6. Ross R, Vogel A: The platelet-derived growth factor. Cell 14;203-210, 1978.
7. Sato G, Reid L: The replacement of serum in cell culture by hormones. in Rickenbert HV (ed): Biochemistry and Mode of Action of Hormones, Baltimore, University Park Press, in press ,1980.
8. Folkman J, Moscona A: Role of cell shape in growth control. Nature 273:345-49, 1978.
9. Stoker M, Macpherson I: Studies on transformation of hamster cells by polyoma virus in vitro. Virology 14:359-370, 1961.
10. Benecke BJ, Ben-Ze'ev A, Penman S: The control of mRNA production, translation and turnover in suspended and reattached anchorage-dependent fibroblasts. Cell 14:931-939, 1978.
11. Stiles CD, Capone GT, Scher CD et al.:Dual control of cell growth by somatomedins and platelet-derived growth factor. Proc. Nat. Acad. Sci. 76:1279-82, 1979.
12. Risser R, Pollack R: A non-selective analysis of SV40 transformation of mouse 3T3 cells. Virology 59:477-89,1974.
13. Pollack R, Risser R, Conlon S, et al: Production of plasminogen activator and colonial growth in semisolid medium are in vitro correlates of tumorigenicity in the immune deficient nude mouse. In Rech E, Rifkin D et al (eds), Protease and Biological Control, New York, Cold Spring Harbor Laboratory, p. 885, 1975.
14. Freedman VH, Shin S: Cellular tumorigenicity in nude mice correlation with cell growth in semi-solid medium. Cell 3:355-359, 1974.
15. Barrett CJ, Crawford BD, Mixter LO, et al: Correlation of in vitro growth properties and tumorigenicity of Syrian hamster cell lines. Cancer Research 39:1504-10, 1979.
16. Pollack R, Lo A, Steinberg B et al: SV40 and cellular gene expression in the maintenance of the tumorigenic syndrome. CSHSQB 44:in press, 1980.
17. Holley RW, Kiernan JA:"Contact inhibition" of cell division in 3T3 cells. Proc. Nat. Acad. Sci. 60:300-4, 1968.
18. Todaro G, Matsuya Y, Bloom S, et al: Stimulation of RNA synthesis and cell division in resting cells by a factor present in serum. The Wistar Symp. Mono. 7:87-101, 1967.
19. Stoker M, O'Neill C, Berryman S, Waxman V:Anchorage and growth regulation in normal and virus-transformed cells. Int. J. Cancer 3:683-693, 1968.
20. Temin H, Rubin H: Characteristics of an assay for Rous sarcoma virus and Rous sarcoma cells in tissue culture. Virology 6:669-88, 1958.
21. Yamada K, Olden K: Fibronectins-adhesive glycoproteins of cell surface and blood. Nature 275:179-184, 1978.

22. Ali IU, Hynes RO: Effects of LETS glycoprotein on cell motility. Cell 14:439-446, 1978.
23. Hynes RO: Alteration of cell-surface proteins by viral transformation and by proteolysis. Proc. Nat. Acad. Sci. 70:3170-3174, 1973.
24. Perkins ME, Ji TH, Hynes RO: Crosslinking of fibronectin to sulfated proteoglycans at the cell surface. Cell 16: 941-952, 1979.
25. Teng NN, Chen LB:The role of surface proteins in cell proliferation as studied with thrombin and other proteases. Proc. Nat. Acad. Sci. 72:413-417, 1975.
26. Koch GLE, Smith MJ: An association between actin and the major histocampatibility antigen H-2. Nature 273:274-278, 1978.
27. Hunter T, Garrels JI: Characterization of the mRNAs for alpha-, beta- and gamma-actin. Cell 12:767-781, 1977.
28. Pollard TD, Weihing RR: Actin and myosin and cell movement. CRC Crit. Rev. Biochm. 2:1, 1974.
29. Spudich, JA, Mockrin SC, Brown SS et al: The organization and interaction of actin and myosin in non-muscle cells. In Cell Shape and Architecture, New York, Alan R. Liss, p. 545, 1977.
30. Tilney LG: Nonfilamentous aggregates of actin and their association with membranes. In Goldman R, Pollard T et al (eds), Cell Motility, New York, Cold Spring Harbor Press, p. 513, 1976.
31. Wang K, Ash J, Singer SJ: Filamin, a new high-molecular weight protein found in smooth muscle of non-muscle cells. Proc. Nat. Acad. Sci. 72:482-86, 1975.
32. Stossel T, Harwig J: Interactions between actin, myosin and an actin-binding protein from rabbit alvoclar macrophages. J. Biol. Chem. 250:5706-12, 1975.
33. Lazarides EJ: Two general classes of cytoplasmic actin filaments in tissue culture cells: the role of tropomyosin. J. Supramol. Struct. 5:531-63, 1976.
34. Goldman RD, Lazarides E, Pollack R, Weber K: The distribution of actin in non-muscle cells. Exper. Cell Res. 90: 333-344, 1975.
35. Buckley IK, Porter KR: Cytoplasmic fibrils in living cultured cells. Protoplasma 64:349-380, 1967.
36. Buckley IK: Three dimensional fine structure of cultured cells: possible implications for subcellular motility. Tissue & Cell 7:51-72, 1975.
37. Buckley IK, Raju T: Form and distribution of actin and myosin in non-muscle cells, a study using cultured chick embryo fibroblasts. J. Microscopy 107:129-149, 1976.
38. Starger JM, Goldman RD: Isolation and preliminary

characterization of 10-nm filaments from baby hamster kidney (BHK-21) cells. Proc. Nat. Acad. Sci. 74:2422-2426, 1977.

39. Heuser JE, Kirschner: Filament organization revealed in platinum replicas of freeze-dried cytoskeletons. J. Cell Biol. 86:212-234, 1980.

40. McNutt NS, Culp LA, Black PH: Contact-inhibited revertant cell lines osolated from SV40 transformed cells IV. Microfilament distribution and cell shape in untransform- ed, transformed and revertant Balb/c 3T3 cells. J. Cell Biol. 56:412-428, 1973.

41. Tucker RW, Sanford KK, Frankel FR: tubulin and actin is paired non-neoplastic cell lines in vitro: fluorescent antibody stains. Cell 13:629-42, 1978.

42. Pollack R, Osborn M, Weber K: Patterns of organization of actin and myosin in normal and transformed non-muscle cells. Proc. Nat. Acad. Sci. 72:994-8, 1975.

43. Edelman G, Yahara I: Temperature-sensitive changes in surface modulating assemblies of fibroblasts transformed by mutants of Rous sarcoma virus. Proc. Nat. Acad. Sci. 73:2047-2051, 1976.

44. Gilula NB: Gap junctions and cell communication. In Brinkley B, Porter K (eds), International Cell Biology. 1976-1977. New York, Rockefeller University Press, pp. 61-69, 1977.

45. Yu J, Branton D: Reconstitution of intramembrane particles in recombinants of erythrocyte protein band 3 and lipid: Effects of spectrin-actin association. Proc. Nat. Acad. Sci. 73:3891-5, 1976.

46. Nicolson GL: The interactions of lectins with animal cell surfaces. Int. Rev. Cytol. 39:89-190, 1974.

47. Ash FJ, Louvard D, Singer SJ: Antibody-induced linkages of plasma membrane proteins to intracellular actomyosin- containing filaments in cultured fibroblasts. Proc. Nat. Acad. Sci. 74:5584-5588, 1977.

48. Bourguignon LYW, Hyman R, Trowbridge I, Singer SJ: Partic- ipation of histocompatibility antigens in capping of mol- ecularly independent cell surface components by their specific antibodies. Proc. Nat. Acad. Sci. 75:2406-10,1978.

49. Bourguignon LYW, Singer SJ: Transmembrane interactions and the mechanism of capping of surface receptors by their specific ligands. Proc. Nat. Acad. Sci. 74:5031-5, 1977.

50. Quigley J, Ossowski L, Reich E: Plasminogen, the serum proenzyme activated by factors from cells transformed by oncogenic viruses. J. Biol. Chem. 249:4306-11, 1974.

51. Burger MM: Cell surface and neoplasia. In Brinkley BR, Porter KR (eds) International Cell Biology. 1976-1977.

New York, The Rockefeller University Press, pp. 131-7,1977.

52. Unkeless JC, Tobia A, Ossowski L et al: An enzymatic function associated with transformation of fibroblasts by oncogenic viruses I. Chick embryo fibroblast cultures transformed by avian RNA tumor viruses. J. Exp. Med. 137 :85-111, 1973.

53. Rohrlich ST, Rifkin DB: Patterns of plasminogen activator production in cultured normal embryonic cells. J. Cell Biol. 75:31-42, 1977.

54. Rifkin D, Pollack R: The production of plasminogen activator by established cell lines of mouse origin. J. Cell Biol. 73:47-55, 1977.

55. Smith J, Martin L: Do cells cycle? Proc. Nat. Acad. Sci. 70:1263-7, 1973.

56. Shields R, Smith JA: Cells regulate their proliferation through alterations in transition probability. J. Cell Physiol. 9:345-6, 1977.

57. Shields R: Further evidence for a random transition in the cell cycle. Nature 273:55-58, 1978.

58. Jacobs S, Chang KJ, Cuatrecasas P: Antibodies to purified insulin receptor have insulin-like activity. Science 200:1283-4, 1978.

59. Kahn CR, Baird K, Flier JS, Jarrett DB: Effects of autoantibodies to the insulin receptor on isolated adipocytes. J. Clinical Invest. 4060:1094-1106, 1977.

60. Kah CR, Baird K, Jarrett DB, Flier JS: Direct demonstration that receptor crosslinking or aggregation is important in insulin action. Proc. Nat. Acad. Sci. 75:4209-13, 1978.

61. Shechter Y, Chang KJ, Jacobs S, Cuatrecasas P: Modulation of binding and bioactivity of insulin by anti-insulin antibody: relation to possible role of receptor self-aggregation in hormone action. Proc. Nat. Acad. Sci. 76: 2720-24, 1979.

62. Shechter Y, Hernaez L, Schlessinger J, Cuatrecasas P: Local aggregation of hormone-receptor complexes is required for activation by epidermal growth factor. Nature 278:835-38, 1979.

63. Smith CJ, Wejksnora PJ, Warner JR et al: Insulin-stimulated protein phosphorylation in 3T3-L1 preadipocytes. Proc. Nat. Acad. Sci. 76:2725-29, 1979.

64. Rifkin D, Pollack R: Tumor promoters induce changes in cytoskeletal organization in chick embryo fibroblasts. Cell 18:361-8, 1979.

65. Wolf BA, Goldberg AR: Rous-sarcoma-virus-transformed fibroblasts having low levels of plasminogen activator. Proc. Nat. Acad. Sci. 73:3613-17, 1976.

66. Rohrschneider LR: Adhesion plaques of Rous sarcoma virus-transformed cells contain the src gene product. Proc. Nat. **Acad. Sci.** 77:3514-3518, 1980.
67. Lane KP, Crawford LV: T-antigen is bound to a host protein in SV40-transformed cells. Nature 278:261-263, 1979.
68. DeLarco J, Todaro GJ: A human fibrosarcoma cell line producing multiplication stimulating activity (MSA)-related peptides. Nature 272:356-58, 1978.

Prevention of Carcinogenesis

INHIBITORS OF CHEMICAL CARCINOGENS

Lee W. Wattenberg, M.D.

Professor of Pathology
Department of Laboratory Medicine & Pathology
University of Minnesota
Minneapolis, Minnesota 55455

An increasing number and diversity of compounds have been found to prevent chemical carcinogenesis. Inhibition can occur at different time points. Some inhibitors, such as ascorbic acid or α-tocopherol, prevent the formation of carcinogens. Investigations bearing on these compounds will be presented by S. Mirvish in this Symposium. Another group of inhibitors prevents carcinogens from reaching or reacting with critical target sites. These compounds are called "blocking agents". They are effective when administered prior to and/or simultaneously with exposure to carcinogens. Inhibition at a later stage is brought about by still other groups of compounds which inhibit or suppress early cellular responses to carcinogenic agents. Retinoids, protease inhibitors, and several anti-inflammatory compounds fall into this category. These inhibitors are dealt with by M. Sporn, W. Troll and their collaborators elsewhere in these volumes.

The present presentation will deal mainly with blocking agents. A wide variety of such inhibitors exist. Some are synthetic but many are naturally occurring constituents of plants (41-43). Blocking agents include: phenols, indoles, flavones, aromatic isothiocyanates, coumarins, disulfiram and related chemicals, as well as a number of other compounds (Figure 1). Three general mechanisms of inhibition of chemical carcinogenesis by blocking agents occur. The first is the direct blocking of enzymatic activation of the carcinogen to its reactive carcinogenic form. The second mechanism of inhibition entails the stimulation of a coordinated detoxification response which results in increased activity of detoxifying enzymes in the microsomes and also the cytosol. At least two subdivisions of this type of mechanism have been found. The

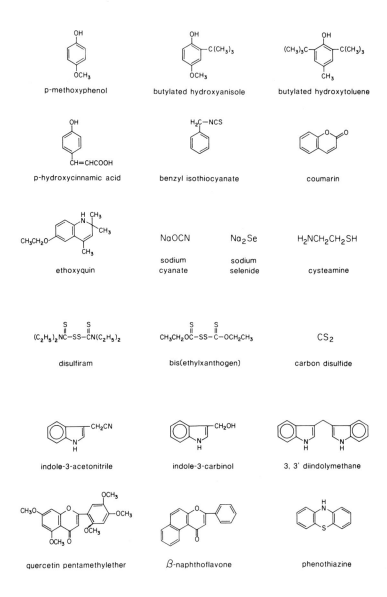

Figure 1.   Some Compounds That Inhibit Chemical Carcinogens.

third general mechanism of carcinogen inhibition entails the direct scavenging of reactive carcinogenic species by the inhibitor.

INHIBITION OF CHEMICAL CARCINOGENESIS BY AGENTS
BLOCKING ENZYMATIC ACTIVATION OF THE CARCINOGEN
TO ITS REACTIVE CARCINOGENIC FORM.

   Disulfiram and related compounds are exceedingly interesting in their effects on carcinogen-induced neoplasia of the
large intestine (39, 47). Disulfiram, diethyldithiocarbamate and bis(ethylxanthogen) when added to the diet profoundly inhibit large bowel neoplasia resulting from subcutaneous administration of symetrical 1,2-dimethylhydrazine
(DMH). Carbon disulfide (CS_2) given by oral intubation likewise inhibits DMH-induced neoplasia of the large intestine
(46a). Work has been carried out with azoxymethane, an oxidative metabolite of DMH. This compound also produces neoplasia of the large intestine. Under comparable experimental conditions to those used with DMH, disulfiram has also
been found to inhibit azoxymethane-induced neoplasia of the
large intestine but to a considerably less extent than with
DMH as the carcinogen (47).
   Studies of the mechanism of inhibition of neoplasia of the
large bowel by disulfiram, diethyldithiocarbamate, bis(ethylxanthogen) and CS_2 have shown that the four compounds all
inhibit the oxidation of DMH in vivo (6). In additional work
using disulfiram and CS_2 as test substances, inhibition of
the in vivo oxidation of azoxymethane was demonstrated. The
inhibitory events described above are shown in Figure 2.
   Investigations have been undertaken on the effects of CS_2
on cytochrome P-450. Incubation of microsomes with CS_2 in
the presence of NADPH results in covalent binding of the
sulfur to the microsomes. There is an accompanying decrease
in cytochrome P-450. Several thiono-sulfur-containing compounds including disulfiram and diethyldithiocarbamate produce a similar decrease in cytochrome P-450 when incubated
with microsomes under comparable conditions (10). This
raises the possibility that thiono-sulfur-containing compounds as a group may have the potential capacity to modify
cytochrome P-450 so as to alter microsomal metabolism in a
manner which decreases the carcinogenicity of DMH and related carcinogens.
   Recent studies have been carried out on the effect of
disulfiram on the carcinogenicity of N-2-fluorenylacetamide
(2-FAA) and N-hydroxy-N-2-fluorenylacetamide (N-OH-2-FAA) for
the rat breast. Disulfiram inhibited 2-FAA but not N-OH-2-
FAA. Consistent with these results was the demonstration of
the inhibitory effect of disulfiram on the metabolic conversion of 2-FAA to N-OH-2-FAA (16). These findings are of

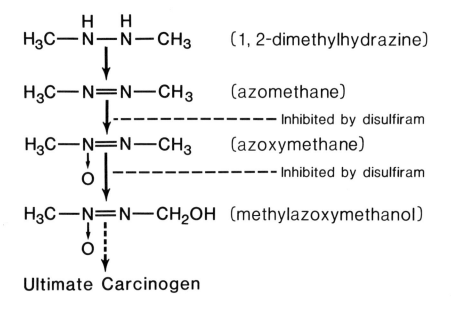

Figure 2.   Inhibition Of 1,2-Dimethylhydrazine Metabolism
            By Disulfiram.

particular interest because, as described above, disulfiram
inhibits, the N-oxidation of azomethane to azoxymethane.
Since a number of nitrogenous carcinogens are activated by
N-oxidation reactions, the capacity of an inhibitor to suppress such reactions could be of importance. Disulfiram has
also been shown to inhibit N-n-butyl-N-(4-hydroxybutyl)-
nitrosamine-induced urinary bladder cancer in the rat (11).

INHIBITION OF CHEMICAL CARCINOGENS BY BLOCKING AGENTS
ENHANCING COORDINATED DETOXIFICATION REACTIONS.

Several inhibitors of carcinogens elicit a coordinated
detoxification response. Such a response entails the enhancement of multiple detoxification systems (25, 26). Two
subdivisions of this type of mechanism have been identified.
One, for which butylated hydroxyanisole (BHA) is a prototype,
shows enhanced activity of conjugating systems in microsomes

and the cytosol but little or no increase in microsomal
mixed function oxidase activity. In contrast, the second
subdivision contains compounds which significantly enhance
microsomal mixed function oxidase activity. Many were originally identified by virtue of their property of inducing
increased aryl hydrocarbon hydroxylase (AHH) activity.

I. Inhibition Of Chemical Carcinogens By
BHA And Related Compounds.

Carcinogen Inhibition Studies

BHA is employed widely as a food additive. This compound
inhibits a broad range of carcinogens and under a variety of
experimental conditions, Table 1. In a typical experiment,
BHA is fed in the diet for about a week prior to an initial
dose of the carcinogen and the feeding is continued until
all doses of the carcinogen have been given. One variation
in this format is for the inhibitor to be given either by
oral intubation or parenterally prior to each administration
of the carcinogen. A second variation is to include both
the inhibitor and carcinogen in the diet (41). All of these
time relationships between inhibitor and carcinogen administrations are those to be expected from inhibitors which
enhance carcinogen detoxification or in some other manner
prevent the active form of the carcinogen from reaching or
reacting with critical cellular target sites.

BHA has been found to inhibit mutagenesis resulting from
administration of known carcinogens and some additional mutagenic compounds in which the capacity to produce neoplasms
has not been established as yet. Two procedures have been
employed, both of which use Salmonella typhimurium tester
strains TA-100 and TA-98 developed by Ames et al. The first
is a host mediated procedure in which the organisms are
introduced into the peritoneal cavity. The test compound is
given either i.m. or p.o. and BHA is added to the diet. An
alternate method entails determination of the effect of dietary BHA on excretion of mutagenic metabolites of test compounds. BHA inhibits host mediated mutagenesis from BP,
hycanthone, metronidazole, metrifonate, praziquental, and
mebenzadole. BHA also reduces the excretion of mutagenic
metabolites of these six compounds as well as diazepam (1).

Other phenolic compounds besides BHA inhibit chemical
carcinogens. The most extensively studied of these is butylated hydroxytoluene (BHT) which has been shown to inhibit
BP, 7,12-dimethylbenz(a)anthracene, FAA, 4-dimethylaminoazo-
benzene, and azoxymethane (31, 34, 41). BHT has noxious
effects, not observed with BHA which detract from its potential usefulness as an inhibitor (23). A study of structure-
activity relationships has been carried out in which the

TABLE 1
Inhibition Of Carcinogen-Induced Neoplasia By BHA

Carcinogen	Species	Site of Neoplasm Inhibited[a]
Benzo(a)pyrene	Mouse	Lung (37)
Benzo(a)pyrene	Mouse	Forestomach (34)
Benzo(a)pyrene-7,8-dihydrodiol	Mouse	Forestomach, lung, lymphoid tissue (46b)
7,12-Dimethylbenz(a)anthracene	Mouse	Lung (37)
7,12-Dimethylbenz(a)anthracene	Mouse	Forestomach (34)
7,12-Dimethylbenz(a)anthracene	Mouse	Skin (27)
7,12-Dimethylbenz(a)anthracene	Rat	Breast (34)
7-Hydroxymethyl-12-methyl-benz(a)anthracene	Mouse	Lung (37)
Dibenz(a,h)anthracene	Mouse	Lung (37)
Diethylnitrosamine	Mouse	Lung (35)
4-Nitroquinoline-N-oxide	Mouse	Lung (35)
Uracil Mustard	Mouse	Lung (37)
Urethane	Mouse	Lung (37)
Methylazoxymethanol acetate	Mouse	Large intestine (52)
trans-5-Amino-3-[2-(5-nitro-2-furyl)-vinyl]-1,2,4-oxa-diazole	Mouse	Forestomach, lung, lymphoid tissue (4)

[a]Numbers denote literature references.

inhibitory effects of 18 synthetic phenolic compounds added to the diet on BP-induced neoplasia of the forestomach of female ICR/Ha mice was determined (45). Seven of the compounds showed suppression of neoplasia. The most potent inhibitors were: p-methoxyphenol, 2-tert-butyl-4-hydroxy-anisole and 3,5-di-tert-butylcatechol. A second group of compounds with a weaker inhibitory activity consists of: 3,5-di-tert-butylphenol, 3-tert-butyl-4-hydroxyanisole, 2-tert-butylhydroquinone and 2-tert-butylphenol. In additional experiments, three naturally-occurring phenolic derivatives of cinnamic acid i.e. o-hydroxycinnamic acid, 3,4-dihydroxycinnamic acid (caffeic acid), and 4-hydroxy-3-methoxycinnamic acid (ferulic acid) were investigated. All three suppressed BP-induced neoplasia of the forestomach.

Studies of Mechanisms Of Carcinogen
Inhibition By BHA

BHA is quite remarkable in terms of the range of electrophiles it inhibits. Studies carried out thus far indicate
that an important mechanism of this inhibition resides in
the capacity of BHA to cause enhanced detoxification. Mice
which have been fed BHA for a period of one to two weeks
under conditions used for carcinogen inhibition experiments
show marked increases in glutathione-S-transferase activity
and also tissue glutathione levels (2, 3a). The activity of
UDP-glucuronyl transferase, a second important conjugating
enzyme is increased (5a). The feeding of BHA also causes an
elevation in epoxide hydratase activity (3a, 5b).

An additional effect of BHA is its capacity to alter the
microsomal mixed function oxidase system. This change is
not accompanied by an increase in AHH activity. The alteration can be demonstrated by incubating BP with liver microsomes, cofactors required for mixed function oxidase activity, and added DNA. Under these conditions, reactive metabolites of BP bind to DNA. If liver microsomes from mice
fed BHA are employed, approximately one half as much binding
of BP metabolites to DNA occurs, as compared to incubation
with control microsomes (30). High pressure liquid chromatography (HPLC) studies of metabolites of BP occurring on
incubating BP with microsomes from mice fed BHA as compared
to controls likewise show changes. Two metabolic alterations are found that could result in inhibition of carcinogenesis. The first is a decrease in epoxidation of BP,
which is an activation process, and the second is an increase in formation of 3-hydroxybenzo(a)pyrene, a metabolite
of detoxification (13, 14). Changes in microsomal metabolism
of BP will occur within 2 hours after administration of BHA
by oral intubation. At that time the microsomal metabolism
of BP to metabolites binding to DNA has been reduced to one-
half that found with microsomes from control animals, a
reduction of the same order of magnitude as in mice fed BHA
for a week or more (29). Changes in the BP metabolite pattern similar to those found after prolonged feeding occur 4
hours after a single dose of BHA, the earliest time interval
studied (13). A point of importance is that no increase in
the overall metabolism of BP, as determined by HPLC, occurs
at any time interval after administration of BHA either by
oral intubation or in the diet. Likewise studies of BP
metabolism using the determination AHH activity do not show
an increase (14, 30).

The work cited above indicates that BHA administration
results in a coordinated detoxification response as shown in
Figure 3. There is a rapid component manifested as an

Coordinated Detoxification Response
to BHA Administration

(a) Alteration in the microsomal monooxygenase system
(occurs by two hours after BHA administration)

(b) Enhanced enzyme activity

BHA
(mechanism not established)

Microsomes   Cytosol
UDP-glucuronyl transferase   Glutathione-S-transferase
Epoxide hydratase

(c) Increased tissue levels of glutathione

Figure 3.   Coordinated detoxification response to BHA
administration.

alteration of the microsomal mixed function oxidase system.
This rapid component is poorly understood. One element
which has been identified is a suppression of epoxidation.
At a later time increases in activity of conjugating enzymes
of the microsomes and cytosol have been found as well as an
increase in epoxide hydratase activity. Enhanced levels of
reduced glutathione also occur. Thus multiple protective
systems are brought into play which overall can inhibit an
electrophilic attack on critical cellular constituents.

Inhibition Of Noxious Effects Of The Cancer
Chemotherapy Agent, Uracil Mustard, By BHA
Agents used in cancer chemotherapy can themselves be
carcinogenic as well as producing toxic reactions (9b). Investigations have been carried out to determine the capacity
of BHA to inhibit the carcinogenicity and acute toxicity of
uracil mustard. In the carcinogenesis study, a diet

containing BHA was fed to mice for 2 weeks prior to initial
challenge with uracil mustard and throughout the course of
subsequent administrations (37). Under these conditions BHA
exerts an inhibitory effect on uracil mustard-induced pulmonary adenoma formation, Table 2. Addition of BHA to the
diet will also reduce the acute toxicity of uracil mustard,
Table 3 (44).

II. Inhibition Of Chemical Carcinogens By Compounds Inducing Increased Microsomal Monooxygenase Activity.

Carcinogen Inhibition Studies

Protection against chemical carcinogens by a variety of
inducers of increased microsomal monooxygenase activity has
been demonstrated. The carcinogens inhibited include BP,
DMBA, FAA, 3'-methyl-4-dimethylaminoazobenzene, 4-dimethyl-
aminostilbene, urethane, aflatoxin and the active agent of
Bracken Fern (41). A wide range of compounds will induce
increased microsomal monooxygenase activity. Inducing
activity also is present in plants including vegetables consumed by man (36, 42). The inducing compounds used for obtaining inhibition in early experiments were polycyclic
aromatic hydrocarbons. Subsequently, inducers with less
noxious properties were found to be effective (41). One
such group of compounds are the flavones. Many flavones
occur naturally in plants. Flavone itself is a moderately
potent inducer. Hydroxylation reduces inducing activity but
corresponding methoxycompounds are active. The vast majority of naturally-occurring flavones are polyhydroxy derivatives. A small number contain only methoxy groups. Two of
these, tangeretin (5,6,7,8,4'-pentamethoxyflavone) and
nobiletin (5,6,7,8,3'4'-hexamethoxyflavone) are active inducers of increased AHH activity (51). Several flavones
have been studied for their effects on BP-induced pulmonary
adenomas formation. The flavones chosen were BNF (5,6-benzo-
flavone), quercetin pentamethyl ether, and rutin (3,3',4',5-
7-pentahydroxyflavone-3-rutinoside). BNF, a synthetic compound, is the most potent flavone found thus far in its
capacity to induce increased AHH activity. Quercetin pentamethyl ether is a moderately potent inducer of increased AHH
activity. This compound is synthetic and was used as a substitute for tangeretin which could not be obtained in sufficient quantity for carcinogen-inhibition studies. Both are
pentamethoxy flavones and have similar inducing capacities.
Rutin is a naturally-occurring compound with very weak AHH-
inducing activity. The three flavones were added to the

TABLE 2

Effects Of BHA In The Diet On Pulmonary Adenoma Formation
In Female A/HeJ Mice Given Uracil Mustard[a]

Additions to the diet	No. of mice	Weight Gain (g)[b]	Lung Tumors	
			No. of mice with tumors	No. of tumors per mouse[c]
None	13	9	13	9.3 ± 0.5
BHA 5 mg/g	12	9	12	3.8 ± 0.5[d]

[a] Uracil mustard given by oral intubation, 0.05 mg x 4 doses.
2 x a week for 2 weeks.

[b] Average weight gain per group during interval between
carcinogen administration and killing of mice.

[c] Mean $\pm$ S.E.

[d] $P < 0.001$

TABLE 3

Effects Of BHA In The Diet On Acute Toxicity Of
Uracil Mustard To Female ICR/Ha Mice[a]

Dose of uracil mustard mg/Kg	Additions to the diet	Number of mice at risk	Deaths by 14 days
1.8	None	45	24
1.8	BHA 5 mg/g	45	2
3.6	None	45	41
3.6	BHA 5 mg/g	45	40

[a] Female ICR/Ha mice were fed powdered Purina Rat Chow with
or without added BHA for 2 weeks prior to administration of
a single i.p. dose of uracil mustard dissolved in 0.1 ml
propylene glycol.

diet fed A/HeJ mice. These animals as well as those fed a control diet were challenged with BP given by oral intubation. BNF caused almost total inhibition of pulmonary adenoma formation, quercetin pentamethyl ether reduced the number of these neoplasms by half. The number of adenomas present in animals fed rutin and the control diet were similar (49). Thus the inhibitory effects on BP-induced neoplasia paralleled the potency of the three flavones in inducing increased AHH activity. In other experiments in which the only flavone employed was BNF, this compound inhibited DMBA-induced mammary tumor formation in the rat, and BP-initiated epidermal neoplasia in the mouse (48, 49).

Indole-3-carbinol, 3,3'diindolymethane and indole-3-acetonitrile occur in edible cruciferous vegetables such as Brussels Sprouts, cabbage, cauliflower and broccoli. The three compounds induce increased AHH activity and also increased monooxygenase activity with other substrates, i.e. phenacetin, 7-ethoxycoumarin and hexobarbital (15, 21, 22). The three indoles have been studied for their effects on BP and DMBA-induced neoplasia in rodents. When added to the diet, all three inhibit BP-induced neoplasia of the forestomach and BP-induced pulmonary adenoma formation. In other experiments, indole-3-carbinol and diindolylmethane was found to inhibit DMBA-induced mammary tumor formation in female Sprague-Dawley rats, but indole-3-acetonitrile the weakest of the three in its AHH inducing capacity, was inactive in this experimental model (50).

Studies Of Mechanisms Of Carcinogen Inhibition By Compounds Inducing Increased Microsomal Monooxygenase Activity

The mechanisms of carcinogen inhibition by inducers of increased microsomal monooxygenase activity is complex. These inhibitors, as indicated by their classification, all induce increased microsomal monooxygenase activity. However in addition, many have also been shown to enhance the activity of major conjugating systems including glutathione-S-transferase and UDP-glucuronyl transferase. An increase in epoxide hydratase activity also occurs. The enhancement of microsomal monooxygenase activity in some instances produces activation reactions as well as detoxification. The classic example of this is with the aromatic amines. With these compounds ring hydroxylation results in detoxification whereas hydroxylation of the nitrogen is an activation reaction (20). In most instances inducers of increased microsomal monooxygenase activity have been found to enhance carcinogen detoxification. The complexity of the microsomal

monooxygenase system is sufficiently great so as to make it
possible that under some circumstances an induction of increased activity of one or more of its cytochrome P-450
species would enhance carcinogenesis. Such may be the case
with safrole. Administration of phenobarbital in the drinking water of rats concurrently fed safrole in the diet results in a greater number of tumors of the liver than in
animals not receiving the phenobarbital (54). However
phenobarbital is a compound with multiple biological actions
which lends an element of uncertainty as to the mechanism by
which it enhances the carcinogenic response to safrole. One
of these biological actions is its capacity to act as a
tumor promoting agent. When phenobarbital is administered
subsequent to the hepatocarcinogens 2-acetylaminofluorene,
diethylnitrosamine and 2-methyl-N,N-dimethyl-4-aminoazo-
benzene, it increases the neoplastic response (12, 23).
Tumor promotion is a hazard which requires evaluation with
respect to other compounds having the capacity to induce
increased microsomal monooxygenase activity. It remains to
be determined whether tumor promotion is a related or unrelated characteristic of a particular class or classes of
inducers.

III.   Comparisons Of Inhibitory Mechanisms Of Blocking Agents Enhancing Coordinated Detoxification Responses.

Compounds enhancing a coordinated detoxification response
comprise the largest category of blocking agents identified
thus far and are also the most complex. Two subdivisions of
this category have been presented previously. For the purpose of further consideration, they are designated type A
and B. To some extent, the subdivisions can be understood
better by considering two classes of enzyme systems proposed
by Williams for the metabolism of noxious xenobiotic compounds (53). The two classes are termed Phase I and Phase
II. Phase I reactions introduce a polar group into the compound. This type of reaction is most frequently carried out
by the microsomal monooxygenase system. The introduction of
a polar group into a lipophilic xenobiotic compound provides
a means by which a subsequent conjugation reaction can occur
leading to excretion. Phase II reactions, for the most part,
are conjugating reactions such as formation of glucuronides,
glutathione conjugates and sulfates. Blocking agents which
have been dealt with in the section entitled "Inhibition Of
Chemical Carcinogens By Compounds Inducing Increased Microsomal Monooxygenase Activity" frequently enhance the

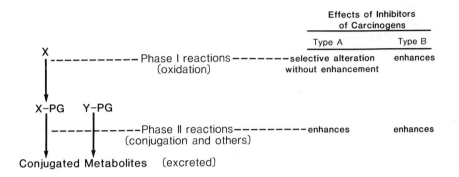

X -Xenobiotic compound lacking a polar group

X-PG -Metabolite of "X" containing a polar group

Y-PG -Xenobiotic compound containing a polar group

Figure 4. Subclassification of blocking agents enhancing a coordinated detoxification response. BHA is a type A inhibitor. β-Naphthoflavone is a type B inhibitor.

activity of both Phase I and Phase II reactions (43). In many instances they enhance oxidation, conjugation and epoxide hydrolysis. Compounds such as BP, lacking a polar group, require both Phase I and Phase II reactions in order to be eliminated from the organism. In Figure 4 inhibitors enhancing both Phase I and Phase II reactions are designated as type B. As has been discussed previously, oxidative reactions can result not only in detoxification but also in activation of a carcinogen to its ultimate reactive form. As a result this group of inhibitors is complex. However they are highly important since they occur in the environment.

Studies with BHA show that carcinogen inhibition can be brought about by a compound which does not enhance Phase I reactions but does enhance the activity of Phase II systems. In Figure 4, inhibitors with the properties of BHA are designated type A. BHA is highly effective in enhancing conjugation reactions and inhibits carcinogens which can be detoxified by these systems. In addition, it also inhibits

carcinogens not containing a polar group and which undergo
oxidative reactions. These oxidations can produce metabolites of the carcinogen which have competing subsequent
pathways, i.e. conjugation (detoxification) or leading to
binding to macromolecules and other cellular constituents
(carcinogenesis or toxicity). Enhancement of Phase II reactions can protect by enhancing the conjugation pathways.

     In addition to its effects on conjugating reactions, BHA
also enhances epoxide hydratase activity (3a, 5b). Epoxides
are reactive compounds which can cause carcinogenic and
other noxious consequences. Rapid destruction of epoxides
can be an important detoxification mechanism. BHA also
diminishes cellular exposure to epoxides by another mechanism, namely suppression of formation of epoxides as has
been demonstrated for the epoxidation of BP and also BP-
dihydrodiols (13, 14). BHA has one further attribute which
merits emphasis. Within a short period after administration,
BHA alters microsomal metabolism so as to enhance carcinogen
detoxification. Relatively little is known about how this
is brought about. However it could be of considerable importance since for an organism to be protected maximally
from noxious agents, a rapid response might be required.

INHIBITION OF CHEMICAL CARCINOGENS
BY TRAPPING AGENTS.

     All chemical carcinogens which have been adequately stud-
ied have been shown to have an ultimate carcinogenic form
which is a highly reactive electrophile (18, 19). Thus the
possibility exists that trapping agents might be employed
which would react directly with these electrophiles and prevent them from reaching or reacting with critical target
sites in the cell. No xenobiotic compound has been defini-
tively demonstrated to inhibit chemical carcinogens in vivo
by this mechanism. For definitive demonstration of a trapping reaction, identification of adducts or products to be
expected from the trapping reaction are required. Cyste-
amine has been postulated to act as a trapping agent but
solid proof for this mechanism of inhibition has not been
put forth (17). Physiological trapping agents exist. A
number of biochemical compounds contain nucleophilic moi-
eties (19). Sulfhydryl groups have been of particular interest. Efforts have been made to increase tissue levels of
nucleophiles by dietary manipulation. In an experiment of
this nature, diets supplemented with·cystine or methionine
or containing large amounts of protein (40% casein) were

reported to inhibit FAA-induced neoplasia of the liver and
ear duct glands (19). In a related type of study, reduction
of the toxicity of nitrogen mustard by i.p. administration
of cysteine has been reported (3b). Inhibitors acting by a
trapping mechanism could be particularly important within
the gastrointestinal tract. An inhibitor which is not
absorbed from the gastrointestinal tract potentially could
have low toxicity and effectively block carcinogens within
the bowel lumen from reaching susceptible targets in adjacent tissues.

DIETARY EFFECTS ON CARCINOGEN METABOLIZING SYSTEMS.

A number of naturally-occurring compounds have the
capacity to inhibit the neoplastic effects of chemical carcinogens. These inhibitors include phenols, flavones, indoles, coumarin and related lactones, organic isothiocyanates and selenium and its salts (38, 40, 42, 49). Vegetables and fruits are a major source of these inhibitors
(33, 36, 42). The importance of naturally-occurring compounds to carcinogen metabolizing systems has been dramatically demonstrated in studies of BP metabolism. Rats fed
typical crude chow diets have substantial AHH activity in
the proximal portion of the small intestine, the liver and
lung. When these animals are fed a semipurified diet, i.e.
casein 27%, starch 59%, corn oil 10%, salt mix 4% and containing a complete vitamin supplement, the AHH activity of
the small bowel and lung almost totally disappears. A
similar effect occurs with starvation for 48 hours. The
AHH activity in the liver does not change significantly
under these conditions. Thus the constituents of the diet
control the AHH activity of tissues of two major portals of
entry, the small bowel and the lung (32). In studies of
another carcinogen metabolizing system it was found that
feeding the semi-purified diet or starvation results in a
marked decrease in 3-MMAB N-demethylase activity in small
bowel and lung. Other microsomal systems have been shown
to respond in a comparable manner. These include O-dealky-
lating of phenacetin and ethoxycoumarin and hydroxylation
of hexobarbital (21).

More recently, investigations have begun on the effects
of dietary constituents on glutathione-S-transferase activity. Mice fed a semipurified diet show a lower glutathione-
S-transferase activity in the small intestine than mice fed
crude diets. Cruciferous vegetables, i.e. Brussels Sprouts

and cabbage enhance the glutathione-S-transferase activity
of the small intestine (28). These data show that the
activity of this important carcinogen detoxification can be
affected by exogenous compounds occuring in the diet.

DISCUSSION

The identification of a substantial number of compounds
having the capacity to inhibit the neoplastic effects of
chemical carcinogens gives rise to two questions. The first
is, "What is the current role that these compounds play in
reducing the impact of chemical carcinogens on man?" The
second is, "What is the optimal role that they could have?"
Evidence suggesting that inhibitors do play a role in man is
of three types: the nature of the inhibitory compounds themselves, mechanisms of inhibition, and epidemiological data.
The inhibitors found thus far are very diverse in chemical
structures. Many of these compounds are consumed by man.
A number occur as natural constituents of vegetables. These
compounds include: indoles, flavones, phenols, coumarins,
selenium salts, and aromatic isothiocyanates. Others such
as BHA are synthetic compounds consumed as food additives.
In addition to those already identified, the great chemical
diversity of inhibitors indicates the likelihood that others
exist.

The available information on mechanisms of inhibition of
chemical carcinogenesis has been discussed above. An important characteristic of these systems is that their activities
are labile and can be changed by xenobiotic compounds occurring in the environment. A dramatic example of this lability
is the observation that in tissues of the major portals of
entry of carcinogens (intestinal tract and lungs), the activity of the microsomal monooxygenase system in metabolizing
at least some carcinogens appears to be largely determined
by exogenous environmental factors. The implication of
these findings is that the nature of the diet, as well as
other environmental exposures, will determine the activity
and characteristics of carcinogen metabolizing systems in
tissues which come into initial contact with chemical carcinogens.

Some support for the possibility that inhibitors of
carcinogens do play a role in man is derived from epidemiological investigations. Several studies have been published
which indicate that consumption of vegetables may diminish
the risk from chemical carcinogens. One of the most dramatic is a case-control study by Saxon Graham _et al_ which

shows an inverse correlation between the magnitude of consumption of cabbage and the occurrence of cancer of the
colon (7). The relative risk in individuals with the highest
consumption of cabbage as compared to those with little or
no intake of this vegetable is about one-third. Several investigations have been published in which an inverse relationship has been found between the magnitude of consumption
of other vegetables including lettuce, celery, and tomatoes
and cancer of the stomach or precursor lesions in that organ
(8, 9a). The reduced incidence of cancer in Seventh Day
Adventists, a group which has a vegetarian diet, is in accord
with the above (24). This group of epidemiological reports
are cited because of the occurrence of inhibitors of chemical carcinogenesis in vegetables. However, these studies
cannot be considered as conclusive.

Considerations of the optimal role that blocking agents
might play in preventing neoplasia entails evaluations of
their deliberate use. At present, it clearly would be premature to undertake such measures. We do not have an adequate base of information. However, at a future time this
course of action might be entertained. Accordingly, there
would be some value in considering factors involved in making decisions concerning the deliberate use of inhibitors of
chemical carcinogenesis. For any normal group of individuals, a critical restraint is the possibility of toxicity.
Inhibitors would have to be taken by individuals for many
years in order to be effective. Even a low toxicity could
outweigh any benefits. However, there are selected situations in which this formidable obstacle might be overcome.
One specific instance is carcinogens within the gastrointestinal tract. In this case, it is conceivable that an
inhibitor might be found which would not be absorbed. Under
these conditions, a compound with little or no toxicity
could be available. The importance of considerations of
this type is made more compelling by recent findings of
mutagenic substances in the feces. If these mutagens are in
fact carcinogens, efforts at finding effective inhibitors
active within the large bowel might be warranted. In other
sites, specific situations amenable to selective approaches
could exist as well.

A conceivable basis for introduction of an inhibitor into
the environment would be the acquisition of favorable data
from epidemiological investigations. Such data should include firm evidence that a population group with a significant intake of a particular inhibitor has a diminished incidence of one or more neoplasms. Mechanistic data relating
the intake of the inhibitor to carcinogen inhibition, i.e.

such as tissues from individuals of the particular population group showing an increased capacity to detoxify carcinogens, would be important. In addition, there should be clear
evidence of lack of toxicity from the inhibitor. Under
these conditions consideration of the use of the material
bringing about the inhibition might be warranted. This, in
essence, is a natural or unplanned type of experiment.
Depending on the magnitude of the inhibition and reliability
of estimates of lack of adverse side effects, convincing
data could be provided for deliberate use of the substance.

There do exist individuals who because of genetic or
acquired characteristics are at increased risk from chemical
carcinogens. Under these conditions, less rigid requirements for lack of toxicity of inhibitors might be justified.
With regard to this possibility, an exceedingly important
prohibition is that inhibitors should not be used as a mechanism for allowing increased exposures to carcinogens or increasing tolerance levels to cancer producing substances.

SUMMARY

A large number of compounds have been found which inhibit
chemical carcinogens when administered prior to and/or
simultaneously with exposure to the carcinogen. These inhibitors are called "blocking agents" since current information indicates that they act by preventing carcinogens from
reaching or reacting with critical target sites.

Blocking agents can be classified into three major categories: 1) Compounds preventing activation of carcinogens to
a reactive species. 2) Compounds enhancing a coordinated
detoxification response. Two subclasses of this category
have been identified and are designated type A and type B.
Type A inhibitors enhance Phase II detoxification systems
(conjugating enzymes and some related entities). Type B
inhibitors enhance both Phase I systems (oxidation) and
Phase II systems. 3) Compounds trapping reactive species of
carcinogens.

Many blocking agents occur in the environment. Systems
enhanced by blocking agents are labile and respond readily
to extrinsic compounds particularly in the diet. These
considerations suggest that blocking agents can be a factor
in determining response to environmental carcinogens.

The considerations entailed in deliberate intervention by
use of blocking agents are discussed.

ACKNOWLEDGEMENTS

Investigations included in this presentation were supported by Public Health Service Grants CA-09599, CA-15638, and CA-14146 from the National Cancer Institute.

REFERENCES

1 Batzinger,R. P., Ou, S. L., and Bueding, E. Antimutagenic effects of 2(3)-tert-butyl-4-hydroxyanisole and of antimicrobial agents. Cancer Res. 12:4478-4485, 1978.
2 Benson, A. M., Batzinger, R. P., Ou, S. L., Bueding, E., Cha, Y. N., and Talalay, P. Elevation of hepatic glutathione-S-transferase activities and protection against mutagenic metabolites by dietary antioxidants. Cancer Res. 12:4486-4495, 1978.
3a Benson, A. M., Cha, Y. N., Bueding, E., Heine, H. S. and Talalay, P. Elevation of extrahepatic glutathione-S-transferase and epoxide hydratase activities by 2(3)-tert-butyl-4-hydroxyanisole. Cancer Res. 39:2971-2977, 1979.
3b Brandt, E. L. and Griffin, A. C. Reduction of toxicity of nitrogen mustard by cysteine. Cancer 4:1030-1035, 1951.
4 Bueding, E., Dunsford, H., and Dolan, P. Personal communication. 1980.
5a Cha, Y. N., and Bueding, E. Effects of 2(3)tert-butyl-4-hydroxyanisole administration on the activities of several hepatic microsomal and cytoplasmic enzymes in mice. Biochem. Pharmacol. 28:1917-1921, 1979.
5b Cha, Y. N., Martz, F. and Bueding, E. Enhancement of liver microsome epoxide hydratase activity in rodents by treatment with 2(3)-tert-butyl-4-hydroxyanisole. Cancer Res. 38:4496-4498, 1978.
6 Fiala, E. S., Bobotas, G., Kulakis, C., Wattenberg, L. W., and Weisburger, J. H. The effects of disulfiram and related compounds on the in vivo metabolism of the colon carcinogen 1,2-dimethylhydrazine. Biochem. Pharm. 26: 1763-1768, 1977.
7 Graham, S., Dayai, H., Swanson, M., Mittelman, A., and Wilkinson, G. Diet in the epidemiology of cancer of the colon and rectum. J. Nat. Cancer Inst. 61:709-714, 1978.
8 Haenszel, W., Correa, P., Cuello, C., Guzman, N., Burbano, L., Lores, H., and Munoz, J. Gastric cancer in Columbia: case-control epidemiological study of precursor lesions. J. Nat. Cancer Inst. 57:1021-1026, 1976.

9a Haenszel, W., Kurihara, M., Segi, M., and Lee, R. K. C.
    Stomach cancer among Japanese in Hawaii. J. Nat. Cancer
    Inst. 49:969-988, 1972.

9b Harris, C. C. The carcinogenicity of anticancer drugs:
    a hazard in man. Cancer 37:1014-1023, 1976.

10 Hunter, A. L. and Neal, R. A. Inhibition of hepatic
    mixed-function oxidase activity in vitro and in vivo by
    various thiono-sulfur-containing compounds. Biochem
    Pharm 24:2199-2205, 1975.

11 Irving, C. C., Tice, A. J. and Murphy, W. M. Inhibition
    of N-n-butyl-N-(4-hydroxybutyl)nitrosamine-induced uri-
    nary bladder cancer in rats by administration of disulf-
    iram in the diet. Cancer Res. 39:3040-3043, 1979.

12 Kitagawa, T., Pitot, H. C., Miller, E. C., and Miller,
    J. A. Promotion by dietary phenobarbital of hepato-
    carcinogenesis by 2-methyl-N,N-dimethyl-4-aminoazo-
    benzene in the rat. Cancer Res. 39:112-115, 1979.

13 Lam, L. K. T., Fladmoe, A. V., Hochalter, J. B. and
    Wattenberg, L. W. Short time-interval effects of buty-
    lated hydroxyanisole on the metabolism of benzo(a)-
    pyrene. Cancer Res. 1980 (in press).

14 Lam, L. K. T., and Wattenberg, L. W. Effects of buty-
    lated hydroxyanisole on the metabolism of benzo(a)pyrene
    by mouse liver microsomes. J. Nat. Cancer Inst. 58:413-
    417, 1977.

15 Loub, W. D., Wattenberg, L. W., and Davis, D. W. Aryl
    hydrocarbon hydroxylase induction in rat tissues by
    naturally-occurring indoles of cruciferous plants. J.
    Nat. Cancer Inst. 54:985-988, 1975.

16 Malejka-Giganti, D., McIver, R. C. and Rydell, R. E.
    Inhibitory effect of disulfiram on rat mammary tumor in-
    duction by N-2-fluorenylacetamide and on its metabolic
    conversion to N-hydroxy-N-2-fluorenylacetamide. J. Nat.
    Cancer Inst. 64:1471-1477, 1980.

17 Marquardt, H., Sapozink, M., and Zedeck, M. Inhibition
    by cysteamine-HCl of oncogenesis induced by 7,12-dime-
    thylbenz(a)anthracene without affecting toxicity. Cancer
    Res. 34:3387-3390, 1974.

18 Miller, E. C. Some current perspectives on chemical car-
    cinogenesis in human and experimental animals. Cancer
    Res. 38:1479-1496, 1978.

19 Miller, E. C. and Miller, J. A. Approaches to the mech-
    anism and control of chemical carcinogenesis. In: Envi-
    ronment and Cancer Twenty-fourth Annual Symposium On
    Fundamental Cancer Research. The University of Texas,
    M. D. Anderson Hospital and Tumor Institute. Williams and
    Wilkins Company, Baltimore, Maryland. 1972, pp. 5-39.

20 Miller, J. A., and Miller, E. C. The metabolic activation of carcinogenic aromatic amines and amides. Prog. Exp. Tumor Res. 11:273-301, 1969.

21 Pantuck, E. J., Hsiao, K. C., Loub, W. D., Wattenberg, L. W., Kuntzman, R., and Conney, A. H. Stimulatory effect of vegetables on intestinal drug metabolism in the rat. J. Pharm. and Exper. Therap. 198:277-283, 1976.

22 Pantuck, E. J., Pantuck, C. B., Garland, W. A., Mins, B., Wattenberg, L. W., Anderson, K. E., Kappas, A., and Cooney, A. Y. Effects of dietary brussels sprouts and cabbage on human drug metabolism. Clin. Pharm. and Therap. 25:88-95, 1979.

23 Peraino, C., Fry, R. J., Staffeldt, E., and Christopher, J. P. Enhancing effects of phenobarbitone and butylated hydroxytoluene on 2-acetylaminofluorene-induced hepatic tumorigenesis in the rat. Food Cosmet. Toxicol. 15:93-96, 1977.

24 Phillips, R. L. Role of life-style and dietary habits in risk of cancer among Seventh-Day Adventists. Cancer Res. 35:3513-3522, 1975.

25 Poland, A., Greenlee, W. F., and Kende, A. S. Studies on the mechanism of action of the chlorinated dibenzo-p-dioxins and related compounds. In: The Scientific Basis for the Public Control of Environmental Health Hazards. Ann N. Y. Acad. Sci. 320:214-230, 1979.

26 Poland, A., and Kende, A. The genetic expression of aryl hydrocarbon hydroxylase activity: Evidence for a receptor mutation in nonresponsive mice. In: Origins of Human Cancer. Cold Spring Harbor Symposium, New York, 1977.

27 Slaga, T. J., and Bracken, W. M. The effects of antioxidants on skin tumor initiation and aryl hydrocarbon hydroxylase. Cancer Res. 37:1631-1635, 1977.

28 Sparnins, V. L. Effects of dietary constituents on glutathione-S-transferase activity. Proc. Am. Assoc. for Cancer Res. 21:80, 1980.

29 Speier, J. L., Lam, L. K. T., and Wattenberg, L. W. Effects of administration to mice of butylated hydroxyanisole by oral intubation on benzo(a)pyrene-induced pulmonary adenoma formation and metabolism of benzo(a)pyrene. J. Nat. Cancer Inst. 60:605-609, 1978.

30 Speier, J. L., and Wattenberg, L. W. Alterations in microsomal metabolism of benzo(a)pyrene in mice fed butylated hydroxyanisole. J. Nat. Cancer Inst. 55:469-472, 1975.

31   Ulland, B. M., Weisburger, J. H., Yammamoto, R. S., and Weisburger, E. K. Antioxidants and carcinogenesis: Butylated hydroxytoluene, but not diphenyl-p-phenylenediamine, inhibits cancer induction by N-2-fluorenyl-acetamide and by N-hydroxy-N-2-fluorenylacetamide in rats. Food Cosmet. Toxicol. 11:199-207, 1973.

32   Wattenberg, L. W. The role of the portal of entry in inhibition of tumorigenesis. Progress in Exp. Tumor Research. 14:89-104, 1970.

33   Wattenberg, L. W. Studies of polycyclic hydrocarbon hydroxylases of the intestine possibly related to cancer. Effect of diet on benzpyrene hydroxylase activity. Cancer 28:99-102, 1971.

34   Wattenberg, L. W. Inhibition of carcinogenic and toxic effects of polycyclic hydrocarbons by phenolic antioxidants and ethoxyquin. J. Nat. Cancer Inst. 48:1425-1430, 1972.

35   Wattenberg, L. W. Inhibition of carcinogenic effects of diethylnitrosamine and 4-nitroquinoline-N-oxide by antioxidants. Fed. Proc. 31:633, 1972.

36   Wattenberg, L. W. Enzymatic reactions and carcinogenesis. In: Cumley, R. D. (Editor): Environment and Cancer, Baltimore, William & Wilkins, 1972, pp. 241-255.

37   Wattenberg, L. W. Inhibition of chemical carcinogen-induced pulmonary neoplasia by butylated hydroxyanisole. J. Nat. Cancer Inst. 50:1541-1544, 1973.

38   Wattenberg, L. W. Inhibition of carcinogenic and toxic effects of polycyclic hydrocarbons by several sulfur-containing compounds. J. Nat. Cancer Inst. 52:1583-1587, 1974.

39   Wattenberg, L. W. Inhibition of dimethylhydrazine-induced neoplasia of the large intestine by disulfiram. J. Nat. Cancer Inst. 54:1005-1006, 1975.

40   Wattenberg, L. W. Inhibition of carcinogenic effects of polycyclic hydrocarbons by benzyl isothiocyanate and related compounds. J. Nat. Cancer Inst. 58:395-398, 1977.

41   Wattenberg, L. W. Inhibitors of chemical carcinogens. In: Klein, G. and Weinhouse, S. (Editors): Advances in Cancer Research, Academic Press, New York, 26:197-226, 1978.

42   Wattenberg, L. W. Naturally-occurring inhibitors of chemical carcinogenesis. In: Naturally-occurring carcinogens-mutagens and modulators of carcinogenesis. Proceedings of the Sixth International Symposium of the Princess Takamatsu Cancer Research Fund. University Park Press, Baltimore, 1979, pp. 315-329.

43 Wattenberg, L. W. Inhibitors of chemical carcinogens.
    In: Environmental carcinogenesis. Emmelot, P. and Kriek,
    E. (eds). Elsevier, New York, 1979, pp. 241-264.
44 Wattenberg, L. W. 1980 (unpublished).
45 Wattenberg, L. W., Coccia, J. B., Lam, L. K. T. Inhibi-
    tory effects of phenolic compounds on benzo(a)pyrene-
    induced neoplasia. Cancer Res. 1980 (in press).
46a Wattenberg, L. W., and Fiala, E. S. Inhibition of 1,2-
    dimethylhydrazine-induced neoplasia of the large intes-
    tine in female CF_1 mice by carbon disulfide. J. Nat.
    Cancer Inst. 60:1515-1517, 1978.
46b Wattenberg, L. W., Jerina, D. M., Lam, L. K. T. and Yagi,
    M. Neoplastic effects of oral administration of (+)-
    trans-7,8-dihydroxy-7,8-dihydrobenzo(a)pyrene and their
    inhibition by butylated hydroxyanisole. J. Nat. Cancer
    Inst. 62:1103-1106, 1979.
47 Wattenberg, L. W., Lam, L. K. T., Fladmoe, A., and
    Borchert, P. Inhibitors of colon carcinogenesis.
    Cancer 40:2432-2435, 1977.
48 Wattenberg, L. W., and Leong, J. L. Inhibition of the
    carcinogenic action of 7,12-dimethylbenz(a)anthracene by
    beta-naphthoflavone. Proc. Soc. Exp. Biol. Med. 128:940-
    943, 1968.
49 Wattenberg, L. W., and Leong, J. L. Inhibition of the
    carcinogenic action of benzo(a)pyrene by flavones.
    Cancer Res. 30:1922-1925, 1970.
50 Wattenberg, L. W., and Loub, W. D. Inhibition of poly-
    cyclic hydrocarbon-induced neoplasia by naturally-occur-
    ring indoles. Cancer Res. 38:1410-1413, 1978.
51 Wattenberg, L. W., Page, M. A., and Leong, J. L. Induc-
    tion of increased benzopyrene hydroxylase activity by
    flavones and related compounds. Cancer Res. 28:934-937,
    1968.
52 Wattenberg, L. W., and Sparnins, V. L. Inhibitory ef-
    fects of butylated hydroxyanisole on methylazoxymethanol
    acetate-induced neoplasia of the large intestine and on
    nicotinamide adenine dinucleotide-dependent alcohol de-
    hydrogenase activity in mice. J. Nat. Cancer Inst. 63:
    219-222, 1979.
53 Williams, R. T. Pathways of drug metabolism. In: Hand-
    book of Experimental Pharmacology. Springer-Verlag, New
    York. 28:226-249, 1971.
54 Wislocki, P. G., Miller, E. C., Miller, J. A., McCoy,
    E. C., and Rosenkranz, H. S. Carcinogenic and mutagenic
    activities of safrole, 1'-hydroxysafrole, and some known
    or possible metabolites. Cancer Res. 37:1883-1891, 1977.

Recent Advances in the Use of Retinoids
for Cancer Prevention

MICHAEL B. SPORN AND DIANNE L. NEWTON

Laboratory of Chemoprevention
National Cancer Institute
Bethesda, Maryland

In several recent reviews, we have described a new biological approach to chemoprevention of cancer and have summarized the use of retinoids (the set of molecules comprised of vitamin A and its synthetic analogs) for this purpose (Sporn, 1977; Sporn et al., 1976, 1981; Sporn and Newton, 1979). In the present article, we will not review this material in detail, but instead will discuss some recent conceptual and practical advances in the use of retinoids for cancer prevention. In addition, we will also discuss some important recent advances in the use of retinoids to induce terminal differentiation in invasive, malignant tumor cells. Although these last findings pertain more immediately to the topic of cancer treatment, rather than cancer prevention, they have obvious implications with respect to cancer prevention and thus will be given a brief review in the present article.

RETINOIDS AND SUPPRESSION OF MALIGNANT TRANSFORMATION

The most important conceptual advance that has occurred recently with respect to retinoids and cancer prevention has been the discovery that retinoids can act directly on cells in culture to suppress the process of malignant transformation, whether it be induced genotypically by either carcinogenic chemicals or ionizing radiation, or phenotypically by polypeptide transforming growth factors. Retinol, retinyl acetate, and retinal (Merriman and Bertram, 1979), as well as several synthetic retinoids (Bertram, 1980) all were effective in suppressing the genotypic transformation of non-neoplastic mouse fibroblastic cells that had been exposed to the polycyclic hydrocarbon carcinogen, 3-methylcholanthrene. The activities of a set of synthetic retinoids in suppressing transformation (Bertram, 1980) correlate well with their ability to control epithelial cell differentiation, as measured in hamster tracheal organ cultures (Newton, Henderson, and Sporn, 1980). Suppression of radiation-induced transformation of murine 10T1/2 cells in culture by an aromatic retinoid has also been reported (Harisiadis et al., 1978); however, a large set of retinoids has not yet been tested in this radiation-induced transformation system. Although the mechanism of action of retinoids in suppressing transformation is not known, recent studies on the interaction between retinoids and polypeptide transforming growth factors (TGF's) suggest that the ability of retinoids to suppress the phenotypic transforming activity of these mitogenic growth factors plays an important role in this regard. TGF's are a class of low molecular weight, acid-stable polypeptides which confer the property of anchorage-independent growth upon normal cells, which ordinarily will not form colonies in soft agar. Furthermore, TGF's release normal cells from density-dependent growth control, and cause morphologic transformation of normal cells, so that their growth pattern resembles that of malignant cells (Todaro and De Larco, 1978; Roberts et al., 1980). The first TGF to have been isolated and characterized is sarcoma growth factor (SGF), which has been obtained from the conditioned medium of virally transformed murine 3T3 cells (De Larco and Todaro, 1978).

The phenotypic transforming effects of low concentrations of SGF on non-neoplastic cells can be blocked by retinoids. When normal rat kidney fibroblasts were treated simultaneously with SGF and nanogram levels of several retinoids (including retinoic acid, retinyl acetate, retinyl methyl ether, and retinylidene dimedone), the transforming effects of SGF were suppressed (Todaro, De Larco, and Sporn, 1978). The molecular mechanism of action whereby the retinoids suppress the activity of SGF is totally unknown, and undoubtedly will have to await the elucidation of the biochemical mechanism whereby the TGF's themselves cause phenotypic transformation. Elsewhere, we have suggested that TGF's should be regarded as ultimate carcinogens; these polypeptides, rather than an exogenous chemical, radiation, or virus may be regarded as the ultimate agents responsible for the phenotypic changes which confer the properties of malignancy upon a transformed cell. As antagonists of transforming growth factors, the retinoids then have a two-fold significance: they may be used as probes to study the biochemical and biological mechanism of malignant transformation, and they may be used in a practical way to suppress transformation and prevent cancer.

COMBINATION CHEMOPREVENTION OF CANCER WITH RETINOIDS

Although there have been numerous studies in which retinoids have been successfully used to prevent epithelial cancer (particularly of the bladder, breast, and skin) in experimental animals, the retinoids themselves do not represent the ultimate in a preventive agent, since they are not effective when a very high level of carcinogenic exposure occurs. Furthermore, although great advances have been made in the design and synthesis of new analogs with more desirable toxicological properties, all retinoids still have some undesirable toxic effects when given chronically in high doses. In this overall context, the possibility of use of retinoids in combination with other chemopreventive agents has been considered by several groups of investigators, to achieve a more potent, synergistic anticarcinogenic effect, as well as to diminish the undesirable toxic effects of retinoids. Although the principle of combination chemotherapy is well established in the area of cancer treatment, combination chemoprevention is a relatively new development (Sporn, 1980). However, several recent studies indicate that this will be a useful area for further investigation. In experiments using the classical two stage model of skin carcinogenesis in the mouse, Verma, Conrad, and Boutwell (1980) showed that combinations of either retinoic acid plus the steroid, dexamethasone, or retinoic acid plus the protease inhibitor, tosyl lysine chloromethyl ketone (TLCK), are markedly synergistic in prevention of skin cancer. In related skin carcinogenesis studies, Verma, Ashendel, and Boutwell (1980) have also shown synergism between retinoic acid and indomethacin (an inhibitor of prostaglandin synthesis) in blocking induction of the enzyme, ornithine decarboxylase, by the tumor-promoting phorbol ester, TPA. Since ornithine decarboxylase activity is believed to be required in this skin system for induction of DNA synthesis, the combination of the retinoid plus the inhibitor of prostaglandin synthesis would be expected to exert a synergistic anti-proliferative effect. However, further in vivo studies will be required to determine whether retinoids and inhibitors of prostaglandin synthesis exert a useful synergistic anti-carcinogenic effect. Synergistic effects of retinoids and another class of chemopreventive agent have also been demonstrated in experimental mammary carcinogenesis. The ergot derivative, bromo-criptine, has previously been shown to suppress prolactin release by the pituitary and to be an effective agent for prevention of experimental mammary cancer (Welsch and Nagasawa, 1977). Likewise, retinyl acetate has been a use-ful agent for prevention of experimental mammary cancer (Moon et al., 1977), although limited in its use because of its hepatotoxic properties. The combination of bromo-criptine and retinyl acetate has recently been shown to be markedly synergistic in preventing mammary cancer in rats treated with the carcinogen, nitrosomethylurea (Welsch et al., 1980). These initial findings in turn suggest further experimentation with less toxic synthetic retinoids, in order to find a practical combination chemopreventive regi-men for women at high risk for development of breast cancer.

COMBINED USE OF RETINOIDS AND INTERFERONS

Another class of molecules that might be considered for combination chemoprevention studies with the retinoids is the set of interferons. Several aspects of the bio-logical activity of interferons make them an attractive choice, particularly from a mechanistic point of view. As discussed by Gresser (1977), interferons have several other important actions in addition to their well known anti-viral activity: 1) interferons inhibit the multiplication of both normal and tumor cells, by a mechanism that is not cytotoxic; 2) interferons enhance specialized, differen-tiated cell functions; and 3) interferons induce altera-tions in the cell surface. All three of these properties of interferons are shared by the retinoids, although there is no evidence that retinoids and interferons exert these effects by identical biochemical mechanisms. However, since all three properties are germane to studies of chemo-prevention, we have begun to explore possible synergisms between retinoids and interferons in cell culture studies which have measured anti-proliferative effects on mouse B16 melanoma cells. Preliminary results with crude mouse fibroblast interferon preparations suggest an additive, possibly a synergistic, effect when the interferon is used together with very low concentrations of all-trans-retinoic acid. However, these results need to be confirmed with highly purified mouse interferon in cell culture studies and then need to be extended into the area of prevention or treatment of malignancy in an experimental animal before they should be considered for any clinical application.

In addition to cell culture studies, experiments are presently under way to determine if the combination of retinoids and synthetic polymers which induce interferons exert
a synergistic effect in prevention of mammary or bladder
carcinogenesis in the rat or mouse.

RETINOIDS AND INDUCTION OF TERMINAL DIFFERENTIATION IN MALIGNANT TUMOR CELLS

For many years, the possibility of control of malignancy by inducing cancer cells to differentiate, rather
than killing them with cytotoxic agents, has been an
appealing prospect (Pierce, Shikes, and Fink, 1978). However, the practical problem of how to achieve this desired
goal has been a very difficult one. The recent demonstration that retinoic acid, in very low concentrations, can
induce terminal differentiation in both murine and human
cancer cells represents an important new finding in this
area. The first report of this phenomenon was made by
Strickland and Mahdavi (1978), who showed that treatment
of mouse F9 teratocarcinoma cell cultures with retinoic
acid caused the carcinoma cells to differentiate into cells
resembling parietal endoderm. Associated with this terminal differentiation were multiple phenotypic changes,
including appearance of new cell surface antigens, elevated
levels of plasminogen activator, and increased synthesis of
collagen-like proteins. Retinoic acid was subsequently
found to be active in vivo when given to mice bearing
transplanted F9 teratocarcinoma cells (Strickland and
Sawey, 1980). Based on these findings, new studies by
Breitman, Selonick, and Collins (1980) have shown that
retinoic acid can induce terminal differentiation in a human
promyelocytic leukemia cell line. Promyelocytic HL-60
cells multiply indefinitely in cell culture, are morphologically relatively undifferentiated, and functionally do not
act as phagocytic granulocytes. When these leukemia cells
are exposed to nanogram levels of retinoic acid, they undergo terminal differentiation. They lose their capacity to
synthesize DNA; they take on the appearance of neutrophilic
granulocytes; and they become capable of phagocytosis of
foreign organisms such as candida. Although this phenomenon
of induction of terminal differentiation of human leukemia
cells by retinoic acid has thus far not been observed in
leukemias other than promyelocytic (Breitman, personal communication), these important findings raise hopes that other
agents will be identified for this purpose. One may again

suggest the possibility that the synergistic action of retinoids, together with other potential inducers of differentiation, may provide a means to control the invasive behavior of a variety of malignant cells, without resort to cytotoxic cell kill. The development of such combined therapies is an important goal for both chemoprevention and chemotherapy of cancer.

ACKNOWLEDGMENTS

We thank Ms. Ellen Friedman for expert assistance with the typescript.

REFERENCES

Bart, R.S., Porzio, N.R., Kopf, A.W., Vilcek, J.T., Cheng, E.H., and Farcet, Y. Inhibition of growth of B16 murine melanoma by exogenous interferon. Cancer Res 1980, 40, 614-619.

Bertram, J.S. Structure-activity relationships among various retinoids and their ability to inhibit neoplastic transformation and to increase cell adhesion in the C3H/10T1/2 CL8 cell line. Cancer Res 1980, 40, 3141-3146.

Breitman, T.R., Selonick, S.E., and Collins, S.J. Induction of differentiation of the human promyelocytic leukemia cell line (HL-60) by retinoic acid. Proc Natl Acad Sci USA 1980, 77, 2936-2940.

De Larco, J.E., and Todaro, G.J. Growth factors from murine sarcoma virus-transformed cells. Proc Natl Acad Sci USA 1978, 75, 4001-4005.

Gresser, I. On the varied biologic effects of interferon. Cellular Immunol 1977, 34, 406-415.

Harisiadis, L., Miller, R.C., Hall, E.J., and Borek, C. A vitamin A analogue inhibits radiation-induced oncogenic transformation. Nature 1978, 274, 486-487.

Lotan, R., and Nicolson, G.L. Effects of β-all-trans-retinoic acid on the growth and implantation properties of metastatic B16 melanoma cell lines. In A.C. Sartorelli, J.R. Bertino, and J.S. Lazo (Eds.) Molecular actions and targets for cancer chemotherapeutic agents. New York, Academic Press, 1981, in press.

Merriman, R.L., and Bertram, J.S. Reversible inhibition by retinoids of 3-methylcholanthrene-induced neoplastic transformation in C3H/10T1/2 CL8 cells. Cancer Res

1979, 39, 1661-1666.

Moon, R.C., Grubbs, C.J., Sporn, M.B., and Goodman, D.G. Retinyl acetate inhibits mammary carcinogenesis induced by N-methyl-N-nitrosourea. Nature 1977, 267, 620-621.

Newton, D.L., Henderson, W.R., and Sporn, M.B. Structure-activity relationships of retinoids in hamster tracheal organ culture. Cancer Res 1980, 40, 3413-3425.

Pierce, G.B., Shikes, R., and Fink, L.M. Cancer - a problem of developmental biology. Englewood Cliffs, N.J., Prentice-Hall, 1978.

Roberts, A.B., Lamb, L.C., Newton, D.L., Sporn, M.B., De Larco, J.E., and Todaro, G.J. Transforming growth factors: Isolation of polypeptides from virally and chemically transformed cells by acid/ethanol extraction. Proc Natl Acad Sci USA 1980, 77, 3494-3498.

Schaeffer, W.I., and Friend, K. Efficient detection of soft agar grown colonies using a tetrazolium salt. Cancer Lett 1976, 1, 259-262.

Sporn, M.B. Retinoids and carcinogenesis. Nutr Revs 1977, 35, 65-69.

Sporn, M.B. Combination chemoprevention of cancer. Nature 1980, 287, 107-108.

Sporn, M.B., Dunlop, N.M., Newton, D.L, and Smith, J.M. Prevention of chemical carcinogenesis by vitamin A and its synthetic analogs (retinoids). Fed Proc 1976, 35, 1332-1338.

Sporn, M.B., and Newton, D.L., Chemoprevention of cancer with retinoids. Fed Proc 1979, 38, 2528-2534.

Sporn, M.B., Newton, D.L., Roberts, A.B., De Larco, J.E., and Todaro, G.J. Retinoids and the suppression of the effects of polypeptide transforming factors - a new molecular approach to the chemoprevention of cancer. In A.C. Sartorelli, J.R. Bertino, and J.S. Lazo (Eds.) Molecular actions actions and targets for cancer chemotherapeutic agents. New York, Academic Press, 1981, in press.

Strickland, S., and Mahdavi, V. The induction of differentiation in teratocarcinoma stem cells by retinoic acid. Cell 1978, 15, 393-403.

Strickland, S., and Sawey, M.J., Studies on the effect of retinoids on the differentiation of teratocarcinoma cells in vitro and in vivo. Devel Biol 1980, 78, 76-85.

Todaro, G.J., and De Larco, J.E. Growth factors produced by sarcoma virus-transformed cells. Cancer Res 1978, 38, 4147-4154.

Todaro, G.J., De Larco, J.E., and Sporn, M.B. Retinoids block phenotypic cell transformation produced by sarcoma growth factor. Nature 1978, 276, 272-274.

Verma, A.K., Ashendel, C.L., and Boutwell, R.K.   Inhibition
    by prostaglandin synthesis inhibitors of the induction
    of epidermal ornithine decarboxylase activity, the accum-
    ulation of prostaglandins, and tumor promotion caused by
    12-0-tetradecanoylphorbol-13-acetate.   Cancer Res 1980,
    40, 308-315.

Verma, A.K., Conrad, E.A., and Boutwell, R.K.   Inhibition of
    mouse skin carcinogenesis by a retinoid, steroid, and pro-
    tease inhibitor.   Proc Amer Assn Cancer Res 1980, 21, 93.

Welsch, C.W., Brown, C.K., Goodrich-Smith, M., Chiusano, J.,
    and Moon, R.C.   Synergistic effect of chronic prolactin
    suppression and retinoid treatment in the prophylaxis of
    N-methyl-N-nitrosourea-induced mammary tumorigenesis in
    female Sprague-Dawley rats.   Cancer Res 1980, 40, 3095-3098.

Welsch, C.W., and Nagasawa, H.   Prolactin and murine mammary
    tumorigenesis: a review.   Cancer Res 1977, 37, 951-963.

Blocking of Tumor Promotion by

Protease Inhibitors

WALTER TROLL

Professor
Department of Environmental Medicine
New York University Medical Center
New York, New York

The occurrence of breast and colon cancer throughout the world
is proportional to fat or meat consumption (Carroll, 1975).
These data confirm the environmental nature of cancer in man
(Cairns, 1975). We, are presented with the dilemma of
explaining it as a causative or preventive phenomenon. Do
meats or some of their components cause cancer, or do
vegetables prevent it? We have looked at prevention of
carcinogens by specific agents as a more useful technique
rather than merely assaying the sea of natural and man-made
carcinogens which surround us as the cause. The removal of
these carcinogens, which include sunlight, ionizing radiation
and aflatoxins among others, may not be possible. We were
encouraged to look for preventive agents after it had been
observed that tumor promotion caused by phorbol-myristate-
acetate (PMA) could be counteracted. The multistep carcinogenesis had its start with two-stage carcinogenesis in mouse
skin, and the concept proliferated to other animal models and

This work was supported by a grant from the National Soil and
Health Foundation, and by U.S. Public Health Service Grant No.
ES 00606 and is part of a Center Program supported by the
National Institute of Environmental Health Sciences, National
Institutes of Health, Grant No. ES 00260. Address reprint
requests to Dr. Walter Troll, Department of Environmental
Medicine, New York University Medical Center, 550 First
Avenue, New York, NY 10016.

to man (Wynder et al., 1978). The purified principle of
croton oil, PMA, has blazed the trail of the non-mutagenic
promoting agent capable of causing the growth of tumors in
mouse skin.

The action of PMA was blocked by a variety of agents
including protease inhibitors, anti-inflammatory hormones and
retinoids (Belman and Troll, 1972; Troll et al., 1970; Verma and
Boutwell, 1977). Here we had the opportunity to branch out
to the breast cancer model where the tumor promoter may be an
ovarian hormone with receptors in breast tissue. The
similarity between PMA and estradiol in inducing protease
and inhibiting estradiol action by protease inhibitors had
beed noted (Katz et al., 1977).

We have recorded significant protection against carcinogenesis in animals which were fed protease inhibitor containing diets (Troll et al., 1979; Troll et al., 1980). In these
experiments, two-stage skin carcinogenesis was used in mice
and Sprague-Dawley rats which had been treated with X rays to
induce breast cancer. These experiments were designed to
support the hypothesis that vegetable protein - in particular
the protease inhibitors occurring in soybeans - consumed by
the Japanese and the Seventh Day Adventists modified cancer
incidence. A casein diet was employed as a control diet
using identical fat composition. Epidemiological investigations have pointed to diet as a factor in cancer occurrence
in man. The supporting data have come from two sources:
first, in examining the occurrence of cancer in migrant
populations, the incidence of cancer changes from that of the
migrant's native country to that of the host country in three
generations. This has been observed with breast cancer in
Japanese and Polish migrants (Haenszel and Kurihara, 1968;
Staszewski and Haenszel, 1965). Second, the incidence of
breast and colon cancers is lower among vegetarian Seventh
Day Adventists than in the general population of the same
geographic area (Phillips, 1975).

The most probable explanation for such differences in
cancer incidence seems to be the differences in diet. The
higher fat content of meat diets has been suggested as a
cause for increased occurrence of breast cancer (Carroll,
1975). However, it appears unlikely that fat is the single
factor in the occurrence of breast cancer. A strong inverse
association was found in the United States between egg consumption and breast cancer mortality in spite of the high fat
content of eggs (Gaskell, 1979). A negative correlation has
also been observed internationally between cereal and legume
consumption and breast cancer (Armstrong and Doll, 1975).

Protease inhibitors are widely distributed in plants
(Richardson, 1977). An especially rich source of protease

inhibitors is seed foods. Soybeans, a major source of protein in vegetarian diets, contain at least five different protease inhibitors capable of inhibiting a variety of serine proteases (Hwang et al., 1977; Ikenaka et al., 1974). Since proteases may be involved in tumorigenesis, the lower incidence of cancer in populations who are vegetarians may be due to the ingestion of protease inhibitors present in the diet.

The mechanism of protease inhibition which causes blocking of tumor promotion remains to be determined. The initial experiments were undertaken after the observation that proteases were induced by the tumor promoter (Troll et al., 1970). The work by the Rockefeller group, headed by Ed Reich, has identified the role of one protease plasminogen activator in carcinogenesis (Ossowski et al., 1973; Quigley, 1976; Reich, 1975; Rifkin et al., 1975; Unkeles et al., 1974). Wigler and Weinstein (1976) demonstrated the induction of the plasminogen activator by PMA. The availability of non-toxic protease inhibitors, isolated by Umezawa from streptomyces, offered further opportunities of studying protease inhibitors in tissue culture systems (Umezawa, 1972). The inhibition of transformation of C3H 10T½ fibroblasts caused by X rays plus PMA reemphasized the action of protease inhibition in blocking tumor promotion (Kennedy and Little, 1978). One of the actions of protease in tumor promotion was considered repression of genes via proteolytic cleavage of protein repressors (Troll et al., 1978). A model for this type of mechanism is the proteolytic cleavage of λ repressor to induce λ prophage (Roberts and Roberts, 1975). These conversion and SOS functions were inhibited by the protease inhibitor antipain (Meyn et al., 1977).

Other protease inhibitor sensitive reactions caused by the tumor promoter are the burst of oxygen consumption and the resultant production of O_2^- and H_2O_2 in leucocyte mast cells (Goldstein et al., 1979). Kunitz soybean trypsin inhibitor and antipain are active antagonists in this test system.

Among the tumor promoter induced responses, the stimulation of superoxide anion radical appears to be a promising injurious response related to tumor promotion. The following observations support this notion: 1) There is a good relationship between tumor promotion and O_2^- promotion (Table 1). The inactive compounds, phorbol diacetate and 4-O-Me-phorbol-myristate acetate, do not give rise to O_2^- while all of the active tumor promoters do (Goldstein et al., 1980). 2) Other known tumor promoters, such as mezerein and teleocidin B (T. Sugimura, personal communication) produce O_2^-. 3) The inhibitors of tumor promotion described above, protease inhibitors, anti-inflammatory hormones and retinoids

TABLE 1

Stimulation of Human Polymorphonuclear Leukocyte Superoxide
Anion Radical (O_2^-) Production by Phorbol Esters

Compound[a]	O_2^- Produced[b], nmoles/min
Phorbol myristate acetate	7.9
Phorbol dibutyrate	4.0
Phorbolol myristate acetate	0.9
4-O-Me-phorbol myristate acetate	0
Phorbol diacetate	0

[a] 5.8×10^{-8} M
[b] 0.71×10^{-6} cells/ml; 0.55 mg cytochrome c/ml

counteract the O_2^- production in leukocytes.

The usefulness of the model cell system, the human leuko-cytes or the macrophage, responding to these tumor promoters has been pointed out (Mastro and Mueller, 1974).

Free oxygen radicals and hydrogen peroxide appear to be common devices used by cells to defend themselves against intruders. A novel example of this is the sea urchin egg which eliminates all but the first sperm by a burst of hydro-gen peroxide (Coburn et al., 1979; Foerder et al., 1977; Sinsheimer et al., 1980). The burst of hydrogen peroxide is caused by the first sperm's entry into the egg. Protease inhibitors and vitamin A inhibit this burst of hydrogen peroxide in the sea urchin egg resulting in polyspermic fertilization.

Thus the action of protease inhibitors and retinoids appears to be similar in preventing the formation of free oxygen radicals. They amplify this effect when used together (Troll et al., 1980), and may also amplify their cancer preventive effect.

The oxygen radical response appears to occur on the cell membrane of a variety of cells. This biological weapon is employed by leukocytes to kill bacteria and by the fertilized egg to eliminate excess sperm. Perhaps the tumor promoter PMA produces this weapon at an inappropriate time causing damage contributing to carcinogenesis. Antioxidants, described by Wattenberg (1980), may not only block the activation of procarcinogens to carcinogens, but may also inhibit tumor promotion by removing one of its active agents, the free oxygen radicals.

REFERENCES

Armstrong, B., & Doll, R. Environmental factors and cancer incidence and mortality in different countries with special reference to dietary practices. International Journal of Cancer, 1975, 15, 617-631.

Belman, S., & Troll, W. The inhibition of croton oil-promoted mouse skin tumorigenesis by steroid hormones. Cancer Research, 1972, 32, 450-454.

Cairns, J. The cancer problem. Scientific America, 1975, 233(5), 64-78.

Carroll, K.K. Experimental evidence of dietary factors and hormone-dependent cancers. Cancer Research, 1975, 35, 3374-3383.

Coburn, M., Schuel, H., & Troll, W. Hydrogen peroxide release from sea urchin eggs during fertilization: importance in the block to polyspermy. Biological Bulletin, 1979, 157(2), 362.

Foerder, C.A., Klebanoff, S.J., & Shapiro, B.M. Hydrogen peroxide production, chemiluminescence, and the respiratory burst of fertilization: Interrelated events in early sea urchin development. Proceedings of the National Academy of Science, USA, 1978, 75, 3183-3187.

Gaskell, S.P., McGuire, W.L., Osborne, C.K., & Stern, M.P. Breast cancer mortality and diet in the United States. Cancer Research, 1979, 39, 3628-3637.

Goldstein, B.D., Witz, G., Amoruso, M., & Troll, W. Protease inhibitors antagonize the activation of polymorphonuclear leukocyte oxygen consumption. Biochemical and Biophysical Research Communication, 1979, 88(3), 854-860.

Goldstein, B.D., Witz, G., Amoruso, M., Stone, D.S., & Troll, W. Stimulation of human polymorphonuclear leukocyte superoxide anion radical production by tumor promoters. Cancer Letters, 1980, in press.

Haenszel, W., & Kurihara, M. Studies of Japanese migrants. I. Mortality from cancer and other diseases among Japanese in the U.S. Journal of the National Cancer Institute, 1968, 40, 43-68.

Hwang, D.L.R., Lin, K.-T.D., Yang, W.-K., & Ward, D.E. Purification, partial characterization and immunological relationships of multiple low molecular weight protease inhibitors of soybeans. Biochimica et Biophysica Acta, 1977, 495, 369-382.

Ikenaki, T., Odani, S., & Koide, T. Chemical structure and inhibitory activities of soybean protease inhibitors. In J. Fritz, H. Tschesche, L.H. Greene, & E. Truscheit (Eds.), Proteinase nhibitors. New York: Springer-Verlag, 1974, 325-343.

Katz, J., Troll, W., Adler, S.W., & Levitz, M. Antipain and leupeptin restrict uterine DNA synthesis and function in mice. Proceedings of the National Academy of Science, USA, 1977, 74, 3754-3757.

Kennedy, A.R., & Little, J.B. Protease inhibitors suppress radiation-induced malignant transformation in vitro. Nature, London, 1978, 276, 825-826.

Mastro, A.M., & Mueller, G.C. Synergistic action of phorbol esters in mitogen-activated bovine lymphocytes. Experimental Cell Research, 1974, 88, 40-46.

Meyn, M.S., Rossman, T., & Troll, W. A protease inhibitor blocks SOS functions in Escherichia coli: Antipain prevents λ repressor inactivation, ultraviolet mutagenesis and filamentous growth. Proceedings of the National Academy of Science, USA, 1977, 74, 1152-1156.

Ossowski, L., Quigley, J.P., Kellerman, G.M., & Reich, E. Fibrinolysis associated with oncogenic transformation. Requirement of plasminogen for correlated changes in cellular morphology, colony formation in agar and cell migration. Journal of Experimental Medicine, 1973, 138, 1056-1064.

Phillips, R.L. Role of life-style and dietary habits in risk of cancer among Seventh-Day Adventists. Cancer Research, 1975, 35, 3513-3522.

Quigley, J.P. Association of a protease (plasminogen activator) with a specific membrane fraction isolated from transformed cells. Journal of Cell Biology, 1976, 71, 472-486.

Reich, E. Plasminogen activator: Secretion by neoplastic cells and macrophages. In E. Reich, D.B. Rifkin, & E. Shaw (Eds.), Proteases and biological control. Cold Spring Harbor, New York: Cold Spring Harbor Laboratory, 1975, 333-342.

Richardson, J. The proteinase inhibitors of plants and microorganisms. Phytochemistry, 1977, 16, 159-169.

Rifkin, D.B., Beal, L.P., & Reich, E. Macromolecular determinant of plasminogen activator synthesis. In E. Reich, D.B. Rifkin, & E. Shaw (Eds.), Proteases and biological control. Cold Spring Harbor, New York: Cold Spring Harbor Laboratory, 1975, 841-847.

Roberts, J.W., & Roberts, C.W. Proteolytic cleavage of bacteriophage lambda repressor in induction. Proceedings of the National Academy of Science, USA, 1975, 72, 147-151.

Sinsheimer, P., Coburn, M., & Troll, W. The toxic effects of vitamin A on sea urchin gametes. Biological Bulletin, 1980, in press.

Staszewski, J., & Haenszel, W.   Cancer mortality among the
    Polish-born in the United States.   Journal of the National
    Cancer Institute, 1965, 35, 291-297.
Troll, W., Belman, S., Wiesner, R., & Shellabarger, C.J.
    Protease action in carcinogenesis.   In H. Holzer, & H.
    Tschesche (Eds.), Biological functions of proteinases.
    Mosbach/Baden, Germany: Springer-Verlag, 1979, 165-170.
Troll, W., Klassen, A., & Janoff, A.   Tumorigenesis in mouse
    skin: Inhibition by synthetic inhibitors of proteases.
    Science, 1970, 169, 1211-1213.
Troll, W., Meyn, M.S., & Rossman, T.G.   Mechanisms of pro-
    tease action in carcinogenesis.   In T.J. Slaga, A. Sivak,
    & R.K. Boutwell (Eds.), Carcinogenesis, Vol. 2.   Mecha-
    nisms of tumor promotion and cocarcinogenesis.   New York:
    Raven Press, 1978, 301-312.
Troll, W., Wiesner, R., Shellabarger, C.J., Holtzman, S., &
    Stone, J.P.   Soybean diet lowers breast tumor incidence in
    irradiated rats.   Carcinogenesis, 1980, 1, 469-472.
Troll, W., Witz, G., Goldstein, B., Stone, D., & Sugimura, T.
    The role of free oxygen radicals in tumor promotion and
    carcinogenesis.   To be presented at the International
    Symposium on Cocarcinogenesis and the Biological Effects
    of Tumor Promoters, October 13-16, 1980, Germany.
Umezawa, H. Enzyme inhibitors of microbial origin.   Tokyo:
    University of Tokyo Press, 1972.
Unkeles, J., Dano, K., Kellerman, G.M., & Reich, E.   Fibri-
    nolysis associated with oncogenic transformation.   Journal
    of Biological Chemistry, 1974, 249, 4295-4305.
Verma, A., & Boutwell, R.K.   Vitamin A acid (retinoic acid),
    a potent inhibitor of 12-O-tetradelanoyl-phorbol-13-
    acetate in mouse epidermis.   Cancer Research, 1977, 31,
    2196-2201.
Wattenberg, L.W.   Inhibition of chemical carcinogenesis by
    antioxidants.   In T.J. Slaga (Ed.), Carcinogenesis, Vol. 5.
    Modifiers of chemical carcinogenesis.   New York: Raven
    Press, 1980, 85-98.
Wigler, M., & Weinstein, I.B.   Tumor promoter induces plas-
    minogen activator.   Nature, 1976, 259, 232-233.
Wynder, E.L., Hoffmann, D., McCoy, D., Cohen, L.A., & Reddy,
    B.S.   Tumor promotion and cocarcinogenesis as related to
    man and his environment.   In T.J. Slaga, A. Sivak, & R.K.
    Boutwell (Eds.), Carcinogenesis, Vol. 2.   Mechanisms of
    tumor promotion and cocarcinogenesis.   New York: Raven
    Press, 1978, 59-77.

Inhibition of the Formation of Carcinogenic
N-Nitroso Compounds by Ascorbic Acid and Other
Compounds

by Sidney S. Mirvish, Ph.D.

Eppley Institute for Research on Cancer,
University of Nebraska Medical Center, Omaha,
Nebraska 68105, U.S.A.

ACKNOWLEDGEMENTS
     I thank Dr. B. Challis (Chemistry Department,
Imperial College, London) for his useful
criticisms and Drs. K. Karlowski, O. Bulay, R.
Runge, and D. Birt, and Mr. J.S. Sams, who col-
laborated in recent work reviewed here. Our
research was supported by grant PO1 CA 25100 and
contract NO1 CP33278 from the National Cancer
Institute, and grant BC-39G from the American
Cancer Society.

Abbreviations: ASC, ascorbic acid and/or
ascorbate; NNO, N-nitroso; DMN, dimethylnitrosamine; NMOR, N-nitrosomorpholine; NPYR, N-nitrosopyrrolidine; MNU, methylnitrosourea; MNNG,
1-methyl-3-nitro-1-nitrosoguanidine.

The use of ascorbic acid (ASC, vitamin C) to inhibit nitrosation was discussed five years ago[1] and will be reviewed in more detail.[2] This presentation will concentrate on ASC, but the phenols and α-tocopherol (vitamin E) will also be discussed.

(1) Chemical and food systems

(a) Studies in acidic aqueous solutions

Most N-nitroso (NNO) compounds, which include nitrosamines and nitrosamides, are carcinogenic in experimental animals. These compounds could be responsible for certain human cancers. Exposure could result because such compounds occurred in the environment or were produced from their precursors (nitrite and amines or amides) in vivo. The acidic stomach contents are a likely site of in vivo nitrosation, because nitrosation is favored by acid.

We investigated the kinetics of NNO compound formation from nitrite and amines or amides[3] and found that the nitrosation of moderately and strongly basic amines proceeds with an optimum rate at pH 3.0-3.4, related to the fact that the acidic dissociation constant (pK_a) of nitrous acid (HNO_2) is 3.4. Amide nitrosation proceeds 10 times faster for each 1-unit drop in pH, without an optimum pH. Amine nitrosation is proportional to nitrite concentration squared, whereas amide nitrosation is proportional simply to nitrite concentration.

In 1972 Dr. Michael Eagen was trying unsuccessfully in my laboratory to reproduce the finding of Dr. W. Lijinsky, that oxytetracycline reacts with nitrite to yield dimethylnitrosamine (DMN). We traced his failure to the fact that we were using a commercial sample of oxytetracycline containing ASC, added as an antioxidant. Accordingly, we studied the effect of ASC in blocking the formation of NNO compounds in simple chemical systems.[4] As an example of our results, Table 1 compares the inhibition of morpholine nitrosation by ASC, urea and ammonium sulfamate.

Table 1. Inhibition of morpholine nitrosation[a]

pH	Time (min)	Yield without inhibitor (%)	Percent inhibition by		
			ASC	Urea	Ammonium sulfamate
1	45	7	–	95	100
2	30	20	98	24	100
3	30	65	100	2	99
4	30	34	100	–	71

[a]Conditions: 25 mM morpholine, 50 mM nitrite, 100 mM inhibitor, 25°C. Data are from ref. 4.

A solution of nitrite was mixed with a solution
containing amine and inhibitor, so that the
inhibitor and amine competed for the nitrite.
ASC inhibited nitrosation effectively from pH
1 to pH 4. The mechanism is simply that ASC
removes the nitrite by reacting with it. The
inhibition was effective for slowly nitrosated
amines, such as dimethylamine (except under one
unusual condition), and for amines nitrosated
at moderate speeds, e.g., morpholine and
piperazine.

The chemical reaction is nitrite reduction
to nitric oxide (NO), linked with ASC oxidation
to dehydro-ASC. Ascorbic acid and ascorbate anion
react with N_2O_3, the active form of nitrous acid
(equations 1-3 and Figure 1).

$$2 \ HNO_2 \rightleftharpoons N_2O_3 + H_2O \quad \dots \dots \dots \dots \dots \dots \dots \dots \dots \dots (1)$$

$$\text{Ascorbic acid } (C_6H_8O_6) + N_2O_3 \quad \xrightarrow{ k_1 }$$

$$\text{dehydro-ascorbic acid } (C_6H_6O_6) + 2 \ NO + H_2O \quad \dots \dots (2)$$

$$\text{Ascorbate } (C_6H_7O_6^-) + N_2O_3 \quad \xrightarrow{ k_2 }$$

$$\text{dehydroascorbic acid } (C_6H_6O_6) + 2 \ NO + OH^- \quad \dots \dots (3)$$

$$R_2NH + N_2O_3 \xrightarrow{ k_3 } R_2NNO + HNO_2 \quad \dots \dots \dots \dots \dots (4)$$

Since the active form of HNO_2 for nitrosamine
formation is also N_2O_3 (equation 4), amines and
ASC compete directly for the same nitrosating
species. If k_1 and k_2 are much greater than k_3,
then ASC will compete successfully with the
amines. According to Dahn et al.,[5] k_2 (equation
3) is 230 x k_1 (equation 2), i.e., ascorbate
reacts with N_2O_3 230 times faster than ascorbic

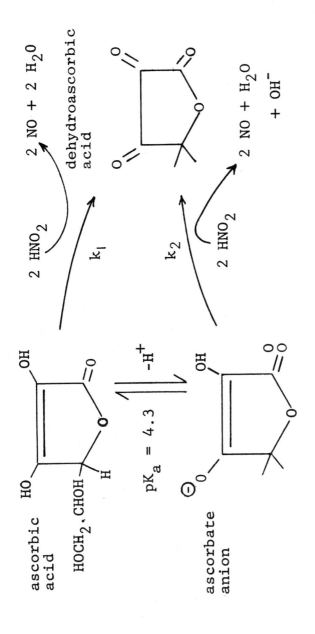

Figure 1: Oxidation of ascorbic acid and ascorbate anion by nitrous acid to give dehydroascorbic acid. The k_2/k_1 ratio is 230:1.

acid. Since the pK_a of ascorbic acid is 4.3, the ASC system is particularly effective around and above this pH. This explains why ASC is effective at pH 3 and 4, where urea and ammonium sulfamate (which react with nitrite most rapidly at highly acidic pH's) are ineffective. The conversion of ASC into dehydro-ASC may proceed via the nitrite ester at the 3 position and probably involves the semiquinone (see Figure 2).[5]

We compared the action of ASC and four other inhibitors, all of which reduce nitrite.[3] For piperazine nitrosation to give mononitroso-piperazine under given conditions, including 20 mM inhibitor, ASC, gallic acid (a polyphenolic component of tannins) and sodium sulfite all blocked the reaction by 100%, but cysteine and tannic acid were less effective. With 5 mM inhibitor, ASC was more effective than the other inhibitors.

Phenols, including polyhydric phenols such as gallic acid, are effective inhibitors of nitrosamine formation under some conditions.[3,6,7] The mechanism is that phenols consume the nitrite, either by the formation of C-nitroso phenols or, in the case of polyphenols, by nitrite reduction to NO (as with ASC), coupled with oxidation of the phenols to quinones (Figure 3). However, under some circumstances, phenols can enhance nitro-samine formation.[8] This is mediated by the C-nitrosophenols, which themselves react with nitrite to form nitrosating species. These species may have the structure shown in Figure 3, which is analogous to the active nitrosating agent, N_2O_3. Similarly, thiols, e.g., cysteine, can inhibit nitrosation because nitrite is used up to form nitrosothiols, RSNO, but these compounds can themselves act as nitrosating agents (Figure 4).[8] These reactions may be important in meat, which contains thiols and phenols as amino acids or (for phenols in smoked meat) as additives.

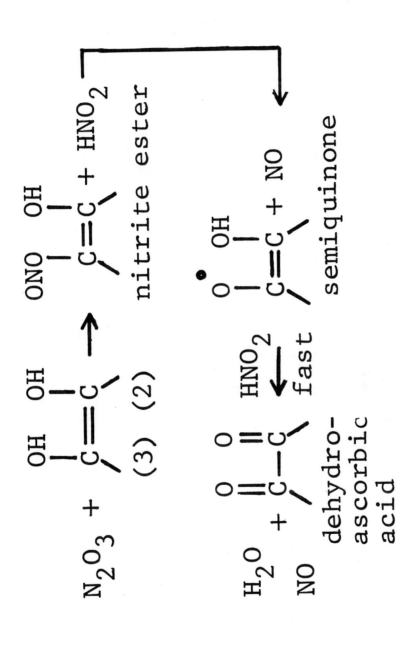

Figure 2: Intermediates in the reaction of nitrous anhydride (N_2O_3) with ascorbic acid. Only carbon atoms 2 and 3 are shown.

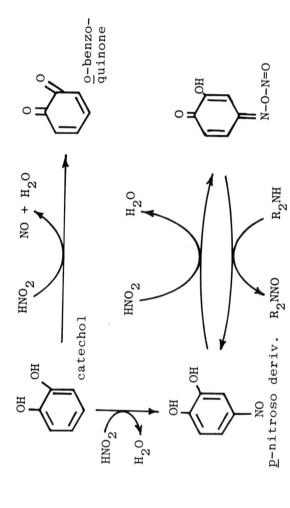

Figure 3: Mechanism whereby phenols can either inhibit nitrosation (by using up the nitrite) or enhance nitrosation (by forming of an active nitrosating species). The reactions shown have not all been demonstrated specifically for catechol.

564

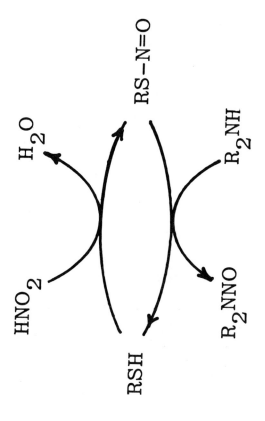

Figure 4: Mechanism whereby thiols can either inhibit or enhance nitrosation.

In our 1972 paper,[4] we proposed that readily
nitrosated drugs, e.g., aminopyrine and
piperazine, should be formulated with sufficient
ASC to block their intragastric nitrosation by
nitrite. [Most nitrite in the human stomach arises
from nitrite produced[9] in the saliva by bacterial
reduction of nitrate.] This proposal seemed
logical, since the pH of gastric contents after
a meal is gradually lowered from 5 to 1. Accordingly, ASC might react with all the nitrite at
the higher pH values, before NNO compounds were
produced. This suggestion has not been widely
adopted. In this connection, research is urgently
needed on the ASC dose required to lower the level
of nitrite normally present in human gastric
juice.[10]

The fate of NO produced from the ASC-nitrite
reaction is of interest. If the gaseous NO does
not escape from the system and excess oxygen is
present, the NO can be oxidized to NO_2, which
then reacts with water to give nitric and nitrous
acids. Hence this cycle (Fig. 5a) regenerates
half the original nitrite, and twice as much ASC
is needed for complete removal of nitrite, when
oxygen is present.[4]

If less oxygen is present, the NO_2 could
react with unoxidized NO to give N_2O_3. This would
be hydrolyzed to regenerate two moles of HNO_2
(Fig. 5b). Under this circumstance, ASC should
not inhibit nitrosamine formation (B. Challis,
personal communication).

Archer et al.[11] studied the effect of oxygen
on ASC inhibition of N-nitrosomorpholine (NMOR)
formation. A solution containing morpholine,
nitrite, and ASC was reacted at pH 3-4. In the
absence of air, 0.5 moles ASC/mole nitrite was
needed to prevent NMOR formation, in accord with
equations 1-4. When air was bubbled into the
solution, 1.0 mole ASC/mole nitrite was needed
to prevent nitrosation. The oxidation of ASC by
nitrite at pH 4 was also studied. One mole of
nitrite oxidized 0.5 moles ASC under anaerobic
conditions, but 1.0 mole ASC when air was bubbled
in. Air alone oxidized only a small amount of
the ASC. Hence, nitrite enables oxygen to oxidize
ASC. This explains why oxygen partly prevented

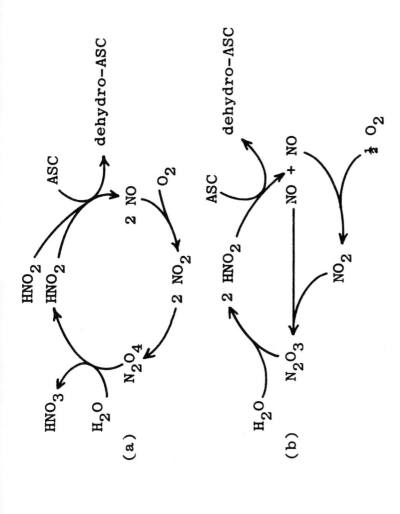

Figure 5: Cycles whereby oxygen could serve to regenerate half (Fig. 5a) or all (Fig. 5b) of the nitrous acid, after its reduction by ASC to give nitric oxide.

ASC from inhibiting NMOR formation. These findings
were attributed to direct oxidation by oxygen
of the ASC semiquinone intermediate (Figure 2)
and perhaps to the mechanism shown in Figure 5a,
which would be less prominent in this open system.
Under conditions where ASC reacted rapidly with
nitrite, amine nitrosation was not observed until
all the ASC was consumed, i.e., there was a lag
period before nitrosation begins.

Nitrosation of a number of drugs has been
shown to be inhibited by ASC. These drugs include
aminopyrine, piperazine, methapyrilene, and the
tetracyclines.[2,3]

(b) Use of ASC in the meat industry

Sodium nitrite ($NaNO_2$) is added to certain
meat products, e.g., frankfurters, bacon and
corned beef, to preserve the meat against contamination by Clostridium botulinum, to improve
the flavor and to give a pink color, due to
nitrosomyoglobin (formed from myoglobin and NO).
Although non-fried, nitrite-preserved meat products do not usually contain nitrosamines (except
for the noncarcinogenic N-nitrosoproline), a few
years ago fried bacon contained up to 100 ppb
of the moderate carcinogen N-nitrosopyrrolidine
(NPYR) and smaller amounts of the strong carcinogen dimethylnitrosamine (DMN). This occurred when
150 ppm $NaNO_2$ was added to the bacon. The nitrosamines are produced during the frying, at around
$180°C$.

ASC was included for many years in some
nitrite-preserved products, to improve the pink
color (which it does by reducing the nitrite to
NO). After our results[4] were presented, Fiddler
et al.[12] showed that ASC inhibited NPYR formation
in fried bacon and related products, and the meat
industry became interested in adding ASC to bacon
as a means of reducing NPYR formation.

It is still unclear whether NPYR in fried
bacon arises by decarboxylation of N-nitrosoproline present in the bacon before it is fried,
or whether pyrrolidine or some other precursor
in the aqueous or lipid phase is nitrosated during
frying to give NPYR. The effectiveness of ASC
or other antioxidants should depend on the
mechanism involved. Whatever this mechanism, since
about 1975 the U.S. meat industry began to use

ASC or erythorbate in bacon, to reduce nitrosamine formation (Erythorbate, i.e., D-ascorbate, is inactive as a vitamin but effective in reducing nitrite.) In current practice, 120 ppm $NaNO_2$ and 500 ppm sodium ascorbate is added to meat products. This reduces NPYR production in fried bacon to about 10 ppb.[13] A current problem is that $NaNO_2$ itself might be a weak carcinogen.[14,15]

(c) Nitrosation in lipids and by nitrogen oxides

Up to this point, we have mainly discussed nitrosation in acidic aqueous solution, for which ASC could be used as an inhibitor. Nitrosation in lipidic media cannot be inhibited by ASC because of its insolubility in these media, and in this case α-tocopherol and other lipophilic antioxidants may be suitable agents. This approach is being studied in the case of fried bacon, where much of the NPYR may be produced in the lipid phase. Bacon was treated with 500 ppm α-tocopherol as a suspension stabilized with a surfactant, in addition to the usual levels of ASC and nitrite. NPYR in the fried bacon was lowered from 10 ppb in the absence of α-tocopherol to 4-6 ppb.[16,17]

The structure of α-tocopherol allows it to be a particularly effective inhibitor.[18] Thus it inhibits nitrosation because it reduces nitrite, while it is oxidized to a quinone-type structure (Figure 6). Since α-tocopherol does not have unsubstituted carbon atoms on the phenolic ring, it cannot form C-nitroso derivatives that might promote nitrosation. In contrast, β, γ, and δ-tocopherol have unsubstituted positions on the phenol ring and are not as effective as α-tocopherol in inhibiting nitrosation, perhaps because they produce nitrosating C-nitroso compounds.[18]

We found that nitrous acid (HNO_2) was partly extracted from acidic aqueous solution by organic solvents, and that nitrosation of lipid-soluble amides, e.g., the pesticide carbaryl, proceeded more rapidly in methylene chloride-water mixtures than in water alone.[19] This nitrosation was attributed to N_2O_3, produced in the organic phase from HNO_2, since reaction rate was proportional to nitrite concentration squared (unpublished

Reaction of α-tocopherol with nitrite

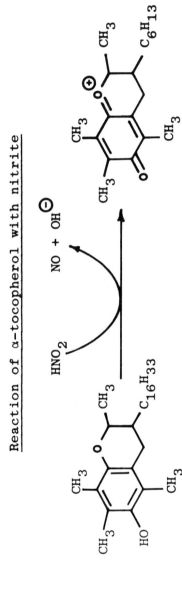

Figure 6:   Reaction of α-tocopherol with nitrite to form α-tocoquinone.

570

results). We also confirmed earlier observations
that nitrosation by the nitrogen oxides (N_2O_4
and N_2O_3) occurs very rapidly at $0°C$ in methylene
chloride solution, in the absence of water. For
example, nitrosation of ethylurea under such
conditions was almost complete in five seconds!
Nitrosation of N-butylacetamide proceeded 31,000
times faster than in water at pH 2. This finding
helps explain why much NNO compound formation
in the environment occurs in lipidic media.

We examined the effect of 3 inhibitors on
N-butylacetamide nitrosation by N_2O_4 in methylene
chloride solution (Table 2). At 15 mM inhibitor,
the effectiveness of the inhibitors was in the
order α-tocopherol > butylated hydroxytoluene
(BHT) > 4-methylcatechol. At 50 mM inhibitor, all
3 compounds were at least 99% effective. At and
below 10 mM, 4-methylcatechol slightly enhanced
the nitrosation, probably by the mechanisms shown
in Figure 3. 4-Methylcatechol was chosen because
it was used by Challis and Bartlett[20] as a model
for chlorogenic acid, a major tannin in coffee.

When N_2O_4 was bubbled into aqueous solutions
of amines under neutral or alkaline conditions,
nitrosamines and nitramines ($R_2N.NO_2$) were
produced.[21] [Nitramines are also carcinogenic.[15]]
This occurred by direct reaction of N_2O_4 with
the amines, and not via hydrolysis to nitrous
acid. The gases N_2O_3 and NOCl behaved similarly.
ASC inhibits this type of nitrosation, but not
as effectively as certain phenols (B. Challis,
personal communication).

Nitrosation in aqueous solution was often
stopped by making the solution alkaline in the
presence of an organic solvent such as methylene
chloride, or else the nitrosamine was extracted
with an organic solvent after the aqueous solution
was made alkaline. In these cases, ASC and phenols
were sometimes found to enhance the nitrosation.
A likely reason is that the ASC-nitrite reaction
produces NO, which dissolves in the organic
solvent and reacts there with oxygen to give NO_2.
This can then nitrosate the amine, especially
if non-ionized amine is extracted into the solvent
from the alkaline solution. Hence the enhancement
may be an artefact. In such experiments, it is
often best to stop the reaction by adding ammonium

Table 2. Effect of α-tocopherol, BHT and 4-methyl catechol on N-butylacetamide nitrosation by N_2O_4 in methylene chloride.[a]

Inhibitor concn. (mM)	Percent inhibition		
	α-Tocopherol	BHT	4-Methyl catechol
50	100	100	99
25	100	97	78
15	93	73	26
12.5	89	34	—
10	53	17	-10
7.5	23	11	-14
3.8	—	—	-18

[a]Conditions: N-butylacetamide, 20 mM; N_2O_4 measured as NOX, 13-24 mM (with BHT) or 17 mM (with other inhibitors); 0°C; reaction time, 45 seconds (BHT) or 5 minutes (other compounds). Nitrosamide yield in the absence of inhibitor, 2.4-3.1 mM (for 45 second reaction) and 8-11 mM (for 5 minute reaction).

sulfamate (which converts nitrite to nitrogen)
at pH 0-2. One should also perform a "zero-time"
experiment, to check that NNO compound is not
produced when the stopping reagent is added to
a solution of nitrite, amine and ASC, just after
they are mixed together.

(2) In vivo studies

(a) Acute toxicity experiments

Kamm[22] has reviewed this subject. When large
single doses of dimethylamine or aminopyrine were
gavaged to rats or mice together with a large
$NaNO_2$ dose, acute liver toxicity develops after
a few days. This effect can be detected by
histological examination and by measuring the
serum transaminases. With both dimethylamine and
aminopyrine, the effect is attributed to intragastric formation of DMN (LD_{50} in rats, 40 mg/kg).
When similar experiments were performed with
aminopyrine, but with ASC added to the amine
solution before gavage, hepatotoxicity was completely prevented.[23] When rats received single
doses of 1500 mg dimethylamine hydrochloride +
125 mg $NaNO_2$ per kg body weight, sodium ASC doses
down to 90 mg/kg completely protected the rats
from necrosis.[24]

A single intragastric dose of DMN produced
acute liver necrosis in rats only when the dose
reached 10 mg/kg.[24] Hence, in the amine + nitrite
experiments, the absence of liver toxicity indicates only that DMN production did not exceed
10 mg/kg body weight. Gavage of rats with an
α-tocopherol suspension in water almost completely
prevented the acute liver toxicity due to aminopyrine + nitrite.[25]

(b) Carcinogenicity experiments

Sander and Bürkle[26] were the first to induce
tumors by feeding nitrite + amines or amides.
The tumors were attributed to in vivo formation
of the NNO compounds, probably in the stomach.
When pregnant rats were gavaged with ethylurea + nitrite, hydrocephalus and nervous system
tumors were induced in the offspring. Both these
effects were prevented when ASC was gavaged
together with the ethylurea.[27]

In our Institute, the induction of lung
adenomas in Swiss or Strain A mice was used to
examine the amine/amide + nitrite system. The

lung adenoma system was convenient because many
adenomas/mouse were induced and they were easy
to count. The amines or amides were administered
in the diet and $NaNO_2$ in drinking water for 20
weeks. The mice were maintained another 10 weeks
and killed, and the lung adenomas were counted.
Tumors were induced by treatment with nitrite + the rapidly nitrosated compounds morpholine, piperazine, N-ethylaniline, methylurea,
and ethylurea, but not by nitrite + the slowly
nitrosated dimethylamine.[28,29] In one experiment
in which morpholine and $NaNO_2$ were administered,
we estimated from the number of induced adenomas
that 0.6% of the morpholine was nitrosated.[30]

When precursor concentrations were varied
in the piperazine + nitrite system, lung adenoma
induction was very approximately proportional
to piperazine dose and to the square of nitrite
dose, in accord with the chemical kinetics for
nitrosamine formation.[31] When ASC was added to
the food together with the amine or urea, and
$NaNO_2$ was added to drinking water, the number
of lung adenomas was reduced, compared to the
position without ASC.[30] Presumably, ASC competed
with the amine or urea for the nitrite and hence
reduced the formation of NNO compounds. With 23 g
ASC/kg food, lung adenoma induction by
nitrite + morpholine or piperazine was inhibited
89-91%. With 5.75 g ASC/kg food, lung tumorigenesis by morpholine + nitrite was inhibited
72%, whereas tumorigenesis by piperazine + nitrite
was inhibited only 37%. Adenoma induction by
methylurea + nitrite was 98% inhibited by 11.5 g
ASC/kg. Gallic acid also strongly inhibited
adenoma induction by morpholine + nitrite.

We examined the effect of ASC on carcinogenesis by morpholine + nitrite in male MRC-Wistar
rats.[32] Morpholine (10 g/kg) was given in the
diet and $NaNO_2$ (3 g/liter) in the drinking water
for two years. Some rats also received sodium
ASC (23 g/kg) in the diet. The incidence of liver
tumors due to morpholine + nitrite was reduced
from 65% in the absence to 49% in the presence
of ASC, and the latent period was nearly doubled,
from 54 to 93 weeks. Hence in vivo NMOR production
was probably about 50% inhibited. Unexpectedly,
the group with morpholine + nitrite + ASC had

a 54% incidence of forestomach tumors, including
an 18% incidence of squamous carcinomas, whereas
no forestomach tumors were seen in the morpholine + nitrite group.

The most likely interpretation of the forestomach results was that ASC lowered the in vivo
production of NMOR. Accordingly, liver tumors
were induced more slowly by the NMOR and the rats
had a longer time to develop forestomach tumors,
which were also induced by NMOR. A less likely
hypothesis was that ASC directly promoted the
development of forestomach tumors.

In recent studies (S.S. Mirvish, R. Runge,
and E. Mahboubi, unpublished work), the experiment
with morpholine, nitrite and ASC was repeated,
but with a $NaNO_2$ level of 2 g/liter drinking
water. The 38 rats treated with morpholine + nitrite showed a 92% incidence of liver tumors
(mostly hepatocellular carcinomas) and a 32%
incidence of forestomach papillomas. In the
morpholine + nitrite + ASC group (29 rats), the
liver tumor incidence was reduced to 38% and the
incidence of forestomach papillomas, was increased
to 72%. In both groups, most forestomachs showed
some acanthosis and hyperkeratosis. The results
for the liver confirmed those of the first experiment. Since, unlike in the first experiment, the
forestomachs of both groups showed tumors and
other lesions, the results indicate that the forestomach tumors were induced by NMOR alone.

(c) Chemical Analysis

A direct way of discovering whether ASC
inhibits in vivo nitrosation is to analyze biological tissues chemically for NNO compounds.
In the experiments by Kamm,[22] ASC inhibited the
acute liver toxicity produced by aminopyrine + nitrite in rats. This paper also reported that
gavage of aminopyrine (125 mg/kg) + $NaNO_2$
(110 mg/kg) produced, 30 minutes later, a serum
DMN level of 1.9 µg/ml. The DMN level was lowered
to 0.7 µg/ml when 18 mg/kg of sodium ASC was
gavaged at the same time, and to zero when
70 mg/kg of sodium ASC was gavaged.[33]

Iqbal et al.[33] studied the effect of inhibitors, given by gavage, on NMOR production in
mice from morpholine + $NaNO_2$ (also gavaged). The
whole mouse was analyzed for nitrosamines, using

the very sensitive Thermal Energy Analyzer. NMOR
formation was inhibited 94–99% by ASC and ammonium
sulfamate, and 55% by α–tocopherol.

We are studying methylnitrosourea (MNU)
formation after administration of ^{3}H–labeled
methylurea + $NaNO_2$, mixed in a 5–g meal.[19] MNU
is determined radiochemically in the stomach contents. When 100 mg methylurea and 4 g $NaNO_2$/kg
commercial diet were administered, and the stomach
contents were analyzed three hours later, the
MNU level corresponded to 0.92% conversion from
methylurea. When 11.5 or 2.9 g sodium ASC/kg was
included in the diet, the gastric MNU levels
corresponded to 0.04 and 0.46% yields from methylurea, respectively. Hence these ASC levels
inhibited MNU formation by 96 and 50%,
respectively.

(3) Possible carcinogenicity and mutagenicity of ASC
If ASC is to be used to inhibit the formation
of carcinogens, it should obviously not itself
cause cancer. Tests for the carcinogenicity of
ASC have yielded negative results, but were not
entirely satisfactory.[30,34,35]

Cupric [Cu(II)] and ferric [Fe(III)] ions
catalyze the oxidation by oxygen (autoxidation)
of ASC, which produces H_2O_2.[36] The influence of
Cu(II) on ASC mutagenicity was examined by Stich
et al.[37] Pre-incubated solutions of ASC and Cu(II)
were mutagenic to S. typhimurium TA 100. An
ASC–Cu(II) mixture caused DNA fragmentation and
repair in cultured human fibroblasts. ASC caused
a dose-dependent increase in sister chromatid
exchanges and an inhibition of DNA synthesis in
mammalian cell cultures.[38] The effects were
partly prevented by adding catalase and were
attributed to free radicals produced from the
H_2O_2.

$$ASC + O_2 \xrightarrow{\text{metal ions}} \text{dehydro–ASC} + H_2O_2 \ldots\ldots\ldots(5)$$

(4) Effects on biological activity of NNO
compounds
ASC did not affect carcinogenesis in the
rat by ethylnitrosourea given transplacentally
and by NMOR.[32,39] We tested the effect of ASC,

given chronically in the diet, on lung adenoma induction by mononitrosopiperazine or NMOR,[30] administered to mice in the drinking water. The ASC groups showed a small (15 to 59%) increase in adenoma yield. This could have been due to a greater intake of nitrosamine-containing drinking water in these groups.

We later tested the effect of sodium ASC (23 g/kg diet) on lung tumorigenesis in Strain A mice by DMN, given as two i.p. injections (Table 3). In this case, the nitrosamine dose could not be affected by the ASC. We also examined the effect of gallic acid (21.8 g/kg diet). The group with ASC showed a significant decrease in DMN tumorigenesis (but with large standard deviations), whereas gallic acid had no effect. Similar results were obtained when ASC was administered from one week before to one week after the DMN injections, or from one week before the first DMN injection for 20 weeks.

Edgar[40] suggested that ASC might inhibit nitrosamine carcinogenesis, because of evidence that ASC shows nucleophilic properties. Hence, ASC might react directly with the alkylating species (carbonium ions) produced during the metabolism of nitrosamines. Guttenplan[41,42] tested the effect of ASC on mutagenesis by NNO compounds, using Salmonella typhimurium TA-1530. ASC inhibited mutagenesis by 1-methyl-3-nitro-1-nitrosoguanidine (MNNG), in the absence of liver microsomes, because the compounds reacted chemically with each other. Both Cu(II) and, less effectively, Fe(III) accelerated the ASC-MNNG reaction, suggesting that ASC oxidation was involved. ASC did not affect mutagenesis by MNU or MNU decomposition. An unidentified direct-acting mutagen produced by the nitrosation of spermidine was also destroyed by ASC.[43]

ASC (2-6 mM) inhibited the microsome-mediated mutagenicity of DMN,[44] and this inhibition was enhanced by Cu(II). It was suggested that ASC reduced an active metabolite of DMN, or that a DMN metabolite alkylated the ASC. The inhibition by ASC of lung adenoma induction due to DMN (Table 3) could be explained by Guttenplan's results.

Table 3. Effect of ASC on lung tumorigenesis by DMN in male strain A mice[a]

Additional treatment	Treatment period (age in weeks)	Effective no. of mice	Lung adnomas/mouse Mean $\pm$ S.D.	$p<$
None	–	33	8.2 ± 8.1	Ref.[b]
Na ASC	10–13	40	4.0 ± 3.3	0.005
Na ASC	10–30	35	5.4 ± 3.4	0.05
Gallic acid	10–13	42	8.5 ± 3.4	N.S.[c]
Gallic acid	10–30	36	9.4 ± 9.6	N.S.[c]

[a]All groups received two i.p. injections of DMN in aqueous solution, given at ages of 11 and 12 weeks. DMN dose was 5 mg/kg body weight/injection. A commercial powdered rodent diet was used, with Na ASC (23 g/kg) or gallic acid (21.8 g/kg) added to the diet as in ref. 30.
[b]Reference group.
[c]Not significant.

(5) Human cancer

Human gastric cancer could be caused by
nitrosoureas or other nitrosamides, produced
intragastrically from amides in food, and nitrite
derived from food or saliva.[44-49] If this
hypothesis is correct, ASC could play a significant role in inhibiting in vivo formation of the
nitrosamides. There is a negative association
between gastric cancer incidence and the consumption of fresh fruit (e.g., citrus) and
vegetables (e.g., lettuce) that contain ASC. This
association has been observed in Holland,
Colombia, U.S.A., Japan, Scandinavia, and
England.[46,47] Hence ASC could reduce the incidence
of gastric cancer by inhibiting nitrosamide
formation in the food and/or in vivo. Other
naturally occurring compounds that react with
nitrite, such as phenols and tannins, could also
play a role here. The incidence of gastric cancer
is falling in the U.S.A. and elsewhere, perhaps
due to the increased consumption of fresh and
frozen fruits and vegetables, in addition to
certain other factors.[48]

If we accept the view that nitrosamides are
likely to be involved in the causation of gastric
cancer, then we should urge that people in areas
at high risk for gastric cancer (e.g., parts of
Japan and Colombia) adopt certain changes in their
diet, including the recommendation that they
should eat more fresh fruit and vegetables, or
pure ASC.

A contributing factor to the high incidence
of nasopharyngeal cancer in southern China may
be the high consumption of salted fish, coupled
with an ASC deficiency.[50] This association could
be due to an NNO compound, whose in vivo formation
was inhibited by ASC.

Esophageal cancer is very common in parts
of Iran, South Africa and China.[51] Nitrosamines
are likely etiologic agents, since certain of
these compounds (e.g., unsymmetric dialkylnitro-
samines) are strong carcinogens for the rodent
esophagus. If nitrosamines were involved, and
especially if they were formed in vivo, then
exposure to ASC should be negatively correlated
with the disease. This may be true in Iran, where

the occurrence of esophageal cancer was correlated
with deficiencies in vitamins A and C and in
riboflavin.[52]

   With respect to colorectal cancer, human
feces may contain nitrite, nitrate, and a
direct-acting mutagen which may be related to
a nitrosamide.[53-55] The mutagen concentration
was reduced by feeding ASC and/or α-tocopherol.
These findings will be discussed by Dr. R. Bruce.

   (6) Summary and Conclusions

   In acidic aqueous solution, ASC inhibits
the formation of nitrosamines and nitrosoureas
from nitrite and the amines or ureas, because
it reduces nitrite to nitric oxide. Ascorbate
anion is more reactive than ascorbic acid and
hence ASC is more effective than most other reducing agents at relatively high pH's of 3-5. In
the presence of oxygen, higher levels of ASC are
needed to inhibit nitrosamine formation; the
mechanism may involve a direct reaction of oxygen
with ASC semiquinone and oxidation of nitric oxide
to regenerate, eventually, some of the nitrite.
Phenols, especially polyphenols, usually inhibit
nitrosation but can, in some circumstances,
enhance this process. Certain nitrogen oxides
readily produce NNO compounds in lipidic media
and lipid-water mixture; in this case, ASC is
inactive but α-tocopherol and other phenols are
effective.

   We suggested that ASC should be administered
with readily nitrosated drugs to inhibit their
in vivo conversion to NNO derivatives, but the
appropriate experimental basis has not been
established in man. ASC is widely used to inhibit
NPYR formation during the frying of bacon.

   In vivo, ASC and α-tocopherol reduced or
abolished the acute toxicity caused by gavage
of nitrite + certain amines. ASC also inhibited
tumor induction by administration of nitrite +
amines or alkylureas in rodents. ASC lowered the
amount of NNO compounds produced in vivo and
determined chemically.

   ASC is apparently not itself carcinogenic
but is mutagenic in the presence of cupric or
ferric ions, perhaps due to hydrogen peroxide
produced by ASC autooxidation. ASC appeared to
inhibit the induction of mouse lung adenomas by

injected DMN and the microsome-mediated mutagenicity of DMN. ASC reacts chemically with MNNG
and hence inhibits its mutagenicity.

Gastric cancer in man may be caused by nitrosoureas or related compounds produced in vivo.
There is a negative association between the
incidence of gastric cancer and the intake of
ASC-containing fresh fruits and vegetables. The
high incidence of nasopharyngeal and esophageal
cancer in certain areas may be due to nitrosamines
and may be correlated with an ASC deficiency.
Human feces contains a mutagen which could be
involved in the genesis of colon cancer and is
reduced in amount by the administration of ASC.

We may draw the following conclusions:

(a) ASC efficiently inhibits N-nitrosation
in acidic aqueous solution from nitrite. Phenols,
especially polyphenols, can act similarly.

(b) α-Tocopherol and some phenols inhibit
lipidic N-nitrosation by nitrogen oxides.

(c) We should establish the conditions under
which ASC and other inhibitors lower intragastric
nitrite levels in man. The inhibitors could then
be administered with readily nitrosated drugs.

(d) Use of ASC by the meat industry is reducing exposure to nitrosamines in fried bacon.

(e) We should encourage an increased consumption of ASC-containing fruits and vegetables,
or of ASC, in areas with high incidences of cancer
of the stomach and, perhaps, cancer of the
nasopharynx and esophagus.

(f) We should explore the connection between
the administration of ASC and α-tocopherol, and
the level of human fecal mutagens.

References
1.   Mirvish SS: Blocking the formation of
     N-nitroso compounds with ascorbic acid in
     vitro and in vivo, in King CG, Burns JJ
     (eds): Second Conference on Vitamin C. Ann
     N.Y. Acad. Sci., 1975, pp. 175-180
2.   Mirvish SS: Ascorbic acid inhibition of
     N-nitroso compound formation in chemical,
     food and biological systems, in Zedeck M,
     Lipkin M (eds): Inhibition of Tumor Induction
     and Development. Plenum Publishing
     Corporation, New York, in press
3.   Mirvish SS: Formation of N-nitroso compounds:
     chemistry, kinetics, and in vivo occurrence.
     Toxicol Appl Pharmacol 31:325-351, 1975
4.   Mirvish SS, Wallcave L, Eagen M, et al:
     Ascorbate-nitrite reaction: Possible means
     of blocking the formation of carcinogenic
     N-nitroso compounds. Science 177:65-68, 1972
5.   Dahn H, Loewe L, Bunton CA: Über die
     oxydation von Ascorbinsaure durch salpetrige
     Säure. Teil VI: Übersicht und Diskussion
     der Ergebnisse. Helvet Chim Acta 43:320-333,
     1960
6.   Challis BC: Rapid nitrosation of phenols
     and its implications for health hazards from
     dietary nitrites. Nature 244-246, 1973
7.   Massey RC, Crews C, Davies R, et al: A study
     of the competitive nitrosations of pyr-
     rolidine, ascorbic, cysteine and P-cresol
     in a protein-based model system. J Sci Food
     Agric 29:815-821, 1978
8.   Davies R, Dennis MJ, Massey RC, McWeeny DJ:
     Some effects of phenol and thiol nitrosation
     reactions on N-nitrosamine formation, in
     Walker EA et al. (eds): Environmental Aspects
     of N-Nitroso Compounds. Lyon, International
     Agency for Research in Cancer, 1978, pp.
     183-198
9.   Tannenbaum SR, Sinskey AJ, Weisman M, et
     al: Nitrite in human saliva: its possible
     relationship to nitrosamine formation. J
     Natl Cancer Inst 53:19-84, 1974
10. Ruddell WS, Blendis LM, Walters CL: Nitrite
     and thiocyanate in the fasting and secreting
     stomach and in saliva. Gut 18:73-77, 1977

11. Archer MD, Tannenbaum SR, Fan TY, et al: Reaction of nitrite with ascorbate and its relation to nitrosamine formation. J Natl Cancer Inst 54:1203–1205, 1975
12. Fiddler W, Pensabene JW, Piotrowski EG, et al: Use of sodium ascorbate or erythorbate to inhibit formation of N-nitrosodimethyl-amine in frankfurters. J Food Sci 38:1084–1085, 1973
13. Birdsall JJ: N-Nitrosopyrrolidine in bacon obtained from 10 commercial bacon production plants, in Linbergen BJ, Krol B (eds): Proc 2nd Int. Symp. Nitrite Meat Prod., Central Agric. Publication Documentation. Wageningen, Netherlands, 1977, pp. 211–213
14. Newberne PM: Nitrite promotes lymphoma incidence in rats. Science 204:1079–1081, 1979
15. Mirvish SS, Bulay O, Runge RG, et al: Study of the carcinogenicity of large doses of dimethylnitramine, N-nitroso-L-proline, and sodium nitrite administered in drinking water to rats. J Natl Cancer Inst 64:1435–1442, 1980
16. Mergens WJ, Kamm JJ, Newmark HL, et al: Alpha-tocopherol: Uses in preventing nitro-samine formation, in Walker EA, Castegnaro M, Griciute L, and Lyle RE (eds): Environ-mental Aspects of N-nitroso Compounds. Lyon, International Agency for Research on Cancer, 1978, pp. 199–212
17. Gray JI, Dugan LR: Inhibition of N-nitro-samine formation model food systems. J Food Sci 40:981–984, 1975
18. Newmark HL, Mergen WJ: Alpha-tocopherol (vitamin E) and its relationship to tumor induction and development, in Zedeck M and Lipkin M (eds): Inhibition of Tumor Induction and Development. Plenum Publishing Corp., New York, in press
19. Mirvish SS, Karlowski K, Sams J, et al: Studies related to nitrosamide formation: nitrosation in solvent:water and solvent systems, nitrosomethylurea formation in the rat stomach, and analysis of a fish product for ureas, in Walker EA, Castegnaro M, Griciute L, Lyle RE (eds): Environmental

Aspects of N-Nitroso Compounds, Lyon, International Agency for Research on Cancer, pp. 161-174

20. Challis BC, Bartlett CD: Possible cocarcinogenic effects of coffee constituents. Nature 254:532-533, 1975

21. Challis BC, Kyrtopoulos SA: Rapid formation of carcinogenic N-nitrosamines in aqueous alkaline solutions. Brit J Cancer 35:693-696, 1977

22. Kamm JJ: Effect of ascorbic acid on amine-nitrite toxicity, in King CG and Burns JJ (eds): Second Conference on Vitamin C, Ann NY Acad Sci 258:169-174, 1975

23. Kamm JJ, Dashman T, Conney AH, et al: Protective effects of ascorbic acid on hepatotoxicity caused by sodium nitrite plus aminopyrine. Proc Natl Acad Sci 70:747-749, 1973

24. Cardesa A, Mirvish SS, Haven GT, et al: Inhibitory effect of ascorbic acid on the acute toxicity of dimethylamine plus nitrite in the rat. Proc Soc Exp Biol Med 145:124-128, 1974

25. Kamm JJ, Dashman T, Newmark H, et al: Inhibition of amine-nitrite hepatotoxicity by alpha-tocopherol. Toxicol Appl Pharmacol 41:575-583, 1977

26. Sander J, Bürkle G: Induktion maligner Tumoren bei Ratten durch gleichzeitige Verfuttenrung von Nitrit und sekindaren Aminen. Z Krebsforsch 73:54-66, 1969

27. Ivankovic S, Preussmann R, Schmähl D, et al: Prevention by ascorbic acid of in vivo formation of N-nitroso compounds, in Bogovski P, Walker EA, (eds): N-Nitroso Compounds in the Environment, International Agency for Research on Cancer, Lyon, 1974, pp. 101-102

28. Greenblatt M, Mirvish SS, So BT: Nitrosamine studies: Induction of lung adenomas by concurrent administration of sodium nitrite and secondary amines in Swiss mice. J Natl Cancer Inst 46:1029-1034, 1971

29. Mirvish SS, Greenblatt M, Kommineni VRC: Nitrosamide formation in vivo: Induction of lung adenomas in Swiss mice by concurrent

feeding of nitrite and methylurea or ethyl-urea. J Natl Cancer Inst 48:1311-1315, 1972

30. Mirvish SS, Cardesa A, Wallcave L, et al: Induction of mouse lung adenomas by amines and ureas plus nitrite and by N-nitroso compounds: Effect of nitrite dose and of ascorbate, gallate, thiocyanate, and caffeine. J Natl Cancer Inst 55:633-636, 1975

31. Greenblatt M, Mirvish SS: Dose-response studies with concurrent administration of piperazine and sodium nitrite to strain A mice. J Natl Cancer Inst 50:119-124, 1973

32. Mirvish SS, Pelfrene A, Garcia, H, et al: Effect of sodium ascorbate on tumor induction in rats treated with morpholine and sodium nitrite, and with nitrosomorpholine. Cancer Lett 2:101-108, 1976

33. Iqbal ZM, Krull IS, Mills K, et al: in Walker EA et al (eds): Analysis and Formation of N-Nitroso Compounds. Lyon, International Agency for Research on Cancer, in press

34. Harman D: Role of free radicals in mutation, cancer, aging and the maintenance of life. Rad Res 16:753-763, 1962

35. Pipkin GE, Schlegel JU, Nishimura R, et al: Inhibitory effect of L-ascorbate on tumor formation in urinary bladders implanted with 3-hydroxyanthranilic acid. Proc Soc Exp Biol Med 131:522-524, 1969

36. Khan MMT, Martell AE: Metal ion and metal chelate catalyzed oxidation of ascorbic acid by molecular oxygen. I. Cupric and ferric ion catalyzed oxidation. J Am Chem Soc 89:4176-4185, 1967

37. Stich HF, Karim J, Koropatnick J, et al: Mutagenic action of ascorbic acid. Nature 260:722-724, 1976

38. Galloway SM, Painter RB: Vitamin C is positive in the DNA synthesis inhibition and sister-chromatid exchange tests. Mut Res 60:321-327, 1979

39. Ivankovic S, Zeller WJ, Schmähl D, et al: Verhinderung der pranatal carcinogenen Wirkung von Äthylharnstoff und Nitrit durch Ascorbinsäure, Naturwissenschaften 60:525, 1973

40. Edgar JA: Ascorbic acid and biological

alkylating agents. Nature 248:136–137, 1974

41. Guttenplan JB: Inhibition by L–ascorbate of bacterial mutagenesis induced by two N–nitroso compounds. Nature 268:368–370, 1977

42. Guttenplan JB: Mechanisms of inhibition by ascorbate of microbial mutagenesis induced by N–nitroso compounds. Cancer Res 38:2018–2022, 1978

43. Kokatnur MG, Murray ML, Correa P: Mutagenic properties of nitrosated spermidine. Proc Soc Exp Biol Med 158:85–88, 1978

44. Mirvish, SS: Kinetics of nitrosamide formation from alkylureas, N–alkylurethans and alkylguanidines: Possible implications for the etiology of human gastric cancer. J Natl Cancer Inst 46:1183–1193, 1971

45. Mirvish SS: N–Nitroso compounds: Their chemical and in vivo formation and possible importance as environmental carcinogens. J Toxicol Environ Health 2:1267–1277, 1977

46. Haenszel W, Correa P: Developments in the epidemiology of stomach cancer over the past decade. Cancer Res 35:3452–3458, 1975

47. Cuello C, Correa P, Haenszel W, et al: Gastric cancer in Colombia. I. Cancer risk and suspect environmental agents. J Natl Cancer Inst 57:1015–1020, 1976

48. Weisburger JH: Mechanism of action of diet as a carcinogen. Cancer 43:1987–1995, 1979

49. Frazer P, Chilvers C, Beral V, et al: Nitrate and human cancer: A review of the evidence. Int J Epidem 9:3–11, 1980

50. Ho JHC: An epidemiologic and clinical study of nasopharyngeal carcinoma. Int J Rad Oncol Biol Biophys 4:183–198, 1978

51. Day NE: Some aspects of the epidemiology of esophageal cancer. Cancer Res 35:3304–3307, 1975

52. Hormozdiari H, Day NE, Aramesh B, et al: Dietary factors and esophageal cancer in the Caspian littoral of Iran. Cancer Res 35:3493–3498, 1975

53. Tannenbaum SR, Fett D, Young VR, et al: Nitrite and nitrate are formed by endogenous synthesis in the human intestine. Science 200:1487–1489, 1978

54. Varghese AJ, Land PC, Furrer R, et al:
     Non-volatile N-nitroso compounds in human
     feces, in Walker EA, Castegnaro M, Griciute
     L and Lyle RW (eds): Environmental Aspects
     of N-Nitroso Compounds. Lyon, International
     Agency for Research on Cancer, pp 257-264,
     1978
55. Bruce WR, Varghese AJ, Wang S, et al: The
     endogenous production of nitroso compounds
     in the colon and cancer at that site, in
     Proceedings of the Ninth International
     Symposium of the Princess Takamatsu Cancer
     Research Fund, University of Tokyo press,
     Tokyo, in press

Reduction in the Formation of Mutagens and Carcinogens in the Large Bowel of Man.

W.R. BRUCE

Research Scientist,
Physics Division,
The Ontario Cancer Institute,
Toronto, Ontario, Canada.

What is it that is wrong with our Western diet? Why do so many of us develop colon cancer and related diseases? Are we eating too much fat, too much protein? Are we eating too little fiber, too few vegetables and fruits, too few vitamins? Or are we cooking our food wrong? All of these suggestions have been made and indeed most of them have the support of epidemiological or animal studies (1-18). Yet it seems unlikely that everything is wrong with our diet. What we need are better ways to define the relation between diet and disease, to sharpen up the hypotheses, to test them efficiently and quickly.

The need for a more specific approach for defining the relation between diet and disease can be answered in two ways. First by measuring the effect of dietary factors on chemicals in the human body that could give rise to colon cancer. And second by measuring the effect of dietary factors on pathological processes in the body that could lead to cancer. Both these methods have advantages and disadvantages. They both take time and the work I will be describing is only a start in these directions.

Chemicals that can give rise to cancer can frequently be identified by their ability to produce mutations (19). We therefore examined extracts of body fluids (feces) for the presence of such compounds (20). Several classes of such chemicals have now been described (21, 22). Our studies to date, however, have centered on only one - a lipid that is directly mutagenic to the Salmonella strain TA-100. This compound is very labile, UV and oxygen sensitive and has a characteristic UV absorbtion at 340 nm. Although the structure of this compound has not been completely worked out, it has been possible to show that it is made in the body and that the level of the compound varies greatly from individual to individual (23) and from population to population (21). Possibly differences in diet led to differences in the amount of the chemical made in the body. It was thus interesting to determine the effects of dietary changes on the levels of fecal mutagens. While these studies are not yet complete, it is clear that several factors do affect the formation of the compound. Effects are seen with ascorbic acid and α-tocopherol at doses of 100 mg/day each together with bran fiber at a dose of 10 grams/day (24).

Before it will be appropriate to interpret this data in terms of cancer causation, it will be necessary to study this compound further and to define the manner in which these dietary changes affect other potential carcinogens in the body. This process will require time for the compounds will probably be present in only small amounts and are likely to be difficult to work with. Nevertheless, work of this type will lead to a better understanding of the chemicals to which the cells of our body are exposed and how this exposure might be modified.

Pathological changes that may lead to cancer can now be examined in the colon with the use of the fiberoptics colonoscope. Previous studies have shown that, in Western Society, many individuals by the age of 70 years have gross colon pathology in the form of colonic polyps (25). Studies utilizing the colonoscope have shown that most, perhaps all, colon cancers develop from adenomatous polyps (26, 27). It is clearly interesting to work out the sequence of events that lead to colon cancer. But it is even more important to determine whether dietary changes from the traditional Western diet can lead to a change in the development of polyps, for if these precursor lesions can be prevented, so can colon cancer.

We have initiated studies of the development of polyps in patients who have had polyps removed. In these studies such patients have been randomized into two groups. One group is being given a placebo while the second receives a dietary intervention (28). We will examine each patient in two years to determine whether there is a difference in the appearance of polyps in the two groups. In the present study the dietary intervention is with ascorbic acid and α-tocopherol. We are initiating studies with fiber and we are

exploring the feasibility of studies with fat reduction.
These studies are quite lengthy and expensive but we hope
they represent a beginning for a series of experiments to the
successful prevention of these precursors. It is possible,
however, that we are beginning our intervention too late and
that we will have to develop strategies for describing
earlier precursor lesions.

Methods for assessing the relation between dietary factors and mutagenic and carcinogenic factors in the body have
thus been developed. They may be used to test hypotheses
relating diet and colon cancer, and to define how our Western
diet can be improved.

REFERENCES

1.   Drassar, B.S., and Irving, D. Environmental Factors and
     Cancer of the Colon and Breast. Br. J. Cancer, 27, 167-
     172, 1973.
2.   Wynder, E.L., and Shigematsu, T. Environmental Factors
     and Cancer of the Colon and Rectum. Cancer, 20, 1520-
     1561, 1967.
3.   Gregor, O., Toman, R., and Prusova, F. Gastrointestinal
     Cancer and Nutrition. Gut, 10, 1031-1034, 1969.
4.   Reddy, B.S., Narisawa, T., and Weisburger, J.H. Effect
     of a Diet with High Levels of Protein and Fat on Colon
     Carcinogenesis in F344 Rats Treated with 1,2-Dimethyl-
     hydrazine. J. Natl. Cancer Inst., 57, 567-569, 1976.
5.   Armstrong, B., and Doll, R. Environmental Factors and
     Cancer Incidence and Mortality in Different Countries
     with Special Reference to Dietary Practices. Int. J.
     Cancer, 15, 617-631, 1975.
6.   Haenszel, W., Berg, J.W., Segi, M., Kurihara, M., and
     Locke, F.B. Large Bowel Cancer in Hawaiian Japanese. J.
     Natl. Cancer Institute, 51, 1765-1779, 1973.
7.   Hill, M., MacLennan, R., and Newcombe, K. Diet and
     Large Bowel Cancer in Three Socioeconomic Groups in Hong
     Kong. Lancet, 1, 436, 1979.
8.   Weisberger, J.H., and Spingarn, N.E. Mutagens as a
     Function of Mode of Cooking of Meats. In: Miller, E.C.,
     et al. (Eds). Naturally Occurring Carcinogens-Mutagens
     and Modulators of Carcinogenesis. Japan Sci. Soc.
     Press., Tokyo/Univ. Park Press, Baltimore, pp. 177-184,
     1979.
9.   I.A.R.C. Microecology Group. Dietary Fibre, Transit-

Time, Fecal Bacteria, Steroids, and Colon Cancer in Two
Scandinavian Populations. Lancet, 2, 207-211, 1977.

10.   Modan, B., Barell, V., Lubin, F., Modan, M., Greenberg,
      R.A., and Graham, S. Low-Fibre Intake as an Etiologic
      Factor in Cancer of the Colon. J. Natl. Cancer Inst.,
      55, 15-18, 1975.

11.   Fleiszer, D., MacFarlane, J., Murray, D., and Brown, R.
      A. Protective Effect of Dietary Fibre Against Chem-
      ically Induced Bowel Tumors in Rats. Lancet, 2, 552-
      553, 1978.

12.   Graham, S., Dayal, H., Swanson, M., Mittelman, A., and
      Wilkinson, G. Diet in the Epidemiology of Cancer of
      the Colon and Rectum. J. Natl. Cancer Inst. 61, 709-
      714, 1978.

13.   Bjelke, E. Epidemiologic Studies of Cancer of the
      Stomach, Colon and Rectum with Special Emphasis on the
      Role of Diet. Scand. J. Gastroenterol. (Suppl.) 9, 1-
      235, 1974.

14.   Sporn, M.B. Prevention of Epithelial Cancer by Vitamin
      A and its Synthetic Analogs (Retinoids). In: Hiatt,
      H.H., Watson, J.D., and Winsten, J.A. (eds.). Origins
      of Human Cancer. New York, Cold Spring Harbor. pp.
      801-810, 1977.

15.   Dion, P.W., Bright-See, E.B., Furrer, R., Eng, V.W.S.,
      and Bruce, W.R. The Effects of Dietary Fat, Ascorbic
      Acid and α-Tocopherol on Fecal Mutagens. Cancer Res.
      (Submitted Feb., 1980).

16.   Cook, M.G., and McNamara, P. Effect of Dietary Vitamin
      E on Dimethylhydrazine-Induced Colonic Tumors in Mice.
      Cancer Res. 40, 1329-1331, 1980.

17.   Wattenberg, L.W. Inhibition of Chemical Carcinogenesis.
      J. Natl. Cancer Inst., 60, 11-18, 1978.

18.   Raicht, R.F., Cohen, B.I., Fazzini, E.P., Sarwal, A.N.,
      and Takahashi, M. Protective Effect of Plant Sterols
      Against Chemically Induced Colon Tumors in Rats. Cancer
      Res., 40, 403-5, 1980.

19.   McCann, J., Choi, E., Yamasaki, E., and Ames, B.N.
      Detection of carcinogens as mutagens in the *Salmonella/*
      microsome test: assay of 300 chemicals. Proc. Natl.
      Acad. Sci. U.S.A. 72: 5135-5139, 1975.

20.   Bruce, W.R., Varghese, A.J., Furrer, R., and Land, P.C.
      A mutagen in human feces. In: Origins of Human Cancer,
      edited by H.H. Hiatt, J.D. Watson and J.A. Winsten. New
      York: Cold Spring Harbor. pp. 1641-1644, 1977.

21.   Ehrich, M., Aswell, J.E., Van Tassell, R.L., and Wilkins,
      T.D. Mutagens in the Feces of 3 South-African Pop-
      ulations at Different Levels of Risk for Colon Cancer.

Mutat. Res. 64, 231-240, 1979.

22. Stich, H.F., and Kuhnlein, U. Chromosome Breaking Activity of Human Feces and its Enhancement by Transition Metals. Int. J. Cancer, 24, 284-287, 1979.

23. Dion, P.W., Bright-See, E.B., Furrer, R., Eng, V.W.S., and Bruce, W.R. The effects of dietary fat, ascorbic acid, and α-tocopherol on fecal mutagens. Submitted.

24. Bruce, W.R., and Dion, P.W. Studies relating to a fecal mutagen. Am. J. Clin. Nutr. 33, 1980.

25. Arminski, T.C., and McLean, D.W. Incidence and Distribution of Adenomatous Polyps of the Colon and Rectum Based on 1000 Autopsy Examinations. Dis. Colon. Rectum, 7, 249-261, 1964.

26. Cole, J.W., and Holden, W.D. Postcolectomy Regression of Adenomatous Polyps of the Rectum. Arch. Surg. 79, 385-392, 1959.

27. Muto, T., Bussey, J.R., and Morson, B.C. The Evolution of Cancer of the Colon and Rectum. Cancer, 36, 2551-2270, 1975.

28. Bruce, W.R., McKeown-Eyssen, G., Ciampi, A., Dion, P.W., and Boyd, N. Strategies for Dietary Intervention Studies in Colon Cancer. Cancer. In press.

Dietary Factors in the Causation and Prevention of Neoplasia

WEISBURGER, J.H., PH.D.

Vice President for Research

REDDY, B.S., PH.D., D.V.M.

Member & Assoc. Chief, Div. Nutrition

FIALA, E. S., PH.D.

Assoc. Chief, Div. Mol. Bio. & Pharmacology

WANG, Y.Y., PH.D.

Div. Nutrition

VUOLO, L.L.

Div. Nutrition

WYNDER, E.L., M.D.

President
American Health Foundation
Valhalla, N.Y. 10595

SPINGARN, N.E., PH.D.

Univ. of Calif.-Los Angeles

Address requests for reprints to J. H. Weisburger, American Health Foundation, Valhalla, N.Y. 10595.
Acknowledgement for grants: Grant support was provided by CA-17613 from NCI, DHEW; and USPHS, NCI grants CA-15400, CA-16382, and CA-24217 through Natl. Large Bowel Cancer Proj.

Many factors have contributed to the great progress made during the last 30 years towards an understanding at the molecular level of the events surrounding the development of cancer, especially through laboratory research in experimental systems (Miller & Miller,1979; Searle, 1976; Slaga et al., 1978; Weisburger & Williams, 1980).

Taking what we have learned about the causes of cancer and the modifying factors that operate in the human setting, it becomes important in our examination to return to man. Reasonably satisfactory data points and arguments relating to many major types of cancer have come from observation of the conditions favoring the development of specific kinds of cancer, and also, from inquiring into the reasons for lower incidences in those cases where higher rates might have been expected. With regard to two of the most important types of human cancer around the world, that is, cancer of the glandular stomach and cancer of the large bowel, sufficient understanding has been gained on causative and modifying factors and the relevant mechanisms underlying these factors, so that these facts can be used as a sound basis for recommendations which may reduce the risk for these neoplasms.

Multidisciplinary efforts on an international basis have contributed to this data base with teamwork efforts by epidemiologists studying the incidence parameters of high and low risk populations, laboratory scientists conducting controlled human studies as to metabolic indicators, experimental animal studies, and in vitro system experiments-- all have strengthened the arguments and interpretations given here.

We have estimated, in accord with Higginson & Muir (1979), that occupationally induced cancers, while preventable through proper engineering, safety controls, and education of management and personnel, account for only a small fraction of all cancers (Weisburger & Williams, 1981; Wynder & Gori, 1977; Table 1).

Most cancers are environmentally caused but have nonoccupational origins that have been obscure until more recently. If each cancer is considered as a separate type (for example, cancer of the lung and cancer of the large bowel), bearing down on the causative and modifying factors for each separate type has resulted in some clarification. Current concepts of their etiology are based on three major approaches and lines of evidence: First, variation in incidence of a specific type of cancer as a function of area of residence and in migrant populations; second, changes in incidence as a function of time; and third, detailed laboratory studies in animal models or in vitro systems (Doll, 1977; Fraumeni, 1975;

Higginson & Muir, 1976; Weisburger et al., 1977; Weisburger et al., 1980a; Wynder and Hirayama, 1977).

When a carcinogen is introduced into the human environment, incidence changes as a function of time (Weisburger et al., 1977), as is readily seen in small population groups with occupational cancers. A more striking case involving large numbers of people is that of cigarette smoking, which became popular among men during World War I and among women about the time of World War II. Twenty to 30 years later, a pronounced upward change in incidence of lung cancer appeared. Thus, introduction of a carcinogen(s) (from smoking) on a large scale results in a striking appearance of neoplastic disease. On the other hand, in the United States, cancer of the glandular stomach has declined considerably over the last 50 years. An obvious conclusion here is that the carcinogenic stimulus must have diminished or that a protective agent was introduced. A decline in the incidence of stomach cancer is now also being observed in those parts of the world where the disease has still had a high incidence--Japan, Iceland, Central and Western Latin America, and Northern and Eastern Europe. Our view on the reasons for this decline will be presented.

TABLE 1.
Causes of Human Cancers*

Related Cause	Cancer Type	% of Total
Occupational	Varied	1- 5
Crytogenic	Lymphomas, leukemias, sarcomas, (cervix?),(viral?)	10-15
Lifestyle		
1) Tobacco-related	Lung,pancreas,bladder,kidney	21
2) Diet-related:		
a)Nitrate-nitrite, low vit. C, mycotoxin	Stomach, Liver	5
b)High fat, low fiber, broiled or fried foods.	Large bowel, pancreas, breast, prostate	45
Multi-factorial		
1) Tobacco & alcohol	Oral cavity, esophagus	5
2) Tobacco-asbestos, tobacco-mining, tobacco-uranium-radium,	Lung, Respiratory tract	5
Iatrogenic-radiation, drugs		1

* Calculated from the 1978 incidence figures published by the American Cancer Society.

With the acquisition of better basic knowledge of specific risk factors for each kind of the important types of neoplastic diseases, it may be possible to design approaches to the inhibition of the entire carcinogenic process, or key portions thereof, as an effective, rational means of cancer prevention. In part, our method of classification of carcinogens into agents operating via genotoxicity, in contrast to those with epigenetic mechanisms, has permitted an improved means of selective inhibition, based on the properties of the several agents involved in cancer causation for each type of neoplasm (Weisburger & Williams, 1980; Williams & Weisburger, 1981).

STOMACH CANCER

Cancer of the glandular stomach is still an important neoplasm and in high incidence in many areas of the world such as Japan, Iceland, mountainous interior regions of Central and Western Latin America, and some Eastern European countries. In contrast, Western Europe, many Anglo-saxon countries (except Wales in the United Kingdom), and the United States have a low incidence. In fact over the last 50 years the gastric cancer rate in the United States has declined appreciably from 30/100,000 for men and 22/100,000 for women to 7.5 and 3.7/100,000 for men and women, respectively.

Dietary risk factors which show positive correlations in high risk populations include the high consumption of dried salted fish, pickled vegetables, smoked fish, and fewer vegetables and a lowered vitamin C intake particularly on a seasonal basis (Bjelke,1974; Stemmerman,1977; Hirayama,1979). Another correlation was reported between elevated levels of nitrate in foods and drinking water due to high levels in the soil and water supply (Zaldivar & Wetterstrand,1978). Crude salt or saltpeter used for preserving certain foods such as fish may also contain nitrate. On the other hand, Hawaiian Japanese with a higher intake of uncooked vegetables such as celery, lettuce, tomato, and fresh fruit juices had a low gastric cancer risk as compared to indigenous Japanese and also the first generation Japanese migrants to Hawaii (Haenszel et al., 1972; Stemmermann,1977; Hirayama,1979).

Glandular stomach cancer mimicking that seen in man has been induced in animal models in a reliable fashion by the use of an alkylnitrosoureido compound such as N-methyl-N'-nitro-N-nitrosoguanidine (MNNG) (Sugimura & Kawachi,1978; Druckrey,1975; Bralow & Weisburger, 1976). Kinetics of the reaction of the nitrosation of alkylamides such as methylurea has been studied by Mirvish (1977) who also made the important discovery that ascorbic acid had a inhibitory effect on the nitrosation of methylurea and alkylamines.

We have demonstrated that treating cooked or raw Sanma mackerel (a fish commonly eaten in Japan) with nitrite at pH 3, mimicking gastric conditions, yields high levels of mutagenic activity for Salmonella typhimurium TA1535, and treatment of beans and borsht with nitrite gave moderate mutagenic activity. Formation of the mutagen was inhibited by the simultaneous presence of vitamin C (Marquardt et al., 1977). When this mutagenic activity from the reaction of nitrite and Sanma was given to Wistar rats by gavage, it proved carcinogenic, inducing in rats adenocarcinomas of the glandular stomach (Weisburger et al., 1980b). The experimental design mimicked the conditions prevailing for migrants living in a high-risk region during the early part of their lives and then spending the rest of their lives in a low-risk region. The nature of the mutagen(s) obtained from the reaction is as yet unknown, but its mode of formation or inhibition, and the mutagenicity/carcinogenicity results suggest it may be an alkylnitrosoureido compound.

Other studies on the formation of gastric carcinogens concern the formation of nitrite from nitrate. Nitrate present in cooked foods is converted to nitrite when such foods are stored at room temperature for 24 hours. This reaction was inhibited by cold storage or refrigeration (Weisburger & Raineri, 1975).

Another source of nitrite is that produced by the bacterial flora in the oral cavity after intake of foods high in nitrate as demonstrated by Tannenbaum et al., 1976,1979.

Current concepts from various lines of evidence (see Reddy et al., 1980 for details) lead to the conclusion that gastric cancer in man may result from the consumption of salted, pickled foods, that the active agent or agents has the properties of alkynitrosoureido compounds formed from nitrite and undefined substrates, that this nitrite may be present in food from reduction of nitrate or may result from reduction of nitrate in the oral cavity, and importantly, that the formation of the carcinogen may be blocked by vitamin C or by vitamin E. Since nitrate is converted in high yield to nitrite when cooked foods stand at room temperature, people who stored leftover foods containing nitrite, as was the practice before the large-scale use of home refrigeration, might have been exposed to sizable amounts of nitrite when consuming leftover foods.

It would seem then that intake of foods containing vitamin C with each meal all year long from childhood onward may inhibit the formation of gastric carcinogens. Indeed, the increased year-round availability of fresh fruits and vegetables - foods containing vitamin C - and the widespread use of refrigeration for food storage may have contributed significantly to the sharp decline in the incidence of gastric cancer in the United States, a decrease beginning in other parts of the world where gastric cancer is still endemic.

Lower salt use would have similar benefits, and also reduce the risk of hypertension. In the MNNG-induced gastric cancer model, Tatematsu et al. (1975) found that salt (sodium chloride had a promoting effect. This test may mimic also human environment, for Joossens et al. (1979) has documented a parallelism in international trends for gastric cancer and for hypertension. The latter, in turn, is associated with salt use (Freis,1976; Meneely & Battarby,1976; Tobian,1978; Trowell,1978).

COLON CANCER

Colon cancer incidence has shown only a slight upward trend in the last 50 years in the United States and exhibits global differences with the highest incidence rates in North America, Australia, New Zealand, and Western and Northern Europe, except for Finland. Low-risk areas are Africa, Asia, Latin America, except Argentina and Uruguay. Japan now shows an increasing incidence, concurrent with the westernization of its diet (Hirayama,1979; Oiso,1975). Further support for environmental influence comes from migrant studies wherein colon cancer incidence is higher in 1st and 2nd generation Japanese immigrants to the United States than in native Japanese (Haenszel et al., 1972; 1976).

An association between colon cancer incidence and total dietary fat consumption has been noted (Reddy et al.,1980) and a worldwide correlation established (Carroll & Khor, 1975). The significant correlation exists between colon cancer and total fat levels, not with animal fat nor vegetable fat alone. Experimental animal studies support this correlation and experiments in a number of laboratories have shown that rats given several types of colon carcinogens had the same high incidence of large bowel cancer whether fed an unsaturated oil such as corn oil at 20% in the diet (corresponding to 40% of calories which is typical of a high fat Western diet) or saturated fat such as lard or tallow. In-

TABLE 2.
Dietary Intake of Various Nutrients and Fecal Excretion of
Various Constituents in Middle-Aged Male Volunteers From
Kuopio (Finland) and New York Metropolitan Area[a]

	Kuopio (15[b])	New York (40)
Dietary constituents		
Total protein	93± 4	89± 2
Total fat	110± 4	115± 3
Saturated fat	59± 3	49± 2
Other fats	51± 3	66± 2
Carbohydrates	320± 4	285± 4
Total fiber	32± 3	14± 2
Fecal constituents		
Fresh feces excreted	277±20	76±12
Fiber	26± 2	9± 1
Fecal dry matter	61± 8	22± 1
Total daily bile acids (mg)	277±22	275±14
Bile acid concentration (mg/gm)	4.59±0.42	11.7±0.54

[a] Averages ± SEM. Units: gm/day
[b] Number of samples.

take of diets containing 5% fat, equivalent to 10% of calories, which mimics a low risk Japanese population, yields a lower incidence of colon cancer (Reddy et al.,1980).

The underlying mechanism between total fat and colon cancer is that, in both people and animals on a high fat intake, the liver, and to a lesser extent, other tissues produce elevated amounts of cholesterol, and dietary cholesterol adds to the total load. Cholesterol, in turn, is metabolized to bile acids, entering the gut via bile, and leading to the excretion of more total primary, and bacterially-produced secondary bile acids in the stools. Also, intake of such high fat regimens yields higher levels of specific secondary bile acids compared to low-risk Japanese or African people, or rats on a 5% fat diet (Mower et al.,1979; Reddy et al., 1980).Bile acids are important since tests in germfree and conventional rats show that they have an appreciable promoting action (by an as yet unknown epigenetic mechanism) in large bowel carcinogenesis (Reddy et al.,1980; Watanabe et al., 1978). Secondary bile acids are more potent than primary bile acids.

Although epidemiological studies show that there is an association between colon cancer and heart disease in various parts of the world,the Finnish people with a diet high in fat (mainly dairy fats), are an exception in that, although their rate of heart disease is high, their colon cancer rate is much lower than that of their Western European neighbors (IARC, 1977; Jensen et al.,1974; Reddy et al.,1978). A partial explanation is that the Finnish people take in higher levels of dietary fiber in the form of whole wheat or rye breads or cereals which contain much bran. A high fiber content in the diet has been thought to have an inhibitory effect, through an increase in stool bulk, lowering the effective concentration of bile acids (Burkitt,1980). Subsequent animal studies with specific fibers such as wheat bran have confirmed this inhibiting effect (Watanabe et al.,1979; Weisburger et al.,1980a.

Epidemiologic studies and geographic comparisons show that high fat and low fiber in the diet are involved in colon cancer carcinogenesis. Since specific carcinogens for human colon cancer are unknown at present (see below), dietary recommendations based on the current data base can concentrate on promoters and protective effects. A diet low in fat (20-35% of calories) with a generous intake of dietary fiber in the form of whole grains might be instrumental in reducing the risk of colon cancer. This applies not only to the general public, but even more so to minimize recurrences in patients with polyps, or successfully treated early colon cancer such as Duke's type A.

MUTAGENS AND MODE OF COOKING

The genotoxic carcinogens responsible for nonoccupational human cancer in the general public in western countries are not known, except for those found in tobacco smoke (Hammond et al.,1977; Wynder & Hoffmann,1979). This is especially so for nutritionally-linked cancers such as colon, breast, or prostate (Reddy et al.,1980).

An important clue as to the nature of such carcinogens came from the demonstration that charcoal broiling of meat or fish yielded mutagenic activity for Salmonella typhimurium TA-98 (Nagao et al.,1978). Since mutagenic activity is often an indicator of carcinogenic activity, the development of mutagenic activity as a function of mode and temperature of cooking was studied under typical realistic cooking conditions (Spingarn & Weisburger,1979). Ground meat, placed in a preheated frying pan has initial browning occurring at 100°C when water boils off and where virtually no mutagenic activity is seen. Subsequently, the temperature rises and sizable mutagenic activity develops and is present in edible

fried meat. Broiling in an electric oven also yields mutagenic activity. Frying meat together with soy protein flour
yielded less mutagenic activity (this Institute, unpublished
data).

One of the products from the pyrolysis of trytophan was a
gamma-carboline derivative, an ortho-methylarylamine type of
compound which so far has been shown to induce liver tumors
and subcutaneous tumors in rats (Kawachi et al.,1979).

Recently, we separated the major mutagenic component of
fried beef into 2 fractions, distinct from any of the known
mutagens from amino acids or protein pyrolysates (Spingarn
et al.,1980). The mutagens from fried fish were more numerous, and included small amounts of compounds such as the
amino acid pyrolysates. However, the main components were
also different (Sugimura et al.1977). One of the main components in fried sardines is identical to one of the mutagens
in beef (Kasai et al.,1980). Its tentative structure,
2-amino-3-methylimidazo[4,5-d]quinoline is similar sterically
and structurally to known homocyclic carcinogenic arylamines,
such as 3,2'-dimethyl-4-aminobiphenyl, which are colon and
mammary gland carcinogens in rodents (Bralow & Weisburger,
1978). The structure of the mutagens to be outlined may not
stem directly from the pyrolysis of amino acids or peptides
but from the formation of heterocyclic compounds from car-
bohydrate components and amino acids.

A model system for browning developed to test this hypothesis showed that reacting sugars with ammonium ion under re-
flux conditions results in the formation of strong mutagenic
activity with similar mobilities on high pressure chromatography systems as those seen in fried meat. These reactions which produce many pyrazine derivatives, are base-cata-
lyzed and can be inhibited by the antioxidant propyl gallate
(Spingarn & Garvie,1979). Thus, the reactions leading to
mutagens during frying may be akin to those that take place
during the browning reactions.

Whether this mutagenic activity is relevant to human disease is the subject of active current research. It is expected that use of this model system may screen compounds to
be used as inhibitors. As noted, the antioxidant propyl
gallate was an effective inhibitor. Soy protein lowered
mutagen formation during frying of meat, and thus may provide
another practical way of reducing mutagen formation which may
be associated with disease risk, a subject of further research.

ANTIOXIDANTS AND INHIBITION OF CARCINOGENESIS

Disulfiram

The late F. Krüger, D. Schmahl, and colleagues noted that
disulfiram (DSF) inhibited the toxicity of dimethylnitroso-
amine (Schmahl & Kruger,1972). An extension led to a study
of possible means of chemoprevention of large bowel neoplasia
caused by exposure to chemical carcinogens. Wattenberg
(1978) found that DSF inhibited 1,2-dimethylhydrazine (DMH)-
induced neoplasia of the large bowel in female CF_1 mice, and
suppressed mammary tumor formation induced by polycyclic hydrocarbons in rats. When DSF was fed concomitantly with a
liver carcinogen, the azo dye 3'-methyl-4-dimethylaminoazo-
benzene (3'-Me-DAB), DSF prevented tumor development
(Fiala,S. et al.,1980).

DSF and other like compounds which act as inhibitors contain a structural carbon disulfide (CS_2) moiety, and a study
of the in vivo metabolism of DMH showed that the CS_2 group
(and CS_2 itself) inhibited a key steps in the metabolic activation of DMH, namely,the N-oxidation of azomethane to azoxymethane and the C-oxidation of azoxymethane to methylazoxymethanol (Fiala, 1979; Wattenberg & Fiala, 1978). This observation provides a useful tool to study the mechanisms of
chemical carcinogenesis whereby inhibition of large bowel
neoplasia might occur. Although knowledge of the mechanism of
action of these inhibitors is at present meager in relation
to the operation of the potential human colon carcinogens,
further research in this area may be of future benefit in the
human situation where such agents might be used to modify
chemically-induced human cancer through chemoprevention.

Butylated Hydroxytoluene(BHT)/Butylated Hydroxyanisole(BHA)

Wattenberg (1978) has reviewed studies in which chemically
induced cancer at several distinct target organs, utilizing
several different carcinogens was inhibited by the antioxidant butylated hydroxytoluene (BHT) and butylated hydroxyanisole (BHA). In most of these studies, based on the original
research of Wattenberg, relatively high dietary levels of antioxidant were utilized, of the order of 0.1-0.75%. Under
these conditions, several studies have demonstrated that one
mechanism whereby carcinogenesis is reduced is through increases in the mixed function oxidases and especially in the
enzymes which conjugate chemicals and drugs with suitable
substituents such as glucuronyl transferase (Daoud & Grif-

fin,1980; Grantham et al.,1973; Irving,1979). Eventually, this results in increased production of detoxified metabolites, especially glucuronides which can be excreted readily. Under these conditions, lowered binding of labelled carcinogen to cellular macromolecules is found, actually reflecting a decreased availability of electrophilic genotoxic metabolites. It is not yet known whether lower levels of antioxidants, mimicking those used in the human diet, would still be effective in the chemoprevention of cancer through mechanisms delineated above, or other modalities associated with the antioxidant function such as trapping of reactive intermediates or even receptor competition.

Selenium and Vitamin E

Selenium in excess can be toxic, especially to the liver. In trace amounts, it is an essential micronutrient. Several epidemiological studies suggest that selenium may have anti-carcinogenic properties since they indicate an increased incidence of several cancers in geographic regions where selenium is deficient (Griffin,1979; Jacobs,1979; Schrauzer,-1979). An association was noted between the amount of selenium in soil and forage crops and cancer mortality rates in the United States and Canada, as well as an inverse relationship between blood selenium levels and the cancer mortality rate. More recently, it was found that selenium intake varied inversely with breast and colon cancer incidence in a wide variety of countries. There have been no epidemiological studies correlating vitamin E consumption and cancer incidence rates, and there is no direct evidence that vitamin E could function as an anticancer agent. However, selenium salts and vitamin E act together as antioxidants. In animals, selenium supplements decreased the incidence of chemically induced mammary and colon tumors (Jacobs et al.,1977). The inhibitory capacity of selenium, and possibly vitamin E, in carcinogenesis has not been studied systematically and mechanistically. Liver carcinogenesis was inhibited because of a decreased formation of electrophilic metabolites from procarcinogens (Daoud & Griffin,1980; Griffin,1980).

Effect of Pyrazole and Similar Compounds

The metabolism of genotoxic carcinogens like alkylnitrosamines and compounds derived from 1,2-dimethylhydrazine eventually involve an intermediate product, the hydroxymethyl derivative. For example, with the prototype dimethylnitros-

amine, Magee (1980), as well as Druckrey (1975), postulated
many years ago an intermediate product of a highly unstable
hydroxymethyl nitrosamine. This would spontaneously release
a methyl carbonium ion as the active product of an alkyl diazonium hydroxide as intermediate. In recent years, several
groups have indeed demonstrated that this original postulate
is true by the synthesis and bioassay of a stable form of the
hydroxymethyl derivative, the acetoxy compound (Frank et al.,
1980; Kleihues et al.,1979; Roller,1975; Weisburger & Williams,1981). Likewise with 1,2-dimethylhydrazine, a key metabolic intermediate is methylazoxymethanol, produced also by
bacterial enzyme-mediated hydrolysis of the plant glycoside,
cyasin, which is methylazoxymethanol-beta-glucoside. For
some years it was thought that this particular metabolite,
methylazoxymethanol, was carcincogenic to the colon because
it, like the hydroxymethyl derivative of dimethylnitrosamine,
yielded a reactive methyl carbonium ion spontaneously. However, this spontaneous decomposition did not seem to account
for the localization of tumors in the small and large bowel,
as well as in several other specific target organs. Inasmuch
as the hydroxymethyl derivative is an alcohol, it was suggested by Schoental (1973), and subsequently demonstrated by
Zedek (Grab & Zedek,1977; Zedek & Tan,1978) and Fiala et al.,
1978 that alcohol dehydrogenase may be involved in the metabolic activation of methylazoxymethanol. One essential element in this demonstration is that an inhibitor of alcohol
dehydrogenase, namely pyrazole, inhibits carcinogenesis in
the intestinal tract. Of collateral interest is the fact
that the synthetic hydroxymethylnitrosamine can also induce
tumors in the intestinal tract, whereas the parent dimethylnitrosamine does not seem to be able to do so. Alcohol dehydrogenase is actually a complex of a number of different isozymes. We have preliminary data that the intestinal localization of alcohol dehydrogenase may involve predominantly one
of these isozymes.

CONCLUSIONS AND PROSPECTS

Current concepts suggest that nutrition and specific nutritional components, as well as dietary habits, in various
parts of the world may play an important role in the causation and development of a number of important cancer types.
It has been calculated that nutrition may impact directly on
30-40% of cancers in men and 50-60% of cancers in women in
the Western World. Because of the rapid westernization of
nutritional customs in Japan, there have been parallel alterations in the incidence of cancers due to this change. These

facts are excellent evidence for the rationale presented in this paper, namely that the mode of cooking and the level of dietary fat and fiber are associated with the occurrence of cancer of the colon, breast, and perhaps of the prostate and pancreas. It is hoped that, as further evidence accumulates from studies in man, through metabolic epidemiology, and in experimental systems, a convincing case can be made for relatively minor alterations in dietary habits, involving mainly a somewhat lower fat intake and a higher fiber consumption. If current research does document further that the mode of cooking, especially frying and broiling, does yield carcinogens for these kinds of cancers, it is hoped that this particular approach would demonstrate ways and means of preventing their formation which would eventually yield a lower risk. Along these lines, research on optimal levels of vitamins, minerals, antioxidants, and other micronutrients in the current diet would provide a broad basis for chemoprevention. Over the last several years, research has provided new perspectives on the causes and modifiers of the main premature killing diseases. Data in the current paper specifically record experimentation designed to yield understanding of underlying mechanisms as a sound reliable basis for prevention of many important kinds of human cancer and for the long-term goals of disease prevention.

TABLE 3.

Long Term Goals for Chronic Disease Prevention	
Action	Preventive Benefit
Stop or control smoking - less harmful cigarette	Coronary heart disease, Cancers of the lung, kidney, pancreas, bladder
Lower total fat intake	Coronary heart disease, cancers: colon, breast, prostate, ovary, endometrium
Lower salt (Na^+) intake balance K^+/Na^+ ratio	Hypertension, cardiovascular disease, stroke
Increase natural fiber	Colon cancer, possibly breast & prostate cancers*
Increase and balance micronutrients, vitamins, minerals	Stomach cancer, possibly heart disease and several other types of cancer*
Lower intake of fried foods	Possibly colon, breast and prostate cancer*

* These disease are under investigation with respect to establishing action-effect relationships.

REFERENCES

Bjelke E: Epidemiologic studies of cancer of the stomach, colon and rectum with special emphasis on the role of diet. Scand J Gastroenterol (Suppl 32) 9:1-235,1974.

Bralow SP, Weisburger JH: Experimental carcinogenesis in the digestive organs. Clin Gastroenterol 5:527-43,1978.

Burkitt DP: Fiber in the etiology of colorectal cancer, in Winawer SJ, Schottenfeld D, Sherlock P (eds.): Colorectal Cancer: Prevention, Epidemiology, and Screening. New York, Raven, 1980, pp 13-18

Carroll KK, Khor HT: Dietary fat in relation to tumorigenesis. Progr Biochem Pharmacol 10:308-53, 1975.

Daoud AH, Griffin AC: Effect of retinoic acid butylated hydroxytoluene, selenium and sorbic acid on azo-dye hepatocarcinogenesis. Cancer Lett 9:299-304,1980

Doll R: Strategy for detection of cancer hazards to man. Nature 265:589-96,1977

Druckrey H: Chemical carcinogenesis on N-nitroso derivatives. GANN Monograph 17:107-132,1975

Fiala ES: Inhibition of carcinogen metabolism and action by disulfiram, pyrazole and related compounds, in Zedek MS, Lipkin M (eds.): Inhibition of Tumor Induction and Development. New York, Plenum, 1981, in press

Fiala ES, Kulakis C, Christiansen G, Weisburger JH: Inhibition of the metabolism of the colon carcinogen, azoxymethane, by pyrazole. Cancer Res. 38:4515-21,1978

Fiala S, Trout EC, Ostrander H, Fiala AE: γ-glutamyltransferase and the inhibition of azo dye-produced neoplasia by concomitant administration of disulfiram. J Natl Cancer Inst 64:267-271,1980

Frank N, Janzowski C, Wiessler M: Stability of nitrosoacetoxymethylmethylamine in in vitro systems and in vivo and its excretion by the rat organism. Biochem Pharmacol 29:383-87,1980

Fraumeni JF,Jr (ed.): Persons at High Risk of Cancer. New York, Academic, 1975, pp 1-544

Freis ED: Salt volume and the prevention of hypertension. Circulation 53:589,1976

Grab DJ, Zedeck MS: Organ-specific effects of the carcinogen methylazoxymethanol related to metabolism by nicotinamide adenine dinucleotide-dependent dehydrogenases. Cancer Res. 37:4182,1977

Grantham PH, Weisburger JH, Weisburger EK: Effect of the antioxidant butylated hydroxytoluene (BHT) on the metabolism of the carcinogens, N-2-fluorenylacetamide and

N-hydroxy-N-2-fluorenylacetamide.   Fd   Cosmet   Toxicol
11:209-217,1973
Griffin AC: Role of selenium in the chemoprevention of can-
cer. Adv Cancer Res 29:419-442,1979
Griffin AC: In vivo intervention of chemical carcinogenesis.
Cancer Bullet 32:143-46,1980
Haenszel W, Kurihara M, Segi M, Lee RK: Stomach cancer among
Japanese in Hawaii. J Natl Cancer Inst 49:969-88,1972
Haenszel W, Kurihara M, Locke FB et al.:   Stomach cancer in
Japan. J Natl Cancer Inst 56:265-74,1976
Hammond EC, Garfinkel L, Seidman H, Lew EA: Some recent
findings concerning cigarette smoking, in Hiatt HH, Watson
JD, Winsten JA (eds.):   Origins of Human Cancer.   Cold
Spring Harbor, N.Y., Cold Spring Harbor Lab., 1977, pp
101-114
Higginson J, Muir CS: The role of epidemiology in elucidat-
ing the importance of environmental factors in human
cancer. Cancer Detect Prev 1:79-105,1976
Higginson J, Muir CS: Epidemiology of Cancer, in Holland JF,
Frei E (eds.):   Cancer Medicine.   Phila., Lea & Febiger,
1979, pp 241-306
Hirayama T: Diet and Cancer.   Nutrit Cancer 1:67-81,1979
IARC Intestinal Microecology Group: Dietary fiber, transit
time, fecal bacteria, and steroids in two Scandinavian
populations. Lancet ii:207-211,1977
Irving CC: Conjugates of N-hydroxy compounds, in Fishman WH
(ed):   Metabolic Conjugation and Metabolic Hydrolysis,
Vol. I. New York, Academic, 1970, pp 53-119
Irving CC, Tice AJ, Murphy WM: Inhibition of N-n-butyl-N-
(4-hydroxybutyl)nitrosamine-induced urinary bladder cancer
in rats by administration of disulfiram in the diet.
Cancer Res 39:3040-43, 1979
Jacobs MM: Effects of selenium on chemical carcinogenesis.
Comparative effects of antioxidants. Biolog Trace Elements
Res 1:1-13, 1979
Jacobs MM, Janssen B, Griffin AC: Inhibitory effects of sel-
enium on 1,2-dimethylhydrazine and methylazoxymethanol
acetate induction of colon tumors. Cancer Lett 2:133-138,
1977
Jensen OM, Mosbech J, Salaspuro M, Jhamaki T: A comparative
study of the diagnostic basis for cancer of the colon and
cancer of the rectum in Denmark and Finland.   Int J
Epidemiol 3:183-86, 1974
Joossens JV, Kesteloot H, Amery H: Salt intake and mortality
from stroke. New Engl J Med 300:1396, 1979

Kasai H, Yamaizumi Z, Wakabayashi K et al.: Potent novel
    mutagens produced by broiling fish under normal condi-
    tions. Proc Japan Acad 56:278-84, 1980
Kawachi T, Nagao M, Yahagi T et al.: Mutagens and carcino-
    gens in food, in Proc 12th Int Cancer Congress, New York,
    Plenum, 1979
Kleihues P, Doerjer G, Keefer, L et al.: Correlation of DNA
    methylation by methyl (acetoxymethyl)nitrosamine with
    organ-specific carcinogenicity in rats. Cancer Res 39:
    5136-40, 1979
Magee P: Metabolism of nitrosamines: an overview, in Coon
    MJ, Conney AH, Estabrook RW et al. (eds): Microsomes, Drug
    Oxidations and Chemical Carcinogenesis, Vol. I. New York,
    Academic, 1980, pp 1087-92
Marquardt H, Rufino F, Weisburger JH: On the aetiology of
    gastric cancer: Mutagenicity of food extracts after incub-
    ation with nitrite. Fd Cosmet Toxicol 15:97-100, 1977
Meneely GR, Battarbee HD: High sodium-low potassium environ-
    ment and hypertension. Am J Cardiol 38:768-81, 1976
Miller JA, Miller EC: Perspectives on the metabolism of
    chemical carcinogens, in Emmelot P, Kriek E (eds): Envi-
    ronmental Carcinogenesis: Occurrence, Risk Evaluation and
    Mechanisms. Amsterdam, Elsevier/No. Holland, 1979, pp
    25-50
Mirvish SS: N-nitroso compounds: Their chemical and in vivo
    formation and possible importance as environmental carcino-
    gens. J Toxicol Environ Health 2:1267-77, 1977
Mower HF, Ray RM, Shoff R et al: Fecal bile acids in two
    Japanese populations with different colon cancer risks.
    Cancer Res 39:328-31, 1979
Nagao M, Honda M, Seino Y et al.: Mutagenicities of smoke
    condensates and the charred surface of fish and meat.
    Cancer Lett 2:221, 1977
Oiso, T: Incidence of stomach cancer and its relation to
    dietary habits and nutrition in Japan between 1900 and
    1975. Cancer Res 35:3254-58, 1975
Reddy BS, Hedges AR, Laakso K, Wynder EL: Metabolic epide-
    miology of large bowel cancer: Fecal bulk and constituents
    of high-risk North American and low-risk Finnish popula-
    tion. Cancer 42:2832-38, 1978
Reddy BS, Cohen LA, McCoy GD et al.: Nutrition and its rela-
    shionship to cancer. Adv Cancer Res 32:237-345, 1980
Roller PP, Shimp DR, Keefer LK: Synthesis and solvolysis of
    methyl(acetoxymethyl)nitrosamine. Solution chemistry of
    the presumed carcinogenic metabolite of dimethylnitros-
    amine. Tetrahedron Letters 2964-68, 1975

Schmahl D, Kruger F: Influence of disulfiram (tetraethyl-thiuramdisulfide) on the biological actions of N-nitrosamines, in Nakahara W, Takayama S, Sugimura T, Odashima S (eds): Topics in Chemical Carcinogenesis, Tokyo, Univ. of Tokyo Press, 1972, pp 199-212
Schoental R: The mechanisms of action of the carcinogenic nitroso and related compounds. Brit J Cancer 28:436-49,1973
Schrauzer GM: Trace elements, nutrition and cancer: Perspectives of prevention. Adv Exp Med Biol 91:323-44,1979
Searle CE (ed): Chemical Carcinogenesis, ACS Monograph 73. Wash., D.C., American Chemical Society, 1976
Slaga TJ, Klein-Szanto A, Fischer SM et al.: Studies on mechanism of action of anti-tumor-promoting agents: Their specificity in two-stage promotion. Proc Natl Acad Sci USA 77:2251-54, 1980
Spingarn NE, Garvie CT: Formation of mutagens in sugar-ammonia model systems. J Agric Food Chem 27:1319-21, 1979
Spingarn NE, Weisburger JH: Formation of mutagens in cooked food. I.Beef. Cancer Lett 7:259-64, 1979
Spingarn NE, Kasai H, Vuolo L et al.: Formation of mutagens in cooked foods. III. Isolation of a potent mutagen from beef. Cancer Lett 9:177-83, 1980
Stemmermann GN: Gastric cancer in the Hawaii Japanese. GANN 68:525-35, 1977
Sugimura T, Kawachi T, Nagao M et al.: Mutagenic principle(s) in tryptophan and phenylalanine pyrolysis products. Proc Japan Acad Sci 53:58-61, 1977
Sugimura T, Kawachi T: Experimental stomach carcinogenesis, in Lipkin M, Good R (eds): Gastro-intestinal Tract Cancer, New York, Plenum, 1978, pp 327-42
Tannenbaum SR, Weisman N, Fett D: The effect of nitrate intake on nitrite formation in human saliva. Fd Cosmet Toxicol 14:459-552, 1976
Tannenbaum SR, Moran D, Rand W et al: Gastric cancer in Colombia. IV. Nitrate and other ions in gastric contents of residents from a high-risk region. J Natl Cancer Inst 62:9-12, 1979
Tatematsu M, Takashashi M, Fukishima S et al.: Effects in rats of sodium chloride on experimental gastric cancers induced by N-methyl-N'-nitrosoguanidine or 4-nitroquinoline-1-oxide. J Natl Cancer Inst 55:101-4, 1975
Tobian L: Salt and hypertension. Ann NY Acad Sci 304:178, 1978
Trowell HC: Hypertension and salt. Lancet II:204, 1978
Watanabe K, Narisawa T, Wong CG, Weisburger JH: Effect of bile acids and neutral sterols on benzo(a)pyrene-induced

tumorigenesis in skin of mice. J Natl Cancer Inst 60: 1501-3, 1978

Watanabe K, Reddy BS, Weisburger JH, Kritchevsky: Effect of dietary alfalfa, pectin, and wheat bran on azoxymethane- or methylnitrosourea-induced colon carcinogenesis in F344 rats. J Natl Cancer Inst 63:141-45, 1979

Wattenberg LW: Inhibitors of chemical carcinogenesis. Adv Cancer Res 26:197-226, 1978

Wattenberg LW, Fiala ES: Inhibition of 1,2-dimethylhydrazine induced neoplasia of the large intestine in female CF_1 mice by carbon disulfide. J Natl Cancer Inst 60:1515-17, 1978

Weisburger JH, Raineri R: Dietary factors and the etiology of gastric cancer. Cancer Res 35:3469-74, 1975

Weisburger JH, Cohen LA, Wynder EL: On the etiology and metabolic epidemiology of the main human cancers, in Hiatt HH, Watson JD, Winsten JA (eds): Origins of Human Cancer. Cold Spring Harbor, NY, Cold Spring Harbor Labs., 1977, pp 567-602

Weisburger JH, Reddy BS, Spingarn NE, Wynder EL: Current views on the mechanisms involved in the etiology of colorectal cancer, in Winawer SG, Schottenfeld D, Sherlock P (eds): Colorectal Cancer: Prevention, Epidemiology, and Screening. Raven, New York, 1980a, pp 19-41

Weisburger JH, Marquardt H, Hirota N et al.: Induction of cancer of the glandular stomach in rats by an extract of nitrite-treated fish. J Natl Cancer Inst 64:163-167,1980b

Weisburger JH, Williams GM: Chemical carcinogenesis, in Doull J, Klaasen C, Amdur M (eds): Toxicology: The Basic Science of Poisons, 2nd ed. New York, Macmillan, 1980, pp 84-138

Weisburger JH, Williams GM: Chemical carcinogenesis, in Holland JF, Frei E (eds): Cancer Medicine, 2nd ed. Phila., Lea & Febiger, 1981a, in press

Weisburger JH, Williams GM: Metabolism of chemical carcinogens, in Becker FF (ed): Cancer: A Comprehensive Treatise, 2nd ed. New York, Plenum, 1981b, in press

Williams GM, Weisburger JH: Systematic carcinogen testing through the decision point approach. Ann Rev Pharmacol Toxicol 21: in press, 1981

Wynder EL, Gori GB: Contribution of the environment to cancer incidence: An epidemiological exercise. J Natl Cancer Inst 58:825-32, 1977

Wynder EL, Hirayama T: Comparative epidemiology of cancers of the United States and Japan. Prev Med 6:567-94, 1977

Wynder EL, Hoffmann D: Tobacco and Health: A societal challenge. New Engl J Med 300:894-903, 1979

Zaldivar R, Wetterstrand WH: Nitrate nitrogen levels in drinking water of urban areas with high and low risk populations from stomach cancer: An environmental epidemiology study. Z Krebsforsch 92:227-34, 1978

Zedek MS, Tan QH: Effect of pyrazole on tumor induction by methylazoxymethanol (MAM) acetate: Relationship to metabolism of MAM. The Pharmacologist 20:174, 1978

I am indebted to Ms. Clara Horn for her dedicated assistance in the writing of this report and preparation of the manuscript.

Advances in Diagnosis

Localized Disease -
The Cure Within Our Grasp

DANIEL G. MILLER, M.D.

Director
Preventive Medicine Institute-
Strang Clinic
New York, New York

The last ten years have seen great strides with regard to the
diagnosis of localized cancer, both conceptually and in practice. Each step brings us closer to the goal on the horizon
- the diagnosis of cancer at an early and curable stage.

There is room for optimism about the role early detection
can play in reducing cancer morbidity and mortality. Both
the promise and the problem are set forth in Figure 1. This
is a tabular representation of end results of treatment in
relation to stage of disease prepared by the Biometry Section
of the National Cancer Institute. Twelve forms of cancer are
shown. These represent 65% of cancer incidence and 85% of
cancer mortality. The results are given in terms of 15-20
year survival rates for localized cancer and disease with
regional spread. Since most unsuccessfully treated cancers
are fatal by ten years from the time of diagnosis, the use of
this long time period largely overcomes the objection that
survival rates as a result of earlier detection may appear
longer but do not change the progression of the disease and
may not reduce mortality rates.

What we see is that for these twelve diseases the survival
rates for patients with localized disease in every case is
80% or greater than that of patients with non-localized
disease. The problem associated with this data is the small
percentage of patients in whom cancer was diagnosed in a
localized stage. Furthermore, if we examine trends in the
detection of localized disease (Table 1) we see that only for
breast, bladder and prostate cancer has there been consistent
improvement, while for cervix and oropharynx cancer, detection of localized disease has actually diminished. The term
"localized disease" has inherent problems. Localized disease
which is in situ will have a different prognosis from localized disease which is invasive. We have no assurance that

615

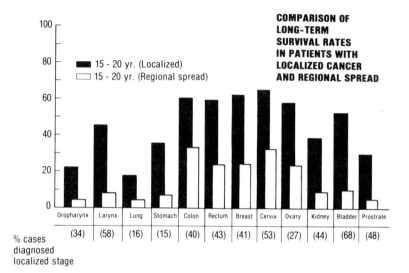

Figure 1

the staging of cancer carried out by the reporting institutions was uniform. The size of the localized tumor, a factor
related to survival, is not included in the reported data;
neither is the pathological grading, another factor related
to malignancy. In addition, our means of estimating microscopic metastases are inadequate, e.g. witness a cumulative
case fatality of 35% or more for all patients with localized
disease. Since the evidence points to cancer as a disease of

TABLE 1

Trends in Diagnosis of Localized Cancer

	1950-54	1955-59	1960-64	1965-69	1970-73
Breast	41	44	47	47	48
Cervix	53	54	54	46	45
Ovary	27	28	29	29	25
Kidney	44	44	48	47	45
Bladder	68	71	80	81	82
Prostate	48	54	61	63	61
Oropharynx	34	32	30	23	20
Larynx	58	59	64	65	62
Lung	16	18	20	18	17
Stomach	15	19	19	19	18
Colon	40	39	42	42	41
Rectum	43	46	47	47	47

monoclonal origin, detection early enough should regularly be associated with cure.[4] However, studies in head and neck cancer and breast cancer have shown that some patients with short duration of symptoms and apparently localized disease have very aggressive cancers, and they have a good chance of passing through the net of early detection examinations.[5,7]

It should also be pointed out that these results were gathered without any special effort at early detection. They represent the experience from conventional medical practice in this country; that is, in most cases the patients initiated medical contact as a result of symptoms or the cancer was a fortuitous finding as a result of an examination for another reason. These results were not the consequence of any deliberate effort at early detection.

However, if we look at deliberate efforts at early detection for the three most common forms of cancer we see that these results may be greatly improved (Table 2).

In the Early Lung Cancer Detection Program which has been conducted by Memorial Sloan-Kettering Cancer Center since 1974, 169 men have been diagnosed with lung cancer out of 10,040 asymptomatic male smokers examined with chest x-rays annually. About one-half of this group had sputum cytology as well. Out of this group of 169 men, 63 or 37% were diagnosed in a localized stage, and only two have died of lung cancer. The statistical estimate of five year survival for these patients with localized disease is over 90%.[2]

In the Breast Cancer Demonstration Project, of 2,500 cancers detected, 70% were in a localized stage; 37% were clinically occult and less than 1 centimeter in size. Studies have shown that the smaller the size of the breast cancer detected, the better the prognosis.[13]

In the colon cancer detection program carried out at Strang Clinic, under the direction of the Department of Gastroenterology of Memorial Hospital, approximately 80% of the colon cancers detected in asymptomatic individuals were localized.[15] Only prolonged observation will determine how many of these patients found with localized disease and

TABLE 2

Comparison of Diagnosis of Localized Cancer in Early Detection Programs and Conventional Experience

	Early Detection	Conventional	Percent Increase
Lung	37%	17%	117%
Breast	70%	48%	45%
Colon	80%	41%	95%

optimally treated will have cures; but the results should
greatly exceed those reported in the NCI end results study.
The point of the above statements is the clearcut demonstration that when a concerted effort is made to find early
cancer, it can be done.

Significant advances have been made in early diagnosis in
terms of technical progress. It is of interest that three of
the most commonly used means of diagnosis, chest x-ray for
lung cancer, Hemoccult slide testing for colon cancer and
mammography for breast cancer represent techniques that were
first used over forty years ago, then downgraded as being of
little value, and are now being used again with success as a
result of the reapplication under conditions which provide
improved results. A new technique which has emerged over the
last ten years has been fiberoptic colonoscopy and broncho-
scopy, which has had an important effect on the early detection of colon and lung cancer. These techniques plus advances in imaging, cytology and immunology will be discussed
in the symposium on advances in diagnosis.

However, after all the technical facilities have been
mobilized into optimal configurations, there will still remain the problem of getting the patient in for medical care
at a time when disease is localized. This requires special
strategies. Screening is one of them.

Screening is a prediagnostic procedure which has as its
endpoint the determination of the probability of the presence
of a disease. In contrast, diagnosis has as its endpoint not
only the determination of whether a disease is present or
not, but the clear delineation of the extent of disease and
the characterization of the disease by pathologic classification. The logic behind screening also differs from that
of diagnosis. In screening one starts with the diagnosis,
defines by deduction the salient features of the disease,
and a determination is made whether or not these features
are present in the individual patient. In the diagnostic
procedure all disease characteristics in a patient are determined and from these the diagnosis is induced. Since staging
is a part of the diagnostic process, a detailed patient
examination is necessary which justifies elaborate diagnostic
procedures since treatment and prognosis will often depend on
the outcome of these procedures. However, in screening
elaborate procedures, those which are expensive and carry a
risk for the patient, may not be justified since the process
of screening involves a population which may be at risk, but
in which most of the patients examined will be asymptomatic
and disease-free. Screening and diagnosis are complimentary
measures in the effort to find cancer in a localized stage.

Screening is one link in the chain of cancer control which extends from prevention to screening to diagnosis, treatment and rehabilitation. A corollary of this is that screening should be part of a total health care delivery system. It should never exist in isolation from that system.

Just as there have been important advances in instrumentation, there have been conceptual advances in early detection. Thomas McKeown of the University of Bristol introduced the concept of primary and prescriptive screening for early diagnosis.[11] Primary screening is simple, risk-free, low-cost, and usually carried out by allied health personnel. Prescriptive, or selective, screening is carried out as a result of risk factors determined by primary screening; it is the beginning of the diagnostic process and may involve invasive procedures such as colonoscopy or other instrumentation. However, since the procedures are used selectively and on indication, there is greater efficiency in detection and the cost effectiveness is increased.

The risk factor approach to screening was systematically formulated by Dr. Alton Sutnick, formerly of the Fox Chase Cancer Center, who developed decision logic and risk factor matrices for cancer screening.[14]

Set theory has been applied to risk factor definition by Larouzé and colleagues.[10] Figure 2 shows how laboratory and epidemiologic data may be used to identify a population at risk for hepatocellular carcinoma. This is a model that may be emulated in other forms of cancer as risk factors are further delineated.

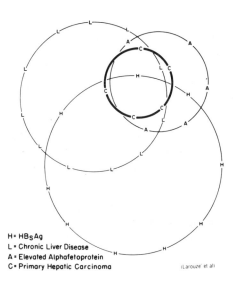

H = HBsAg
L = Chronic Liver Disease
A = Elevated Alphafetoprotein
C = Primary Hepatic Carcinoma

Figure 2   (Larouze' et al)

However, there is an important limitation in the risk
factor approach. This may be exemplified by epidemiologic
considerations in breast cancer. It is possible to identify
3% of the female population with risk factors which causes
this subset to have about 10% of all breast cancer and this
group deserves special attention. But 90% of all cases of
breast cancer will occur in females who do not have as yet
determinable risk factors other than age. Does this mean we
abandon this universe and concentrate exclusively on the high
risk group because it would be most cost effective to do so?
Is cost-effectiveness the only criterion, or is it even the
proper criterion to use in determining the selection of a
test which may be lifesaving? This is one of the problems
in value judgement that comes up repeatedly when one has to
establish policies regarding screening.

Another advance in screening is the developing role of
allied health professionals in conducting these examinations.
The results of screening of 1,000 consecutive female patients
at the Preventive Medicine Institute-Strang Clinic by a
nurse clinician and a physician showed a high degree of concordance in the findings.[12] The nurse clinician had more
positive findings, but there were no significant false negative findings in this trial. It has been our experience
that the well trained nurse clinician is a superb screening
examiner. In addition to screening examinations, nurse
clinicians are now conducting flexible proctosigmoidoscopy
examinations at PMI-Strang.

The occasion of screening for the early detection of
cancer has come to mean more than an examination and the
performance of tests. The importance of using this encounter
for personalized health education should be stressed.
Giving out a pamphlet or showing someone a sign is not
education. If it were, then no one would smoke and everyone
would use seat belts. Education is an individualized process
that results in a change in knowledge, attitude and most
important, a change in practice. The screening encounter
must provide an opportunity with regard to health education
for smoking cessation, breast self-examination, and the
evaluation of environmental hazards. The use of these principles allows for the development of low-cost, non-invasive,
primary screening facilities. Virtually any community would
have the resources to develop such a cancer screening
activity.

Despite the above mentioned advances in instrumentation
and concepts, a significant impact of early detection has
yet to be made. For this one must look to the future. In
this regard three points should be made.

1. Cancer screening is not enough for an optimal early detection and prevention program. One should not separate the delivery of cancer detection services provided periodically from the needs of an individual at any time during the year that cancer suspicious symptoms develop. Cancer detection and prevention must be an all year-round program. The current practice is to recommend cancer detection for asymptomatic individuals only, with the expectation that as soon as symptoms develop patients will apply for medical care. But we know this is not so; there is a vast literature on patient delay in cancer diagnosis. Delay is a universal phenomenon.[6] There is a large difference between a patient having to decide if a chronic symptom is important enough to seek medical care, whom he should consult and when, and a situation in which the patients are told repeatedly through the year which symptoms are important, how they can be seen without inconvenience, without delay and without financial barriers. The all year-round nature of cancer detection and prevention must be stressed. The periodic examination has to be just one part of an ongoing comprehensive program.

There have been a number of studies showing that the screening examination tends to pick up the slow growing tumors, those with a longer detectable asymptomatic stage and a longer duration of symptoms.[5,7] Because of its periodicity, the screening examination may miss the rapidly developing interval cases. Austin and Dunn put it this way:

> It is possible to distinguish between the term "early detection" and the term "screening". Early detection may be considered to be a generalized concept denoting a means of bringing all or most cancers to diagnosis in a curable state. It connotes a continuous state of observation or heightened awareness toward the possibility of a malignancy and hence, in practical terms, a condition of each individual. In contrast, cancer screening is an intermittent, site-specific search for malignancy using technical procedures administered by trained technicians and professionals. Screening is aimed at identifying cancers at a stage prior to that detectable by an acutely aware host, but it is aimed at specific points in time, seldom oftener than annually. Thus, the screening program exerts its effects through repetitive intermittent "snapshots" in time, while early detection may be accomplished through continuous host awareness to early tumor symptoms.

Austin DF, Dunn JE: Cancer symptoms, clinical stage, and survival rates. Am J Pub H 70:5, 474-475, 1980.

2. The periodic screening examination represents fragmentation of medical care unless it is part of a continuum of
medical services. This is particularly true for cancer.
Prevention and early detection must be part of a comprehensive cancer control program. Only in this way will there be
adequate follow-up and end result evaluation, proper statistical and epidemiologic analyses. If there is no uniformity
in diagnosis and treatment, it is virtually impossible to
determine the impact of screening on treatment outcome.
3. An enrolled and motivated population is essential. In
order to make cancer prevention and early detection most
effective, to achieve the cure within our grasp, is going to
require a degree of motivation of the public that has not
been accomplished so far. In the so-called "war against
cancer" we have enlisted everyone except the troops. The
war is being carried out in laboratories and hospitals. In
addition, we need a guerrilla war fought in the streets and
in homes. We need the assistance of social scientists as
well as medical scientists until we have a motivated constit-
uency for early detection and prevention. Until that occurs
the necessary collaborative effort between the public and
the health professions to achieve community-wide cancer control will never take place.

There are important trials going on at present to evaluate
site-specific, early detection programs. We have to know the
best ways to use the tools we have, what their limitations
are, their risks and their benefits. However, when these
programs are completed, they will have to be delivered to the
public in a way that will have an impact on cancer related
morbidity and mortality rates. In this regard there are
three programs which merit attention as potential models or
prototypes for effective cancer prevention and detection
activities. The first is the CANSCREEN Program. This is a
voluntary association of nonprofit clinics, all of which apply the aforementioned principles of low-cost, non-invasive,
primary screening carried out by allied health professionals
with strong emphasis on health education and prevention. All
participating clinics employ the same decision logic, share
a common record-keeping system, and pool data for quality
control and epidemiologic study. There are ten such clinics
operating currently throughout the country, under diverse
auspices such as comprehensive cancer centers, community
hospitals, a health maintenance organization and major cor-
poration and labor unions. These are as follows in Table 3.
The Kaiser-Permanente Foundation's preventive medicine programs, directed at cancer and other diseases is another example.[3] It has been ongoing for sixteen years to members of

TABLE 3

Clinics Participating in The National CANSCREEN Program

Sponsoring Institution	Location
PMI/Strang Clinic - Memorial Sloan-Kettering Cancer Center	New York, N.Y.
Fox Chase Cancer Center	Philadelphia, Pa.
Evanston Hospital	Evanston, Ill.
Marshfield Health Maintenance Organization	Marshfield, Wis.
Northwestern Indiana Cancer Detection Center	Merrillville, Ind.
Daniel Freeman Hospital	Inglewood, Cal.
Samuel Merritt Hospital	Oakland, Cal.
Community Cancer Corporation of Luzerne County	Wilkes-Barre, Pa.
General Motors Corporation - UAW Cancer Detection Program	Detroit, Mich.

a health maintenance organization. Participating and control populations have been evaluated for the impact on postponable deaths. There has been a statistically significant improvement in the overall mortality rate in the preventive medicine group, and specifically a statistically significant improvement in colorectal cancer mortality. The ability to carry out this program demonstrates the advantages of a pre-paid enrolled population with regard to education, motivation and communication for the purposes of preventive medicine.

There is an additional example that is worthy of study. It occurs in another society, another culture, under vastly different circumstances. Much of it is not transferrable to the United States. Nevertheless, there are lessons to be learned. This is a program funded by the U.S. Agency for International Development in Southeast Asia. It is called the Lampang Health Development Project and serves 600,000 people in rural Thailand.[8,9] It has won international acclaim for the innovations it has made in health care delivery.

The Lampang Health Development Project starts on the village level--no doctors, no nurses, no clinics. The first step in implementing this program has been to develop cadres of voluntary community health workers. The interface between the population and the health care system is carried out by a group of health communicators, one for each ten families, to provide a network of advice, referral services and health information to every household for which they are responsible.

Each village also has a village health volunteer who is
trained to provide personalized health education, advise on
the use of non-prescriptive drugs, provide first aid and
facilitate proper referral of patients with problems identified by the volunteer health communicators. This diminishes
delay in seeking medical care and provides preventive services according to individual needs. The next level of
health care is carried out at a subdistrict health center
staffed by trained physician's assistants carrying out functions which independent nurse practitioners do in this country and barefoot doctors carry out in China. They are
trained in midwifery, certain categories of curative medicine, family planning and preventive medicine. Patients are
referred from the subdistrict health center to the district
hospital. This is a dispensary and infirmary staffed by a
physician with the assistance of allied health professionals.
Patients requiring major surgery or specialized care are sent
to the provincial hospital. Further referral for highly
specialized services such as radiation therapy and chemotherapy would be to university hospitals.

    While it should be emphasized that much of this system is
not transferrable to other societies, it is also not difficult to visualize the benefits that such an organized health
care system would bring to cancer control. An integrated
approach to prevention, early diagnosis and treatment, based
on the Lampang model is shown in Figure 3. Health communicators and community health volunteers could provide person-

AN INTEGRATED APPROACH TO PREVENTION, EARLY DIAGNOSIS, AND TREATMENT

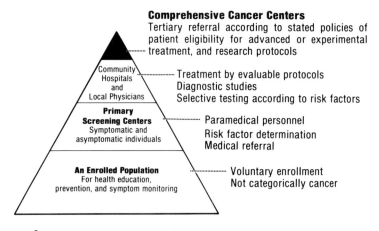

Figure 3

alized health education for smoking cessation, provide classes for breast self-examination and hold these classes at
regular intervals to see that this practice takes hold.
Monitoring for environmental health hazards is easier to
carry out on the community level. Local problems with regard
to the needs of special groups of individuals who are at high
risk by virtue of age, ethnic background, or personal practices can be identified and responded to. Periodic screening
can be carried out by allied health professionals effectively
with appropriate referrals made for positive findings according to appropriately designed clinical algorithms. Once cancer is identified, protocols for extent of disease workup and
staging would be done and treatment carried out according to
protocols designed for end result evaluation. The importance
of such a system for follow-up cannot be overestimated since
the patient will again be returning to his "village equivalent", i.e. community where again the health communicator
could assist in compliance with medical recommendations,
follow-up visits and monitoring the patient's quality of
life, providing needed psychological support on a local
level, and assuring that the patient returns for needed
medical follow-up.

The implication of cooperation between a population anx-
ious to improve its health status, and health professionals,
broadly defined, is worthy of study. The idea of a three
pronged attack on cancer with health education, primary
screening and symptom monitoring in an all year-round program, this is something we can do. This would not require
a great deal of funding, but it would require a great deal of
planning. It could be an effective way of enlisting the concerned segment of a population in the war against cancer, and
avoid the feeling of passivity and fatalism so many people
have about the disease.

Cancer prevention and detection work. The potential for
reducing cancer related morbidity and mortality is real. The
epidemiologic data showing the improved results of treatment
of localized disease provides a challenge that must be translated into action programs. Such programs do not depend on
new discoveries. We have the ability right now to seize this
cure within our grasp.

REFERENCES

1. Austin DF, Dunn JE: Cancer symptoms, clinical stage, and survival rates. Am J Pub H 70:5, 474-475, 1980.
2. Beattie EJ: Memorial Sloan-Kettering Cancer Center Statement Regarding ACS Report on Cancer Related Health Checkups, March 21, 1980.
3. Dales LG, Friedman GD, Collen MF: Evaluating periodic multiphasic health checkups: A controlled trial. J Chron Dis 32:385-404, 1979.
4. Fialkow PJ: Clonal origins of human tumors. Ann Rev Med 30:135-143, 1979.
5. Heuser L, Spratt JS, Polk HC Jr.: Growth rates of primary breast cancers. Cancer 43:1888-1894, 1979.
6. Kalmer H (ed.): Reviews of research and studies related to delay in seeking diagnosis of cancer. Health Ed Mono, Vol. 2, No. 2, 1974.
7. Kaufman S, Grabau JC, Lore JM Jr.: Symptomatology in head and neck cancer: A quantitative review of 385 cases. Am J Pub H 70:5, 520-522, 1980.
8. Lampang Health Development Project - A Thai Primary Health Care Approach. Ministry of Public Health, Royal Thai Government, Thailand. Amarin Press, Bangkok, Thailand, 1978.
9. The Lampang Health Development Project - Thailand's Fresh Approach to Rural Primary Health Care. International Council for Educational Development. Essex, Connecticut, U.S.A., 1979.
10. Larouzé B, Blumberg BS, London WT et al.: Forecasting of the development of primary hepatocellular carcinoma of the use of risk factors: Studies in West Africa. J Natl Cancer Inst 58:1557-1561, 1977.
11. McKeown T, Know EG: The framework required for validation of prescriptive screening, in Screening in Medical Care, Reviewing the Evidence, A Collection of Essays, London, Oxford University Press, 1968, pp 159-173.
12. Miller DG: What is early diagnosis doing? Cancer 37:426-432, 1976.
13. Report of the Working Group to Review the National Cancer Institute - American Cancer Society Breast Cancer Detection Demonstration Projects. September 6, 1977, Office of Cancer Communications, National Institutes of Health, Bethesda, Maryland.
14. Sutnick AI, Miller DG, Samson B, et al.: Population cancer screening. Cancer 38:1367-1372, 1976.
15. Winawer SJ, Andrews M, Flehinger B, et al.: Progress report on controlled trial of fecal occult blood testing for the detection of colorectal neoplasia. Cancer 45:2959-2964, 1980.

Biochemical and Immunologic
Diagnosis of Cancer

MORTON K. SCHWARTZ

Chairman
Department of Biochemistry
Memorial Sloan-Kettering Cancer Center
New York, New York

In many types of cancer there is a better prognosis if
the disease is diagnosed and treated at an early stage.
During the past decade the dramatic rise in the performance
of laboratory tests at Memorial Hospital is in part an
indication of the clinicians need for assistance beyond the
history and physical examination in achieving early diagnosis.
The potential role of biochemical and/or immunochemical tests
in early detection and diagnosis is emphasized by the reality
that about two-thirds of patients who present themselves with
clinical symptoms of cancer already have metastases. The
recent development of newer techniques which permit measurement of nanogram or even femtomole (10^{-15}) concentrations of
proteins and other metabolites has given great hope that
tumor specific (related to a single cancer) or tumor
associated (related to cancer in general) materials might be
discovered which could be measured in biological fluids and
allow early detection and diagnosis of cancer before clinical
symptoms were present and at a time before metastases had
occurred.

The potential role of marker measurement has been
discussed by numerous workers. The ultimate use of these
assays would be in screening and detection of individuals
with cancer as well as those with a high risk to eventually
develop the disease. In addition the marker can assist in
diagnosis and staging of the cancer, be used in predicting
the success of therapy or in following the growth or regression of tumor burden and finally in predicting prognosis
at an early stage of the disease. Any marker assay should be
based on measurement of material released directly from the
tumor or by a reaction of the cancer on the surrounding tissue
which in turn causes a release of the substance into the

circulation. The factors of sensitivity, specificity,
analytical precision and the time and ease of performance as
well as the cost of the test should all be taken into account
in evaluating a tumor marker.

There are a few cancers which are characterized by
snythesis of detectable amounts of tumor specific materials
which are useful as diagnostic and/or prognostic aides.
These include α-fetoprotein(α-FP) in hepatocellular carcinoma,
α-FP and chorionic gonadotropin in germ cell tumors,monoclonal
λ-globulins in myelomas, alkaline phosphatase in osteogenic
sarcoma, vanilmandelic   acid (VMA) and catecholamines in
neuroblastoma and pheochromacytoma.   However markers are not
yet available which are specific for those cancers which in
1980 in the United States will account for more than 60% of
the cancer deaths (lung, 90,500;   colon and rectum, 51,592;
breast, 34,481;   prostate, 20,790;   ovary and uterus, 21,495;
pancreas, 10, 938;   and stomach, 8,688).

The most important points to consider in the evaluation
of a tumor marker is the specificity and sensitivity of the
procedure. By sensitivity is meant the ability of the test
to detect all patients with cancer. Thus a test with 75%
sensitivity will detect 75 of 100 patients with cancer and
demonstrate 25 false negatives. Specificity refers to the
ability of the test to discriminate those individuals who do
not have the disease. A test with 90% specificity will yield
in 100 normal individuals, 10 false positive results. A
specificity of less than 95% creates great difficulty in the
use of the test in screening.   If a test has 95% specificity
and 75% sensitivity (very few tests achieve this capability)
and if a population of 100,000 is screened in which there is
a prevalence of 100 patients with cancer, the following
results will be obtained: seventy five of the 100 cancer
patients will be detected (25% false negative) and in the
remaining 99,900 individuals there will be 4,995 false
positive results. Thus 75 cancers will be detected, but these
will be included in a group of 5,070 persons with positive
results. The frustration, cost and difficulties in
identifying the 2% of the individuals in this group who have
cancer is obvious. It should be kept in mind that this represents a best-case situation and that most tests exhibit
much less than 95% specificity.

I wish to discuss the role of several markers currently
in use in patient evaluation and in screening.

Acid Phosphatase. Serum acid phosphatase has been used
as a cancer marker for 40 years [11] . However, it is now well
documented that the assay of the enzyme by traditional
chemical catalytic methods will indicate the presence of
prostatic cancer in 65 to 90% of patients having bony metastases, but in only 30% of patients without metastases to bone
and only 5 to 10% of men who have early prostatic carcinoma
confined to the gland itself. Since acid phosphatases occur
in many tissues, attempts have been made to improve the sensitivity and specificity by use of "prostate specific" substrates such as β-glycerol phosphate, α-napthyl phosphate and
thymolphalein monophosphate. Although these substrates
apparently eliminate elevations in certain nonspecific
diseases such as Gaucher's disease and breast cancer, they do
not improve the percentage pickup of early cases of prostatic
cancer. The use of specific prostatic acid phosphatase inhibitors such as L-tartrate also has not been successful in
sharpening the diagnostic utility of serum acid phosphatase
assays. As early as 1964 it was reported that antibodies
could be raised to acid phosphatase in prostatic fluid. The
antiserum gave a precipitin reaction with prostatic fluid
acid phosphatase but not with extracts from other tissues or
normal serum. Within the last several years these findings
have extended and a solid phase radioimmunoassay has been
developed for the assay of serum prostatic acid phosphatase
[3] . With this technique all of 50 normal patients had
values less than 6.6 ng/ml. Five of 36 patients (14%) with
benign prostatic hypertrophy (BPH) had values greater than
this as did 14/83 (17%) of patients with non-prostate
cancer and 2/20 (10%) of persons with gastrointestinal disease.
If 8.0 ng/ml was used as the cutoff point (mean + 4 SD), only
2/36 (6%) of BPH patients were elevated as were 9 of 83
patients with other forms of cancer and 1 of 20 patients with
gastrointestinal disorders. When the higher cutoff point was
used in the patients with cancer, elevations were observed in
8/24 (33%) of patients with Stage I disease (tumor not
detectable by rectal examination); in 26/33 (79%) of
patients with Stage II disease (tumor confined within the
prostatic capsule); in 22/31 (71%) of patients with Stage III
disease (tumor locally extended beyond capsule, but no lymph
node involvement or positive bone scan or survey); and in
23/25 (92%) of patients with Stage IV disease (bone metastases
and possible metastases to other organs). According to the
authors, the most promising aspect of the test is the
detection of large numbers of patients with Stage II disease.

In another immunochemical approach a counter immunoelectrophoresis method has been used to measure serum
prostatic acid phosphatase. In preliminary data with this
technique the serum acid phosphatase was not detected in one
patient with Stage A disease (confined to prostate and not
palpable); in 6/30 (25%) of patients with Stage B disease
(confined to capsule but palpable); in 27/49 (55%) of
patients with Stage C disease (local extension of tumor); and
in 98/125 (80%) patients with Stage D disease (distant metastases to bone or soft tissue). The assay could detect
20 ng/ml or more of prostatic acid phosphatase and enzyme was
not detected in any of 19 patients with benign prostatic
hypertrophy or 107 normal individuals. The National Prostatic
Cancer Project is now carrying out a large trial to compare a
radioimmunoassay method with the counter immunoelectrophoresis
technique. Griffiths has also evaluated the RIA method and
has observed elevations in 9% of patients with benign
prostatic disease, 12% of those with Stage I cancer, 32% with
Stage II, 47% with Stage III and 86% with Stage IV. With a
catalytic method only 5% of Stage I and 20% of Stage II were
detected.[6] It has been reported that bone marrow acid phosphatase assays may be helpful in staging and monitoring
patients receiving therapy. Cooper, Foti and Herschman used
the RIA method and concluded that low titer elevations of bone
marrow phosphatase are observed inclinically understaged,
Stage III and may indicate in fact Stage IV disease. In
therapeutically responsive patients both serum and bone
marrow acid phosphatase decrease in activity [2] .

Carcinoembryonic Antigen. Carcinoembryonic antigen (CEA)
is the term applied in 1965 by Gold and Freedman to a protein
found in intestine, liver and pancreas of the fetus during
the first 6 months of gestation and in human cancerous colon,
liver or pancreas   . It was not detected in normal adult
human tissues or tissue from patients with benign disease of
the colon. In 1969 Thompson et al used a radioimmunoassay
able to detect as little as 1 ng of CEA per ml of serum and
reported values greater than 2.5 ng/ml in 35 of 36 patients
with adenocarcinoma of the colon. Values less than this were
found in patients with colon cancer who had their tumor removed surgically, patients with other forms of cancer, and
all normal persons or those with non-malignant diseases. Subsequent studies by other workers have not confirmed these
original observations, and CEA elevations have been observed
in patients with a wide variety of cancers [12] .

The most complete study is a collaborative effort by
Hansen and his associates in which 35,000 samples from more
than 10,000 patients and healthy subjects were analyzed [7] .
Levels less than 2.5 ng/ml were observed in 88.5% of 1,425
healthy subjects and values less than 5.0 ng/ml in 98.7% of
these persons. In 2,107 other healthy subjects in whom a
smoking history was obtained, 865 of 892 nonsmokers, 592 of
720 smokers and 219 of 235 former smokers had levels less than
2.5 ng/ml. Of 576 patients without clinical evidence of
cancer who underwent barium enema examination, 23 were found
to have colon cancer, and of these, CEA values greater than
2.5 ng/ml were detected in 18 and greater than 5.0 ng/ml in
15. Forty-six other patients with positive CEA values had
acute inflammatory disease of the colon or a variety of
metabolic diseases. An important observation was that in a
third of the "false" positive group, normal values were
obtained upon assay of a second sample.

Similar findings have been obtained in our laboratory in
a study of plasma CEA values in 1341 adult patients admitted
to Memorial Hospital or seen in the Out-Patient Clinic over
a three-month period. Non-malignant conditions were found in
467 patients. Elevations were observed in about 20% of these
individuals. Of 74 patients with leukemia, lymphoma, Hodgkins
disease or multiple myeloma, only 14 (26%) had plasma CEA
levels of 5 ng/ml or greater. Similar patterns of elevation
were seen in patients with malignant melanoma, 9/57 (16%) had
sarcoma, 9/48 (19%). In these patients, there was no
correlation between plasma CEA concentrations and the extent
of disease.

In the remaining patients, all of whom had carcinoma, the
percentage of patients with elevated CEA was related to the
extent of disease. Overall, elevations were seen in more than
30% of patients with cancer of the liver or pancreas, colon-
rectum, lung, breast, head and neck, bladder, cervic and
prostate.

CEA is obviously not an organ specific indicator of
cancer, nor can it be as a screening test for early diagnosis.
In colon-rectal cancer and perhaps in breast and lung cancer,
initial values appear to be a good indicator of prognosis.
However, an important use of CEA is serial assays in assessing
the status of patients during therapy. Persistent elevations
may be indicative of therapeutic failure whereas following
successful surgery or chemotherapy the levels will fall toward
normal levels and remain at that level until a recrudescence

of the disease occurs. In a prospective study of 102 patients
who had no clinically detectable disease following colorectal
surgery, CEA levels became elevated in 12 patients. Six of
these developed recurrent cancer 0 to 29 months after the
elevated CEA was detected. The other 6 patients did not
develop a recurrence, and in 2 patients recurrence was
observed despite normal CEA.

We examined the relation of carcinoembryonic antigen
levels to time, site and extent of recurrence in 358 patients
with colorectal cancer. The recurrence rate was higher in
patients with Dukes' B and Dukes' C lesions who had preoperative levels higher than 5 ng per milliliter. There was
a linear inverse correlation between preoperative levels and
estimated mean time to recurrence in patients with Dukes' B
and C lesions, ranging from 30 months for a level of 2 ng/ml
to 9.8 months for a level of 70 ng/ml. In patients with
Dukes' C lesions the median time to recurrence was 13 months
if preoperative levels were higher than 5 ng per milliliter,
and 28 months if they were lower. Preoperative carcinoembryonic antigen levels in patients with resectable Dukes' B
and C cancer provided an additional criterion for assigning
these patients to groups at high or low risk for recurrence
[15] [14].

Chorionic Gonadotropin. In trophoblastic neoplasms, the
quantitative assay of urinary and/or serum chorionic gonadotropin (hCG) is essential for initial diagnosis and then for
following the course of the disease. For many years a bioassay which did not differentiate between human pituitary
leutenizing hormone and gonadotropin from non-pituitary
sources was used. The development by Vaitukaitis and her
associates of a specific radioimmunoassay for the determination of the β-subunit of hCG has permitted its assay without any interference from other hormones [13]. In an
evaluation of the assay in serum of normal individuals, no
hCG was observed in samples from 115 control patients. In
our laboratory, values below 2 ng/ml are considered within
normal limits. Although the assay is primarily useful in
monitoring therapy in trophoblastic tumors, elevations have
been reported in other cancers. Griffing and Vaitukaitis
have found elevations in from 11% of patients with lung cancer
to 35% of patients with pancreas cancer [5]. The role of
ectopically produced hormones as cancer markers will not be
discussed here. In embryonal cell carcinoma of the testes
the serum hCG may dramatically reflect the clinical course of
the patient. In a study by Jones, Lewis and Lehr, serum hCG

levels were monitored in 10 women during chemotherapeutic
treatment of gestational trophoblastic disease. These assay
values in serum were compared to those obtained by a bioassay
of hCG in urine. The authors concluded that tumor activity
can be detected by the β-subunit assay at a time when biologic
activity in the urine (both hCG and leutenizing hormone)
indicate remission. These workers continued chemotherapy on
the basis of the serum hCG assay in patients in whom therapy
would have been discontinued until a re-evaluation in urinary
hCG occurred. In patients treated in this way, remission was
defined as no detectable hCG in the serum. In the patients
in whom remission on this basis was achieved, there has been
no recurrence of tumor in observation periods ranging from 2
to 13 months. [9]

The use of α-FP and β-hCG permits a laboratory classification of germ cell tumors [8]. In adult type embryonal
carcinomas there is an elevation of both α-FP and β-hCG
whereas in endodermal sinus tumors there is only elevation of
α-FP. In choriocarcinoma there is only an elevation of β-hCG
and in seminoma and teratoma usually neither is elevated.

Galactosyl transferase. Bhattacharya measured a UDP-
galactose: glycoprotein galactosyl transferase in serum and
tissue of patients with ovarian cancer [1]. In ovarian
tissue the enzyme level was 3 to 5 times higher than that in
normal tissue in the presence or absence of fetuin. In 10
normal controls the serum activities ranged from 147 to 179
pmoles galactose transferase/10 μl serum/60 min (165 + 10.6)
and did not seem to vary with blood type. Significant
elevations were seen in patients with ovarian cancer. In 11
patients the activity ranged from 227 to 519 pmoles. In each
case in which there was a post-operative specimen a fall of
13 to 20% was observed. In serial studies increasing levels
preceded subsequent clinically confirmed relapse.

Podolsky and his associates studied an isoenzyme of
galactosyl transferase (galactosyl transferase II) in colon
cancer [10]. They found in early studies that the isoenzyme
was not detectable in normals or patients with benign colon
disease but was elevated in serum of 13 to 17 patients with
colon cancer. The levels in patients with local disease was
2.0 + 0.5 units and in patients with metastases, 6.1 + 3.0
units. Elevations were not observed in Dukes' A disease or in
benign disease but in 8 of 9 (89%) patients with Dukes' B, 24
of 32 (75%) with Dukes' C and 14 of 19 (74%) patients with
distant metastases. They also reported that levels of the

enzymes reflected the course of the disease. This marker
deserves further study. However, the test as now performed
is lengthy and laborious. Clinical utility will probably
not be possible until an immunochemical method is developed
for the assay.

    Conclusion. The introduction of powerful analytical
tools, immunochemical and competitive equilibrium techniques
has made possible quantitation of proteins and other constituents in serum and plasma at the picogram and femtomole
levels. The current interest in α-FP, CEA, hCG and acid
phosphatase and other markers will undoubtedly lead to
evaluation of a large series of different antigens and other
markers. Success in the search for cancer specific markers
will be a function of the ability to separate and purify
individual constituents in sufficient amounts for use in
reagent preparation and introducing sophisticated analytical
procedures. Well organized clinical trials will then be
needed to establish the true role of the marker and both its
clinical and economic utility.

                              REFERENCES
1. Bhattacharya, M., Chatterjee, S.K. and Barlow, J.J.:
Uridine 5'-diphosphate gàlactose: glycoprotein galactosyltransferase activity in the ovarian cancer patient. Cancer
Res. 36:2096-2101 (1976).
2. Cooper, J.F., Foti, A., and Herschman, H.: Combined
serum and bone marrow radioimmunoassays for prostatic acid
phosphatase. J. Urol. 122:498-502 (1979).
3. Foti, A.G., Cooper, J.F., Herschman, H., and Malvaez, R.S.
Detection of prostatic cancer by solid-phase radioimmunoassay
of serum prostatic acid phosphatase. N. Eng. J. Med. 297:
1357-1361 (1977).
4. Gold, P., and Freedman, S.Q.: Demonstration of tumor-
specific antigens in human colon carcinomata by immunological
tolerance and absorption techniques. J. Exptl. Med. 122:
467-481 (1965).
5. Griffing, F. and Vaitukaitis, J.L.: Hormone secreting
tumors in cancer markers S. Sell,(ed), Humana Press, New
Jersey, 1980, p. 169-190.
6. Griffiths, J.: Prostate-specific acid phosp atase: Re-
evaluation of radioimmunoassay in diagnosing prostatic
disease. Clin. Chem. 26: 433-436 (1980).
7. Hansen, H.J., Snyder, L.J., Miller, E., et al: Carcinoembryonic antigen (CEA) assay. A laboratory adjunct in the
diagnosis and management of cancer. Human Path. 5:139-147
(1974).

8. Jaradpuur, N.: Biologic tumor markers in management of testicular and bladder cancer. Urology 12:177-183 (1978).

9. Jones, W.B., Lewis, J.L. Jr., and Lehr, M.: Monitor of chemotherapy in gestational trophoblastic neoplasms by radioimmunoassay of the β-subunit of human chorionic gonadotropin. Am. J. Obst. Gynecol. 121:669-673 (1975).

10. Podolsky, D.K., Weiser, M.M., Isselbacher, et al: A cancer-associated galactosyltransferase isoenzyme. New Eng. J. Med. 299:703-705 (1978).

11. Schwartz, M.K.: Laboratory aids to diagnosis-enzymes. Cancer 37:542-548 (1976).

12. Thompson, P., Krupey, P., Freedman, S. and Gold, P.: The radioimmunoassay of circulating carcinoembryonic antigens of the human digestive system. Proc. Nat. Acad. Sci. U.S. 64:161-170 (1969).

13. Vaitukaitis, J.L., Braunstein, G.D., and Ross, G.T.: Radioimmunoassay which specifically measures human chorionic gonadotropin in the presence of human luteinizing hormone. Am. J. Obst. Gynecol. 113:751-758 (1972).

14. Wanebo, H.J., Rao, B., Pinsky, C.M., et al: Preoperative carcinoembryonic antigen level as a prognostic indicator in colorectal cancer. New Eng. J. Med. 299:448-451 (1978).

15. Wanebo, H.J., Stearns, M.W. and Schwartz, M.D.: Use of CEA as an indicator of early recurrence and as a guide to a selected second-look procedure in patients with colorectal cancer. Ann. Surg. 188:481-492 (1978).

Advances in Nuclear Imaging

HENRY N. WAGNER, JR., M.D.

Professor
Departments of Medicine, Radiology
and Environmental Health Sciences
The Johns Hopkins Medical Institutions
Baltimore, Maryland

From the beginning nuclear imaging has been concerned with
the detection of cancer. The first application of the recti-
linear scanner invented by Cassen in 1950 was to image the
thyroid gland and determine whether palpable nodules accumulated radioactive iodine (Cassen et al, 1951). Demonstration
that a nodule was functional decreased the likelihood that it
was cancer. The first studies of the brain by Moore between
the years 1947 and 1953 were concerned with the localization
of brain tumors (Moore, 1953; Moore, 1947).

The goal was to be able to inject a radioactive tracer
that would accumulate in localized neoplasms and make them
detectable by nuclear imaging devices, in a sense, a "magic
bullet". The closest we have been able to come up to now
has been the use of ionic gallium-67. Using this radiotracer
as a bone-imaging agent, Edwards and Hayes in 1969 observed
its accumulation in lymphomatous tissue and realized its
potential in cancer diagnosis (Edwards et al, 1969). In 1972
Lomas, Dibos and Wagner reported on the use of gallium-67 in
the differential diagnosis of lesions detected in liver scanning with technetium-99m sulfur colloid (Lomas et al, 1972).

It was soon found that gallium-67 accumulation was not
specific for neoplasms, since it was found to accumulate even
more avidly in sites of inflammation, particularly infections.
Nevertheless, nuclear imaging with gallium-67 is useful in
patients with suspected or proven cancer, as will be described
subsequently. Although the search continues for a better
agent, gallium-67 citrate remains the most widely used diagnostic agent in nuclear oncology (Hoffer et al, 1978).

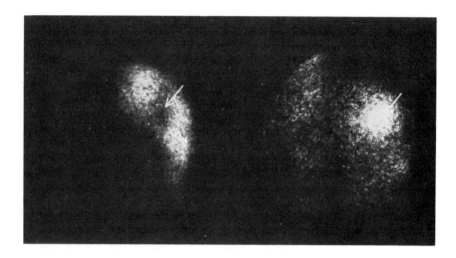

Figure 1. Left, solitary filling defect in a technetium-
sulfur colloid scan of the liver (posterior view). Right,
avid uptake of gallium-67 by the lesion.

NUCLEAR ONCOLOGY

The current and potential use of nuclear imaging in oncology
can be summarized as follows:

(1) Detection of premetastatic cancer
(2) Diagnosis of symptomatic cancer
(3) Determination of location and extent of involvement
(4) Aid in planning treatment
(5) Aid in prognosis
(6) Aid in monitoring response to treatment
(7) Elucidation of the cause of cancer

   An example of the usefulness of nuclear imaging is shown
in Figure 1. The asymptomatic patient was found to have an
elevated serum alkaline phosphatase. The technetium-99m
sulfur colloid scan of the liver revealed a round defect in
phagocytic activity, indicated by the arrow. Gallium-67

accumulated avidly in the lesion as seen in the image on the right. This indicated the serious nature of the lesion and led to surgery; it proved to be a resectable lymphoma.

In contrast, the patient whose liver scan with technetium-99m colloid is shown in Figure 2 also was found to have large areas of impaired phagocytic activity (left image), but the distribution of gallium-67 corresponded to the areas of phagocytic activity. The absence of accumulation of gallium-67 supported the diagnosis of cirrhosis of the liver without superimposed hepatoma. Characteristically, hepatomas accumulate gallium avidly and this observation aids in their diagnosis (Standalnik et al, 1978).

GALLIUM-67 IN CHEST DISEASE

To illustrate how gallium-67 is used in cancer diagnosis, we will consider chest disease as an example. Gallium-67 administered in the form of gallium citrate has been found to accumulate in the following lesions:

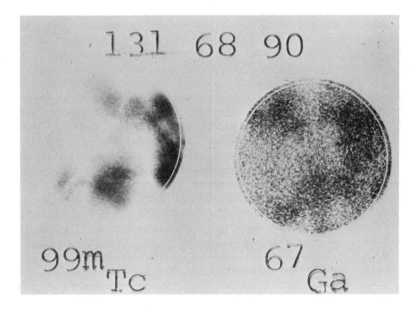

Figure 2. Left, defects in distribution of technetium-sulfur colloid liver scan. Right, distribution of gallium-67 corresponded to the phagocytic activity, supporting diagnosis of cirrhosis.

(1) Bronchogenic carcinoma
(2) Lymphoma
(3) Leukemia
(4) Infection
(5) Sarcoidosis
(6) Pneumoconiasis
(7) Bleomycin toxicity
(8) Radiation pneumonitis

Although the accumulation of gallium-67 is not completely specific for neoplasm, it is relatively specific for neoplasm or inflammatory sites. Its uses can be summarized as follows:

(1) Evaluation of focal lesions
(2) Prediction of resectability
(3) Aid in prognosis
(4) Avoidance of unhelpful thoracotomy
(5) Aid in locating lesions
(6) Evaluation of response to treatment

Several groups have found gallium-67 imaging to be very sensitive in the detection of mediastinal node involvement in patients with bronchogenic cancer (Alazaraki et al, 1978; DeLand et al, 1974; DeMeester et al, 1978; Lesk et al, 1978). They use this procedure to decrease the number of patients who are found at thoracotomy to have inoperable carcinoma of the lung. McNeil et al (1977) reported that 18% of patients who have thoracotomies are found to have unresectable lesions and that the post-operative mortality is 10%. She believes that preoperative evaluation for metastases can eliminate 45-80% of the thoracotomies that are not therapeutically effective. Alazaraki has proposed the following preoperative strategy (Alazaraki et al, 1978):
If the patient has evidence of mediastinal involvement in the chest radiograph, the patient should have mediastinoscopy. If the chest radiograph does not reveal mediastinal nodes, the patient should have a gallium-67 scan. If the primary lung lesion accumulates gallium-67 and the mediastinal nodes do not, the patient goes to thoracotomy without mediastinoscopy; if the mediastinal nodes show evidence of gallium accumulation, the patient has mediastinoscopy. An example of a patient with mediastinal nodes that accumulate gallium-67 is shown in Figure 3.

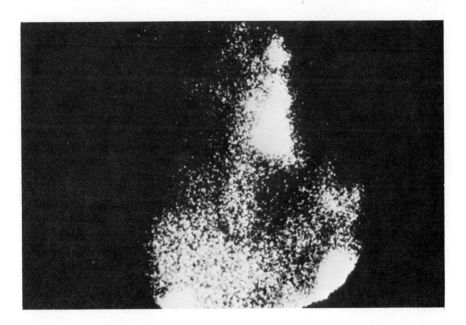

Figure 3. Uptake of gallium-67 in mediastinal nodes of a
patient with metastatic carcinoma of the lung. (Published
with permission of Waxman from Cedars-Sinai Hospital in
Los Angeles.)

    The mechanism of gallium accumulation in neoplasms remains
uncertain. Several proposed mechanisms are as follows:

(1) Hyperpermeability of cell membranes (Hayes et al, 1973)
(2) Binding to calcium or magnesium binding sites (Anghileri
     et al, 1977)
(3) Binding by tumor lactoferrin (Hoffer et al, 1979)
(4) Binding by tumor transferrin (Larson et al, 1979;
     Sephton et al, 1974)

    Tsan et al have investigated the mechanisms of gallium-67
accumulation in inflammation, some of which may be important
in cancer (Tsan et al, 1979; Tzen et al, 1980):

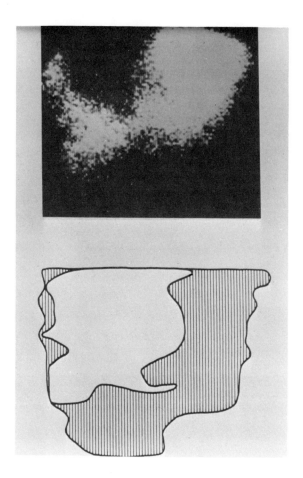

Figure 4. Upper, technetium-sulfur colloid scan of the liver
in a patient with a hepatoma seen as the defect in the upper
part of the liver. Lower, volume reconstruction of the lesion
from 16 computed tomographic sections.

(1) Increased capillary permeability
(2) Expanded extracellular space
(3) Damaged polymorphonuclear neutrophil membranes
(4) Bacterial uptake
(5) Protein binding by lactoferrin and other proteins
     in situ

NEW "MAGIC BULLETS"

Several groups have taken an immunological approach to the
detection of cancer (Kim et al, 1980; Levine et al, 1980).
Using radioiodinated anti-carcinoembryonic antigen (CEA)
purified by adsorption and affinity chromatography, these
investigators have found imaging a sensitive means of detecting pulmonary neoplasms. Levine et al have recently developed monoclonal anti-tumor antibodies derived from hybridomas.
At present these are derived from mouse myeloma clones, but
in the future, they may be available from human myeloma cells.
To date, they have been able to identify teratocarcinomas in
mice.

At our institution, Order and his colleagues have developed radioiodinated antiferritin antibodies and investigated
their accumulation in rat neoplasms and patients with hepatoma (Order et al, 1980). Nuclear imaging with technetium-99m
sulfur colloid (Figure 4, upper) and quantified computed
tomography (Figure 4, lower) are used to monitor the size of
the lesions. The uptake of ^{131}I anti-ferritin, superimposed
over the technetium-99m sulfur colloid is shown in Figure 5.

BREAST CANCER

Katzenellenbogen and his colleagues at the University of
Illinois, working with Welch and others at Washington University in St. Louis, have successfully labeled estradiol
with the positron-emitting radionuclide, bromine-77 or fluo-
rine (Katzenellenbogen et al, 1980). They have demonstrated
masked accumulation of this new agent in the uterus of immature and mature rats, as well as in mammary tumors in rats.
Further development of such agents may permit extension of
work done in tissue samples with tritiated estrogens to
in vivo studies in patients with proven or suspected breast
tumors.

While the search for tumor specific radiotracers continues,
the most widely used nuclear imaging procedure in breast
cancer remains the bone scan with technetium-99m phosphorus

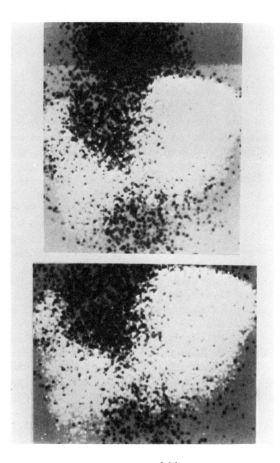

Figure 5. Superimposition of an ^{131}I anti-ferritin image
showing uptake by a hepatoma at the superior and inferior
border of the liver on top of a technetium-sulfur colloid
image (white area). The upper image includes the heart as
well.

compounds. In our hospital, we have found the yield of
abnormal bone scans proved to be metastatic disease in
patients with Stage I and Stage II cancer of the breast is
too low to warrant routine preoperative bone scanning of
these patients unless they have bone pain or other reason to

suspect metastatic disease (Baker et al, 1977). On the other hand, in Stage III breast cancer we routinely perform bone scans because the yield of positive findings has been great even in patients without bone pain.

LUNG CANCER

Measurement of regional ventilation and perfusion by nuclear imaging in patients with lung cancer is useful in helping predict post-operative lung function, in predicting the resectability of the lesion and in prognosis.

In our experience in the use of nuclear imaging in the early detection of lung cancer in heavy smokers, we did not find the nuclear techniques particularly helpful in making the diagnosis of lung cancer, primarily because of the severe underlying focal disease even in patients who did not have lung cancer (Katz et al, 1980).

THYROID CANCER

Technetium-99m pertechnetate is widely used for thyroid imaging because of the following:

(1)   It has an excellent gamma energy of 140 keV;
(2)   There is a very low radiation dose;
(3)   Images may be obtained 20 minutes after injection; and
(4)   The tracer is inexpensive.

Several comparisons of $^{99m}TcO_4^-$ and ^{131}I have found the accuracy of the scan findings comparable (Alderson et al, 1976; Strauss et al, 1970). It must be remembered, however, that ^{99m}Tc-pertechnetate reflects only the trapping process of the gland, and the technetium uptake may be high when organification of iodide to tryosine is abnormal, as in Hashimoto's thyroiditis or congenital defects. In these cases, radioiodine, preferably ^{123}I, should be used to evaluate function.

The accumulation and visualization of a radioactive tracer, or lack of accumulation, in the thyroid gland can answer several questions about a solitary thyroid nodule. First, it tells whether the nodule is "hot", functioning, or "cold", nonfunctioning. The incidence of cancer in functioning nodules is low and these are seldom treated surgically. The cold nodule, however, is a more difficult problem since most malignant nodules are cold, but only about 15% to 25% of cold nodules are malignant (Groesbeck, 1959; Hoffman et al, 1972; Kendall et al, 1969). The incidence of thyroid cancer in patients without a history of prior irradiation whose scans show more than one nonfunctioning lesion is 5% or less (Alderson et al, 1976), but in patients who have previously been treated with neck irradiation, usually in childhood, the occurrence of cancer even in a multifocal gland may be as high as 30%. The thyroid scan--when interpreted with a knowledge of the patient's age, sex, history of prior radiation, and thyroidal function data--by providing functional information about a nodule, helps to determine the probability of cancer.

Localization of functioning metastases in patients with proven thyroid carcinoma is performed routinely after operative removal of the gland or after ablation with therapeutic doses of ^{131}I. A whole body scan is performed 24 to 72 hours after radioiodine is administered. Either ^{99m}Tc or radioiodine may be used following surgical resection of the gland to establish the presence or absence of residual thyroid tissue. A scan should always be done before removal of a sublingual mass to determine whether it is a sublingual thyroid and whether it is the only thyroid tissue present. In most patients, it usually is.

Recently Japanese physicians have found whole body imaging after administration of thallium-201 has been more sensitive in detecting metastatic cancer of the thyroid than has the use of radioiodine (Tonami et al, 1980).

BONE TUMORS

Whole body bone imaging with ^{99m}Tc labeled phosphonate complexes is a sensitive means of detecting regions of active bone metabolism, reflecting an increased blood supply and new bone formation. Although the visualization of bone function does not give the structural detail of a roentgenograph, it is usually an earlier indicator of bone disease and skeletal involvement by disease of all types, including metastatic disease. Since a positive bone scan indicates increased mineral turnover, not neoplastic cells per se, the bone scan is not a specific test for cancer, although it is the most sensitive test for detecting bone metastases, including those from breast, prostate, lung, and kidney. When correlated with regional radiographs and measurement of serum calcium or alkaline phosphatase, the findings at specific sites can be interpreted with greater accuracy (Belliveau et al, 1975). Recent trauma, old fracture, arthritis, degenerative disease, or infection must be ruled out before a "hot spot" on a bone scan is diagnosed as a metastatic lesion. A single focal lesion is less likely to indicate metastases than multiple lesions.

SUMMARY

Nuclear imaging is widely used in patients with breast, prostate, lung and liver cancer, as well as in patients with lymphomas and leukemia. They are useful in detection of lesions, both primary and secondary as well as in assessment of the regional function of organs directly or indirectly involved by cancer or by the treatment of cancer. An example of the latter is the use of nuclear techniques to assess cardiac toxicity resulting from adriamycin treatment.

Advances are being made:

(1) in the development of new tracers, a most promising example being the development of estradiol labeled with bromine-77 for detection of breast tumors containing estrogen receptors; and

(2) in the use of tomography, both for single photon tracers labeled with technetium-99m (Figure 6) or iodine-123, and in positron-emitting tracers, labeled with carbon-11, fluorine-18 and nitrogen-13.

The technology of nuclear imaging in both chemistry and instrumentation has advanced to a point where we can obtain more quantitative data than was possible in the past. The future of nuclear oncology can be summarized as better chemistry, better quantification and better physiology, especially regional physiology.

REFERENCES

Alazaraki N, Ramsdell JW, Taylor A, et al: Reliability of gallium scan and chest radiography compared to mediastinoscopy evaluating for mediastinal spread in lung cancer. Am Rev Respir Dis 117: 415-420, 1978.

Alderson PO, Sumner HW, Siegel BA: The single palpable thyroid nodule. Cancer 37: 258-265, 1976.

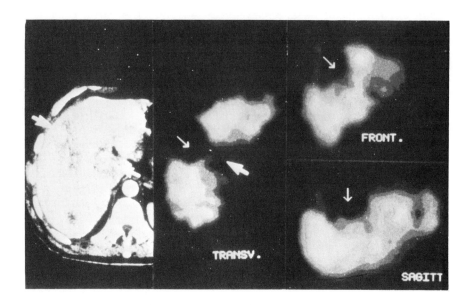

Figure 6. Transmission (left) and emission (right)
computed tomography of the liver of a patient with
multiple metastases.

Anghileri LJ, Heidbreder M: On the mechanism of accumulation
    of ^{67}Ga by tumors. Oncology 34: 74-77, 1977.
Baker RR, Holmes ER, Alderson PO, Khouri NF, Wagner HN jr:
    An evaluation of bone scans as screening procedures for
    occult metastases in primary breast cancer. Ann Surg 186:
    363-368, 1977.
Belliveau RE, Spencer RP: Incidence and sites of bone lesions
    detected by ^{99m}Te-polyphosphate scans in patients with
    tumors. Cancer 36: 359-363, 1975.
Cassen B, Curtis L, Reed C, Libby R: Instrumentation of I^{131}
    used in medical studies. Nucleonics 9: 46, 1951.
DeLand FH, Sauerbrunn BJL, Boyd C, et al: ^{67}Ga-citrate imag-
    ing in untreated primary lung cancer: preliminary report
    of cooperative group. J Nucl Med 15: 408-411, 1974.
DeMeester TR, Bekerman C, Joseph JG, et al: Gallium-67 scan-
    ning for carcinoma of the lung. J Thorac Cardiovasc Surg
    72: 699-708, 1976.
Edwards CL, Hayes RL: Tumor scanning with ^{67}Ga citrate.
    J Nucl Med 10: 103-105, 1969.

Groesbeck P: Evaluation of routine scintiscanning of non-toxic thyroid nodules. I. The preoperative diagnosis of thyroid carcinoma. Cancer 12: 1-5, 1959.

Hayes RL, Carlton JE: A study of the macromolecular binding of Ga-67 in normal and malignant tissues. Cancer Res 33: 3265-3272, 1973.

Hoffer, P. B., Bekerman, C., & Henkin, R.E. Gallium-67 Imaging. New York: John Wiley and Sons, Inc., 1978, 114.

Hoffer PB, Miller-Catchpole R, Turner DA: Demonstration of lactoferrin in tumor tissue from two patients with positive gallium scans. J Nucl Med 20: 424-426, 1979.

Hoffman GL, Thompson NW, Heffron C: The solitary thyroid nodule: a reassessment. Arch Surg 105: 379-385, 1972.

Katz RD, Alderson PO, Tockman MS, et al: Ventilation-perfusion lung scanning in patients with early lung carcinoma. Radiology, submitted for publication, 1980.

Katzenellenbogen JA, Carlson KE, Heiman DF, Goswami R: Receptor-binding radiopharmaceuticals for imaging breast tumors: estrogen-receptor interactions and selectivity of tissue uptake of halogenated estrogen analogs. J Nucl Med 21: 550-558, 1980.

Kendall LW, Condon RE: Prediction of malignancy in solitary thyroid nodules. Lancet 1: 1070-1073, 1969.

Kim EE, DeLand FH, Domstad PA, et al: Radioimmunodetection of lung cancers using radiolabeled antibodies to carcino-embryonic antigen (CEA), alpha-fetoprotein (AFP) and human chorionic gonadotropin (HCG). J Nucl Med 21: 54, 1980 (abstract).

Larson SM, Rasey JS, Allen DR, Granbaum Z: A transferrin-mediated uptake of gallium-67 by EMT-6 sarcoma. II. Studies in vivo (BALB/C mice). J Nucl Med 20: 843-846, 1979.

Lesk DM, Wood TE, Carroll SE, Reese L: The application of ^{67}Ga scanning in determining the operability of broncho-genic carcinoma. Radiology 128: 707-709, 1978.

Levine G, Ballou B, Reiland J, et al: Tumor imaging in mice with I-131 labeled monoclonal antibody. J Nucl Med 21: 54, 1980 (abstract).

Lomas F, Dibos PE, Wagner HN jr: Increased specificity of liver scanning with the use of ^{67}Ga citrate. N Engl J Med 286: 1323-1329, 1972.

McNeil BJ, Collins JJ jr, Adelstein SJ: Rationale for seeking occult metastases in patients with bronchial carcinoma. Surg Gynecol Obstet 144: 389-393, 1977.

Moore, G. E. Diagnosis and Localization of Brain Tumors: A Clinical and Experimental Study Employing Fluorescent and Radioactive Tracer Methods. Springfield, Illinois: Charles C. Thomas, 1953.

Moore GE: Fluorescein as an agent in the differentiation of
  normal and malignant tissues.   Science 106:   130, 1947.
Order SE, Klein JL, Ettinger D, et al: Phase I-II Study
  of radiolabeled antibody integrated in the treatment of
  primary hepatic malignancies.   Int J Radiat Oncol Biol 6:
  703-710, 1980.
Sephton RG, Harris AW: Gallium-67 citrate uptake by
  cultured tumor cells, stimulated by serum transferrin.
  J Natl Cancer Inst 54:   1263-1266, 1974.
Standalnik RC, DeNardo GL: Isotope imaging in the diagnosis
  of primary and secondary tumors of the liver, in Ariel IM
  (ed):   Progress in Clinical Cancer, Volume V.   New York:
  Grune & Stratton, Inc., 1978.
Strauss HW, Hurley PJ, Wagner HN jr: Advantages of ^{99m}Tc-
  pertechnetate for thyroid scanning in patients with
  decreased radioiodine uptake.   Radiology 97:   307-310,
  1970.
Tonami N, Hisada K, Aburano T, Seto H: Tl-201 scintigraphy
  in post-operative patients with thyroid cancer.   J Nucl
  Med 21:   33, 1980 (abstract).
Tsan MF, Scheffel U: Gallium-67 accumulation in inflammatory
  lesions.   J Nucl Med 20:   173, 1979.
Tzen KY, Oster ZH, Wagner HN jr, Tsan MF: Role of iron-
  binding proteins and enhanced capillary permeability on
  the accumulation of gallium-67.   J Nucl Med 21:   31-35,
  1980.

Early diagnosis of liver cancer and its preceding stage through AFP serology

Sun Tsung-tang

Chairman
Department of Immunology
Cancer Institute
Chinese Academy of Medical Science
Beijing, China

Chu Yuan-yun

Vice Director
Qidong Liver Cancer Institute
Kiangsu, China

Liver cell cancer, one of the commonest human malignancies, remains to be a very grave disease. Early detection might constitute an important component of the strategy of approach, directed toward secondary and primary prevention of the cancer (Sun et al, 1980). Since alphafetoprotein (AFP) was found to be a good marker of liver cell cancer (Abelev, 1971), and its positivity rate was high among areas of increased incidence, usually heavily populated, it is worthy to explore the potential of a early detection program through AFP serology. Studies along this line appear to be encouraging, as being demonstrated by the results of field trials carried out chiefly in China in the recent years (CGRLCC, 1974, 1978; Chu, 1980).

1. Early diagnosis of liver cell cancer:

Early diagnosis means the definition of the cancer at a stage during which proper intervention will lead to the cure of patients with relatively high probability (Sun et al, 1979). This depends primarily on whether there exists a stage during which the liver cell cancer is still remaining localized to enable complete surgical removal, yet detectable through presently available serological means. This critical

issue, challenged by the prevalent concept of multifocal
occurrence of liver cancer, could only be partially resolved
at the present. As a result of joint collaborative effort
(CGRLCQ, 1975) a series of 27 patients detected early by AFP
survey and having their liver cancer resected, have survived
over 4 years without any sign of recurrence. Of these, the
majority have been over 5 years, which hopefully places them
in the category of long term survivors. To reduce the possibility of severe hepatic decompensation, the amount of liver
tissue removed with the tumor was usually restricted to less
than one fourth or even one sixth of the total liver mass.
The tumor nodules, single or sometimes multiple occurring in
vicinity, were found mostly in the right lobe, which formed
the bulk of the organ. Microscopically, minute satellite
cancer foci were frequently seen nearby the main tumor nodule,
and cancer thrombi sometimes observed in the surgical specimens excised. These facts demonstrated that liver cells cancers in these patients were still confined within the relatively small regions resected at the time of surgery, and that
the tendency of intrahepatic dissemination from the main cancer focus had already started even at this early phase. The
27 patients just mentioned were mostly asymptomatic, being
still in the subclinical stage. The 3 year disease free survival of subclinical cancers were found to be around 40% (Chu,
1980; Sun et al, 1980). Field trials had also shown that majority of liver cell cancer patients could be detected at
their subclinical stage through AFP sero-surveys performed
twice a year (Chu, 1980; Ji et al, 1979). It was thus estimated that in about one third of the patients their liver cancers could be found in the localized state and hence be completely resected. In the other two thirds of the liver cell
cancers, their growth status in the early phase remains to be
clarified.
      The real possibility of early diagnosis of liver cell
cancer through AFP serology was demonstrated by the mass-
screening and sequential follow-up trials, conducted in Qidong
and Shanghai areas of China since 1974 (CGRLCC, 1978; Chu,1980)
The AFP serology had been shown to play important role in 3
links. The first one was to detect those sero-positive individuals from the general population through mass-survey. Sensitive and relatively simple techniques, such as reverse pas-
sive hemoagglutination (Lo et al, 1975) and radio-rocket electrophoresis autography (Sun et al, 1975), had been used for
this purpose. The positive individuals, having their serum
AFP exceeding 25 or 50 ng/ml, were then followed. Special
attention was paid to follow those individuals with AFP in the
range below 1,000 ng/ml, since candidates of early liver can-

cer most probably fell in this group. However, they were
usually outnumbered in several folds by the nonmalignant
patients, mostly suffering from chronic liver diseases.
Therefore, the second important role of AFP serology was to
provide reliable information for differential diagnosis.
The pattern, characterized by the steadily rising concentrations of serum AFP in sequential follow-up for 2 or more
months, was found to be the reliable serological expression
of the presence of liver cell cancer, provided that embryonic
cancers could be excluded (CGRLCQ, 1975; Sun et al, 1978).
The general rising trend was usually modulated by fluctuations of varying amplitude and its doubling time was mostly
in the range of 20 to 50 days. Over 90% of cases presenting
this pattern were found to be liver cancer patients
(Sun et al, 1980). The pattern observed probably reflected
the progressive expansion of tumor cell population at this
stage of development, and the complete removal of the cancer
was invariably followed by rapid decline of AFP to low levels.
The third role of AFP serology was explored to see whether it
could provide the quantitative information for the timely
handling of the critical moment to start radical treatment.
The 3 year survival data for a group of patients operated
before their serum AFP had exceeded 1,000 ng/ml was found to
be around 40%, whereas patients operated above this level had
a significantly lower survival rate (Sun et al, 1980). The
latter fact was consistent with the relatively low survival
data obtained in previous trials using less sensitive screening techniques (Chu, 1980). These facts indicated the probability of finding AFP positive liver cancers in localized
state was significantly reduced when the tumor marker had
exceeded the level of 1,000 ng/ml. However, the proper handling of the critical moment to start early treatment on individual cases of liver cancer could not be simply solved by
the AFP serology alone.

Even though the majority of liver cell cancers could be
diagnosed at their early phase, only 40% of the patients at
this stage could receive real benefit from the early treatment by surgery. In the remaining 60% of the patients, surgical approach was unsuccessful. The tumor had either grown
to a stage beyond resection, or it could not be found in the
surgical exploration. The potential thus provided by AFP
detection program could not be better utilized without the
introduction of other effective diagnostic techniques which
might define the extent and location of the suspected cancer
early in the course of serological follow-up (Sun et al, in
press). It had been claimed that hepatic angiography was the
technique of choice for identifying the small liver cancers

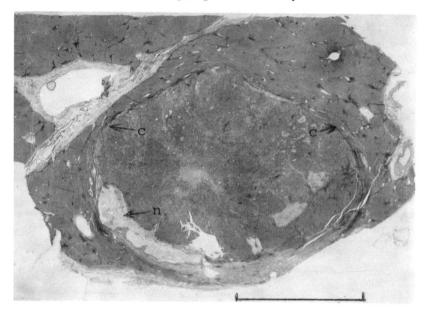

Fig. 1 Pathological Section of an early liver cell cancer
   c: capsule   n: necrosis area
   Scale: 1 cm   paraffin section, H. E. staining

(Okuda, 1979; Tang et al, 1979). Alternative approach using
non-traumatic techniques is also worthy to be explored. The
reassessment of the pathological features of early liver cell
cancers resected indicates such possibility. As shown in
Table 1, the apparent difference in consistency between early
liver cancer and their surrounding media including the
fibrous capsule may be reflected in the difference of relevant physical parameters which determines the contrast. The
characteristics of their size, shape and contour (see also
Fig. 1) may also facilitate the identification of the target
(Sun et al, in preparation). Our preliminary results from a

Table 1. Some pathological features of early liver cell
          cancers.

Diameters	1.0 to 4.5 in most cases
Shape	round or oval
Contour	relatively smooth
Consistency	less dense than surrounding media
Cell density	$2.50 \pm 1.04 \times 10^8$ cells/cm^3

(Based on the analysis of 25 surgical specimens)

recent collaborative study demonstrated that in a serologically diagnosed patient a translucent oval area of 2 cm diameter in the left liver was shown by computerized tomography. Surgical resection, followed by rapid fall of serum AFP, confirmed the presence of liver cell cancer in the location identified. The abundance of lipid content of the small cancer shown by Sudan staining partly explained the relatively lower absorbance of the tumor tissue. In another patient, a similar clear area indicating the presence of tumor in the depth of right lobe shown by CT was not confirmed by surgical exploration. Studies are still under way to clarify this situation. Obviously, if the progress in spatial identification of subclinical liver cancers could be made in the majority of cases through non-traumatic approach, an impact on the survival rate of liver cell cancer patients in the high incidence field studied would be reasonably expected.

2.   Definition of the preceding stage of liver cell cancer:

Since AFP could be elaborated by the regenerating liver cells following hepatic injury (Abelev, 1971), and the increased turnover of hepatic cells in experimental animals had been found to make these cells more vulnerable to the effect of hepato-carcinogens (Craddock, 1976), it was logical to investigate whether people in the high incidence field presumed to have increased exposure to hepato-carcinogens were more prone to exhibit increased level of AFP, and hence to have higher incidence of liver cell cancer. AFP sero-survey program for early diagnosis of liver cancer offered such unique opportunity to address this important issue.

The screening of the general population above 15 years of age in the high incidence field had detected a group of sero-positives, mostly in the range of 25 to 200 ng/ml. They constituted around 0.6% of the population not including pregnant women. Their AFP pattern exhibited fluctuations, sometimes falling to normal levels. The pattern was followed for one year or more for its definition in order to differentiate them from the serologically detectable liver cancer patients at the intial rising phase. Cancer incidence data collected since second year of follow-up demonstrated that these groups of people were indeed at high risk to subsequent development of liver cell cancer. The cancer incidence among such groups was found to be 3 to 6 per annum (Table 2), being much more risky than the serologically negative counterparts in the same area.

TABLE 2.

Liver Cancer Incidence Among The High Risk Groups In The
Field

No. of Patients	Years of Follow-up	LCC Found	Incidence Rate
25	2nd to 5th yr.	6	6% *
233	2nd to 3rd yr.	14	3% **

*   Ji and Sun; unpublished observations
** Chu Yuan-yun; in preparation

      The characteristic AFP pattern seen in the high risk
group just described was found to be closely associated with
chronic liver diseases, having prominent hyperplasia of hepatic cells. This association was established according to
evidences obtained in studies along two lines. First, liver
specimens removed with cancer showed invariable presence of
chronic hepatitis with prominent liver cell hyperplasia.
Serological follow-up of 15 patients after the resection of
localized tumor demonstrated that 10 of them indeed expressed
a similar pattern of elevated AFP in the course of years
(Sun et al, 1979). These patients are still well 5 years
after surgery, without any sign of tumor recurrence. The
observed AFP pattern obviously was not associated with cancer,
most likely it reflected the waves of proliferation of hepatic cells as a component of chronic inflammatory process of
the liver. Along another line, there were 10 individuals
identified in the field as members of the high risk groups
according to the serological criteria just mentioned. They
were all traced to the eventual development of liver cell ca
expressing a shift of the low level fluctuating AFP pattern
to a steadily rising one. In 5 of them, pathological diagnosis was made. Chronic liver pathology with prominent hyperplasia was in each case, thus confirming the association of
the pathological background with the serological expression.
      The definition of high risk group and its pathological
basis appears to be important in many respects. First of all,
it allows us to know more about the natural history of the
development of human liver cancer, the occurrence of which is
usually preceded by a stage having defined pathological basis
and serological expression (Sun, et al, 1980). A few members
of the high risk groups were also found to develop AFP negative ca in follow-up years. The definition of the high risk
group also offers research opportunities for expanding

secondary prevention trials to patients in the premalignant stage. The existence of two important quantitative markers, AFP and HB_SAg, greatly fascilitates the rapid assessment of the effect of any intervention installed. Studies along this direction have been under way.

Works on early diagnosis of liver cancer and its preceding stage had also provided evidences, indicating the possible influences of host factors on the development of liver cancer in different directions. First, epidemiological data showed that significant risk was imposed on the local people in the field by environmental factors. However, only those individuals who appeared to have increased susceptibility to develop persistent liver cell hyperplasia in responding to the common assault suffered the highest risk to liver cancer occurence (Sun et al, in press). On the other hand, there are also evidences indicating the possible existence of host resistance against the development of liver cancer. As shown in Table 3 which is the extension of previously reported data (Sun et al, 1980), the patients after their localized liver cancer had been surgically removed had significantly lower incidence of developing liver cancer de novo even though their liver disease background and serological expressions were comparable to those of the high risk group served as control. This phenomenon resembles the concomitant immunity observed in experimental systems. The existence of host effect, if confirmed in subsequent studies, will provide additional approach to the secondary prevention of human liver cell cancer besides its theoretical implications.

The early detection program through AFP serology also promotes the development of primary prevention studies. Thus, it had fascilitated the establishment of local anti-cancer network and registration system, the increase of public awareness to cancer control, and also the identification of possi-

TABLE 3

Occurence Of LCC In Groups Having Similar Liver Pathology

	High Risk Group	LCC Resected
No. of patients studied	29	29
Total person-years	124	151
No. of LCC occured	7	1
Cancer Incidence	5.6%	0.99%*

*2/3 of this group expressed AFP pattern similar to control, LCC incidence/100 person-yr was corrected accordingly.

ble etiological factors.As a matter of fact, preventive trials directed toward the control of human liver cell cancer, both secondary as well as primary in nature, have been on the way in the high incidence fields of China. It should be noted that immunology plays an active role in this multi-disciplinary approach.

REFERENCES

Abeleb, G.I. Alpha-fetoprotein in ontogenesis and its association with malignant tumors. Advances Cancer Res, 1971, 14:295-358.

Chu Yuan-yun. AFP sero-survey and early diagnosis of liver cell cancer in the Qidong field. Chin J Oncology, 1980, 2(4), in press

Chu Yuan-yun. Follow-up analysis of 233 cases exhibiting increased serum AFP at low level. in preparation

Coordinating Group for Research on Liver Cancer, China. Studies on human AFP. Res Cancer Control, 1974, (4);277-286.

Coordinating Group for Research on Liver Cancer, China. Studies on human AFP; further study in the application of AFP assay in mass screening for liver cancer. Nat Med J China, 1978, 58:586-588

Coordinating Group for Research on Liver Cancer in Qidong. Experience on early diagnosis and surgical treatment of primary liver cancer. Res Cancer Control, 1975, (1):1-5.

Craddock, V.M. Cell proliferation and experimental liver cancer. In H.M.Cameron et al (eds), Liver cell cancer. Netherland: Elsevier, 1976, 153.

Ji Shen, Sun Zongtang, Wang Laiqi et al. Characteristics of AFP serology in early PHC and the high risk group. Chin J Oncology, 1979, 1(2):96-100.

Lo Gin-han, Chu Yuan-yun, Cheng Ming et al. Preliminary report on the use of hemoagglutination test for serum AFP in mass survey of hepatocellular carcinoma. Res Cancer Control 1975, (1):6-12.

Okuda, K. & Nakashima, T. Hepatocellular carcinoma: A review of the recent studies and developments. In H.Popper & F.Schaffner(Eds), Progress in liver diseases. Vol.V. New York: Grune & Stratton, 1979, 639-650.

Sun Tsung-tang, Wang Lai-che. Radio-rocket electrophoresis autography in assaying serum AFP. Res Cancer Control, 1975, (1):12-16.

Sun Tsung-tang, Wan Lai-che, Chang Yu-lan et al. Radio-rocket electrophoresis autography through labelled antigen for AFP assay and its application in sero-epidemiological investi-

gation on primary hepatocellular carcinoma. Nat Med J
China, 1978, 58(11):649-658.

Sun Zongtang, Wang Nengjun, Xia Qiujie et al. Pathological
and serological investigation on early primary hepatocellular carcinoma and its liver disease background.
Chin J Oncology, 1979, 1(1):13-19.

Sun Zongtang, Chu Yuan-yun, Wang Laiqi et al. Immunological approach to natural history, early diagnosis and
etiology of human hepatocellular carcinoma. 7th Cold
Spring Harbor Conference on Cell Proliferation, 1980,
in press.

Sun Tsung-tang, Tang Zhao-you, & Chu Yuan-yun. Epidemiology, early diagnosis and treatment of liver cell cancer.
In J.J.DeCosse & P.Sherlock (Eds.), Gastro-intestinal
Malignancies. Vol.1. Netherland: Martinus Nijhoff, in
press.

Sun Zongtang, Wang Nengjun & Xia Qiujie. Further studies
on pathological features of early liver cell cancer.
in preparation.

Tang Zhao-you, Yang Binghui & Zhou Xinda. Advances in
early diagnosis of primary liver cancer in China. Chin
J Oncology, 1979, 1(3):233-235.

ADVANCES IN DIAGNOSIS OF
GASTROINTESTINAL NEOPLASMS

H. WORTH BOYCE, JR., M.D.
Professor of Medicine and Director
Division of Digestive Diseases and Nutrition
University of South Florida College of Medicine
Tampa, Florida

The exciting and clinically relevant developments in fiber-optic endoscopy dramatically have increased the diagnostic accuracy for gastrointestinal cancer over the past decade. Carcinomas of the esophagus, stomach, duodenum, colon and rectum reliably are diagnosed by inspection, biopsy and cytology in over 90% of cases.[2] The diagnostic capability of endoscopy is being further improved by new accessory procedures for localization and sampling of diseased tissue.

Diagnostic success rates of endoscopy in cancer of the gastrointestinal tract now are being approached by the endoscopic techniques used for study of the pancreas, and liver. Accuracy here exceeds 70% for pancreas and 90% for metastatic cancer of the liver.[7,20]

There is a tragedy associated with these remarkable technical and clinical developments, i.e., the fact that many endoscopic diagnoses are made in patients with symptoms in whom the cancer unfortunately is sufficiently advanced to prevent cure by present treatments. Hopefully, the increased use of endoscopy for diagnosis of many gastrointestinal disorders will allow us to recognize and correlate early changes of malignancy with characteristic symptoms.

Screening methods (biochemical, immunological, scanning and radioisotope) currently are being evaluated for detecting malignancies at an early, potentially curable stage. Endoscopy will be a primary method for evaluating the sensitivity and specificity of these noninvasive screening tests. In certain high risk groups endoscopy is proving valuable both for diagnosis and therapy of early malignant and premalignant lesions.

Advances in Instrumentation

The basic design and construction of current fiberoptic endoscopes are similar to those of earlier instruments. The important recent changes have been a significant reduction in diameter, improved distal tip control and, in some models, the addition of a second channel for accessories and suction. A better quality of fiberoptics in the viewing bundle and improved light transmission allow better resolution of the image for visual diagnosis, photography and television recording. A teaching device is available to permit simultaneous observation by a second person.

Biopsy forceps now have a pin between the jaws that permits the operator to fix the tissue directly in the proper axis as the forceps jaws are closed. Relief ports in the forceps jaws allow removal of a larger specimen than otherwise would be possible. The cytology brush has been enclosed in an outer sheath that eliminates the problem of cytology specimen loss occurring when the bare brush is extracted through the full length of the operating channel.

Large mucosal and lesion biopsies as well as polypectomy are possible by using wire loop snares and electrosurgical units that provide coagulation, cutting or blended currents. Transendoscopic lasers are being used for coagulation of bleeding lesions and for cancer therapy in some centers.

Procedural Innovations For Cancer Diagnosis

Biopsy, brush cytology and electrosurgical snare excision are the primary and most reliable accessory diagnostic procedures.[2,21] In an effort to improve visual recognition of focal neoplastic changes several innovations currently are under investigation.

Mucosal staining or dye scattering methods appear to have value in localizing surface changes that help the endoscopist precisely direct the forceps and cytology brush to areas that previously showed no significant changes.[9,13] Dyes may assist by outlining topographical aberration, by their absorption into certain epithelial cells, by color reaction based on pH at the cell surface and by fluorescence. Both upper and lower intestinal fiberoptic endoscopes with 30 power magnification also are being evaluated for a possible role in endoscopic diagnosis.

Endoscopic methods allow the clinician to obtain gastrointestinal, biliary and pancreatic secretions for cytology, biochemical testing and analysis for certain tumor markers.[5,10] Pancratic fluid collection can be enhanced by administration of the hormone secretin while a cannula is placed into the main pancreatic duct via the duodenoscope.

Japanese investigators have developed a minute (3 mm diameter) endoscope for examination of the common bile duct and pancreatic duct. This instrument is passed through a channel in a side viewing duodenoscope. Although this "baby scope" can be passed by experts into bile and pancreatic ducts there presently are enough technical problems to prevent the method from gaining wide use.

Transendoscopic intramural and transmural needle biopsy and aspiration methods are meeting with some success. The "thorny" needle has been successfully used to evaluate the histology of submucosal connective tissue neoplasms.[1] Two of three leiomyosarcomas were correctly diagnosed preoperatively by this technique and tumor cells were obtained from 9 of 12 submucosal myogenic tumors. Transmural biopsy by fine needle is being used for diagnosis of pancreatic lesions.

Reliability Of Endoscopic Diagnosis

During the past decade the clinical standards for practice of gastrointestinal cancer diagnosis have evolved along with the technological developments in instrumentation. Most patients who undergo operations for cancer of the gastrointestinal tract now have a confirmed histological diagnosis prior to surgery. The surgeon can use the information provided by endoscopy to make decisions on proper timing and the type of operation. The radiation therapist uses the endoscopist's report on precise location and extent of a malignant lesions in determining the proper field for irradiation therapy. Hepatic or other distant metastases may be confirmed or denied by some endoscopic methods thereby enhancing the assessment required to make judgements on curative or palliative therapy. The following discussion will review recent experiences in diagnosis of primary and metastatic malignancies by endoscopy.

Esophagus

Diagnosis of "early", i.e. non-metastatic, esophageal carcinoma among the general population of this country is exceedingly rare. Esophageal cancer like those of stomach, pancreas and colon, usually is discovered too late for cure to be achieved. At this stage diagnostic accuracy, using endoscopy plus biopsy and cytology, approaches 100% while the chance for cure remains low. The stenosis produced by the typical squamous cell carcinoma may reduce the diagnostic accuracy of endoscopic guided biopsy because the endoscopist may not be able to satisfactorily position the forceps. A cytology brush can be passed into the stenosis segment to obtain adequate tissue.

Winawer et al. reported 97% accuracy for directed brush cytology in esophageal cancer and a significantly lower (66%)
accuracy for forceps biopsy.[22] Combined biopsy and cytology
yielded 100% diagnostic accuracy. Some clinicians have used
the iodine staining characteristic of normal esophageal mucosa
and the lack of staining by malignant cells to aid in tissue
sampling by forceps or cytology brush.[13]

Esophagoscopy assists in therapy by providing a means for
passing a guide wire for esophageal dilation and in placement
of a peroral polyvinyl prosthesis to palliate dysphagia.[3]

Esophagoscopy, biopsy and cytology may prove useful in surveillance of patients with a columnar lined esophagus that is
believed to be a predisposing factor in devlopment of adenocarcinomas of the esophagus. The incidence of adenocarcinoma
of the esophagus in these individuals ranges from 2.0% to 8.5%
It has been reported that over half of the patients with adenocarcinoma of the esophagus will have an associated columnar
lined esophagus. On the basis of this relationship annual
examination by endoscopy with biopsy and cytology is recommended. There is yet no evidence that this practice will lead
either to a significant yield for diagnosis or improvement in
the current dismal prognosis for adenocarcinoma of the esophagus.

                              Stomach

The most heralded accomplishment for upper gastrointestinal
endoscopy in cancer diagnosis is related to the Japanese experience with "early" gastric cancer in their high risk population. In Japan approximately 50% of all cancer deaths are
due to gastric carcinoma.

A sixfold increase in the number of cases of early gastric
cancer over a 10 year period was reported from Japan by
Kidokoro.[11] In this report early gastric cancer accounted for
5.7% of all resectable cases of gastric cancer in 1961 compared to 34% in 1969. The excellent review of Quizilbash and
Stevenson emphasizes the pathological features and increased
recognition of early gastric cancer in institutions where
special diagnostic effort has been made.[16] The report of
Seifert et al. from Germany demonstrates the improvement in
diagnosis that can result from a diligent diagnostic effort.[19]
In their clinic early gastric cancer among all gastric cancer
increased from 10% in 1970 to 22% in 1978. Several reports
indicate that cancer will be found in about 5% of otherwise
typical benign gastric ulcers and that as many as 70% of early
gastric cancers occur in association with an ulcerated lesion.

Nowhere is the need for a systematic and thorough endoscopic
examination more important than in the search for early cancer.

To diagnose such early lesions the endoscopist has learned to identify subtle changes in surface texture and color. The earliest signs of stomach cancer appear to be redness, small polypoid lesions, flat mucosa with slight unevenness and small depressed lesions. Kobayashi et al. have emphasized that as many as 27% of early gastric cancers by inspection, i.e. without biopsy or cytology will be diagnosed as benign lesions.[12] In their report of 369 patients 95.1% of early cancers were diagnosed by the first set of biopsies; this increased to 98.1% after the second examination and 98.6% after three endoscopies with biopsy.

Excellent diagnostic results now are achieved by endoscopy with biopsy and cytology in patients who are examined for the usual symptomatic gastric cancer. It clearly has been shown that neither a positive nor a negative barium contrast study of the stomach in symptomatic patients is a conclusive examination for carcinoma, lymphoma or benign gastric ulcer. In one report, conventional barium radiography was incorrect in 36.7% of patients with gastric cancer.[14] Consequently, present practice standards dictate that visual examination of the entire gastric mucosa is essential in patients with negative radiographic studies as well as those with questionable or obvious radiographic abnormalities. The "definite" lesion seen on barium contrast study either may be a false positive finding or impertinent to the patient's symptoms that in reality are due to a lesion seen only by gastroscopy.

Endoscopic diagnosis of gastric lymphomas has been less reliable than that for adenocarcinoma. This lower diagnostic accuracy probably is due to the common submucosal location of many lymphomas until late in their course when mucosal ulceration provides access to tumor cells. Using both brush cytology and biopsy forceps technique gastric lymphoma now can be confirmed in about 80% of patients.

The value of gastroscopy for cancer screening of those with conditions potentially at higher risk for gastric cancer, such as pernicious anemia, gastric tubular adenomas and those with gastric resection and Billroth II anastomosis of over 10 years duration has yet to be determined.

Colon And Rectum

Rectal examination with the classical rigid proctoscope remains a reliable, generally available, safe and inexpensive method. However, in most clinics this instrument frequently is not inserted to its full 25 cm length because of the normal angulation of the rectosigmoid junction and patient discomfort. Since many sigmoid and all rectal polyps and carcinomas are within its reach it will remain the method most widely available for examination of the rectosigmoid for years to come.

The value of routine proctoscopy as a screening procedure clearly has been shown by the work of Gilbertsen and co-workers.[8] They showed that proctoscopic screening and regular removal of all adenomatous polyps significantly reduced the predicted incidence of subsequent rectosigmoid cancer.

Recently flexible fiberoptic proctosigmoidoscopes have been evaluated for their diagnostic potential as screening instruments. These short (60 cm) versions of the fiberoptic coloscope have gained favor among many physicians. In some clinics these instruments are now preferred for proctosigmoidoscopic examinations and are resulting in better patient acceptance and improved diagnosis compared to the rigid, shorter open tube proctosigmoidoscope. The distance achieved for examination significantly exceeds that of the rigid proctoscope since the fiberoptic sigmoidscope permits examination to 25 cm in 98% of patients and to 50 cm in 46%.[23] As expected this greater distance for examination produced more positive diagnoses of neoplastic colon lesions. In 108 patients there were 5 cancers found by flexible sigmoidoscopy but only 1 by the rigid proctoscope; 20 polyps larger than 5 mm were found by flexible compared to 2 by the rigid endoscope. The proper role for fiberoptic proctosigmoidoscopy in diagnosis of colon neoplasms is yet to be defined but the present consensus is that this instrument is best used for screening examinations by fully trained physicians preferably in conjunction with air contrast barium enema.

As the fiberoptic instruments have been improved, access to the entire colon has become an expected goal of every examination. Present coloscopes vary from 110 to 180 cm in length, are about 13 mm in diameter, have differential flexibility decreasing from distal to proximal end, excellent optical systems and either one or two channels for accessory instruments, air inflation, water injection and suction. A properly trained and experienced clinician will reach the cecum in 80 to 90% of patients with current instruments.

Detection of adenomas and their removal by snare polypectomy and forceps hold promise of reducing the risk of cancer later developing in this high risk patient group. Patients with previous colon cancer and adenomatous polyps should be placed under surveillance because of their particularly high risk of developing further polyps or cancer. Brady et al. recently reported their preliminary results in a group of patients who had had surgery for colon cancer.[4] Although their 62 patients had been followed periodically by rigid proctoscopy and standard column barium enema, 6 (10%) were found to have second carcinomas and 40 adenomatous polyps were found and removed. It is important to note that only 4 of the 6 cancers produced occult blood in the stool, 4 of 6 were above 25 cm and only 4 of 6 were diagnosed subsequently by air contrast barium enema. The consensus is that the best procedure for following such patients is air contrast barium enema and total fiberoptic coloscopy.

Fiberoptic coloscopy is indicated prior to surgery for colon cancer found by barium enema or proctoscopy. This is important because occasionally the barium enema gives a false positive result and needless surgery may be prevented by a negative endoscopy or proof of a benign lesion. A common occurrence is the finding of adenomatous polyps in 20-50% of patients with a colon cancer and a second, synchronous cancer in 4% to 7%.[24]

Most pathologists and clinicians agree that adenomas of the colon are premalignant lesions. It is believed that their detection and removal likely will reduce the expected incidence of cancer just as occurred in the study of rectosigmoid polyps by Gilbertsen.[8] Diagnosis and removal of adenomas and early carcinomas by coloscopy offers promise of significant improvement in survival and reduction of cancer risk, in addition to providing a large volume of tissue to aid in further study of the adenoma-carcinoma sequence.

Fiberoptic coloscopy and proctosigmoidoscopy are being used as a means of surveillance in patients with chronic ulcerative pancolitis of over 10 years duration who are recognized to be at a high risk of developing cancer.[25] A dysplasia of the colon mucosa has been found in these patients and this change is gaining acceptance as a precancerous lesion that may be used as a marker for those persons at highest risk.[17] The optimum surveillance procedure currently appears to be biopsy sampling throughout the colon. This is only possible by fiberoptic coloscopy.

Pancreas

Adenocarcinoma of the pancreas generally defies diagnosis during its curable stages because of its lack of symptom production. About 85 to 90% of pancreatic cancers have extended beyond the pancreas by the time of diagnosis. With each new diagnostic procedure developed there is hope for earlier cancer diagnosis but any "earlier" diagnosis realized for pancreatic cancer thus far has not improved survival statistics.

Endoscopic retrograde cholangiopancreatography (ERCP) has provided a means for recognizing the pancreatic and common bile duct changes caused by carcinoma and provides a correct diagnosis in 75% to 90% of patients.[7,18] However, the relatively high number (10%-25%) of false negative diagnoses make it an insensitive screening method. The skilled endoscopist can introduce the side-viewing endoscope into the duodenum, locate the papilla or Vater, insert a small cannula into the desired duct about 90% of the time, inject contrast media and obtain radiographs of the ductal system(s) in about fifteen minutes. The complication rate overall is about 2.2% and the mortality rate 0.13% in one report of 3,884 examinations.[15] Both are quite acceptable rates based on the diagnostic bene- fit derived.

In spite of its failure to assist in diagnosis of cancer early enough for cure, ERCP has provided a means to rapidly confirm a suspected diagnosis of pancreatic cancer and to de- fine the biliary and pancreatic ductal anatomy. The informa- tion provided concerning location of ductal involvement, whether pancreatic, common bile or both ducts are involved and the capability for histologic confirmation by cytology of pan- creatic juice, ductal brush cytology and aspiration biopsy permits a positive tissue diagnosis preoperatively in most cases.[5,10] Research is underway to evaluate the presence of tumor markers such as oncofetal antigens in pancreatic juice as a means for screening and diagnosis.

Liver And Peritoneum

Exploratory laparoscopy has been used in many countries to determine the presence of malignant neoplasms of liver and peritoneum as well as other organs. It has proven to be the most accurate method for the diagnosis of hepatic metastases short of laparotomy. In combination with guided liver biopsy the accuracy for hepatic metastases is approximately 90%.[20] About 10% of patients with metastases in the liver will not have evidence of lesions on the hepatic surface, hence the reason for the 10% false negative rate for laparoscopy.

Primary hepatic carcinoma is more likely to be deep within liver substance and either may be invisible or manifest only by an alteration in surface contour. In one series 84% of patients had positive identification of hepatocellular carcin- oma by laparoscopic inspection.[6] The combined use of liver scanning methods to detect deep intrahepatic lesions and di- rected biopsy during laparoscopy can reduce the false negative rate even further. Another advantage for laparoscopy is the clinician's ability to recognize and biopsy peritoneal metas- tases and thereby spare the patient any risk of liver biopsy. Brush cytology from surface lesions or touch cytology made from needle biopsy specimens may be used to enhance diagnostic accuracy.

Radioisotope liver scans, sonography and computerized tomo- graphy of the liver are not reliable procedures for diagnosis of hepatic metastases unless the lesions are large or exten-

sive. Blind percutaneous liver biopsy will be diagnostic
of metastases only in about 50% of patients. Blind biopsy
will miss most cases with small or few metastases associated
with a normal sized liver and normal liver tests. When the
selection of proper therapy is dependent upon knowledge of
whether hepatic metastases are present, laparoscopy is a most
accurate method with a 10% false negative rate similar to exploratory laparotomy.

Laparoscopy has proven of value in the staging of ovarian
carcinoma. The identification of metastases by this method
provides a followable finding upon which important decisions
on chemotherapy can be based dependent upon the response noted
at a subsequent or "second look" examination. Laparoscopy has
been shown to be of value in staging patients with carcinoma
of the esophagus, lung, breast, and Hodgkin's disease and non-
Hodgkin's lymphoma.

Future Prospects

The truly remarkable technical and clinical achievements of
gastrointestinal endoscopy over the past decade are just now
being made available to a large enough segment of the population to have a significant impact on the diagnosis and therapy
of cancer. These methods make the various screening tests
more meaningful and provide the long awaited capability to
confirm or deny the existence of malignant disease. Endoscopy
with biopsy and cytology can provide histologic confirmation
of a diagnosis of gastrointestinal cancer in nearly 100% of
cases. Accessory procedures presently being investigated will
further enhance the diagnostic and therapeutic potential of
gastrointestinal endoscopy during the next decade.

REFERENCES

1.   Asaki S, Sato A, Wakui K: New device for diagnosis of
     gastric submucosal tumor: endoscopic biopsy using thorny
     needle. Tohoku J Exp Med 127:257-264, 1979.
2.   Bemvenuti G A, Hattori K, Levin B, et al: Endoscopic
     sampling for tissue diagnosis in gastrointestinal malig-
     nancy. Gastrointest Endosc 21:159-161, 1975.
3.   Boyce H W Jr, Palmer E D: Techniques of Clinical Gastro-
     enterology. Springfield, Thomas, 1975.
4.   Brady P G, Frank B A, Daly J M: The role of colonoscopy
     following partial colon resection for adenocarcinoma.
     Gastrointest Endosc 26:64, 1980.
5.   Cotton P B, Denyer M E, Kreel L, et al: Comparative
     clinical impact of endoscopic pancreatography, grey-scale

ultrasonography and computed tomography (EMI scanning) in pancreatic disease: preliminary report. Gut 19:679-684, 1978.

6. Etienne J P, Chaput J-C, Feydy P, et al: La laparoscopie dans le cancer primitif du foie l'adulte. Ann Gastroenterol Hepatol (Paris) 9:49-56, 1973.

7. Fitzgerald P J, Fortner J G, Watson R C, et al: The value of diagnostic aids in detecting pancreas cancer. Cancer 41:868-879, 1978.

8. Gilbertsen V A: Proctosigmoidoscopy and polypectomy in reducing the incidence of rectal cancer. Cancer 34:936-939, 1974.

9. Kawai K, Sasaki Z, Misaki F, et al: Endoscopic diagnosis of intestinal metaplasia of the stomach and its evaluation as a precancerous lesion. Front Gastrointest Res 5:140-148, 1979.

10. Kawanishi H, Pollard H M: Endoscopic evaluation of cancer of the pancreas. Sem Oncol 6:309-317, 1979.

11. Kidokoro T: Frequency of resection, metastasis and five year survival rate of early gastric carcinoma in a surgical clinic, in Murakami T (ed): Early Gastric Cancer. Baltimore, University Park Press, 1971, p. 45.

12. Kobayashi S, Kasugai T, Yamazaki H: Endoscopic differentiation of early gastric cancer from benign peptic ulcer. Gastrointest Endosc 25:55-57, 1979.

13. Mandard A M, Tourneux J, Gignoux M, et al: In situ carcinoma of the esophagus. Macroscopic study with particular reference to the Lugol test. Endoscopy 12:51-57, 1980.

14. Moshakis V, Hooper A A: The accuracy of endoscopic diagnosis of gastric carcinoma and the conventional barium meal. Clin Oncol 4:359-368, 1978.

15. Nebel OT, Silvis S E, Rogers G, et al: Complications associated with endoscopic retrograde cholangiopancreatography. Gastrointest Endosc 22:34-36, 1975.

16. Qizilbash A H, Stevenson GW: Early gastric cancer. Pathol Ann 14:317-351, 1979.

17. Riddell R H, Morson B C: Value of sigmoidoscopy and biopsy in detection of carcinoma and premalignant change in ulcerative colitis. Gut 20:575-580, 1979.

18. Rohrmann C A, Silvis S E, Vennes J A: Evaluation of the endoscopic pancreatogram. Radiology 113:297-304, 1974.

19. Seifert E, Butke H, Gail K: Diagnosis of early cancer. Am J Gastroenterology 71:563-567, 1979.

20. Van Waes L, D'Haveloose J, Demeulenaere L: Diagnostic accuracy of laparoscopy in the detection of liver metastases. A prospective study. Belgium Gastroenterology 74 (5, part 2):1107, 1978.

21. Winawer S J, Melamed M, Sherlock P: Potential of endoscopy, biopsy and cytology in the diagnosis and management of patients with cancer. Clin Gastroenterol 5:575–595, 1976.
22. Winawer S J, Sherlock P, Belladonna J A: Endoscopic brush cytology in esophageal cancer. JAMA 232:1358, 1975
23. Winawer S J, Leidner S D, Boyle C: Comparison of flexible sigmoidoscopy with other diagnostic techniques in the diagnosis of sectocolon neoplasia. Dig Dis and Sci 24:277–281, 1979.
24. Wolff, W I: Colonoscopy updated. Adv Surg 13:145–168, 1979.
25. Yardley J H, Bayless T M, Diamond M P: Cancer in ulcerative colitis. Gastroenterology 76:221–224, 1979.

Index

673

674

Cervical cancer, *continued*
  smoking and, 76
Chemical carcinogens, 428
  detection of, 281–290
    biochemical assay systems, 283
    cell transformation systems,
      286–287
    conceptual outline of the
      carcinogenic process, 281–282
    cytogenetic assay systems, 286
    in vivo target organ systems,
      287–288
    mammalian mutagenesis systems,
      285–286
    metabolic activation, 288
    promotor detection systems, 288
    regulatory process and short-term
      tests, 289–290
    submammalian assay systems,
      283–284
  inhibitors of, 517. *See also* Blocking
    agents
  metabolic activation of, 269–277
    bioassay systems of, 288
    cancer prevention and, 275–277
    electrophilic metabolites, 270–275
    general aspects of, 271
    initiation and promotion, 269–271,
      382–383
    somatic mutation hypothesis and,
      382–383
Chemoprevention, 259
  with retinoids, 541, 543–545
Childhood cancer
  radiation exposure *in utero* and, 39,
    188–189, 223–227
  thyroid cancer, in thymus-irradiated
    children, 199, 203, 205
Children, 12
China, nasopharyngeal cancer in, 8
Cholesterol, colon cancer and, 601
Chorionic gonadotropin, 632–633
Chromosomal aberrations, 383–385
Chromosomal abnormalities, 407–415
  in acute lymphocytic leukemia
    (ALL), 410–411
  in acute non-lymphocytic leukemia
    (ANLL), 408–410

  in Burkitt's lymphoma, 411–412
  in chronic myelogenous leukemia,
    408
  in embryonic carcinomas, 412–414
  in leukemia, 424
  in non-Hodgkin's lymphomas,
    411–412
  in retinoblastoma, 412–414
  in Wilms' tumor, 413–414
Chromosome 14
  acute lymphocytic leukemia and, 433,
    434, 438
  Ataxia-Telangiectasia and, 433,
    438–439
  in Burkitt's lymphoma, 434, 439–441
  benign and malignant breakpoints in,
    439
  chronic lymphocytic leukemia (CLL)
    and, 438
  diffuse histiocytic lymphomas
    (DHL), 435–437
  Hodgkin's disease and, 437
  mechanism of action of, 439–441
  multiple myelomas and plasma cell
    leukemias, 437–438
  mycosis fungoides and, 437
  non-Burkitt's lymphomas, 435
  in normal cultured lymphocytes, 439
Chromosome 15 trisomy, 90
Cigarette smoke, 13
Cigarette smoking, 8. *See also* Smoking
Cirrhosis, primary hepatocellular
  carcinoma and, 165, 167
Clinical research, expenditures on, 3–4
Colectomy, prophylactic, 429
Colon cancer
  carcinoembryonic antigen as a
    marker for, 630–632
  diet and, 73–74, 589–591, 600–602
  genetic predisposition to, 385
  heart disease and, 601–602
  hereditary, 423, 429
  incidence of, 56
  prophylactic colectomy for, 429
Colorectal cancer, nitrosamines and,
  580
Coloscopy, 667
Comprehensive Cancer Centers, 5

676

677

678

Flavones, 525
Focal nodular hyperplasia (FNH), 66
Fujinami sarcoma virus (FSV), 112,
119–122

Galactosyl transferase, as cancer
marker, 633–634
Gallium-67, nuclear imaging with,
637–643
Gardner's syndrome, 423
Gastric cancer
dietary factors and, 598–600
endoscopic diagnosis of, 664–665
nitrosoureas or other nitrosamides
and, 579, 581
Gastrointestinal neoplasms
endoscopic diagnosis of, 661–669
advances in instrumentation, 662
esophageal cancer, 663–664
gastric cancer, 664–665
liver and peritoneal cancers,
668–669
pancreatic cancer, 667–668
procedural innovations for,
662–663
rectal cancer, 665–666
reliability of, 663
Genetic epidemiology, 397–404
breast cancer, 397–398
definition of, 397
linkage analysis and, 398–404
statistical models of disease
susceptibility, 398–399
Genes, cancer, 383, 384, 389–392
Genetic counseling, 429
Genetic linkage, 388–389
Genetics (genetic cancers), 381–392.
See also Chromosomal
abnormalities; Genetic
epidemiology
clinical features and management of,
421–430
germinal mutations, 385–389
initiating mutations, 389–392
somatic mutation hypothesis,
381–385

Germinal mutations, 385–389, 422
Granulocyte-macrophage colony
stimulating factor (GM-CSF),
myeloid leukemia and, 465–471

HBeAG, 167
HBsAG, 162, 163, 165, 167
Heart disease, and colon cancer,
601–602
Hepatitis B virus (HBV), 94
liver cancer (primary hepatocellular
carcinoma), 32, 94, 161–178
in Africa and Asia and, 8, 13
evidence to support connection
between, 163–171
model for the relation of, 173–174
maternal transmission of, 167,
171–172
nomenclature of components and
serology of, 162
other viruses similar to (ICRONS),
178–180
prevention of infection with, 171–172
Hepatitis, chronic, primary
hepatocellular carcinoma and,
165, 167
Hepatomas, 66
Herpes viruses, 84, 86, 92. *See also*
Epstein-Barr virus
Hodgkin's disease, chromosome 14
and, 437
Hr-T mutants, polyoma virus and,
104–108
Hyperparathyroidism, 429

Iatrogenic cancer, 8
ICRONS, 163, 178–180
Immunology, 309–376
Immunopotentiators, 322–323
Immunoregulation, cancer-induced,
336–340
Immunotherapy, non-specific,
322–323
Incidence of cancer, trends in, 55–56

Individual susceptibility, 13–14
Indoles, 527
Initiating mutations, 389–392
Initiation of carcinogenesis, 269–270, 389–392
Initiators, 13
Interferons, 324–326, 367–376
  in animals, 368–369
  combination chemoprevention with retinoids, 544–545
  fibroblast, 370–371
  future prospects in cancer therapy, 373–376
  immune reactions and, 373
  leukocyte, 369–371
  in man, 369–372
  mechanisms of antitumor activity, 372–373
Interleukin 1 (IL-1), 325–326
Iran, precancerous mucosal lesions in, 8

Japanese-Americans, breast cancer among, 57–60
Japanese women. *See also* Atomic bomb survivors
  breast cancer in, 210, 216

Kaiser-Permanente Foundation, prevention medicine programs of, 622–623

Lactation, breast cancer and, 213
Lampang Health Development Project, 623–625
Latent period, 10
Leukemia. *See also* Myeloid leukemias
  acute lymphocytic, chromosome 14 and, 433, 434, 438
  acute non-lymphocytic, chromosome abnormalities in, 408–410
  in ankylosing spondylitis patients, 230–231

in atomic bomb survivors, 188, 232–235, 237
avian acute, 119–122
bovine, 92
in children, 188
chromosomal aberrations in, 383–385
chromosome 15 trisomy and, 90–91
chronic lymphocytic, chromosome 14 and, 438
chronic myeloid, 383, 384, 408
feline, 92
gross (murine), 82–83
lymphocytic, 410–411
myeloblastic, 384
myelogenous, 409
plasma cell, chromosome 14 and, 437–438
promyelocytic, 384–385, 409
radiation-induced, 188–189
  breast cancer and, 217–218
T-cell, 83, 90–91
thymus-derived, 90–91
Leukemia cells, antigens on, 312–315
Leukemia viruses
  C-type, 90, 92
  directly transforming, 88–89
  feline, 137–143, 356–357
  without direct transforming effect, 89–90
Lifestyle factors, 11, 16, 71–77
  diet and nutrition, 72–75
  future research on, 19
  modification of, 17
  sexual reproductive habits, 75–76
  socio-economic status, 71–72
Linkage analysis, 388–389
  genetic epidemiology and, 398–404
Liver cancer
  dietary factors and, 75
  early diagnosis of, with AFP serology, 651–658
  preceding stage of liver cell cancer, 655–658
  endoscopic diagnosis of, 668–669
  hepatitis B virus and, 32, 94, 161–178. *See also* Hepatitis B virus

681

National Cancer Act, 2–4
National Cancer Institute, 2, 3
  virology and, 4
National Institutes of Health, 2
Nitrosamines, 9, 73, 262
  stomach cancer and, 53–54, 598–600
Nitrosation
  ascorbic acids and other agents used
    to inhibit, 558–581
    in vivo studies, 573–576
    nitrosation in lipids and by nitrogen
      oxides, 569–573
    studies in acidic aqueous solutions,
      558–568
    use of A SC in the meat industry,
      568–569
Nuclear imaging, 637–647
  of bone tumors, 646–647
  of breast cancer, 643–645
  current and potential uses of,
    638–639
  with gallium-67, 637–643
  of lung cancer, 645
  of thyroid cancer, 645–646

Occupational cancer (or carcinogens),
    8, 16, 596, 597. *See also*
    Environmental cancer
  epidemiological studies of, 11–12
  lifestyle factors and, 11, 16–17
  population-based tumor registries in
    the identification of, 291–298
  radiologists and other radiation
    workers, 241–253
Occupational Safety and Health
    Administration (OSHA), 289
Oncornaviruses, 87–91
  directly transforming, 87–89, 95
  without direct transforming effect,
    89–90
Onc genes, 111–128
  carcinogenetic role of, 128
  cellular chromosomal sequences and,
    125–128
  definition of, 116–117
  designs of, 123–124

multiple, 124–125
  of replication-defective oncogenic
    viruses, 117–123
Oophorectomy, prophylactic, 429
Oracon, endometrial cancer and, 27–28
Oral contraceptives
  endometrial cancer and, 27–28, 32
  liver tumors and, 65–66
  ovarian cancer and, 32
Osteosarcoma, interferon in treatment
    of, 369–370
Ovarian cancer, 429
  galactosyl transferase as marker for,
    633–634
  oral contraceptives and, 32

Pancreatic cancers, endoscopic
    diagnosis of, 667–668
Papovaviruses, 84, 101–103
Peritoneal cancer, endoscopic diagnosis
    of, 668–669
Phenobarbital, 528
Phenols, as inhibitors of nitrosamine
    formation, 562
Phenotype
  evolution of, in mammary neoplasms,
    455–462
    alternative pathways to mammary
      neoplasms, 456
    heterogeneity of primary tumors,
      450–461
    modulation of expression of the
      neoplastic phenotype, 458–459
    modulation of expression of the
      preneoplastic transformed state,
      456–457
Phenotype of the cancer cell, 446–450
Philadelphia chromosome, 383–385
Phorbol-myristate-acetate (PMA),
    549–551
Plasmocytomas, murine, 91
Polycyclic aromatic hydrocarbons, 262
Polyoma virus, 84
  cell transformation by, 103–108
    early region of the viral genome and
      its products, 105–107

a
b
c
d
e
f
g
h
1 i
8 2 j